Clinical Nutrition and Dietetics

Clinical Nutrition and Dietetics

Frances J. Zeman, Ph.D., R.D.
Professor of Nutrition
University of California, Davis

With contributions by Robert J. Hansen, Ph.D., Sushma Palmer, D.Sc., Robert B. Rucker, Ph.D., Bruce M. Wolfe, M.D., and Wayne I. Yamahata, M.D.

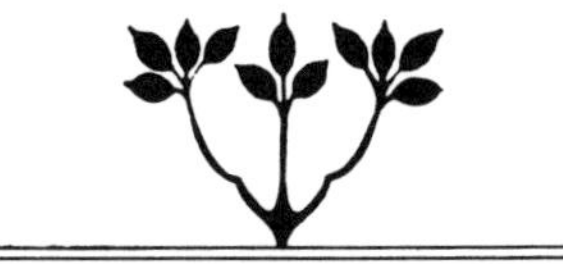

The Collamore Press
D.C. Heath and Company
Lexington, Massachusetts
Toronto

Every effort has been made to ensure that drug-dosage schedules and indications are correct at time of publication. Since ongoing medical research can change standards of usage, and also because of human and typographical error, it is recommended that readers check the *PDR* or package insert before prescription or administration of the drugs mentioned in this book.

Published simultaneously in Canada
Printed in the United States of America
International Standard Book Number: 0-669-05234-5
Library of Congress Catalog Card Number: 81-70162

Library of Congress Cataloging in Publication Data

Zeman, Frances J.
Clinical nutrition and dietetics.

Includes bibliographies and index.
1. Nutrition disorders. 2. Diet therapy.
3. Diet in disease. I. Title [DNLM: 1. Dietetics. 2. Nutrition. WB 400 Z526c]
RC620.5.Z45 1983 616.3'9 81-70162
ISBN 0-669-05234-5

Contributors

Robert J. Hansen, Ph.D.
Associate Professor of Physiological Sciences
School of Veterinary Medicine
University of California, Davis

Sushma Palmer, D.Sc., R.D.
Executive Director
Food and Nutrition Board
Commission on Life Sciences
National Academy of Sciences
Assistant Professor of Pediatrics
Georgetown University School of Medicine
Washington, D.C.

Robert B. Rucker, Ph.D.
Professor of Nutrition
University of California, Davis

Bruce M. Wolfe, M.D.
Associate Professor of Surgery
School of Medicine
University of California, Davis
Attending Surgeon
University of California, Davis, Medical Center
Sacramento

Wayne I. Yamahata, M.D.
Department of Surgery
School of Medicine
University of California, Davis
Surgery Resident
University of California, Davis, Medical Center
Sacramento

Contents

Preface and Acknowledgments

In recent years, dietitians have participated to an increasing extent in patient care. In order to become properly prepared to discharge these greater responsibilities, it is necessary for dietitians not only to be knowledgeable in the fields of physiology and biochemistry but also to have a background in related biologic sciences, such as anatomy, immunology, genetics, and pathology.

This book was written primarily for the dietetics student who has already completed rigorous courses in biochemistry and normal physiology. It attempts to integrate the theoretical basis for nutritional care with these sciences and with other relevant biologic sciences in order to provide the student with the background for increasing independence in planning nutritional care. This book also provides the background information that will serve as a basis from which the student may continue to learn and advance in the field. Therefore, it provides less emphasis on current usage of specific diets. With few exceptions, examples of diets are not included, and a diet manual should accompany this book when it is used as a text.

It is hoped that this book will be instrumental in helping students of clinical dietetics to function as full members of a health care team.

Instructors of diet therapy may wish to arrange their courses in a sequence different from the chapters in this book. To this end, cross-references to other chapters containing related material are included throughout the text. Case studies and additional references are included at the ends of chapters to provide flexibility for the instructor who chooses to use them.

This book may also be useful as a desk reference for dietitians and public health nutritionists. It might also be of interest to the many pharmacists, medical students, residents, and practitioners in medicine who have an interest in nutrition. The term *nutritional care specialist,* although somewhat cumbersome, has been used throughout to indicate more accurately the function of the dietitian in nutritional care and to include the growing numbers of practitioners of medicine with expertise in clinical nutrition.

In order to be competent in planning for nutritional care, nutritional care specialists must be familiar with the recent literature and new advances in the field. Although students in clinical dietetics have usually been introduced to the scientific literature in their courses in normal nutrition, they frequently are not familiar with the literature of the health professions. At the end of Chapter 2, useful journals of general interest to the nutritional care specialist are listed. In the succeeding chapters, journals that are relevant to the specific subject matter are appended. A nutritional care specialist should make it a habit to read, on a regular basis, those journals that are most useful in his or her particular position. The alert professional will find that reading the abstract section of the *Journal of the American Dietetic Association* is an efficient way to become informed of new articles of interest.

Thanks are due to the dietitians of the University of California Hospitals and Clinics, San Francisco, and of the Sutter Community Hospitals, Sacramento, who reviewed many of the chapters. My appreciation also goes to the nutritionists of the Alta California Regional Center, Sacramento, for many valuable comments concerning the last chapter, to Mary Ann Berkman, R.D., for her helpful review of the chapter on cardiovascular disease, and to Judith Stern, Sc.D., R.D., for reviewing the material on obesity.

Many thanks also are extended to Robert B. Rucker, Ph.D., for reviewing the material with concern for its clarity to those not specifically versed in dietetics and for his encouragement throughout. Others who were helpful in various ways were Ruth E. Shrader and Nathaniel Clark, R.D.

I wish particularly to express my appreciation for comments expressing the students' point of view from our graduate students, Bruce Rengers, R.D., Cynthia Payne, R.D., Denise Ney, R.D., Joyce Hayashi, R.D., and Kurt Miller, and from undergraduates too numerous to mention. However, Ashley Owen and Marcia Stieber deserve special mention for their thoughtful comments.

Last, I am grateful to Nancy Mata and Ann Huffaker for their dedicated typing and great endurance and to Adele Hipps for her untiring care in the preparation of the figures.

F.J.Z.

I. Introduction

1. Introduction to Pathology

A knowledge of the effect of disease on body tissue and its reaction to injury is fundamental to an understanding of the basis for nutritional care of patients. Therefore, this text will begin with a brief review of the fundamentals of pathology. By definition, *pathology* is "that branch of medicine which treats the essential nature of disease, especially of the structural and functional changes in tissues and organs of the body which cause or are caused by disease."[1]

NORMAL TISSUES AND TISSUE CHANGES

The body develops from the union of the ovum and the sperm. In succeeding steps, a single new cell is produced which has the properties of other single cells. It is capable of movement by flow of its cytoplasm (*diapedesis*), ingestion of solids (*phagocytosis*) or liquids (*pinocytosis*), and cell division for reproduction (*mitosis*). As the fertilized ovum divides, the cells diversify and acquire individual characteristics. This process is known as *differentiation.* As cells differentiate, they undergo morphological changes—that is, they change in form and structure.

During the early development of the embryo, there is a stage during which the embryo consists of three germ layers. One of these is the *ectoderm* (outer layer), which differentiates to form the nervous system, including the eye and ear, and the epidermis (skin) and related structures such as hair, nails, and the glands of the skin. Another layer is the *endoderm* or *entoderm* (inner layer), which forms the lining of the gut, respiratory system, and urinary tract. The *mesoderm* (middle layer) lies between the other two germ layers and gives rise to muscle, connective tissue, cartilage, bone, blood cells, adipose cells, lymphoid tissue, and the linings of the major body cavities, joint cavities, and blood vessels.

Normal Morphology and Function

All body cells arise from one of these germ layers. The body also contains intercellular substances, which are formed by the cells and body fluids. Cells of the same type that together perform a special function are called a *tissue.* There are four primary tissues in the body and these are, of course, derived from the three germ layers. They are epithelium, muscle, nervous tissue, and connective tissue. Each body cell is included in one of these four classifications.

Epithelium

Epithelial cells are closely apposed and have very little cementing substance between them. Many are arranged as sheets of tissue called *membrane,* which cover or line surfaces. The mucous membrane in the mouth and the peritoneal membrane lining the abdominal cavity are examples. These membranes may be arranged in a single layer (*simple epithelium*) or in multiple layers (*stratified*). The cells may be very flat and wide (*squamous*), tall and narrow (*columnar*), or of equal height and width (*cuboidal*), or there may be variations of these (Fig. 1-1). Some epithelial cells are specialized further and have *cilia* (hairs) or *microvilli* (minute, fingerlike protrusions) on their surfaces.

The epithelial membranes lie on a *basal lamina* or *basement membrane,* which separates the epithelium from the underlying connective tissue. There are no blood or lymph vessels in epithelial membranes, so nutrients must be obtained by diffusion through the basal lamina from the underlying connective tissue.

Endothelium, originating from the mesoderm, is a special subclassification of epithelium. Endothelial cells line the cavities of the heart, blood vessels, and lymph vessels. The *mesothelium* is a thin flat layer of cells, also derived from mesoderm, that covers the surface of the peritoneum (lining of the abdominal and pelvic cavities and covering their contained organs), the pericardium (sac enclosing the heart), and the pleura (lining of the thoracic cavity and covering for the lungs). Endothelium and mesothelium are capable of some functions different from those of simple squamous epithelium, which they resemble. They are less differentiated and can form *fibroblasts,* a primitive type of connective tissue cell. They are also phagocytic.

Some epithelial cells are specialized further and have a secretory function. In certain locations, they invaginate the underlying connective tissue. In some cases, the site of the invagination is maintained as a duct system and the structure is known as an *exocrine gland.* The secretory products of exocrine glands pass into the ducts and then to a body surface. Exocrine glands may be very simple tubes or very complex in structure. They may be branched, coiled, or have compound structures with multiple branches. Some glands lose their connection with the epithelial surface of their origin and have no duct system. These are the *endocrine glands,* which release their secretions directly into the blood or lymph.

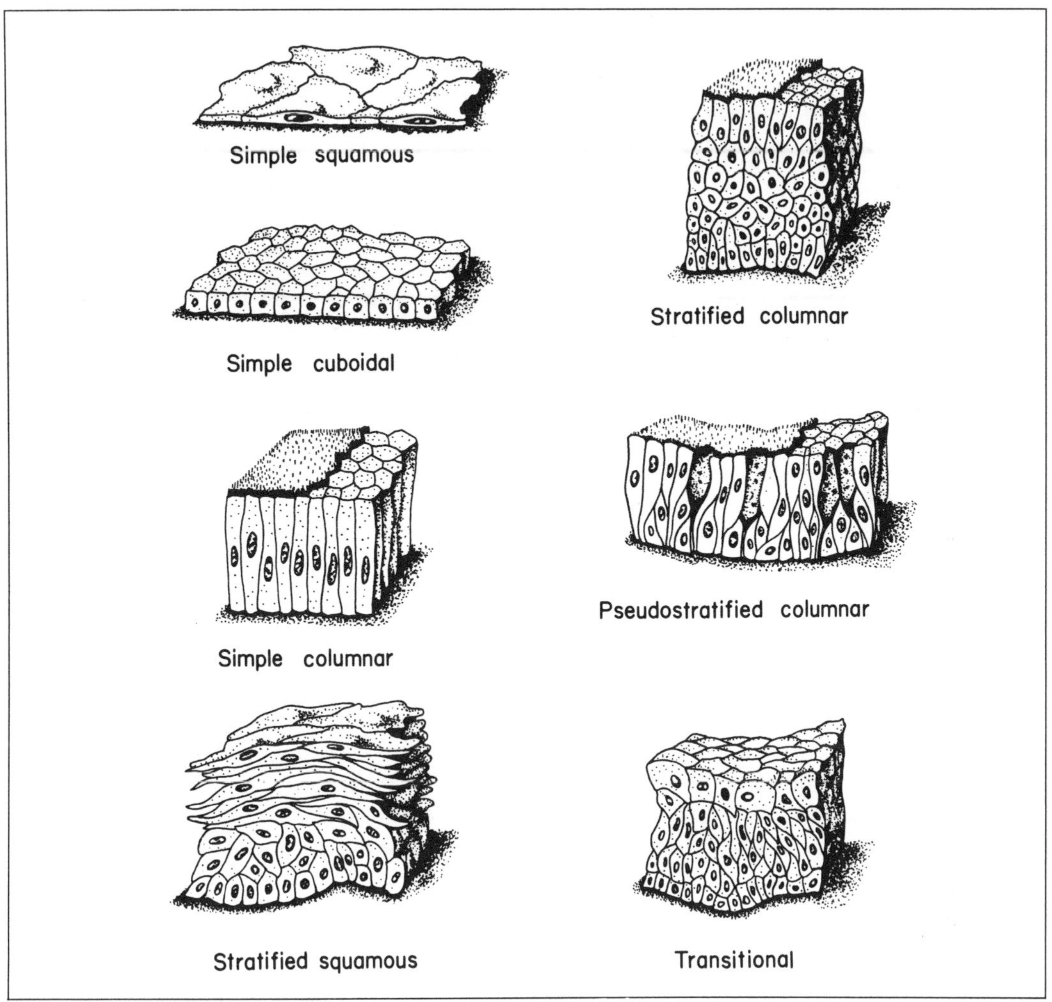

Figure 1-1. The shape and arrangement of cells in the principal types of epithelia. (Reprinted with permission from Bloom, W., and Fawcett, D.W., A Textbook of Histology, *10th ed. Philadelphia: W.B. Saunders, 1975, p. 85.)*

The main functions of epithelial tissue are protection, absorption, and secretion. Further details of the structure and function of epithelial cells are included in later chapters related to individual organ systems.

Muscle Tissue

The purpose of muscle tissue is to produce movement of the body or its parts. This is accomplished by *contractions* of the muscle cells or fibers. The cells are long and narrow and usually are grouped in bundles. A rich network of blood vessels provides nutrients and oxygen and removes waste products. These, together with nerve fibers, are carried among the muscle cells by connective tissue which binds the muscle fibers together and finally harnesses the muscle to other structures such as bone.

There are three types of muscle. *Smooth* muscles (also known as *involuntary* or *nonstriated* muscles) are found in areas of involuntary movement such as in the digestive system, arteries, and veins. *Skeletal* muscles (also known as *voluntary* or *striated* muscles) have a striped or striated appearance under the microscope. They also have rich blood vessel and nerve supplies supported by connective tissue. *Cardiac* (heart) muscle is striated but involuntary. It has less connective tissue, its own intrinsic contractility, and a unique blood supply, in that all arteries are end arteries with no overlap into adjacent areas.

Nervous Tissue

Anatomically, the nervous system consists of two parts. The *central nervous system* (CNS) is composed of the brain and spinal cord, and the *peripheral nervous system* is composed of all other nervous system structures. The CNS receives nervous impulses from within and from outside of the body and generates nervous impulses, whereas the peripheral nervous system interconnects other parts of the body with the CNS.

The major functioning cell of the nervous system is the *neuron.* Neurons often include in their structures long threadlike processes called *nerve fibers* or *axons,* which conduct impulses from the cell body. Neurons also possess one or more *dendrites,* processes that carry impulses to the cell body. The point of contact between the axon of one neuron and the dendrite of another is the *synapse.* The basic functions of the neurons are irritability, by which electrical impulses are carried to the neuron, and conduction, by which electrical impulses are carried from the neuron.

In addition to neurons, other types of cells are included in the nervous system. Many nerve fibers are surrounded by a layer of *Schwann* cells, the plasma membranes of which are known as *myelin.* In the CNS, there are a variety of connective tissue cells called *glial cells.* They form myelin, provide valuable metabolic and nutritive functions, act as supporting structures, and are phagocytic.

The brain and spinal column are protected by strong connective tissue membranes and are bathed by cerebrospinal fluid (CSF). The CSF, formed from the blood by a filtration process, serves protective and metabolic functions.

Connective Tissue

The mesoderm layer is the source of a meshwork of embryonic connective tissue known as *mesenchyme.* Mesenchymal cells can differentiate along various lines and can produce many different kinds of cells; therefore, they are pluripotential cells. They serve as the source of connective tissue proper and also of blood cells, bone, cartilage, and adipose tissue. Fig. 1-2 summarizes the possibilities.

Intercellular Material. Connective tissues produce abundant amounts of intercellular material so that the cells themselves are widely separated. The intercellular material or *matrix* includes fibers and an amorphous ground substance. The intercellular substances are nonliving materials that form the structure in which the body's cells live. They also act as a medium through which tissue fluid diffuses from blood to cells.

The fibrous or formed intercellular materials are proteins in long chains of three types. *Collagen* is secreted by fibroblasts and forms the meshwork of fibrillar material present in the stroma (structure) of all organs. In more concentrated form, it makes up tendons and fascia (bands or sheets connecting muscles). *Reticular fibers,* formed by primitive reticular cells similar to mesenchymal cells, create a fine supporting network around other cells. *Elastin* is an elastic material that, in fibrillar form, is associated with collagen in connective tissue. It also forms sheetlike layers in the walls of blood vessels.

The basal lamina serves as the boundary between connective tissue and other cells (Fig. 1-3). Its source is unknown, but it presumably is produced by either the adjacent epithelial or connective tissue cells.

Amorphous intercellular materials often exist in the form of stiff gels. They provide support and strength and are a medium through which nutrients and waste products must diffuse. There are two types: ground substance, which is relatively soft, and cement substance, which is quite firm. Both

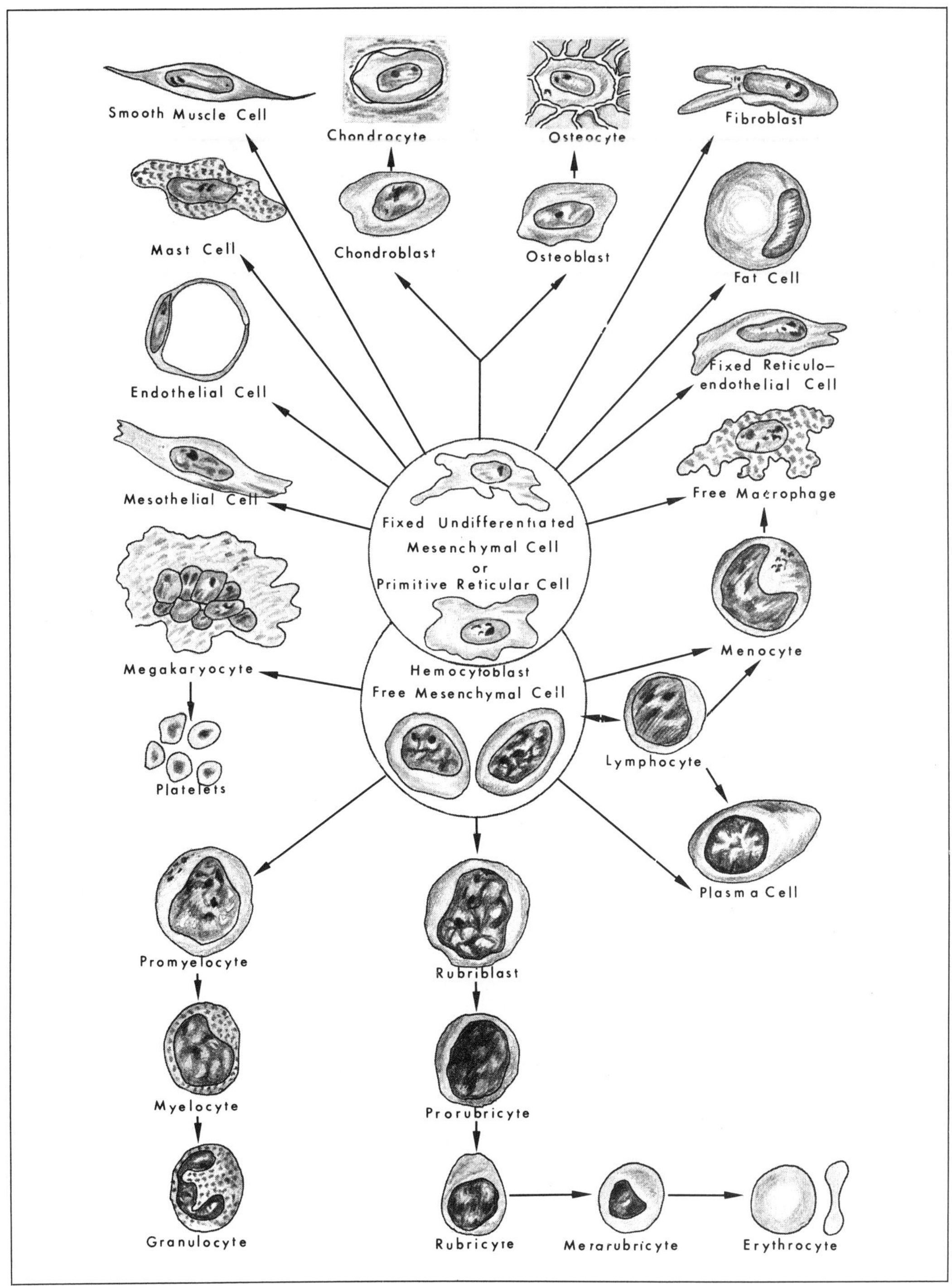

Figure 1-2. The interrelationships between cells of blood and connective tissues. (Reprinted with permission from Leeson, C.R., and Leeson, T.A., Histology, *3rd ed. Philadelphia: W.B. Saunders, 1976, p. 179.)*

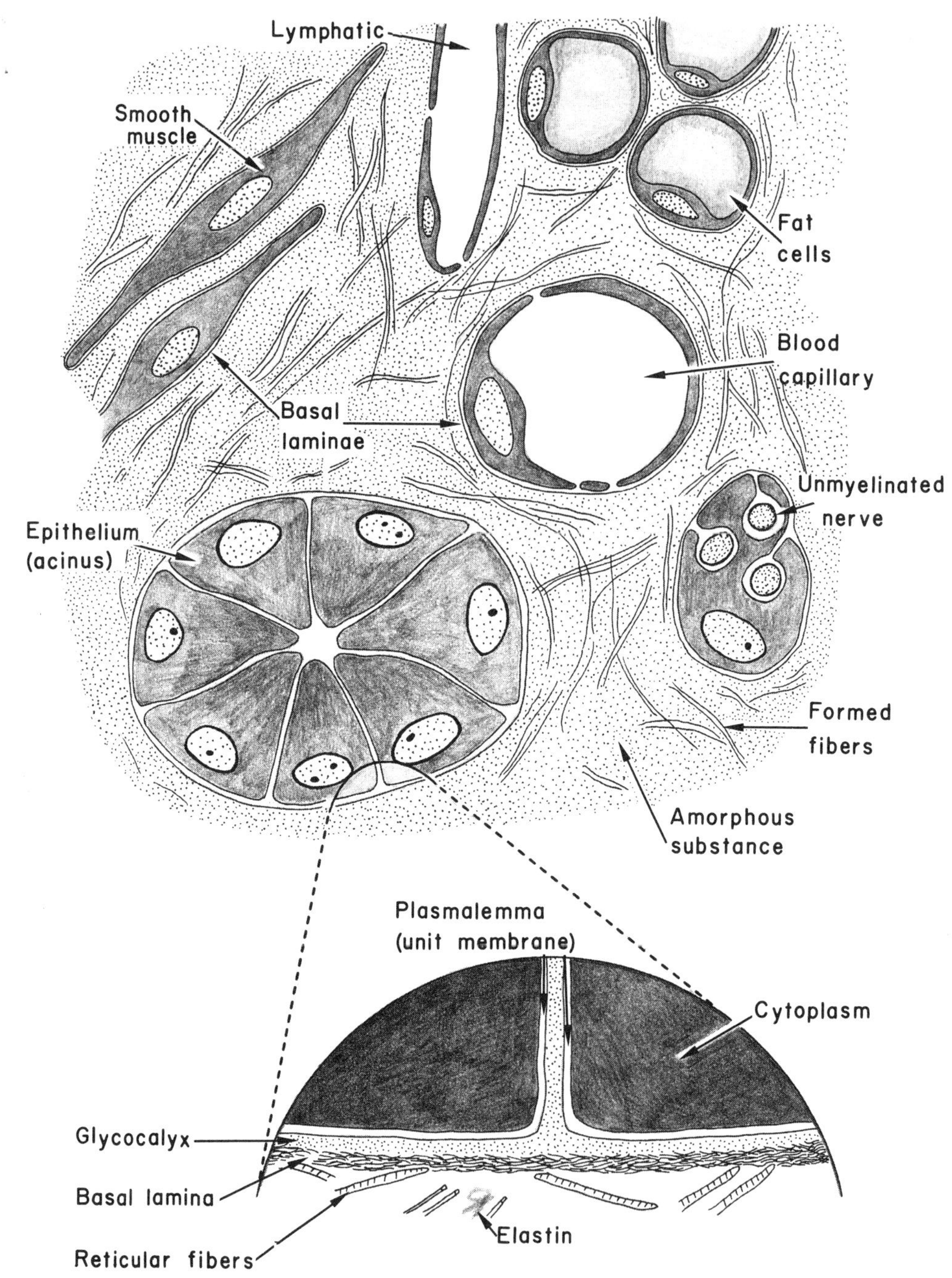

Figure 1-3. Basal laminae. Note that the connective tissue space is "limited" by basal laminae but the lymphatic capillary lacks a basal lamina. Below, the components of the basal lamina are shown. Probably periodic acid–Schiff stains the glycocalyx, basal lamina itself (mucopolysaccharide component), and associated reticular fibers. (Reprinted with permission from Leeson, C.R., and Leeson, T.S., Histology, *3rd ed. Philadelphia: W.B. Saunders, 1976, p. 85.)*

are synthesized by connective tissue cells and contain collagen and other proteins, mucopolysaccharides, carbohydrates, lipids, water, and other materials.

Cells of the Connective Tissue Proper. There are a number of different types of cells that make up the connective tissue proper. Fibroblasts are very numerous. They are believed to secrete the various connective tissue fibers and most or all of the amorphous ground substance. They retain, throughout their lives, a capacity for growth and regeneration and also are capable of some movement. *Macrophages* are also connective tissue cells. Their formation and function are described in Chapter 4. *Adipose cells* (fat cells) occur singly or in clumps. If present in large numbers, they form adipose tissue, the formation and metabolism of which are discussed in Chapter 15.

The nature of the connective tissue in the body varies greatly. It generally is divided into two categories. *Loose (areolar) connective tissue* is a loosely arranged, somewhat elastic tissue that binds various organs to each other but still allows the organs to move. Fibroblasts and macrophages, as well as collagen and a few elastin fibers, are distributed within it, and ground substance occupies its little spaces or *areolas.* Adipose tissue also forms within loose connective tissue. *Dense connective tissue* has closely packed fibers with few cells. In some structures, the fibers lie in parallel, forming tendons and ligaments. The parallel structure provides great tensile strength. Where tensions occur in all directions, irregularly arranged fibers provide strength. The fibers are interwoven to form structures such as the dermis of the skin, capsules of various organs, and most fascias.

Cartilage and Bone. Cartilage and bone are structures of the skeletal system. These tissues consist of cells, fibers, and ground substance, as do other body tissues, but their matrix (intercellular substance) is much more rigid.

Blood Cells. The blood cells, or formed elements of the blood, also are differentiated forms of connective tissue. The formation and function of *erythrocytes* (red blood cells) are described in Chapter 14. *Leukocytes* (white blood cells) are discussed in Chapter 4.

Physiologic Changes in Cells

Differentiated cells vary in their ability to reproduce. In some tissues, there is a constant turnover of cells. These cells are very *labile*—that is, they proliferate continuously throughout life. For example, simple squamous epithelial cells on surfaces are shed and replaced from cells in deeper layers, red and white blood cells die and are replenished from undifferentiated stem cells, and cells lining the lumen of the intestinal tract are sloughed and replaced continuously. In many other tissues, cells can be replaced by division of adjacent cells. These cells are *stable* and proliferate very little in adult life unless stimulated by tissue injury. There is great variability within the category of stable cells. Liver cells, for example, have an extensive replacement capability and will replace a whole lobe of liver. In contrast, renal glomerular cells will proliferate to some extent but will not do so sufficiently to develop new glomeruli. *Permanent cells* are highly specialized cells such as neurons and cells in the heart and some glands, which do not replicate in postnatal life.

Some cells are capable of increases in size or activity when appropriately stimulated. The increase in muscle size with increased activity is an example, as is the increase in adrenal function in stress.

GENERAL PRINCIPLES OF PATHOLOGY

Diseases are abnormalities of the structure or function of the body or any of its parts. The study of the causes of disease in general is known as *etiology,* but when a specific disease-producing agent is referred to, it is said to be a *cause* rather than an etiology; for example, the tubercle bacillus is the *cause* of tuberculosis. The causes of many diseases are unknown but are generally one of three types. *Biologic* causes include microorganisms and antibodies. Among *physical* causes are heat, cold, radiation, and similar phenomena. *Chemical* causes include materials such as acids, alkalies, and poisons. The *pathogenesis* of a disease is the response of the body to injury, since it is these reactions, rather than the injury, that produce the manifestations of disease. It is important to understand that, in response to injury, no new biochemical or physiologic mechanisms are created. Cellular reactions to injury occur by increasing or decreasing the rate of existing reactions.

Types of Abnormalities

An abnormality may occur in a cell, a tissue, or an entire *organ* ("a somewhat independent part of the body that performs a specialized function of functions"[1]), such as the liver, pancreas, or brain. The abnormality may be *structural* (a broken leg, for example) or *functional* (such as the inability to produce enough insulin). Structural abnormalities are called *lesions* and may be anatomic, such as a missing hand, or *morphological*, a large number of dead cells in the liver, for example.

Manifestations of Disease

The detectable indications of the presence of disease are its manifestations. They include both structural and functional abnormalities and may be classified into one of three categories:

1. *Symptoms* are manifestations verbalized by the patient (e.g., "I have a pain in my chest").
2. *Signs* are observations by a qualified examiner (e.g., The physician observes an apparent reaction to pain [tenderness]).
3. *Laboratory abnormalities* (e.g., High blood urea levels).

Diagnosis

Under ideal circumstances, the diagnosis will indicate the cause of the abnormal condition and define the reactions that are producing the manifestations of the disease. If a single manifestation is specific for a certain disease and if a positive accurate diagnosis can be made on the basis of the existence of that manifestation, then that manifestation is said to be *pathognomonic* for that disease. However, most diseases have nonspecific manifestations. Pain, fever, swelling, or rash, for example, occur in association with many diseases.

Cellular Responses To Injury

Although there are many specific agents that can injure the body, there are only a limited number of possible cellular responses. These are (1) growth disturbances, (2) abnormal development, (3) inflammation and repair, (4) cell degeneration, and (5) cell death.

Growth Disturbances

The process by which an organ completely fails to develop is known as *aplasia* or *agenesis*. Given a differentiated tissue or organ, disturbances of growth can be controlled or uncontrolled. In controlled changes, a stimulus can cause an increase in cell number (*hyperplasia*) or cell size (*hypertrophy*). In some circumstances, the absence of normal stimuli may result in *hypoplasia* (the failure to achieve normal development or size), whereas removal of the stimuli causes a decrease in the size of a tissue or organ (*atrophy*). Atrophy may result from a decrease in cell number or size or both.

In uncontrolled growth (*neoplasia*), cell replication does not cease when the original stimulus is removed. It involves an increase in the number of cells. This increase differs from normal physiologic growth in that it involves a change in the heredity of the cells, which produces a line of cells that are less subject to the normal regulatory mechanisms. Nutritional care of patients with neoplastic diseases is described in Chapter 13.

Developmental Disorders

A developmental abnormality is a structural or functional abnormality that results from the prenatal action of an injurious agent. Injuries occurring during birth are not included. The injury can become apparent before, during, or after birth. Thus, some developmental abnormalities are not observed until years after birth.

Developmental abnormalities can be classified four ways, including the following:

By cause of the abnormalities: A chemical, physical, or biologic agent may be the injurious factor. These may affect the genes or chromosomes or may injure the developing embryo or fetus directly. However, most causes are unknown.

By type of onset: The onset may be congenital or noncongenital. A congenital condition is one that is present at birth. It is important to recognize the distinction between genetic and congenital. A genetic disease is inherited and reflects the DNA structure that is passed from one generation to the next. Some abnormal genes produce disease whereas others do not. If a disease is produced, it may be congenital—that is, detectable at birth—or it may be noncongenital and become evident later in life.

By pathogenic mechanism: Developmental abnormalities may be caused by intrauterine injury or by genes or chromosomes. Chromosomal diseases may be related to autosomes or to sex chromosomes. Autosomal changes involve gross structural abnormalities evident at birth and therefore are congenital, whereas sex chromosome changes may produce abnormalities that become evident during later sexual maturation. Other conditions, such as maternal infections during pregnancy, can cause congenital abnormalities that are not genetic. Some cause an injury that is not apparent until sometime after birth and therefore are not congenital; however, it still may be a developmental abnormality but difficult to identify as such. A *familial disease* is one that affects more than one member of an extended family. Some, but not all, are genetic.

By type of structural or functional abnormalities: Structural and functional abnormalities can be subclassified as (1) *gross body deformities,* evident on physical examination; (2) *gross organ deformities* having obvious structural defects which are evident if the organ can be examined directly; and (3) either *diffuse* or *focal tissue reactions,* which occur in many developmental degenerative or inflammatory lesions and which can be seen with a microscope. Physiologic or biochemical defects are abnormalities detectable with physiologic or biochemical tests. Those in which nutritional care is important are discussed in Chapter 10.

Embryonic and Fetal Abnormalities. During the embryonic period, after some differentiation has occurred, one type of differentiated cell can affect other cells by a "message," probably a chemical stimulus. The process is called *induction.* The stimulus causes the induced cells to grow (increase in number or size), differentiate, or involute (decrease in number or size). Newly differentiated cells cause further induction leading to orderly development.

One period of differentiation is called *organogenesis,* the formation of the organs and limbs. *Involution* removes tissues that are not needed once they have served their purpose during development (for example, webbing between the digits). Prenatally, the organism is most susceptible to injury during germ layer formation, cell differentiation, and organogenesis.

Fertilization commonly occurs approximately 2 weeks following the mother's last menstrual period. The germ layers form during the fifth week after the menstrual period, whereas cell differentiation and organogenesis take place in weeks 6 through 10. Injuries early in embryogenesis produce grotesque anomalies and abortions with few survivors to birth. Gross organ malformations probably are due to injuries that occur somewhat later in development. Embryonic abnormalities often are called *congenital anomalies.* The anomalous organogenesis produces organ or body deformities that are present at birth.

The fetus differs in many ways from the adult. It has a high growth rate with large amounts of active DNA replication. It has underdeveloped immune mechanisms and conjugation mechanisms (see Chapter 3). Damage to the fetus may be the result of infection, immune mechanisms, drugs and toxins, radiation, malnutrition, or metabolic abnormalities in the mother.

Genetic Abnormalities. Theoretically, genetic defects produce abnormalities that can be logically associated with the protein that corresponds to the defective gene. They can cause structural defects or can affect enzyme proteins and cause metabolic defects. Those in which nutritional care is particularly useful are described in Chapter 10.

Most frequently, genetic diseases are multifactorial and clear lines of inheritance are difficult to establish. Some genetic diseases vary in *penetrance* (frequency with which the trait is manifested by individuals carrying the gene) or *expressivity* (extent to which the trait is manifested by the individual carrying the gene). The most common inherited disease is diabetes mellitus, which is discussed in Chapter 9.

Chromosomal Abnormalities. Many more genes are involved in chromosomal abnormalities than in genetic disorders, and the consequences of chromosomal disorders are less predictable. Most autosomal disorders cause spontaneous abortions. The most common chromosomal disorder in live-born children is mongolism or Down's syndrome. Nutritional care of these patients is discussed in Chapter 16.

Inflammation

Inflammation is a vascular and cellular response produced when cells are injured or destroyed by biologic, chemical, or physical agents (Table 1-1). It can occur anywhere in the body. Signs and symptoms are pain, heat, redness, and swelling. It is distinct from infection in which there is invasion of the body by pathogenic microorganisms. The reactions to infection may include inflammation, but degeneration or necrosis, described later in this chapter, also may occur.

Vascular Response. When cells are injured or killed, chemical mediators and acids are released. The chemical mediators cause the dilation of the nearby capillaries and increase their permeability (see Table 1-1). *Histamine,* released from mast cells and basophils, initiates the vascular response, but is short-acting. Long-acting responses are mediated by plasma *kinins,* released from the plasma protein alpha-2-globulin, and the blood-clotting mechanism. The capillary dilation increases the blood in the area and causes heat and redness. Increased capillary permeability allows fluids, protein, and blood cells to exude into the surrounding tissue and causes swelling. The material escaping from the capillaries under these conditions is an *exudate.* An exudate must be distinguished from a *transudate,* which is fluid that is forced out of the capillaries as a result of increased pressure.

Inflammations produce various kinds of exudates. The type is determined by the duration of the inflammation, the nature of the

Table 1-1. Summary of the Inflammatory Response

Events	Site	Morphologic Alteration	Mediator or Mechanism
Hemodynamic alterations	Arterioles	Vasodilation	Neurogenic Chemical: Histamine, prostaglandins E and F
	Venules	Vasodilation	Chemical: Histamine, kinins, complement fractions, lysosomal products
	Capillaries	Vasodilation and opening of inactive channels	
Permeability changes			
Early	Venules	Dilation, congestion, and widening of endothelial junctions	Physical: Increased hydrostatic pressure Chemical: Histamine, kinins, complement fractions, lysosomal products, prostaglandin E(?)
Late	Capillaries	Dilation, congestion, and endothelial injury	Physical: Increased hydrostatic pressure, direct endothelial injury Chemical: Prostaglandins(?), SRS-A(?)[a]
White blood cell events			
Margination and pavementing	Venules and capillaries	Peripheral orientation and adherence to endothelial surfaces	Interruption of laminar flow Chemotactic factors(?)
Emigration	Venules and capillaries	Escape from vessels	Chemotactic factors(?)
Chemotaxis		Accumulation at site of injury	Chemotactic factors *For neutrophils:* Complement fractions, fibrin fractions, components of kinin system, bacterial products *For macrophages:* Bacteria, complement fractions, neutrophil fractions, lymphocyte factors
Phagocytosis		Engulfment of bacteria and debris	Lymphokines Opsonins Complement

Reprinted with permission from Robbins, S.L., Angell, M., and Kumar, V., *Basic Pathology,* 3rd ed. Philadelphia: W.B. Saunders, 1981, p. 40.

[a] SRS-A = Slow-reacting substance of anaphylaxis.

injurious agent, the severity of the condition, and the tissues affected. A *serous exudate* may be formed in a mild inflammation when the increase in capillary permeability is moderate. Serous exudate is a watery fluid resembling blood serum and contains small-molecule proteins. It forms from blood serum and from secretions of serosal cells of the linings of the body cavities. When inflammation is severe or sustained, capillary dilation is greater and fibrin (the protein in serum that is essential for blood clotting) escapes in the exudate, forming a *fibrinous exudate. Suppurative* or *purulent exudate* (pus) contains large amounts of dead and living cells, especially neutrophils and pyogenic (pus-producing) bacteria. *Catarrhal exudates* are similar to serous exudate but contain large amounts of mucus. They are produced in inflammations of mucous membranes. When a mucous membrane is attacked by a very toxic agent, the fibrinous exudate combines with necrotic cells and inflammatory cells to form a false membrane, a process called *pseudomembranous inflammation.* When red blood cells also escape from damaged vessels, the exudate is *hemorrhagic.*

An exudate can cause further cell damage. It also causes pain by irritation of the local nerve endings through fluid pressure and the presence of kinins and acids released from dead cells.

Cellular Response. As fluid exudes from the capillaries, the flow of blood slows and certain white blood cells (neutrophils and monocytes) emigrate into the damaged area (see Table 1-1). They attack and ingest or digest the offending agents and remove the killed cells in preparation for repair. Digestion makes the debris soluble so that it can be carried away by plasma.

Other cells important in the inflammatory response occur in the tissues. Macrophages, similar to and derived from the monocytes in the blood, also are phagocytic. They multiply rapidly when tissues are injured. Giant cells form from the fusion of macrophages or by amitotic division to ingest large pieces of debris. Lymphocytes and plasma cells also participate in the body's defenses. Their actions are described in Chapter 4.

Systemic Manifestations. Some inflammations are localized and others are diffuse. When they are diffuse, they cause a number of systemic manifestations. Chemical agents called *pyrogens,* some of which are released from certain types of cells, including bacteria, affect the thermoregulatory center in the brain and produce a fever. Fever also occurs in infections, tissue necrosis, hemorrhage, some neoplasms, and other conditions. It increases the metabolic rate and often is accompanied by loss of appetite. As a result, there may be depletion of body tissue, with muscle wasting and loss of body fat. Fluid losses may lead to dehydration. The nutritional consequences of fever are described in Chapter 12.

Fluid and protein that escape from the capillaries are taken up by the lymphatics and carried to the lymph nodes. These become enlarged and painful, a condition known as *lymphadenitis.*

Factors Modifying the Inflammatory Response. Inflammations vary in duration, location, degree of localization, and type of exudate. These are influenced by the amount of the damaging agent, the duration of exposure, and the *pathogenicity* of the agent (its inherent ability to cause disease and its ability to invade the tissue).

Several factors in the host also modify the inflammatory response. One of these is the general health of the host. It is generally accepted that advanced age, poor nutrition, and the presence of preexisting disease are negative influences. In addition, the immunity of the host (see Chapter 4) modifies the inflammatory response.

The vascularity of the injured tissue and its location also have an effect. The spread of disease is reduced in dense compact tissue such as bone, and the defensive response is poor when blood supply is poor.

The duration of inflammation is classified as *acute* (hours to weeks), *subacute* (weeks to a month), or *chronic* (months to years). The term *acute* sometimes is used to suggest great severity instead of duration. Inflammations persist only as long as damaging agents are present. Chronic inflammations must be caused, then, by agents that persist. These agents must be (1) resistant to phagocytosis or digestion, (2) continually produced in the body, or (3) present in the environment and therefore make exposure constant. The inflammation also tends to persist when host defenses are poor such as in impaired immune function or decreased blood supply. In chronic inflammation, the inflammatory response is less pronounced than is the case in acute conditions. Fibroblasts proliferate and may cause scarring, adhesions, or obstructions. Some injurious agents induce a response called *chronic granulomatous inflammation,* in which some microorganisms or foreign materials that are resistant to phagocytosis or digestion become surrounded by macrophages, thus causing small nodules or granulomas to develop, walling off the injurious agent.

Necrosis

Cell death is the irreversible permanent cessation of the vital functions such as respiration, maintenance of homeostasis, and protein synthesis. Two types of irreversible changes indicative of cell death are *rupture of the cell membrane* and *nuclear changes.* These can be seen with a microscope.

The death of the patient is *somatic death. Necrobiosis* or *physiologic cell death* occurs as part of normal turnover. *Necrosis,* on the other hand, refers to the abnormal death of cells within a living body. It does *not* include either the gradual death of some cells in the aging process or cell death that occurs after the patient has died.

When a portion of the body becomes necrotic, the surrounding area becomes congested and inflamed. Under these circumstances, necrosis and inflammation coexist.

Mechanisms of Necrosis. There are four general modes of action by which necrosis is produced:

Anoxia. Anoxia (lack of oxygen) is the most common cause. It is produced by interference at any step in the process of supplying oxygen and therefore may be local, regional, or systemic. In some circumstances, the alteration is metabolic. In others, there is a localized functional or mechanical interference with the blood supply known as *ischemia.* When ischemia results in the death of all cells in an area, the lesion is called an *infarct.*

Some organs have components that are more susceptible to injury than others. When anoxia is systemic or regional rather than localized, these susceptible portions are more likely to be injured, even if the anoxia is not sufficiently severe to kill all the cells. The result is called *selective necrosis.* These same cells often are also easily injured by toxic compounds. In the kidney, for example, the resulting condition is called *acute tubular necrosis* (see Chapter 7). In mild, prolonged regional ischemia, there is a reduction in organ size (*ischemic atrophy*).

Protein precipitation. Some toxic substances cause necrosis by precipitating proteins in cells with which they come in contact. An example is ingestion of caustic chemicals.

Osmotic injury. Three mechanisms can disrupt the maintenance of osmotic homeostasis by the cell membrane: (1) physical trauma that disrupts the cell membrane; (2) exposure to hypertonic or hypotonic solutions in excess of the cell's ability to adjust, resulting in cell shrinkage or bursting; and (3) antigen-antibody reactions on cell surfaces with possible complement activation leading to lysis of the membrane (see Chapter 4).

Accumulation of certain metabolic products. Excess production of some metabolic products or reduced ability to remove metabolic wastes can result in cell death by interfering with the normal metabolism of the cell.

In the various disease processes, the methods by which cell necrosis is produced is often a combination of these four mechanisms. In some disorders, cell necrosis is caused by digestion of the cells by enzymes. For example, pancreatic digestive enzymes can digest the pancreatic protein itself and that of surrounding tissues. When large numbers of neutrophils are attracted to an area of infection by pyogenic bacteria, their enzymes may kill surrounding healthy tissue also. In some patients, such as diabetics (see Chapter 9), gas gangrene develops in dead tissue killed by anoxia. The causative organisms, *Clostridium perfringens,* liberate enzymes that can kill adjacent tissue. In another example, allergic reactions (see Chapter 4) may cause necrosis by such effects as damaging cell membranes and by releasing histamine which causes swelling that then interferes with blood flow.

Types of Necrosis. The specific nature of necrotic lesions varies with the type of tissue and the injurious agent. They can be distinguished through a microscope by a pathologist, but the distinction usually is not important to the nutritional care specialist. One exception is the existence of gangrene.

Gangrene is a subtype of necrosis. It usually is caused by ischemia, with secondary invasion by putrefactive bacteria which do not invade live tissue since they are anaerobic. Gangrene has three subtypes: wet, dry, and gas gangrene. *Dry gangrene* usually occurs in extremities that are infarcted. The affected area dries up and turns black from the liberation of bacterial hydrogen sulfide. The invasion by putrefactive bacteria is slow and so the infection spreads slowly. *Wet gangrene* occurs in moist tissues that become necrotic. The bacterial invasion occurs rapidly. It occurs in abdominal organs most commonly but can occur in the extremities. If it leads to perforation of abdominal organs, the spread of infection can be rapid. *Gas gangrene* is the most dangerous form. It usually is associated with wounds. Certain types of clostridia release a toxin that causes more necrosis and liberate gas that causes bubbles in the necrotic tissue. The dead tissue must be removed (*debrided*) very quickly.

Degeneration

Degeneration, in contrast to necrotic changes, refers to detrimental cellular alterations that are potentially reversible. Often, however, degenerative changes precede cell death, and there is a continuous progression from reversible degeneration to irreversible loss of function to irreversible changes to death.

Classification. Acute degenerations generally are caused by milder forms of the same factors that cause necrosis, anoxia being the most common. In *chronic degeneration,* a variety of substances accumulate within the cell or extracellularly. Deposited materials may be protein, fat, carbohydrate, or minerals. The materials deposited usually are inert; otherwise, they would cause necrosis. They may be intracellular or interstitial deposits or consist of alterations of existing interstitial materials. As extracellular deposits accumulate, normal cells often atrophy.

Some degenerations are processes in which the accumulated materials are produced locally and are referred to as *accumulation* or *storage.* In others, the material is brought to the tissue and is referred to as a *deposit* or *infiltration.*

Degeneration Involving Water. Acute degenerations due to increased cellular water content with increased cell size is called *cloudy swelling* if mild or *hydropic degeneration* if more severe. In cloudy swelling, organ weight increases; the organ increases in opacity or cloudiness and may be pale. There is tension on organs with nonelastic capsules such as the kidney. Cloudy swelling occurs in most tissues following mild injury.

Chronic degeneration with intracellular water accumulation is unknown. Water that accumulates between cells (*edema*) is classified as a hemodynamic disorder, not a form of degeneration.

Degeneration Involving Carbohydrate. There are two types of carbohydrate involved in degenerations. *Glycogen* accumulates in cells in some inherited metabolic disorders. For example, in some of the glycogen storage diseases, enzymes involved in glycogen breakdown are deficient and glucose mobilization is poor. As a result, glycogen accumulates in the tissue. In contrast, in diabetes mellitus, glucose utilization is defective, resulting in high glucose levels in blood and urine. Glucose is converted to glycogen and accumulates in renal tubule cells and hepatic nuclei. Diabetes mellitus is discussed in detail in Chapter 9.

In a different form of carbohydrate degeneration, the materials that accumulate are *carbohydrate-protein complexes.* These materials are found in extracellular ground substance and in mucus-secreting epithelial cells. Their accumulation is not considered to be a degeneration in the narrow sense of the term. Rather, the term *mucin degenerations* is loosely used to include:

1. Plugged excretory ducts from which mucin cannot be removed. (This condition occurs in cystic fibrosis of the pancreas, which is discussed in Chapter 6.)
2. Mucin-producing cancers, which spill mucin into connective tissue. (Nutritional care of cancer patients is discussed in Chapter 13.)
3. Myxomas, connective tissue tumors that produce ground substance.
4. Atrophy of connective tissue with a *relative* increase in ground substance.

Degeneration Involving Lipids. Lipids involved in degenerations may occur as liquid droplets, protein-bound complexes, or cholesterol crystals. They are found within the cell except for the cholesterol crystals and accidentally inhaled oils. The extracellular lipids are removed by macrophages, if possible. Otherwise, the area is walled off by fibrous tissue. If adipose tissue is accidentally injured, the triglyceride escaping from ruptured adipose cells is removed by macrophages.

Degenerations involving triglyceride accumulation may occur in adipose tissue cells or in *hepatocytes* (functional cells of the liver). Accumulation of triglyceride (*adiposity*), which takes the form of a general and severe increase in lipid content of adipose tissue cells, is called *obesity.* The nutritional treatment of obesity is discussed in Chapter 15.

Another form of adiposity is the replacement of *parenchymal tissue* (functional cells) by normal-appearing adipose tissue. Some adiposity occurs in the heart muscle and pancreas with aging but is not considered to be important clinically. Adipose tissue cells are not found in the parenchyma of the brain, lung, liver, kidney, or spleen.

Fatty metamorphosis of the liver is seen in many patients who come to the attention of the nutritional care specialist. This condition consists of the accumulation of globules of neutral lipid within the hepatocytes which then resemble adipose tissue cells. Thus, the response of the liver to fat accumulation is fatty metamorphosis, not adiposity. The liver may receive lipids from the intestine or plasma or may manufacture it from carbohydrate or protein. It uses the lipid for energy or exports it in the form of lipoprotein or triglyceride coated with lipoprotein (see Chapters 8 and 11). The main export is to adipose tissue. Factors promoting fatty metamorphosis in the liver are (1) increased lipid input, (2) decreased utilization of lipid for energy, and (3) inability to export it due to defective lipoprotein synthesis.

Increased input of lipid may be dietary or result from excessively rapid release of lipid from adipose tissue. This rapid release can occur in circumstances such as acute starvation or insulin deficiency. Decreased utilization of lipid by the liver may result from deprivation of carbohydrate to "feed" the tricarboxylic acid cycle or anything that interferes with oxidative metabolism. Inability to export triglyceride is due to defective synthesis of lipoprotein. This can occur in protein or choline deficiency or as a toxic reaction to alcohol, carbon tetrachloride, and some phosphorus compounds.

Mild to moderate fatty metamorphosis can be transient or prolonged. It is associated with many diseases but usually is not accompanied by detectable changes in liver function. Severe fatty metamorphosis, however, is likely to be prolonged and associated with liver enlargement, changes in function, and sometimes jaundice (high bilirubin levels in the blood, skin, and mucous membrane with a yellow appearance in the patient). It tends to be chronic in alcoholism (Chapter 11), prolonged protein deficiency, and diabetes (Chapter 9).

Xanthomas consist of localized collections of *histiocytes* (large phagocytic cells) containing cholesterol. They often are associated with elevated serum cholesterol and usually are found in the skin. Histiocytes containing cholesterol sometimes are called *foam cells* or *xanthoma cells.*

Lipidoses are rare genetic diseases associated with storage of lipoprotein complexes.

Atherosclerosis is characterized by lipid deposits in the walls of large and medium-sized arteries. The lesions are called *atheromas.* In early formation, they consist largely of foam cells containing much cholesterol. These cells later break down and cholesterol crystals are formed. This condition and its extensive consequences are described in Chapter 8.

Degeneration Involving Protein. Accumulations of protein or proteinlike materials may be extracellular or intracellular. *Hyaline* is an adjective used to describe protein deposits that are homogeneous and transluscent in appearance under the microscope. The material deposited is called *hyalin.* Most hyaline deposits are composed of collagen, fibrin, *amyloid* (a homogeneous, transluscent glycoprotein), edema fluid with a high protein content, some foreign bodies, and compacted platelets. Fibrin masses are associated with inflammatory lesions where fibrin has time to accumulate. The presence of collagen is considered a degeneration only when dense masses of old acellular scar tissue accumulate.

Amyloid is thought to be produced by plasma cells (see Chapter 4). It therefore is associated with inflammations and malignant tumors of plasma cells (malignant myeloma). It occurs in the walls of small blood vessels, between muscle fibers of all three types of muscle, and between cells of such organs as liver, spleen, kidney, and adrenal glands. The condition is called *amyloidosis,* a term that refers to a group of rare, slowly progressing conditions in which a material composed of alpha and gamma globulins and glycoproteins is deposited. It may be *primary* (no previous cause known) or *secondary* to other diseases. It also may occur in the form of amyloid tumors, usually in the upper respiratory tract. Secondary amyloidosis occurs in patients who have long-standing inflammations such as rheumatoid arthritis, but the amyloid deposits occur in organs remote from the site of the inflammations, commonly in the liver, kidneys, spleen, or adrenal glands. Primary amyloidosis commonly affects cardiac muscle, smooth muscle of the small blood vessels and gastrointestinal tract, and skeletal muscle of the tongue.

Degeneration Involving Calcium. Degeneration may involve deposits of calcium, phosphorus, iron, or unidentified crystals. The most common of these is calcification. In *dystrophic calcification,* the deposits occur at sites of tissue necrosis or degeneration but the metabolism of calcium itself is normal. In *metastatic calcification,* calcium metabolism has been affected by a disease process and serum calcium levels are elevated. Calcium then precipitates at sites such as the kidney, gastrointestinal tract, or lung, and can cause disease in these organs.

HEALING

Healing is the process by which normal structure and function are restored following injury. Complete restoration is not always possible, but the attempt to do so is a form of healing.

Healing Processes

The processes involved in healing include:

1. *Resolution:* The resorption of exudates and liquefied debris
2. *Sloughing:* The separation of dead tissue or exudate from an internal or external surface

3. *Repair.* The replacement of dead or injured tissue by new parenchymal (functional) or stromal (structural) cells

Resolution occurs as part of the cellular response to inflammation. Resolution and sloughing may precede or accompany repair.

Parenchymal cells are much more susceptible to injury than are stromal cells. When parenchymal cells are killed, there may be permanent loss of function following resolution, even if the stroma is intact.

The kind of repair that occurs is determined primarily by the proliferative capacity of the cells involved. *Regeneration* is replacement of lost cells by proliferation of the remaining parenchymal cells. The lost cells must, then, be labile or stable cells. Regeneration is not possible if the lost cells are permanent cells, such as neurons in the brain. The types of cells in each category are listed in Table 1-2. In contrast to regeneration, connective tissue repair or *organization* consists of replacement of the lost cells by proliferation of the connective tissue (stroma) of the organ. In scarring, the replacement is with collagenous tissue in its entirety, with no significant parenchymal replacement.

As a general rule, parenchyma of glandular organs such as renal tubules, secretory glands of the digestive tract, and endocrine organs, and most mesenchymal tissues, such as stroma, bone, cartilage, adipose tissue, and glia, contain stable cells. Muscle tissue varies in its regenerative capacity. Smooth muscle is capable of some regeneration whereas cardiac muscle is not. In striated muscle and in nerves, if the *sarcolemma* (sheath covering the muscle fiber) or *neurilemma* (sheath covering myelinated nerves) is intact, and if the nucleus is intact, the cell can regenerate the injured portion.

Regeneration can be *orderly* and thus restore normal structure and function, but it is *disorderly* in some circumstances—that is, the regeneration is a combination of parenchymal regeneration and connective tissue repair resulting in disorganized structure and loss of function. A fibrotic liver (Chapter 11) is an example of disorderly regeneration. The type and severity of injury are important in determining the type of regeneration that will occur, if any. First, there must be some remaining parenchymal tissue to regenerate. Second, if the stroma is intact, orderly regeneration is more likely to occur. If the stroma also is damaged, disorderly regeneration will ensue. In summary, for orderly regeneration to occur, there must be labile or stable cells, some living parenchyma, and an intact stroma.

Table 1-2. Regenerative Capacities of Tissues and Organs

Labile cells
Epithelium of skin, gastrointestinal and genitourinary tracts, renal tubule, exocrine gland ducts
Red blood cells, white blood cells, platelets in bone marrow
Liver parenchyma
Lymphoid tissues
Endothelium
Bone
Peripheral nerves
Stable cells
Skeletal and smooth muscle
Lung parenchyma
Renal glomeruli
Endocrine glands
Gonadal parenchyma
Permanent cells
Cardiac muscle
Neurons of central nervous system
Retinal tissue and other special sense organs
Permanent teeth

Organization or connective tissue repair is the invasion and replacement of dead cells and exudate by new cells originating from the stroma of the organ. Typically, there is growth of capillaries and fibroblasts. Later, fibrous tissue forms. This process can occur in any organ to provide strength when it is permanently injured. When exudates are organized, there is an unnecessary loss of normal structure and function.

The invading reparative tissue produced early in organization is called *granulation tissue.* It consists primarily of fibroblasts and

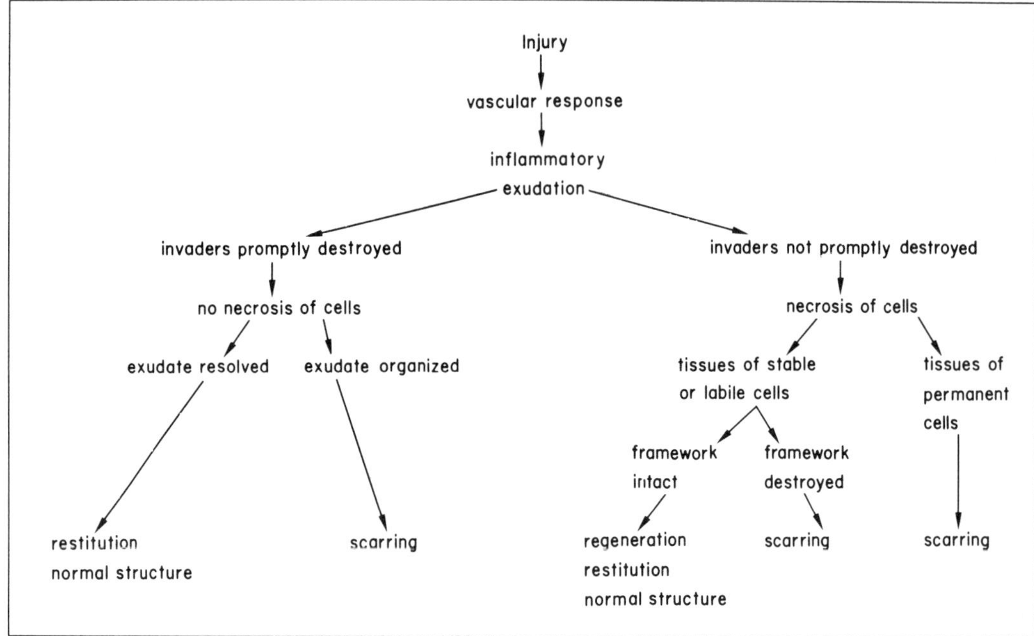

Figure 1-4. Pathways of reparative response. (Reprinted with permission from Robbins, S.L., Angell, M., and Kumar, V., Basic Pathology, *3rd ed. Philadelphia: W.B. Saunders, 1981, p. 57.)*

endothelial cells and results in formation of a scar. Granulation tissue has many cells and a rich blood supply. In time, collagen is laid down and rearranged; the wound is contracted and, thus, smaller, and the blood vessels are pinched off. Cellularity and vascularity thereby are reduced. Scar formation is familiar on the skin, but it also can occur in internal organs with consequent permanent loss of function. Under some circumstances, *adhesions* are formed in positions that create an abnormal union between previously separate parts, restricting their movement. The reparative response is summarized in Fig. 1-4.

Factors That Affect Healing

Three factors are necessary for rapid wound healing: good apposition of the margins of the wound, a minimum of necrotic tissue, and minimum infection. If these conditions are not met, the early healing may break down and then heal more slowly with a larger scar. The repair rate is influenced by the blood supply and temperature of the damaged tissue; tissues with a poor blood supply heal slowly. Deficiencies of nutrients (especially protein and vitamin C), old age, corticosteroid medications, and the presence of debilitating illness also interfere with healing.

References

1. Dorland's Illustrated Medical Dictionary (26th ed.). Philadelphia, Penn.: W.B. Saunders Company, 1981.

Bibliography

Bloom, W., and Fawcett, D.W. *A Textbook of Histology,* 10th ed. Philadelphia: W.B. Saunders, 1975.

Frohlich, E.D., Ed. *Pathophysiology. Altered Regulatory Mechanisms in Disease,* 2nd ed. Philadelphia: J.B. Lippincott, 1976.

Ham, A.W. *Histology,* 8th ed. Philadelphia: J.B. Lippincott, 1979.

Hill, R.B., Jr., and LaVia, M.F., Eds. *Principles of*

Pathobiology, 3rd ed. New York: Oxford University Press, 1980.
Junqueira, L.C., Carneiro, J., and Contopoulos, A.N. *Basic Histology,* 3rd ed. Los Altos, Calif.: Lange Medical, 1980.
Robbins, S.L., and Angell, M. *Basic Pathology,* 2nd ed. Philadelphia: W.B. Saunders, 1976.
Sodeman, W.A., and Sodeman, T.M. *Pathologic Physiology. Mechanisms of Disease,* 6th ed. Philadelphia: W.B. Saunders, 1979.
Weiss, L., and Greep, R.O. *Histology,* 4th ed. New York: McGraw-Hill, 1977.
Widmann, F.K. *Pathobiology: How Disease Happens.* Boston: Little, Brown, 1978.

2. General Principles of Nutritional Care

- I. Essentials of Nutritional Care
- II. Documentation of Nutritional Care
  - A. Problem-oriented medical record
    - 1. Data base
    - 2. Problem list
    - 3. Initial care plans
    - 4. Progress notes
    - 5. Other pertinent information
  - B. Source-oriented record
- III. Nutritional Assessment
  - A. Assessment procedures
    - 1. Measurements of muscle mass and subcutaneous fat
    - 2. Measurement of visceral protein
    - 3. Cell-mediated immune function
    - 4. Nitrogen balance
    - 5. Basal energy expenditure
    - 6. Other laboratory tests
    - 7. Clinical observations
    - 8. Dietary assessment
      - a. methods to obtain data
        - (1) twenty-four-hour recall
        - (2) food frequency lists
        - (3) food records
        - (4) dietary history
        - (5) food preference questionnaire
        - (6) direct observation
      - b. evaluation of the diet
        - (1) estimates of nutrient content of the diet
        - (2) comparison of nutrient content to requirements
  - B. Evaluation of nutritional status
    - 1. Diagnosis of protein-calorie malnutrition
    - 2. Estimate of clinical risk
- IV. Identification of Problems
- V. Planning Nutritional Care
- VI. Implementation of the Nutritional Care Plan
  - A. Procedures in feeding patients
    - 1. Normal nutritional base
    - 2. Adaptations for disease
      - a. purposes of therapeutic diets
      - b. types of therapeutic diets
        - (1) routine diets
        - (2) modified diets
        - (3) test diets
        - (4) quantitative and qualitative diets
        - (5) parenteral and enteral feeding
    - 3. Adaptations for individual characteristics
  - B. Education and other forms of intervention
- VII. Evaluation of Patient Care
- VIII. Case Study

The most important function of the nutritional care specialist is to assure that all patients, regardless of specific diagnosis, are adequately nourished, either by the actual provision of nutrients or by counseling patients in their own food choices. Not only must the normal nutritional requirements of healthy persons be considered, but also the increased needs mandated by the nature of the patient's illness must be met. In addition, the individual characteristics and preferences of the patients cannot be disregarded. In providing for the patients' needs, nutritional care specialists must integrate their own activities with those of other members of the health care team.

This chapter will provide an overview of the nutritional care process, without regard to specific diagnosis, and a discussion of the means of documenting that care. Later chapters will consider nutritional care in diseases of the various organ systems.

ESSENTIALS OF NUTRITIONAL CARE

In practice, an initial evaluation, applied to all patients, identifies those who require nutritional care. Nutritional care, then, consists of four basic steps:

1. *Assessment* to identify the patient's specific nutritional problems
2. *Planning* for care
3. *Implementation* of the plans for care
4. *Evaluation* of the results of care

Evaluation involves reassessment, making nutritional care a cyclic process.

All steps in nutritional care should be documented in the medical record; therefore, it is important that the nutritional care specialist be familiar with the recording procedures used.

DOCUMENTATION OF NUTRITIONAL CARE

There are two formats of medical records in common use, the *problem-oriented medical record* (POMR) and the *source-oriented medical record* (SOMR). The problem-oriented record is the newer system and is thought by many to be superior.[1,2]

Problem-Oriented Medical Record

The POMR, in which all aspects of patient care are documented, provides a vehicle for recognition of all the patient's problems and for coordination of the activities of all members of the health care team. It consists of four major parts: the data base, a problem list, the initial care plan, and progress notes.[3] In addition, the record will include flow sheets and a discharge summary.

Data Base

The data base is established at the time that care is initiated. It includes a *patient profile*—that is, a description of the patient along with relevant environmental, social, and family factors—the patient's perception of his purpose in seeking care (the chief complaint), medical history and family medical history. It also contains the *review of systems,* a series of focused screening questions arranged by organ systems, the results of physical examination, the results of laboratory tests and other diagnostic procedures, and the nutrition history. The original nutritional assessment is included in the data base. A list of commonly used abbreviations is given in Appendix A.

Problem List

Based on the data, a master problem list is established by the physician. A problem is anything that requires diagnostic procedures or management. Problems may be symptoms, an abnormal physiologic or laboratory test result, a diagnosis, or social, nutritional, or psychiatric factors. *Current problems* are those for which an initial plan will be written, whereas *inactive problems* are those that require no further management. New problems are added to the current list as they become known and those that are resolved are moved to the inactive list.

Allergies, sensitivities, and intolerances to foods and drugs, such as gluten intolerance, milk allergy, or penicillin allergy, should be included in the problem list. Problems related to previously prescribed diets or drugs also are listed. These might include the diabetic patient who does not follow a given diet, for instance.

The problem list is kept at the front of the patient's chart and acts as a table of contents, with each problem bearing its own number. In most institutions, only the physician adds items to or removes an item from the problem list.

Initial Care Plans

Plans for dealing with each problem are written by the physician in a standardized format containing the following elements, known by the acronym SOAP:

Subjective data: Any information obtained from the patient or the patient's family that is pertinent to the listed problem is recorded, including the patient's perception of how he or she feels and his or her description of symptoms and other concerns (e.g., "I get diarrhea every time I drink milk").

Objective data: Data obtained from tests, analyses, or observations made by members of the health care team that can be confirmed by others are listed (e.g., blood or urine analyses, roentgenograms, diet analysis, measures of intake or output, observations of behavior).

Assessment: The physician gives the interpretation (diagnosis), if known, or his or her impression of the significance of the problem.

Plan: Specific plans are stated for dealing with each problem.

For each problem, plans may be of several types. If the diagnosis is unknown, plans are made to obtain further information leading to diagnosis. Specific treatment plans, including nutritional care such as a modified diet, may be instituted. Referral to the nutritional care specialist may be made at this time. Patient education, including nutritional counseling of the patient or significant other may be employed. (*Significant other* is a sociologist's term referring to important persons in the individual's social system. In nutrition, this usually means those with whom the patient lives and shares meals or other close family members.)

Progress Notes

Once the initial problem list is established, the continuing care of the patient is documented chronologically in the POMR by those involved in that care. Progress notes, marked with the number of the problem to which they are related, are contributed by the physician, nursing staff, nutritional care specialist, physical therapist, occupational therapist, social worker, or any other professional involved in the care of that patient. The type of note (for example, nutrition note, nutrition consult, or dietitian's note) is stated also. Within the record, the actual nutritional care provided must be documented, including the type of diet, adjustments for intolerance to the diet, and diet instructions given by the nutritional care specialist.

Progress notes are written in SOAP format. In this fashion, all members of the health care team are aware of the functions, contributions, and activities of all the others. Coordination and cooperation thus are fostered. It should be obvious that, since thought processes must be documented, the POMR also is an educational tool for the health professionals who read these notes.

Using the example of a particular male patient, some items appropriate to narrative notes might be:

S: A statement from the patient that reflects changes in his symptoms, concerns, and feelings. *Example:* "I felt very hungry and light-headed yesterday afternoon."

O: Data that indicate the patient's response to treatment and education. *Example:* Blood glucose level in midafternoon measured 40 mg/dl.

A: Information that reveals the patient's progress and the causes of new problems. *Example:* The subjective and objective data suggest hypoglycemia in the mid-afternoon.

P: Suggestions for formulation of new or revised plans based on the new assessment. Plans may be directed toward obtaining of more information, treatment, or education. *Examples:* Redistribute carbohydrate in the diet to provide a midafternoon snack that will prevent hypoglycemia. Instruct the patient on the change in his diet.

Other Pertinent Information

Two other items of interest to the nutritional care specialist are also contained in the medical record. *Flow sheets* are records of data that are obtained periodically. Some examples of this type of data are temperature, pulse, respiration, medications, and nutrient intake. These may accompany or follow the progress notes. The *discharge summary* includes a note in SOAP format on each problem and summarizes the level of resolution of that problem at the time the patient is discharged. This is written by a physician.

Source-Oriented Medical Record

The SOMR is organized so that similar types of information from similar sources are filed together. There may or may not be a problem list. The components of the SOMR are patient identification data, admission notes, physician's orders, laboratory reports, medication records, consents, consultations, operating room records, progress notes, and flow sheets. The patient identification data and admission notes contain the same information as the data base of the POMR.

NUTRITIONAL ASSESSMENT

The first step in the nutritional care process is the assessment of the patient's current status. A great deal of evidence in recent years has shown that protein-calorie malnutrition is distressingly prevalent in hospital patients[4-7] and that patients often deteriorate during hospitalization.[6] The evidence also indicates that aggressive nutritional care with promotion and maintenance of good nutritional status results in more rapid wound healing and decreased incidence of infections and other complications, with a decreased mortality rate.

It is possible, but rare, for vitamin and mineral deficiencies to exist in hospitalized patients in the absence of coexisting protein or calorie deficits.[8] In addition, vitamin and mineral deficiencies can be more rapidly treated than can protein-calorie malnutrition. As a result, assessment of protein and calorie nutritional status is given highest priority. An important function of nutritional assessment, therefore, is to identify patients who are protein-calorie malnourished or who have exceptionally high needs and are likely to become protein-calorie malnourished (Table 2-1). Once identified, these patients can be provided with special nutritional support. It is obvious from Table 2-1 that many patients are potential candidates for special attention.

Conditions resulting from protein and calorie malnutrition were once thought to be confined to underdeveloped countries, but marasmus (or cachexia) or a kwashiorkorlike syndrome, or a combination of these two syndromes has been found in hospitalized patients.[9] The detection and differentiation of these conditions have been shown to be important in the further treatment of the patient.

These findings have led to a more general appreciation of the importance of good nutrition in the care of patients and greater participation by nutritional care specialists in that care. At the same time, financial limitations require that nutritional support be directed to those patients whose need for such support is greatest.

Assessment Procedures

There is no good single test that provides a measure of nutritional status. Instead, a variety of somewhat nonspecific indicators are used to provide the basis for evaluation.[10] Those in current use will be described. Further study should provide more precise procedures in the future.

The assessment process consists of datagathering followed by an interpretation of the data for the identification of the problems. The methods used to gather the data necessary to assess nutritional status are

Table 2-1. Conditions Suggesting Nutritional Risk

Inadequate nutrient intake (quantity or quality)
- Alcoholism
- Drug addiction
- Avoidance of specified food groups (meat, eggs, milk; fruits and vegetables; grains)
- Constipation, hemorrhoids, diverticulosis
- Poor dentition
- Food idiosyncrasies
- Poverty; isolation
- Anorexia (from disease process, drugs, emotional problems)
- Recent weight loss or gain
- Allergies
- Inappropriate food choices from lack of information
- Following head or neck trauma, gastrointestinal surgery
- Loss of senses of taste or smell
- Ill-fitting dentures

Inadequate nutrient absorption
- Related to drug use (antacids, anticonvulsants, laxatives, neomycin, cholestyramine)
- Malabsorption (diarrhea, steatorrhea)
- Intestinal parasites
- Gastrointestinal surgery (gastrectomy, intestinal resection)
- Pernicious anemia
- Pancreatic disease

Decreased nutrient utilization
- Inborn errors of metabolism
- Alcoholism
- Related to drug use (anticonvulsants, antimetabolites, oral contraceptives, isoniazid)

Increased nutrient losses
- Abnormal metabolism (selected hepatic, renal, and endocrine disorders)
- Alcoholism
- Blood loss
- Ascitic and pleural taps (*centesis*)
- Diarrhea
- Draining abscesses, fistulas, and wounds
- Diabetes (uncontrolled)
- Peritoneal dialysis or hemodialysis
- Recurrent vomiting
- Exudative enteropathy

Increased nutrient requirements
- Fever
- Hyperthyroidism
- Athetosis
- Surgery, trauma, burns, infections
- Tissue hypoxia
- Normal physiologic stresses (infancy, adolescence, pregnancy, lactation)
- Malignancy

Other
- Radiation treatment
- Aging
- Conditions related to overnutrition (excessive vitamin intake; obesity)
- Mental illness
- Hypertension
- Hyperlipemia

classified as anthropometric, biochemical, clinical, and dietary. These sometimes are referred to as the ABCDs of nutritional assessment.

In practice, a stepwise procedure is used to ensure the most efficient use of resources. A routine screening process, consisting of some of the simpler methods, should be applied to all patients to identify those in need of further study. In addition, the routine screening establishes baseline values for use in later evaluation. Candidates for complete assessment include those with conditions that place them at risk (see Table 2-1) and those whose preliminary assessment show the following:

Serum albumin less than 3.2 g/dl
Total lymphocytes less than 1,500/mm^3
Nonvoluntary weight loss
A history of nutritional deficiency
A statement from the patient of change in appetite

Patients who are hospitalized for lengthy periods should be reevaluated at intervals.

For convenience in assessment of protein-calorie status, the body proteins are considered to exist in two compartments — the *somatic proteins* (in skeletal muscle) and the *visceral proteins,* consisting of all others. A measure of *cell-mediated immunity,* a subdivision of the visceral protein compartment, has been found to be especially important in indicating the potential for infection. Other parameters of value include an estimate of fat stores and a nutritional history. These data currently are used in nutritional assessment in many institutions. Their limitations as well as their functions will be discussed.

Measurements of Muscle Mass and Subcutaneous Fat

Anthropometric measurements may offer some useful information, but many of the anthropometric standards used for evaluation were not based on measurements of Americans but were recommended for use in developing countries. Therefore, the measurements may be most useful when repeated on the same patient so that the *direction* of change can be evaluated.

Several anthropometric measurements are useful if they are done carefully. For routine screening, the patient's *height* in centimeters (1 in. = 2.54 cm), *weight* in kilograms (1 kg = 2.2 lb.), and *sex* are obtained. The percentage of change from usual to present body weight can be calculated using the formula:

$$\frac{\text{Usual weight} - \text{present weight}}{\text{Usual weight}} \times 100 = \text{Percent of weight change} \quad \textbf{(1)}$$

Interpretation of the change in weight is given in Table 2-2. If 20 percent of a patient's body weight is lost, that patient's risk of mortality increases.[11,12]

If the patient is unable to provide information on his or her usual weight, ideal body weight (IBW) may be obtained from height-weight tables (see Appendix B), or may be quickly estimated, based on height, using one of the following formulas:

For men: 106 lb.
+ 6 lb. for each inch over 60 = IBW **(2)**

For women: 100 lb.
+ 5 lb. for each inch over 60 = IBW **(3)**

The use of ideal rather than usual body weight has many limitations. If an obese patient has lost weight but is still obese or is at ideal weight, the results of the calculations based on ideal weight are not valid. Height-weight relationships are also invalid if the patient is retaining fluid and has edema. An additional problem arises when ideal weights are related to individual frame size. Some tables give weights for small, medium, and large frames, but these terms are poorly defined. A procedure for differentiating frame size is given in Appendix B.

Table 2-2. Evaluation of Weight Change

Time	Significant Weight Loss (% of change)	Severe Weight Loss (% of change)
1 wk	1–2	>2
1 mo.	5	>5
3 mo.	7.5	>7.5
6 mo.	10	>10

Reprinted with permission from Blackburn, G.L., Bistrian, B.R., Maini, B.S., et al., Nutritional and metabolic assessment of the hospitalized patient. *J.P.E.N.* 1:15, 1977.

For patients who require further assessment, two additional measurements may be made, the *thickness of the skinfold over the triceps muscle* and the *circumference of the mid-upper arm* using the side opposite from the arm of predominant use. Although it often is recommended that these measurements be made with the patient standing,[13,14] measurements made on supine patients have also been found to be acceptable.[15] The *triceps skinfold* (TSF) is measured with calipers. A tape measure may be used to measure midarm circumference. From these values, the *arm muscle circumference* (AMC) is derived using the formula:

$$\text{AMC (cm)} = \text{Arm circumference (cm)} - (0.314 \times \text{TSF [mm]}) \quad \textbf{(4)}$$

The AMC is correlated with and provides an estimate of somatic protein or muscle mass,[13,16,17] whereas the thickness of the TSF gives an indication of subcutaneous fat

Table 2-3. Standards for Anthropometric Measurements

Sex	Triceps Skinfold (mm)	Arm Circumference (cm)	Arm Muscle Circumference (cm)
Male	12.5	29.3	25.3
Female	16.5	28.5	23.2

Reprinted with permission from Blackburn, G.L., Bistrian, B.R., Maini, B.S., et al., Nutritional and metabolic assessment of the hospitalized patient. *J.P.E.N.* 1:15, 1977.

and is considered an index of stored energy.[13,18–22] It is important to realize that these values contain sources of error and therefore are *estimates,* not precise measurements. They do not take into account, for example, any variability in the diameter of the bone.

These values are compared with the reference values (Table 2-3) using the following formula:

$$\text{Percent of standard} = \frac{\text{Measurement obtained}}{\text{Standard}} \times 100 \quad \textbf{(5)}$$

However, it must be kept in mind that the "standards" used are not true standards. Sometimes the terms *reference data* or *reference values* are considered preferable. Interpretation of the values obtained is given in Table 2-4. A review of the basis for these standards indicates that new data are needed based on a larger population that is more typical of the population from which the patients are drawn. The establishment of percentile standards is suggested.[23] Measurements of fat layers at sites in addition to the triceps area also may increase accuracy.

An additional test of somatic protein requires the collection of a 24-hour urine sample, a procedure that must be ordered by the attending physician. From this sample, the amount of creatinine excreted is determined by chemical analysis. Creatinine normally is formed in an amount proportionate to muscle mass, and its urinary excretion is related to the amount of skeletal muscle. In patients of ideal body weight, the *creatinine coefficient* is 23 mg/kg ideal body weight for men and 18 mg/kg ideal body weight for women. These values have been used to make a table of ideal creatinine excretions for patients whose weights and body compositions are ideal for their height (Table 2-5). Comparison of the actual urinary creatinine excretion per 24 hours and the expected excretion of a person of the same height and sex provides a

Table 2-4. Interpretation of Nutritional Assessment Values[a]

	Deficit			
Observation[a]	None	Mild	Moderate	Severe
TSF (% of standard)	>90	90–51	50–30	<30
AMC (% of standard)	>90	90–81	80–70	<70
CHI (% of standard)	>90	90–81	80–71	70–60
Serum albumin (g/dl)	>3.5	<3.5–3.2	<3.2–2.8	<2.8
Transferrin (mg/dl)	>200	<200–180	<180–160	<160
TIBC (μg/dl)	>214	<214–182	<182–152	<152
Total lymphocytes (per mm³)	>1,500	1,500–1,201	1,200–800	<800

Values compiled from Blackburn, G.L., Bistrian, B.R., Maini, B.S., et al., Nutritional and metabolic assessment of the hospitalized patient. *J.P.E.N.* 1:11–22, 1977; and Blackburn, G.L., Nutritional assessment: An overview. *Clin. Consult. Nutr. Support* 1:10, 1981.

[a] TSF = thickness of triceps skinfold; AMC = arm muscle circumference; CHI = creatinine-height index; TIBC = total iron-binding capacity.

Table 2-5. Ideal Urinary Creatinine Values Relative to Height

Men[a]		Women[b]	
Height (cm)	Ideal Creatinine (mg)	Height (cm)	Ideal Creatinine (mg)
157.5	1,288	147.3	830
160.0	1,325	149.9	851
162.6	1,359	152.4	875
165.1	1,386	154.9	900
167.6	1,426	157.5	925
170.2	1,467	160.0	949
172.7	1,513	162.6	977
175.3	1,555	165.1	1,006
177.8	1,596	167.6	1,044
180.3	1,642	170.2	1,076
182.9	1,691	172.7	1,109
185.4	1,739	175.3	1,141
188.0	1,785	177.8	1,174
190.5	1,831	180.3	1,206
193.0	1,891	182.9	1,240

Reprinted with permission from Blackburn, G.L., Bistrian, B.R., Maini, B.S., et al., Nutritional and metabolic assessment of the hospitalized patient. *J.P.E.N.* 1:15, 1977.

[a] Creatinine coefficient = 23 mg/kg of ideal body weight.

[b] Creatinine coefficient = 18 mg/kg of ideal body weight.

creatinine-height index (CHI). This calculation provides a sensitive measurement of somatic protein:

$$\text{CHI} = \frac{\text{Actual urinary creatinine}}{\text{Ideal urinary creatinine for height}} \times 100 \qquad \textbf{(6)}$$

The measurement can be used to obtain an estimate of lean body mass compared to ideal body mass with the formula:

$$\text{Percent of standard} = \frac{\text{Actual CHI}}{\text{Ideal CHI}} \times 100 \qquad \textbf{(7)}$$

Values for interpretation are provided in Table 2-4. These standards are based on a small number of patients and apply only to patients with normal renal function.[23] Since the test correlates well with AMC, it may be unnecessary duplication of information.[23] Also, since 24-hour urine samples are difficult to obtain, this test rarely is done.

Measurement of Visceral Protein

Serum albumin concentration (measured in grams per deciliter) is used in preliminary screening as an indication of visceral protein, that is, all protein other than structural protein. Normal concentration is 3.5 to 5.0 g/dl. Synthesis requires an adequate supply of amino acids and adequate hepatic function. Since albumin has a half-life of 20 days,[24] a deficit is considered an indication of impairment in protein synthesis in the liver due to a deficiency in quantity or quality of substrate, provided the patient does not have diagnosed liver disease, renal disease, congestive heart failure, or inflammation.[24,25] This value, obtained from a test ordered by the physician, is routinely available to nutritional care specialists from the patient's medical record. The severity of any deficit may be measured by comparison of the actual value and the values in Table 2-4. Total serum protein is not an adequate substitute, since variation in serum globulin levels, which make up part of total protein, may introduce a large error.

As an alternative to serum albumin, the measurement of *total iron-binding capacity* (TIBC) sometimes is used. *Serum transferrin* can be calculated from TIBC but, since the values vary proportionately, the calculation probably is not necessary. Direct measurement of transferrin is not done often. Transferrin is synthesized in the liver and has a half-life of 8 to 10 days.[24] Normal concentration is 170 to 250 mg/dl. Normal concentration of TIBC is 250 to 410 μg/dl. A deficit in transferrin is believed to be a more sensitive indicator of visceral protein than is serum albumin because of its shorter half-life.[26-28] However, transferrin levels are affected by hepatic and renal disease, congestive heart failure, and inflammation, as is serum albumin, limiting the usefulness of either measure in these conditions. In addition, transferrin concentration is influenced by iron status. The possible use of prealbumin[29] or of retinol-binding protein[30] as an alternative to serum albumin is being investigated since each of these has an even shorter half-life, but the normal range of values has not been firmly established.

Cell-Mediated Immune Function

The *total lymphocyte count* is used in the preliminary screening to provide an estimate of immune function (see Chapter 4). A *complete blood cell count* (CBC) is ordered routinely on admission of most patients and provides the total number of white blood cells (white blood cell count; WBC) per cubic millimeter of blood. It also provides a *differential count,* which states the percentages of the different types of white blood cells that make up the total. For assessment purposes, total lymphocyte count is obtained by the following calculation:

$$\text{Total lymphocyte count} = \frac{\%\ \text{lymphocytes} \times \text{total WBC/mm}^3}{100} \quad \textbf{(8)}$$

A lymphocyte count of more than 1,500/mm^3 is considered adequate. Values may be interpreted in comparison to those in Table 2-4, but consideration should be given to the fact that conditions other than nutrition, such as viral infections, may have an effect.

For those patients requiring further assessment, *recall antigen skin testing* (*delayed hypersensitivity*) for cell-mediated response to various injected substances sometimes is used.[31] This procedure usually is done by a nurse but occasionally may be the responsibility of the nutritional care specialist. Typically, several antigens are injected intradermally in the forearm and the amount of induration (hardening due to inflammation) in millimeters is measured in 48 hours. An induration of less than 5 mm of all three tests (mumps; *Candida,* and streptokinase/streptodornase [SK/SD]) commonly is interpreted to be a negative reaction (*anergy*), indicating that the patient has an inadequate immune response. Indurations of less than 10 mm is interpreted as a moderate deficit, whereas a value of more than 10 mm on any one test indicates immune competence. The physiologic basis for this procedure is explained in Chapter 4.

Many questions have arisen concerning the use of this measurement. A number of other factors affect cell-mediated immune response such as chemotherapy, sepsis, age, and injury.[32] Antibody-producing capacity also is affected in protein-calorie malnutrition, but less severely. Ongoing research may find a more accurate and sensitive indicator of immune competence.

Nitrogen Balance

The measurement of urea in the collected urine sample, when combined with protein intake data, can be used to give a rough estimate of *nitrogen balance,* the difference between nitrogen intake and output. When patients have high rates of protein catabolism, the increased losses of nitrogen are reflected in increased urinary excretion of urea,[33] which therefore is considered a good indicator of nitrogen excretion.[34] An additional 4 g/day is added to account for nonurea nitrogen in the urine and the nitrogen losses in the feces and through the skin. This value is relatively stable except in patients with diarrhea. Thus, the formula for estimation of nitrogen balance is:

$$\text{Nitrogen balance} = \frac{\text{Protein intake (g)}}{6.25} - (\text{urinary urea nitrogen} + 4) \quad \textbf{(9)}$$

in which grams of protein, which is 16 percent nitrogen, are converted to grams of nitrogen by dividing by 6.25. This formula estimates the degree of catabolism in relation to the patient's protein intake and is useful for planning nutritional care and evaluating the adequacy of that care by estimating nitrogen retention or loss.

Basal Energy Expenditure

Concurrent with the calculations of nitrogen balance, an estimate of basal energy expenditure (BEE) may be calculated from anthropometric data and compared with energy intake. Basal energy expenditure is obtained by use of one of the following formulas:

$$\text{For men: BEE} = 66 + (13.7 \times W) + (5 \times H) - (6.8 \times A) \quad \textbf{(10)}$$

$$\text{For women: BEE} = 655 + (9.6 \times W) + (1.7 \times H) - (4.7 \times A) \quad \textbf{(11)}$$

where W = kg body weight, H = height in centimeters, and A = age in years.

The caloric intake can be evaluated in relation to BEE:

$$\text{Caloric intake as a percentage of BEE} = \frac{\text{Caloric intake}}{\text{BEE}} \times 100 \quad \textbf{(12)}$$

Calculation of BEE also is useful in estimating kilocalorie need when planning nutritional care.

Other Laboratory Tests

The protein-calorie malnourished patient may be deficient in other nutrients. Guidelines for interpretation of some of the values obtained from tests involving these other nutrients are given in Table 2-6.

Clinical Observations

Many clinical signs of malnutrition are nonspecific (Table 2-7). They may result from deficiencies of more than one nutrient or from causes unrelated to nutrition. Nevertheless, they may be useful to indicate which patients need further evaluation. Many of these signs will be noted on the patient's chart by the physician. When interviewing patients, as well as when reviewing the medical record, the nutritional care specialist should be alert to their presence.

Dietary Assessment

A dietary evaluation is an important part of the nutritional assessment, as is observation of the current intakes of the hospitalized patient. The process most often involves interviewing the patient. Skilled interviewing is important in many steps of patient care but is beyond the scope of this text. Excellent information on interviewing techniques is available elsewhere.[35-38]

Methods to Obtain Data. The procedure chosen to obtain the data varies with the circumstances. It is important to use a method that provides as much (*but not more*) detailed information as is required to achieve the purpose. Commonly used procedures include the following.

Twenty-four-hour recall. The patient is asked to describe the food eaten in the previous 24 hours or on a "typical day." Although in some illnesses the recent diet may be atypical, it often is important to be aware of this. A frequently used technique is to ask the patient about activities in a typical day and explore the content of meals and snacks in the context of a day's usual activities. Questioning may begin with, "What time do you usually get up in the morning?" Later questions include, "When do you eat first?" and "What kinds of food do you usually eat then?" Information on the amount, preparation, form, and other details are obtained for each food. Sometimes, pictures or food models are helpful to the patient in describing the size of portions. It is important to elicit information on consumption of alcoholic beverages, coffee, candy, soft drinks, chewing gum, other snack foods, and vitamin and mineral medications.

Table 2-6. Current Guidelines for Criteria of Nutritional Status for Laboratory Evaluation

		Criteria of Status		
Nutrient and Units	Age of Subject (yr)	Deficient	Marginal	Acceptable
Hemoglobin (g/dl)[a]	6–23 mo.	Up to 9.0	9.0–9.9	10.0+
	2–5	Up to 10.0	10.0–10.9	11.0+
	6–12	Up to 10.0	10.0–11.4	11.5+
	13–16 M	Up to 12.0	12.0–12.9	13.0+
	13–16 F	Up to 10.0	10.0–11.4	11.5+
	16+ M	Up to 12.0	12.0–13.9	14.0+
	16+ F	Up to 10.0	10.0–11.9	12.0+
	Pregnant (after 6+ mo.)	Up to 9.5	9.5–10.9	11.0+
Hematocrit (packed cell volume in %)[a]	Up to 2	Up to 28	28–30	31+
	2–5	Up to 30	30–33	34+
	6–12	Up to 30	30–35	36+
	13–16 M	Up to 37	37–39	40+
	13–16 F	Up to 31	31–35	36+
	16+ M	Up to 37	37–43	44+
	16+ F	Up to 31	31–37	33+
	Pregnant	Up to 30	30–32	33+
Serum albumin (g/dl)[a]	Up to 1		Up to 2.5	2.5+
	1–5		Up to 3.0	3.0+
	6–16		Up to 3.5	3.5+
	16+	Up to 2.8	2.8–3.4	3.5+
	Pregnant	Up to 3.0	3.0–3.4	3.5+
Serum protein (g/dl)[a]	Up to 1		Up to 5.0	5.0+
	1–5		Up to 5.5	5.5+
	6–16		Up to 6.0	6.0+
	16+	Up to 6.0	6.0–6.4	6.5+
	Pregnant	Up to 5.5	5.5–5.9	6.0+
Serum ascorbic acid (mg/dl)[a]	All ages	Up to 0.1	0.1–0.19	0.2+
Plasma vitamin A (μg/dl)[a]	All ages	Up to 10	10–19	20+
Plasma carotene (μg/dl)[a]	All ages	Up to 20	20–39	40+
	Pregnant		40–79	80+
Serum iron (μg/dl)[a]	Up to 2	Up to 30		30+
	2.5	Up to 40		40+
	6–12	Up to 50		50+
	12+ M	Up to 60		60+
	12+ F	Up to 40		40+
Transferrin saturation (%)[a]	Up to 2	Up to 15.0		15.0+
	2–12	Up to 20.0		20.0+
	12+ M	Up to 20.0		20.0+
	12+ F	Up to 15.0		15.0+
Serum folic acid (ng/ml)[b]	All ages	Up to 2.0	2.1–5.9	6.0+
Serum vitamin B_{12} (pg/ml)[b]	All ages	Up to 100		100+
Thiamine in urine (μg/g of creatinine)[a]	1–3	Up to 120	120–175	175+
	4–5	Up to 85	85–120	120+
	6–9	Up to 70	70–180	180+
	10–15	Up to 55	55–150	150+
	16+	Up to 27	27–65	65+
	Pregnant	Up to 21	21–49	50+

Table 2-6. Current Guidelines for Criteria of Nutritional Status for Laboratory Evaluation (continued)

Nutrient and Units	Age of Subject (yr)	Criteria of Status: Deficient	Marginal	Acceptable
Riboflavin in urine (μg/g of creatinine)[a]	1–3	Up to 150	150–499	500+
	4–5	Up to 100	100–299	300+
	6–9	Up to 85	85–269	270+
	10–16	Up to 80	70–199	200+
	16+	Up to 27	27–79	80+
	Pregnant	Up to 30	30–89	90+
RBC transketolase-TPP effect (ratio)[b]	All ages	25+	15–25	Up to 15
RBC glutathione reductase–FAD effect (ratio)[b]	All ages	1.2+		Up to 1.2
Tryptophan load (mg xanthurenic acid excreted)[b]	Adults (Dose: 100 mg/kg body weight)	25+ (6 hr)		Up to 25
		75+ (24 hr)		Up to 75
Urinary pyridoxine (μg/g of creatinine)[b]	1–3	Up to 90		90+
	4–6	Up to 80		80+
	7–9	Up to 60		60+
	10–12	Up to 40		40+
	13–15	Up to 30		30+
	16+	Up to 20		20+
Urinary N′methyl nicotinamide (mg/g of creatinine)[a]	All ages	Up to 0.2	0.2–5.59	0.6+
	Pregnant	Up to 0.8	0.8–2.49	2.5+
Urinary pantothenic acid (μg)[b]	All ages	Up to 200		200+
Plasma vitamin E (mg/dl)[b]	All ages	Up to 0.2	0.2–0.6	0.6+
Transaminase index (ratio)[b]				
EGOT	Adult	2.0+		Up to 2.0
EGPT	Adult	1.25+		Up to 1.25

Reprinted with permission from Christakis, G., Ed., Nutritional assessment in health programs. *Am. J. Public Health* (Suppl.) 63:34–35, 1973.

M = male subjects; F = female subjects; RBC = red blood cells; TPP = thiamine pyrophosphate; FAD = flavin adenine dinucleotide; EGOT = erythrocyte glutamic oxaloacetic transaminase; EGPT = erythrocyte glutamic pyruvic transaminase.

[a] Adapted from the Ten-State Nutritional Survey.

[b] Criteria may vary with different methodology.

Food frequency lists. The patient is asked how often he or she eats foods in each of a number of groups on a standardized list. For example, "How many times in a day (or week) do you drink milk?" The results can be used as a cross-check on the information obtained in the 24-hour recall; therefore, these two methods often are used together.

Food records. Occasionally, a patient may be asked to keep a record of his or her food intake for a specified period, usually 3 or 7 days. This is a technique more often used in nutritional consulting with ambulatory patients than with hospitalized patients. It is important to recognize, when evaluating the diet, that the process of keeping the record

Table 2-7. Clinical Nutrition Examination

Clinical Findings	Possible Deficiency	Possible Excess
Hair, nails		
Flag sign (transverse dyspigmentation of hair)	Protein, copper	
Hair easily pluckable	Protein	
Hair thin, sparse	Protein, biotin, zinc	Vitamin A
Nails spoon-shaped	Iron	
Nails lackluster, transverse ridging	Protein calorie	
Skin		
Dry, scaling	Vitamin A, zinc, essential fatty acids	Vitamin A
Erythematous eruption (sunburnlike)		Vitamin A
"Flaky paint" dermatosis	Protein	
Follicular hyperkeratosis	Vitamins A, C; essential fatty acids	
Nasolabial seborrhea	Niacin, pyridoxine, riboflavin	
Petechiae, purpura	Ascorbic acid, vitamin K	
Pigmentation, desquamation (sun-exposed area)	Niacin (pellagra)	
Subcutaneous fat loss	Calorie	
Yellow pigmentation sparing sclerae (benign)		Carotene
Eyes		
Angular blepharitis	Riboflavin	
Band keratitis		Vitamin D
Corneal vascularization	Riboflavin	
Dull, dry conjunctiva	Vitamin A	
Fundal capillary microaneurysms	Ascorbic acid	
Papilledema		Vitamin A
Scleral icterus (mild)	Pyridoxine	
Perioral area		
Angular stomatitis	Riboflavin	
Cheilosis	Riboflavin	
Oral area		
Atrophic lingual papillae	Niacin, iron, riboflavin, folate, vitamin B_{12}	
Glossitis (scarlet, raw)	Niacin, pyridoxine, riboflavin, vitamin B_{12}, folate	
Hypogeusesthesia (also hyposmia)	Zinc, vitamin A	
Magenta tongue	Riboflavin	
Swollen, bleeding gums (if teeth present)	Ascorbic acid	
Tongue fissuring, edema	Niacin	
Glands		
Parotid enlargement	Protein	
Sjögren's syndrome	Ascorbic acid	
Thyroid enlargement	Iodine	
Heart		
Enlargement, tachycardia, high-output failure	Thiamine (wet beriberi)	
Small size, decreased output	Calorie	
Sudden failure, death	Ascorbic acid	

(*continued*)

Table 2-7. Clinical Nutrition Examination (continued)

Clinical Findings	Possible Deficiency	Possible Excess
Abdomen		
Hepatomegaly	Protein	Vitamin A
Muscles, extremities		
Calf tenderness	Thiamine, ascorbic acid (hemorrhage into muscle)	
Edema	Protein, thiamine	
Muscle wastage (especially temporal area, dorsum of hand, spine)	Calorie	
Bones, joints		
Beading of ribs (child)	Vitamins C, D	
Bone and joint tenderness (child)	Ascorbic acid (subperiosteal hemorrhage)	Vitamin A
Bone tenderness (adult)	Vitamin D, calcium, phosphorus (osteomalacia)	
Bulging fontanelle (child)		Vitamin A
Craniotabes, bosselation (child)		Vitamin D
Neurologic considerations		
Confabulation, disorientation	Thiamine (Korsakoff's psychosis)	
Decreased position and vibratory senses, ataxia	Vitamin B_{12}, thiamine	
Decreased tendon reflexes, slowed relaxation phase	Thiamine	
Drowsiness, lethargy		Vitamins A, D
Ophthalmoplegia	Thiamine, phosphorus	
Weakness, paresthesias, decreased fine tactile sensation	Vitamin B_{12}, pyridoxine, thiamine	
Other		
Delayed healing and tissue repair (e.g., wound, infarct, abscess)	Ascorbic acid, zinc, protein	
Fever (low-grade)		Vitamin A

Reprinted with permission from Weinsier, R.L., and Butterworth, C.E., Jr., *Handbook of Clinical Nutrition.* St. Louis: C.V. Mosby, 1981, pp. 30–31.

may cause an alteration in the intake. Patients may be stimulated to change their diets when required to give more thought to their meals. Others may alter the record to avoid embarrassment.

Dietary history. A dietary history is a more complete assessment. It usually includes the 24-hour recall plus the food frequency list. In addition, it includes information about other factors that influence food intake, nutritional needs, and nutritional adequacy. Some of these factors are the patient's financial resources, occupation, physical activity, allergies, medications, dental health, handicaps, home life and living conditions, cultural background, and other socioeconomic factors. Obtaining a useful and accurate dietary history requires a great deal of skill in interviewing.

Food preference questionnaire. Using a special questionnaire, the patient provides information about his or her preferences for various types of foods, indicating those he or she refuses to eat and those he or she likes and eats frequently, and rating others on a scale between these extremes. This type of questionnaire is useful in nutritional counseling but not for assessment since no quantities are obtained.

Observations of food intake. When a patient is hospitalized, most of his or her current intake may be determined by direct observation. It is important, in addition, to inquire about consumption of foods brought to the patient by visitors or given to the patient by a roommate. The nursing staff is helpful in providing such information. Nursing records provide information on fluid intake and output.

When greater precision is needed, foods may be weighed before being put on the tray and foods not eaten may then be weighed when the tray is returned. Again, the degree of precision varies with the purpose. A graduated cylinder and spring balance are sufficiently accurate for most purposes. Some patients, however, are subjects for research projects and are housed in a research unit. Their nutrient intake is measured with precision if the research protocol so requires.

Other methods, such as determination of "household consumption," which is used in population surveys, generally are not useful for application to individuals.

Evaluation of the Diet. Any of these data-gathering methods can provide valuable information if the nutritional care specialist is skillful, but the information still requires interpretation. An estimate of the nutrient content of the foods eaten may be obtained and compared to the patient's requirements.

As a practical matter in clinical practice, the translation from food intake to nutrient content often is not done in great detail for two reasons. First, the diet information obtained usually is approximate. The patient may not recall eating some items,[39-41] his or her estimates of quantities frequently are inaccurate, and the content of many mixtures is unknown. Second, our knowledge of the individual's nutrient requirements also is approximate. Under these circumstances, precision in evaluation is not possible. In addition, other demands on the time of the nutritional care specialist usually do not permit detailed calculations. The most common types of quantitative data obtained are the intake of sodium, amount and type of carbohydrate, and the intake of saturated fat when they are related to the specific disease state. The number and timing of meals is recorded for obese patients or patients with diabetes mellitus.

A common practice in diet evaluation is to compare the diet with guidelines such as the Daily Food Guide, familiar to all nutritionists as the "basic four," but the limitations of this guide must be recognized. A recent study demonstrated that the basic four provides only 60 percent or less of the National Research Council's (NRC) 1974 Recommended Dietary Allowances for energy, vitamins E and B_6, magnesium, zinc, and iron.[42] A modification is suggested that can be used in evaluation of diets. It includes:

Two servings milk and milk products
Four servings protein foods (two animal protein and two legumes and/or nuts)
Four servings fruits and vegetables, including one serving vitamin C–rich and one serving dark green
Four servings whole grain cereal products
One serving fat or oil

When more detail is required, the protein, fat, and carbohydrate content of the diet may be calculated using so-called exchange lists. The procedure is described in Chapter 9.

Even greater detail can be provided by using extended tables of food values. These contain information on a broad spectrum of nutrients.[43-47] Other tables contain data on single nutrients.[48-51] Commercial manufacturers often provide data on nutritive values of their products, and many research papers give information on individual items. However, these tables of food values also are limited in accuracy. They represent average values obtained from laboratory determinations sometimes performed with varying methods and in different places. The foods analyzed can differ in variety, geographic source, season of the year, and subsequent processing and storage, all of which can affect their nutritive content. The nutritional value of the foods the individual patient eats also is influenced by the preparation methods in the home and the recipes used.

Given the many sources of error in the data and the time constraints placed on the nutritional care specialist in practice, only limited use is made of calculations in the detail provided in this type of table, unless the patient is the subject of research. Recently, however, nutrient information has been housed in some computer data banks.[52] If the nutritional care specialist has access to such a system, more detailed diet analyses are possible.

Once the nutrient content of the diet is determined, it must then be compared to the patient's needs. In this process, the NRC table of Recommended Dietary Allowances[53] or the Dietary Standard for Canada[54] often is used as a starting point, even though neither was designed to be applied to individuals. When the amount of a nutrient consumed by an individual falls below the amounts given in either of these tables, it cannot be assumed that the individual is deficient.[53,55] The effect of the patient's disease and of any medications or other treatment must also be considered. These matters require knowledge and experience and will be discussed in the remaining chapters of this text.

Evaluation of Nutritional Status

With the collective data obtained from the previously outlined procedures, the patient's nutritional status is evaluated. The more severe forms of protein-calorie malnutrition often are considered to be analogous to primary protein deficiencies in childhood. Thus, the terms *marasmus* and *kwashiorkor* commonly are used, but it is important to remember that many patients, even if depleted, will be less severely affected than the use of these terms implies.

Diagnosis of Protein-Calorie Malnutrition

Marasmus or *cachexia* results from a calorie deficit that often has extended over months or years. The patient experiences severe wasting of fat and muscle. Arm muscle circumference and skinfold thickness are diminished, indicating loss of muscle tissue and of fat stores. The patient also has reduced immune function. Serum proteins may be moderately reduced or normal. The *prognosis* is good if the patient is provided with adequate oral nutritional support, but with additional stress, the patient can develop marasmic kwashiorkor very rapidly.

A *kwashiorkorlike syndrome* develops much more rapidly than does marasmus, sometimes within weeks, as a consequence of a protein deficit concurrent with severe stress, such as those described in Chapters 12 and 13. In these patients, fat reserves and muscle mass tend to be normal and may even be above normal; however, laboratory tests will indicate severely depressed serum albumin and transferrin and depressed immune function. The patient may be edematous and have delayed wound healing. Aggressive nutritional support is needed, sometimes by means other than simply supplying the patient with a tray of food. Prognosis is poor compared to the patient with marasmus.

Marasmic kwashiorkor is the combined form of protein-calorie malnutrition that occurs when a stress is superimposed on a chronically starved patient. The prognosis is very poor. Mortality rate increases as a result of increased infections and poor wound healing.

Evaluation of the patient's diet can be used to confirm a diagnosis obtained from anthropometric and biochemical parameters. Dietary data also provides information basic to planning for nutritional intervention. Nutritional assessment, repeated at intervals, also is used to evaluate the efficacy of nutritional support during treatment.

Estimate of Clinical Risk

A *prognostic nutritional index* (PNI) has been developed that provides a quantitative estimate of risk of anergy, sepsis, and death.[12] It is expressed as a percentage and is calculated from the following formula:

$$\text{PNI} = 158 \text{ percent} - [(16.6 \times \text{ALB}) - (0.78 \times \text{TSF}) - (0.2 \times \text{TFN}) - (5.8 \times \text{DH})] \quad \textbf{(13)}$$

where ALB = serum albumin concentration (in grams per deciliter); TSF = triceps skinfold (in millimeters); TFN = transferrin (in grams per deciliter); and DH (delayed hypersensitivity) = grade of reactivity to any of three antigens (mumps, *Candida*, or SK/SD). Reactivity is graded as *nonreactive* if induration equals 0, *1* if induration is less than 5 mm, and *2* if induration is greater than or equal to 5 mm.

The following comparative values of a well-nourished and a malnourished patient are exemplary:

	Well-Nourished Patient	
ALB	4.7 g/dl × 16.6 =	78.0
TSF	15.0 mm × 0.78 =	11.7
TFN	245 g/dl × 0.2 =	49.0
DH	2 × 5.8 =	11.6
Total		150.3
PNI	158 − 150.3 = 7.7%	

	Malnourished Patient	
ALB	2.8 g/dl × 16.6 =	46.5
TSF	10.2 mm × 0.78 =	8.0
TFN	160 g/dl × 0.2 =	32.0
DH	1 × 5.8 =	5.8
Total		92.3
PNI	158 − 92.3 = 65.7%	

According to this method, the malnourished patient has eight and one-half (65.7/7.7) times the risk of complications as does the well-nourished patient.

IDENTIFICATION OF PROBLEMS

The data base for identification of nutritional problems, which includes a nutritional assessment with anthropometric, biochemical, clinical, and dietary data, together with psychologic, social, economic, and educational factors, must be carefully evaluated to assure that all the needs of the patient will be met. This requires skillful integration of the biologic and social science knowledge of the nutritional care specialist plus practice and experience in application.

An estimation of the patient's immediate nutritional needs and comparison with intake are required. The patient's nutrient needs are affected by (1) current nutritional status, (2) current or projected stress factors, and (3) the method of feeding. There is no condition in which malnutrition is a desirable goal of treatment. The patient who is protein malnourished must have a sufficient supply of nutrients for anabolism to occur in order to replace lost tissue. If he or she is well nourished, the patient's needs are for maintenance. Some general recommendations for protein and energy intake are given in Table 2-8.

In addition, problems related to the patient's food choices, education, and financial problems, and any other factor influencing the patient's nutritional state must be identified. The influence of these factors is unpredictable, and the nutritional care specialist must judge their relevance in each case.

PLANNING NUTRITIONAL CARE

When problems have been identified, the next step is to establish goals and objectives for dealing with each one. A *goal* states the general purpose of the effort, whereas an *objective* states a specific measurable and verifiable step toward achieving the goal. For procedures for implementation and evaluation to follow logically, it is necessary that the objectives be patient-centered. They

Table 2-8. Nutritional Therapy

Energy requirements		*Kilocalories required/24 hr*	
Parenteral anabolic therapy		1.75 × BEE	
Oral anabolic therapy		1.50 × BEE	
Oral maintenance therapy		1.20 × BEE	
Prescriptions for anabolism[a]	*Protein (g/day)*		*Calories (kcal/day)*
Oral protein-sparing therapy	1.5 × weight[b]		
Total parenteral nutrition	(1.2 to 1.5) × weight[b]		40 × weight[b]
Oral hyperalimentation	(1.2 to 1.5) × weight[b]		35 × weight[b]

Reprinted with permission from Blackburn, G.L., Bistrian, B.R., Maini, B.S., et al., Nutritional and metabolic assessment of the hospitalized patient. *J.P.E.N.* 1:17,1977.

BEE = basal energy expenditure.

[a] Levels of protein intake are to be adjusted according to blood urea nitrogen values and nitrogen balance.

[b] Weight = actual weight in kilograms.

should be stated in terms of what the patient will achieve if the objective is met and should be stated in quantitative terms whenever possible. Here is an example:

Problem No. 1: Patient lacks knowledge of the principles of a gluten-free diet.
Goal: Understanding of and ability to apply the principles of the gluten-free diet.
Objective: Patient will demonstrate understanding of and the ability to apply the principles of his gluten-free diet by selecting proper foods from the hospital menu on Tuesday, Wednesday, and Thursday of this week.

There may be more than one goal per problem and more than one objective necessary to reach each goal.

IMPLEMENTATION OF THE NUTRITIONAL CARE PLAN

When the objectives related to each problem have been determined, the procedure to be used to help the patient to reach these objectives must be established. The general types of activity or interventions that are used in nutritional care are: (1) prescription of a diet, (2) provision of food and supplements, (3) nutrition education, and (4) referrals for public aid, nutrition follow-up, or other social services. Each intervention should be related to one of the established objectives and should be stated in specific terms. On the patient's chart, the nutritional care specialist must state what was done, where, when, how, and why, along with the results.

Procedures in Feeding Patients

A person's *diet* is defined as that person's intake of food and drink. The term does not necessarily imply that the patient's usual food intake has been altered in any way. For many patients a normal unrestricted intake is an adequate diet, but for others, an important aspect of nutritional intervention is an alteration in their usual diets.

Normal Nutrition Base

In planning for the diet of patients, it is important to use the normal unrestricted diet as the starting point whenever possible. Only those alterations are made that are required to achieve the objectives. This procedure has several advantages. It makes for easier planning for nutritional adequacy; shows as clearly as possible to the patients the relationship to a normal diet and reduces a sense of alienation, of being "different"; clarifies and simplifies the procedures for providing meals either in an institution or in the home; and reduces the number and variety of special items that must be prepared.

Adaptations for Disease

Purposes of Therapeutic Diets. The patient's diet may be modified for one or more of the following reasons:

1. To maintain or restore good nutritional status. This should be an objective in feeding all patients.
2. To rest or relieve an affected organ (e.g., a soft or liquid diet in gastritis).
3. To adjust to the body's ability to digest, absorb, metabolize, or excrete (e.g., a low-fat diet for fat malabsorption).
4. To adjust to tolerance of food intake by mouth (e.g., a liquid diet for sore throat, tube feedings for patients with cancer of the esophagus, or parenteral feeding for patients with severe short bowel syndrome).
5. To adjust to mechanical difficulties (e.g., a soft diet for the patient without teeth).
6. To increase or decrease body weight (e.g., a 1,200-calorie diet for obesity).

It is important to realize that modification of the diet does not, except in nutrient deficiency disease and perhaps in simple obesity, cure any disease. The diet may reduce symptoms, make the patient more comfortable and, in some circumstances, prolong life, but nutrients are curative only in nutrient deficiency diseases. A diabetic diet, for example, does not cure diabetes, but it may be instrumental in prolonging the patient's life and improving the quality of that life.

Types of Therapeutic Diets. The diets served in institutions commonly are classified as standard, modified, or test diets. These categories are established for convenience and efficiency of service and are explained in detail in the diet manual of each institution.

Routine diets. The *standard, routine,* or *progressive diets* are a group of diets used in all acute care hospitals and usually are served to relatively large numbers of patients. The foods included in these diets are fairly consistent from one institution to another, but the terminology varies. Some of the alternative terms are indicated here. All of these diets are based on the normal adequate diet, but they differ in consistency.

The *clear liquid diet* is the most limited of the routine diets. It is used to relieve thirst, to provide some fluid for the prevention of dehydration, to minimize stimulation of the gastrointestinal tract, and to serve as the initial feeding when a patient is returned to oral feeding following surgery or a period of intravenous feeding. Foods commonly included are listed in Table 2-9. The diet may contain 600 to 900 kcal/day, primarily from carbohydrate. A small amount of incomplete protein is obtained from gelatin. Since the diet is nutritionally inadequate, it seldom is used for more than 1 or 2 days. For patients requiring a residue-free liquid diet for longer periods, a commercial low-residue feeding may be added (see Appendix L).

The *full liquid diet* (see Table 2-9) is the next in the progression to the unrestricted diet. It provides food for the patient who is unable to chew, swallow, or digest more solid foods. It is given to postoperative patients, those with gastrointestinal inflammations and those with pathologic conditions of the head and neck. It is composed of those foods allowed on the clear liquid diet plus others that are liquid at body temperature (37°C.) or at any lower temperature and includes a large amount of milk and milk products. The caloric density (kilocalories per milliliter) is low, and feedings between meals often are included to increase the nutritive content. As usually served, the diet is adequate for maintenance. It can be modified for an increase in calories and protein, to reduce the sodium content, and to fit into a

Table 2-9. Summary of Routine Hospital Diets

Food Group	Clear Liquid	Full Liquid	Puréed	Soft	House
Soup	Broth, bouillon (fat-free)	Broth, bouillon (fat-free), strained cream soups	Broth, bouillon (fat-free), strained cream soups	Broth, bouillon (fat-free), strained cream soups	All
Cereal		Refined or strained in gruels	Refined or strained	Refined cooked, cornflakes, rice, paste products	All
Bread			White bread	White breads, rolls, crackers	All
Meat and substitutes		Pasteurized eggs in milk drinks, eggs in custards; strained meat or poultry in soup	Eggs, ground meats, or poultry, white fish (not fried); no pork	Eggs, milk, cheese, tender beef, lamb, veal, bacon, poultry (not fried)	All
Milk		Milk, milk drinks, cream, plain yogurt	Milk, milk drinks, cream, plain yogurt	Milk, milk drinks, cream, plain yogurt	All
Vegetables		In strained cream soups only; vegetable juices	Potatoes (not fried); strained or puréed bland cooked vegetables	Potatoes (not fried); whole tender or chopped bland cooked vegetables	All
Fruits	Bland clear juices; fruit ades	All juice	All juice; puréed bland cooked fruit	All juice; whole bland cooked fruit; raw banana; oranges and grapefruit sections (no membrane)	All
Desserts	Plain gelatin desserts; fruit ices; popsicles	Foods from preceding column, plus plain ice cream, sherbet, custard, pudding	Foods from preceding columns, plus plain cake	Foods from preceding columns, plus plain cookies	All
Miscellaneous	Soft drinks; decaffeinated coffee, tea; cereal beverage; sugar, honey; hard candy; salt; low-residue defined formula (on prescription only in some institutions)	Foods from preceding column; butter, margarine, oil in cream soups; honey, syrup; cocoa, chocolate syrup	Foods from preceding columns, plus salt, pepper, jelly	Foods from preceding columns, mayonnaise or similar dressing	All

diabetic diet. Cholesterol level is high; iron is low. The diet is also fiber-free.

In some institutions, the full liquid diet is modified further into *medical liquid diet, surgical liquid diet,* or other variations. The details of these diets, designed to meet the needs of patients in a particular institution, are found in the diet manuals of those institutions.

The *soft diet* is more solid than the liquid diet and is made up of easily digested foods without strong seasoning and containing a limited amount of fiber. It may be subdivided into two subcategories. In one, allowed meats, fruits, and vegetables are served whole. In the other, the meat is ground and vegetables and fruits are pureed (see Table 2-9). In this form, the diet sometimes is called the *purẽed diet* or *strained soft diet.* The soft diet is used for patients with difficulties in chewing and swallowing, acute infections, or some gastrointestinal disturbances, and as a transitional step from the liquid to an unrestricted diet in postoperative patients. The diet is nutritionally adequate.

The *light diet* consists of foods prepared very simply but is less restricted than the soft diet. It provides for mechanical ease of eating and ease of digestion. It is low in fiber and often is useful for patients without teeth or with ill-fitting dentures. Foods usually omitted are fried foods, rich pastries and other high-fat foods, foods containing bran, nuts, most raw vegetables and raw fruits. The diet is nutritionally adequate. Not all institutions include the light diet as one of their progressive diets since it closely resembles the soft diet; therefore, it is not included in Table 2-9.

The *house diet* (see Table 2-9) is also known as the *general, regular,* or *full diet.* It is an adequate normal diet, used for patients whose food intake can be unrestricted in kind or amount and who do not need additional nutritional support. As served in most institutions, it provides 2,000 to 2,500 kcal with 60 to 80 g protein, 80 to 100 g fat, and 200 to 300 g carbohydrate for adults. Some institutions use instead the "prudent diet" recommended by the American Heart Association (see Chapter 8). Most institutions allow the patients to select their meals from a list of available items known as the *selective menu.* Those that have a pediatrics unit have a series of diets adjusted for the ages of the children.

Some patients elect to follow a *vegetarian* diet, and it is necessary for the nutritional care specialist to be familiar with these diets. There are four main categories of vegetarian diets. Some patients are *partial vegetarians* who elect to use only selected meats. Commonly, partial vegetarians will eat fish and poultry but not beef, pork, or lamb. The *lactoovovegetarian* includes dairy products and eggs in the diet. The *lactovegetarian diet* contains milk products but not eggs, whereas the *vegan* accepts only foods of purely plant origin. Adequate lactoovovegetarian and lactovegetarian diets are fairly easy to plan. A modification of the basic four for vegetarian diets has been suggested by King et al.[42] and includes four servings of milk, two servings of legumes, and one serving of nuts along with six servings of whole grain or enriched cereals. In addition, three servings of vitamin C–rich fruits and vegetables, one and a half dark green and three other fruits and vegetables are included, for a total of seven and a half servings of fruits and vegetables.

The vegan diet requires more careful planning. It lacks concentrated sources of proteins of high biologic value and is limited in calcium, iron, riboflavin, and vitamin B_{12}. In order to plan for an adequate supply of amino acids to support normal growth and maintenance, a simplified system has been described.[56] It recommends the use *at each meal* of whole grains and cereals. In addition, at each meal a supplementary protein should be added. This may be provided by legumes or vegetables, or by a combination of nuts and seeds. Enriched grains will provide iron, the absorption of which can be increased by including a source of ascorbic acid in each meal. Dark green vegetables and some nuts provide calcium, and cereal products provide riboflavin. Vitamin B_{12} may be obtained by vegans from B_{12}-fortified soy milk or meat analogues.

The diets of vegetarians should be monitored carefully in the presence of risk factors such as a history of weight loss, use of laxatives and enemas, fasting, fluid restriction, pregnancy, lactation, or infancy.

Modified diets. The *modified diets* are available for patients needing diets that differ from the routine diets. There is a wide variety of alterations that can be made. In general, each modified diet is used for a much smaller number of patients and often requires more individualized planning. For convenience, they have been classified according to the types of alterations:

1. Kilocalories (e.g., high-calorie or low-calorie).
2. Consistency (e.g., low-fiber, high-fiber, soft, or liquid).
3. Single constituents or balance among nutrients (e.g., low-fat, sodium-restricted, low-fiber, diabetic, low-protein).
4. Method of preparation (e.g., soft).
5. Specific food restriction (e.g., milk-free).
6. Number, size, and frequency of meals (e.g., six small meals per day).

As is apparent from this list, some diets fit into more than one of these categories. It also is seen that the routine diets can be included in this classification, particularly in the category of changes in consistency.

Test diets. Test diets are single meals or diets lasting only 1 or a few days that are given to patients in connection with certain laboratory tests. They are used when the results of a test are affected by variations in food intake. For example, for the fecal fat excretion test, a consistent amount of fat, 70 to 100 g daily for 5 days preceding the test, is given. Test diets are not always nutritionally adequate, but this is not a matter of concern if they are used for a very brief period.

Quantitative and qualitative diets. An additional type of diet categorization which sometimes is useful is the division into *quantitative* and *qualitative diets.* Qualitative diets are any of those in which the patient may have any amount of the allowed foods that he or she desires. In quantitative diets, the amount of allowed foods is restricted. The diabetic diet and the calorie-restricted diet are the most common of the quantitative diets.

Parenteral and enteral feeding. Most of the diets previously described are eaten by or fed to the patient from a tray. Other patients are fed by a tube into the gastrointestinal tract (*enteral feeding*) or receive nutrients via the circulatory system, bypassing the digestive system (*parenteral feeding*). Although nutritional care specialists have traditionally been associated with providing meals on a tray, recent developments have increased the importance of knowledge of these alternative methods and of nutritional supplements. These procedures are described in detail in Chapters 5 and 12.

Adaptations for Individual Characteristics

In addition to the modifications required for the patient's disease, it is necessary to adapt the diet to the individual characteristics of the patient. Even if the patient is receiving a house diet, that patient's personal preferences, habits and cultural background must be considered if it affects his or her food acceptance. For patients who must follow a diet after discharge from the hospital or for those who are being treated on an outpatient basis, ability to prepare the food and availability of required special items must be considered in addition to the economic and cultural factors. The integration of all these factors requires skill, understanding, and patience, as well as a thorough knowledge of the biologic and social sciences.

Education and Other Forms of Intervention

An additional aspect of nutritional care is the education of the patient. Some patients need counseling on normal nutrition but, in actual practice, this rarely is done in hospitals. Many patients need information on a modified diet, food purchasing and preparation, or other matters that affect his or her nutritional status. In some circumstances, patients are given information on food stamps or other forms of aid or are referred to other community agencies. Follow-up in clinics, such as those for diabetic and cardiovascular disease patients, sometimes is made part of the nutritional care plan. This allows for continuing patient education and can improve patient compliance with the diet.

It is obvious that the nutritional care specialist must be skilled in techniques in education and knowledgeable of community resources. These generally are the subject of courses in nutrition education and community nutrition and are not included in this book. Some references are provided in the Bibliography at the end of this chapter.

EVALUATION OF PATIENT CARE

The evaluation of the effectiveness of the nutritional care of an individual patient is very simple if the objectives and interventions have been stated in measurable terms. The extent to which a patient's nutritional requirements are being met may be stated in terms of a *nutritional index* (NI) using the following formula:

$$NI = \frac{\text{Actual intake} - \text{desirable intake}}{\text{Desirable intake}} \times 100 \quad \textbf{(14)}$$

The patient's food and fluid intake must be monitored in order to use this formula. Other activities in evaluation include monitoring changes in the anthropometric, biochemical, and clinical values and monitoring changes in food intake or food choices.

Nutritional knowledge and the results of counseling are best evaluated by observation of changes in patient behavior. When the patient selects his or her own meals from a selective menu, for example, changes in nutrition knowledge may be evaluated by observation of the choices made.

Case Study: Nutritional Assessment

V.W., a 70-year-old retired man, was admitted to the hospital complaining of abdominal pain and diarrhea of 3 days' duration. The medical record states that the patient lives alone and does his own shopping and cooking. His only family member is a son who lives out of town. His income from a private pension fund and Social Security seems to be adequate for his needs. His only previous medical history was an appendectomy at age 14. He has a full set of dentures which fit comfortably.

The medical record provides the following information:

Height	178 cm
Weight	55 kg
WBC	4,500/mm³
Lymphocytes	23 percent
Glucose	114 mg/dl
Cholesterol	145 mg/dl
Serum albumin	3.5 g/dl
BUN	16 mg/dl

Anthropometric measurements yielded the following additional information:

TSF	9.5 mm
AMC	23 cm
Wrist	7.2 in.

The patient's 24-hour dietary recall included the following items:

¾ c. corn flakes
½ c. milk
Coffee, black
12 oz. soft drink

Tuna fish sandwich
  Approximately 2 oz. tuna
  1 Tbsp. mayonnaise
  2 slices white bread
2 eggs, scrambled
5 saltines
½ glass milk
2 canned peach halves in heavy syrup

The patient tells you this is typical of the last 3 days. Prior to his illness, he would have lunch at a nearby senior citizen center 3 days each week. Breakfasts remained the same. In the evening, he would have a "beer and a T.V. dinner." He rarely ate between meals.

Exercises

1. Calculate:
   Percent of ideal body weight
   Percent of standard of TSF
   Percent of standard arm circumference
   Percent of standard arm muscle circumference
   Total lymphocyte count
   Kilocalorie intake for the previous day
2. Compare the total lymphocyte count to the normal value.
3. Assess the patient's nutritional status and make recommendations for nutritional care in the form of a SOAP note.

References

1. Atwood, J., Mitchell, P.H., and Yarnall, S.R. The POR: A system for communication. *Nurs. Clin. North Am.* 9:229, 1974.
2. Fowler, D.R., and Longabaugh, R. The problem-oriented record. Problem definition. *Arch. Gen. Psychiatry* 32:831, 1975.
3. Weed, L.L. *Medical Records, Medical Education and Patient Care.* Chicago: Year Book Medical Publishers, 1969.
4. Bistrian, B.R., Blackburn, G.L., Hallowell, E.H., and Heddle, R. Protein status of general surgical patients. *J.A.M.A.* 230:858, 1974.
5. Bistrian, B.R., Blackburn, G.L., Vitale, J., et al. Prevalence of malnutrition in general medical patients. *J.A.M.A.* 235:1567, 1976.
6. Weinsier, R.L., Hunker, E.M., Krumdieck, C.L., and Butterworth, C.E., Jr. Hospital nutrition: A prospective evaluation of general medical patients during the course of hospitalization. *Am. J. Clin. Nutr.* 32:418, 1979.
7. Bollet, A.J., and Owens, S.D. Evaluation of nutritional status of selected hospitalized patients. *Am. J. Clin. Nutr.* 26:931, 1973.
8. Blackburn, G.L., and Bistrian, B.R. Nutritional care of the injured and/or septic patient. *Surg. Clin. North Am.* 56:1195, 1976.
9. Weinsier, R.L., and Butterworth, C.E., Jr. *Handbook of Clinical Nutrition.* St. Louis: C.V. Mosby, 1981.
10. Blackburn, G.L., Bistrian, B.R., Maini, B.S., et al. Nutritional and metabolic assessment of the hospitalized patient. *J.P.E.N.* 1:11, 1977.
11. Studley, A.O. Percentage of surgical risk in patients with chronic peptic ulcer. *J.A.M.A.* 106:458, 1936.
12. Mullen, J.L., Buzby, G.P., Waldman, M.T., et al. Prediction of operative morbidity and mortality by preoperative nutritional assessment. *Surg. Forum* 30:80, 1979.
13. Jelliffe, D.B. *The Assessment of the Nutritional Status of the Community.* Geneva: World Health Organization, 1966.
14. Ruiz, L., Colley, J.R.T., and Hamilton, P.J.S. Measurement of triceps skinfold thickness—and investigation of sources of variation. *Br. J. Prev. Soc. Med.* 25:165, 1971.
15. Jenson, T., Dudrick, S., and Johnston, D. A comparison of triceps skinfold and arm circumference values measured in standard and supine positions. *J.P.E.N.* 3:513, 1979.
16. Standard, K.L., Wills, V.G., and Waterlow, J.C. Indirect indicators of muscle mass in malnourished infants. *Am. J. Clin. Nutr.* 7:271, 1959.
17. Reindorp, S., and Whitehead, R.G. Changes in serum creatinine kinase and other biological measurements associated with musculature in children recovering from kwashiorkor. *Br. J. Nutr.* 25:273, 1971.
18. Fomon, S.J. *Nutritional Disorders of Children: Prevention, Screening and Follow-up.* D.H.E.W. Publication No. (HSA) 78-5104. Washington, D.C.: U.S. Government Printing Office, 1978.
19. Brozek, J. Physique and nutritional status of adult men. *Hum. Biol.* 28:124, 1956.
20. Tanner, J.M. The measurement of body fat in man. *Proc. Nutr. Soc.* 18:148, 1959.
21. Ward, G.M., Krzywicki, H.J., Rahman, D.P., et al. Relationship of anthropometric measurements to body fat as determined by densitometry, potassium-40 and body water. *Am. J. Clin. Nutr.* 28:162, 1975.
22. Cahill, G.F. Starvation in man. *N. Engl. J. Med.* 282:668, 1970.

23. Gray, G.E., and Gray, L.K. Anthropometric measurements and their interpretation: Principles, practices, and problems. *J. Am. Diet. Assoc.* 77:534, 1980.
24. Guyton, A.C. *Basic Human Physiology: Normal Function and Mechanism of Disease,* 2nd ed. Philadelphia: W.B. Saunders, 1977.
25. Wallach, J.B. *Interpretation of Diagnostic Tests: A Handbook Synopsis of Laboratory Medicine,* 3rd ed. Boston: Little, Brown, 1978.
26. Reeds, P.J., and Laditan, A.A.O. Serum albumin and transferrin in protein energy malnutrition. *Br. J. Nutr.* 36:255, 1976.
27. Kaminski, M.V., Fitzgerald, M.J., Murphy, R.J., et al. Correlation of mortality with serum transferrin and anergy. *J.P.E.N.* 1:27A, 1977.
28. Mullen, J.L., Gertner, M.H., Buzby, G.P., et al. Implications of malnutrition in the surgical patient. *Arch. Surg.* 114:121, 1979.
29. Ingenbleek, Y., DeVisscher, M., and DeNayer, P. Measurement of prealbumin as index of protein-calorie malnutrition. *Lancet* 2:106, 1972.
30. Ingenbleek, Y., Van Den Schrieck, H.G., DeNayer, P., and DeVisscher, M. The role of retinol-binding protein in protein-calorie malnutrition. *Metabolism* 24:633, 1975.
31. Meakins, J.L., Pietsch, J.B., Bubenick, O., et al. Delayed hypersensitivity: Indicator of acquired failure of host defenses in sepsis and trauma. *Ann. Surg.* 186:241, 1977.
32. Blackburn, G.L., and Thornton, P.A. Nutritional assessment of the hospitalized patient. *Med. Clin. North Am.* 63:1103, 1979.
33. Cuthbertson, D.P. The disturbance of metabolism produced by bony and non-bony injury with notes on certain abnormal conditions of bone. *Biochem. J.* 24:1244, 1930.
34. Kaminski, M.K., Jr. Enteral hyperalimentation. *Surg. Gynecol. Obstet.* 143:12, 1976.
35. Mason, M., Wenberg, B.G., and Welsch, P.K. *The Dynamics of Clinical Dietetics.* New York: John Wiley and Sons, 1977.
36. Froelich, R.E., and Bishop, F.M. *Medical Interviewing.* St. Louis: C.V. Mosby, 1969.
37. Bernstein, L., and Dana, R.H. *Interviewing and the Health Professions.* New York: Appleton-Century-Crofts, 1970.
38. Bird, B. *Talking with Patients,* 2nd ed. Philadelphia: J.B. Lippincott, 1973.
39. Campbell, V.A., and Dodds, M.L. Collecting dietary information from groups of older people. Limitations of the 24-hr recall. *J. Am. Diet. Assoc.* 51:29, 1967.
40. Madden, J.P., Goodman, S.J., and Guthrie, H.A. Validity of the 24-hr recall. Analysis of data obtained from elderly subjects. *J. Am. Diet. Assoc.* 68:143, 1976.
41. Beal, V.A. The nutritional history in longitudinal research. *J. Am. Diet. Assoc.* 51:426, 1967.
42. King, J.C., Cohenour, S.H., Corruccini, C.G., and Schneeman, P. Evaluation and modification of the basic four food guide. *J. Nutr. Educ.* 10:27, 1978.
43. Food and Nutrition Service, Agriculture Research Service. *A Daily Food Guide.* FNS-13. Rev. July 1975. Washington, D.C.: U.S. Department of Agriculture, 1975.
44. Watt, B.K., and Merrill, A.L. *Composition of Foods—Raw, Processed, Prepared.* Rev. U.S.D.A. Handbook No. 8. Washington, D.C.: U.S. Department of Agriculture, 1976.
45. Consumer and Food Economics Research Division, Agriculture Research Service. *Nutrition Value of Foods.* S1, rev. U.S.D.A. Home and Garden Bull. No. 72. Washington, D.C.: U.S. Department of Agriculture, 1971.
46. Pennington, J., and Church, H.N., Eds. *Food Values of Portions Commonly Used,* 13th ed. New York: Harper and Row, 1980.
47. Adams, C.F. *Nutritive Value of American Foods in Common Units.* U.S.D.A. Handbook No. 456. Washington, D.C.: U.S. Department of Agriculture, 1976.
48. Food and Agriculture Organization of the United Nations, Food Policy and Food Science Service. *Amino Acid Content of Foods and Biological Data on Proteins.* Rome: Food and Agriculture Organization, 1970.
49. Orr, M.L. *Pantothenic Acid, Vitamin B_6 and Vitamin B_{12} in Food.* U.S.D.A. Home Economics Research Report No. 36. Washington, D.C.: U.S. Department of Agriculture, 1969.
50. Orr, M.L., and Watt, B.K. *Amino Acid Content of Foods.* U.S.D.A. Home Economics Research Report No. 4. Washington, D.C.: U.S. Department of Agriculture, 1957.
51. Toepfer, E.W., Zook, E.G., Orr, M.L., and Richardson, L.R. *Folic Acid Content of Foods.* U.S.D.A. Handbook No. 29. Washington, D.C.: U.S. Department of Agriculture, 1951.
52. Hoover, L.W. Computers in dietetics: State-of-the-art. *J. Am. Diet. Assoc.* 68:39, 1976.
53. Food and Nutrition Board, National Research Council. *Recommended Dietary Allowances,* 9th rev. ed. Washington, D.C.: National Academy of Sciences, 1979.
54. Committee for Revision of the Canadian Dietary Standard, Bureau of Nutritional Sciences, Health and Welfare Canada. *Dietary Standards for Canada,* rev. ed. Ottawa: Information Canada, 1975.

55. Sabry, Z.I. The Canadian dietary standard. *J. Am. Diet. Assoc.* 56:195, 1970.
56. Pemberton, C.M., and Gastineau, C.F., Eds. *Mayo Clinic Diet Manual.* Philadelphia: W.B. Saunders, 1981.

Bibliography

Banathy, B.H. *Instructional Systems.* Palo Alto: Fearon, 1968.

Bloom, B.S., Ed. *Taxonomy of Educational Objectives: The Classification of Educational Goals. Handbook I: Cognitive Domain.* New York: David McKay, 1956.

Cyrs, T.E., Jr. *You, Behavioral Objectives and Nutrition Education.* Chicago: National Dairy Council, 1975.

Davis, R.H., Alexander, L.T., and Yelon, S.L. *Learning System Design.* New York: McGraw-Hill, 1974.

Grant, A. *Nutritional Assessment Guidelines,* 2nd ed. Seattle: Anne Grant, 1979.

Grant, J.P., Custer, P.B., and Thurlow, J. Current techniques of nutritional assessment. *Surg. Clin. North Am.* 61:437, 1981.

Hackney, H., and Cormier, S.N. *Counseling Strategies and Objectives,* 2nd ed. Englewood Cliffs, N.J.: Prentice-Hall, 1979.

Jensen, T., and Dudrick, S.J. Implementation of a multidisciplinary nutritional assessment program. *J. Am. Diet. Assoc.* 79:258, 1981.

Kibler, R.J., Barker, L.L., and Miles, D.T. *Behavioral Objectives and Instruction.* Boston: Allyn and Bacon, 1970.

Krathwohl, D.R., Bloom, B.S., and Masia, B.B. *Taxonomy of Educational Objectives: The Classification of Education Objectives. Handbook II: Affective Domain.* New York: David McKay, 1964.

Mager, R.F. *Developing Attitude Toward Learning.* Belmont, Calif.: Fearon, 1968.

Mager, R.F. *Goal Analysis.* Belmont, Calif.: Fearon, 1972.

Mager, R.F. *Measuring Instructional Intent.* Belmont, Calif.: Fearon, 1973.

Mager, R.F. *Preparing Instructional Objectives,* 2nd ed. Belmont, Calif.: Fearon, 1975.

McAshan, H.H. *The Goals Approach to Performance Objectives.* Philadelphia: W.B. Saunders, 1974.

Popham, W.J., and Baker, E.L. *Planning an Instructional Sequence.* Englewood Cliffs, N.J.: Prentice-Hall, 1970.

Sources of Current Information

American Journal of Clinical Nutrition
Annals of Internal Medicine
Annual Review of Nutrition
Archives of Internal Medicine
Human Nutrition: Applied Nutrition
Human Nutrition: Clinical Nutrition
Journal of the American Dietetic Association
Journal of the American Medical Association
Journal of the Canadian Dietetic Association
Journal of Human Nutrition
Journal of Nutrition
Journal of Nutrition Education
JPEN. Journal of Parenteral and Enteral Nutrition
Medical Clinics of North America
New England Journal of Medicine
Nursing Clinics of North America
Nutrition Abstracts and Reviews
Nutrition and Metabolism
Nutrition Research
Nutrition Reviews
Nutrition Today
Pediatric Nutrition and Gastroenterology
Postgraduate Medicine
World Review of Nutrition and Dietetics

3. Drugs and Nutritional Care

- I. General Principles of Pharmacology
  - A. Mechanisms of drug action
  - B. Factors influencing rate and magnitude of drug effects
    - 1. Drug dosage
    - 2. Methods of administration
    - 3. Absorption
      - a. solubility
      - b. concentration
      - c. properties of the drug molecule
        - (1) size of molecules
        - (2) lipid solubility
        - (3) ionization
      - d. effect of gastric emptying
      - e. blood supply at injection site
    - 4. Distribution
      - a. volume of distribution
      - b. blood supply to target organ
      - c. plasma protein binding
      - d. concentration in adipose and other tissues
      - e. blood-brain barrier
      - f. placental barrier
      - g. inflammation
  - C. Drug metabolism and excretion
    - 1. Excretion
    - 2. Drug biotransformations
      - a. nonsynthetic reactions
      - b. synthetic reactions
      - c. factors influencing rate of metabolism
  - D. Drug safety and effectiveness in individuals
    - 1. Factors modifying drug effects in individuals
    - 2. Individual variations in drug response
    - 3. Drug interactions
  - E. Classification and terminology
- II. Nutrition-Drug Interrelationships
  - A. Effects of drugs on nutrition
    - 1. Drug effects on taste, appetite, and food intake
      - a. anatomy of taste and odor
      - b. effect of disease on taste and odor perception
      - c. drug effects on taste and odor perception
      - d. drug effects on appetite and food intake
    - 2. Drug effects on nutrient absorption
    - 3. Drug effects on nutrient metabolism
      - a. protein
      - b. lipids
      - c. carbohydrates
      - d. vitamins and minerals
  - B. Effects of food and nutrients on drugs
    - 1. Effects of food on drug absorption
      - a. food in the digestive tract
      - b. specific nutrients
    - 2. Effects of nutritional status on drug metabolism and excretion
      - a. protein
        - (1) drug-protein binding
        - (2) effects on drug metabolism
      - b. lipids
      - c. minerals
      - d. vitamins
    - 3. Detrimental systemic food-drug interactions
      - a. vasoactive compounds and monoamine oxidase inhibitors
      - b. alcohol and drugs
        - (1) disulfiram
        - (2) hypoglycemic agents

The existence of interrelationships between nutrition and drugs has become increasingly clear in recent years. At the same time, the need has grown for practitioners in the health professions to have a knowledge of these interrelationships. In order to provide appropriate nutritional care to patients receiving drugs, to work as a member of a health care team, and to understand advances in this important field of knowledge, an appreciation of some basic principles of pharmacology and a command of current knowledge of drug-nutrient interrelationships is required. This chapter provides an introduction to the fundamentals of pharmacology, followed by a discussion of drug-nutrient interrelations. In later chapters, the effects of drugs on nutrition in specific disease states will be reviewed.

GENERAL PRINCIPLES OF PHARMACOLOGY

Pharmacology is the study of the activity and effects of chemicals in living matter. One of its branches is *pharmacy*, the preparation and dispensing of these chemicals for therapy. As used in medicine, a *drug* is any chemical used in the prevention, diagnosis, or treatment of disease.

Mechanisms of Drug Action

Drugs do not create new metabolic processes. Instead, they act by increasing or decreasing a naturally occurring process. They may inhibit an enzyme, facilitate enzyme action by acting as a coenzyme, activate an inactive part of the DNA molecule to stimulate synthesis of a protein, alter membrane permeability, or act as a chelator.

The usual mode of drug action requires the formation of a drug-receptor complex, which then produces one or more reactions. The amount of the response depends on the number of drug-receptor reactions which, in turn, depends on the concentration of the drug near the receptor. A few drugs do not form a drug-receptor complex. An example is sodium bicarbonate, which neutralizes gastric acidity by direct reaction with the gastric hydrochloric acid. Another example is a chelating compound such as penicillamine, which chelates copper and is useful in the treatment of Wilson's disease.

Usually a drug can bind to more than one type of receptor and thereby produce more than one effect. Any effects other than those the drug was intended to produce are its *side effects*. These vary in nature and degree of severity. As a general rule, serious side effects are acceptable only when there is no equally effective alternative drug and the disease being treated also is serious. For example, more severe side effects are acceptable in the drug treatment of cancer than in the treatment of a less serious disease. Side effects are frequently a major concern in nutritional care, since they very often include nausea, vomiting, diarrhea, and other symptoms that influence nutritional status.

Factors Influencing Rate and Magnitude of Drug Effects

Drug Dosage

The rate and magnitude of drug effect is influenced, first of all, by the dosage of the drug. The drug dose varies in amount and frequency and is influenced by the maximum effect of which the drug is capable. A basic tool for determining the *amount* of a drug necessary to produce a given effect is the *logarithmic dose-response curve* (Fig. 3-1). In that part of the curve marked *A*, there is a small increase in dose and a small increase in response. The dose at which a response is first measured is the *threshold dose*. In part *B* of the dose-response curve, there is a large increase in response in proportion to the increase in dose. It is in this part of the curve that the minimum dose necessary to produce a maximum response is found. In part *C*, there is no further response regardless of the amount of increase in dose. At this dose level, receptor sites are saturated and no further response is possible. It usually is in part *C* that toxic side effects occur. In some drugs, such as anticancer drugs, toxic side effects may occur in part *B* of the curve. The nutritional significance of this action in cancer patients is discussed in Chapter 13.

The duration of action of the drug must be considered in determining the *frequency* of dose administration. A few drugs may be given only once. Prolonged action of some drugs is needed, and so they must be given repeatedly. The size and frequency of the

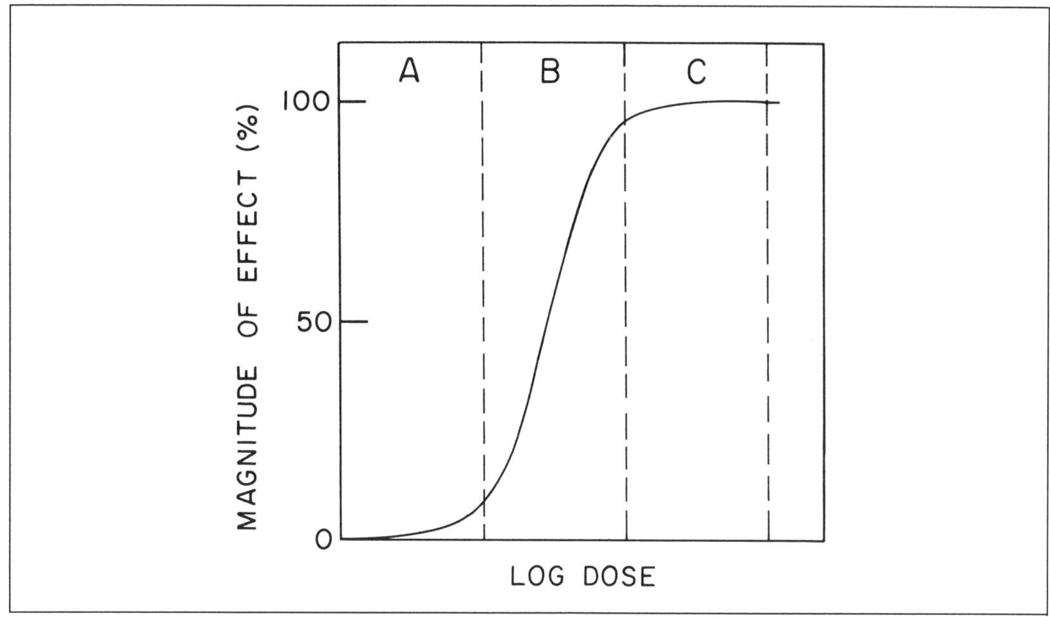

Figure 3-1. Logarithmic dose-response curve.

dose is established at a level to maintain concentration of the drug above its threshold but below its toxic level. The frequency of administration is affected by the rate at which the drug is excreted or inactivated; rapidly excreted drugs must be given more frequently.

The *power* or *efficacy* of a drug refers to its maximum effect. A more powerful drug has a greater maximum effect.

Methods of Administration

The route by which a drug is administered affects the rate at which it is transferred to the vicinity of its receptor sites. Some drugs, such as ointments, liniments, powders, paints, eye drops, and nose drops, are used for a local effect on the skin or mucous membranes. This is called *topical* administration. However, most drugs have more general or *systemic* effects or an effect at a site other than the site of administration.

Systemic administration of drugs has been divided into two categories. One of these is *enteral* administration, that is, via the gastrointestinal tract. More specifically, this can include giving medication by mouth (p.o.), sublingually by allowing it to dissolve under the tongue, or by a tube into the stomach or intestines. Drugs may also be given rectally in the form of suppositories. It is estimated that approximately 80 percent of all drugs are taken by mouth. The other major category of systemic administration is *parenteral* (outside of the gastrointestinal tract). This includes injecting medication (1) *subcutaneously* (s.c.) or under the epidermis, (2) *intradermally,* or into the dermis just below the epidermis, (3) *intramuscularly,* or into a muscle (i.m.), (4) *intrathecally,* or into the spinal fluid, and (5) *intravenously* (i.v.), or into a vein. In addition, a few drugs can be administered by *inhalation.* Probably the most familiar example of drugs that are inhaled are certain anesthetics.

Regardless of the means of administration, the drugs must then be absorbed and transported to their site of action. Those given enterally or by inhalation must cross the epithelial cells of the gastrointestinal tract or lungs. They also must cross the endothelial cells of the capillaries to reach the bloodstream, as must drugs given subcutaneously, intradermally, or intramuscularly. After they reach the bloodstream, most drugs, including those given intravenously, must again cross endothelial cells of the capillaries to reach the target cells. When a drug is given intravenously, it can be expected to cause a more rapid response than if it is given intramuscularly or subcutaneously, because the latter must be absorbed into the bloodstream first. The absorption is slowed down even further if the site of administration has a poor blood supply.

Absorption

The rate and magnitude of a drug effect also is influenced by factors affecting its absorption. We shall use the term *absorption* to include the processes by which a drug is transferred from the lumen of the gastrointestinal tract, the muscles, dermis, or similar site to the blood or lymph. These processes, defined and described in elementary biochemistry and physiology texts, are *passive transfer* by simple diffusion or filtration, *specialized transport* by facilitated diffusion or active transport, and *pinocytosis*. They apply to transfer to and from the capillaries, into and out of target cells, and into excretory pathways (such as into the urine), as well as to absorption from the gastrointestinal tract. Many properties of drugs affect their absorption.

Solubility. Drugs may be administered in the form of solutions, suspensions, capsules, or tablets. If a drug is not in solution, it must be dissolved before it can be absorbed. This process will affect the rate at which it will be absorbed. The structure of the drug can often be manipulated to affect the speed of solubility. For example, protamine sulfate is added to insulin to form a suspension and decrease its rate of absorption. Food in the stomach or taken concurrently affects the solubility of some drugs taken orally.

Concentration. Absorption of most drugs from the gastrointestinal tract is by diffusion, and the rate is proportionate to the concentration. Thus, larger more frequent doses will result in higher concentrations and more rapid absorption. The concentration of drugs taken by mouth may be decreased by dilution with gastric contents if the drug is taken with or immediately following meals.

Properties of the Drug Molecule. Several properties of drugs affect the rate at which they are transported across membranes and thereby affect their absorption.

Size of molecules. Smaller molecules generally are absorbed more rapidly than large molecules. The rate of absorption of a drug can therefore be slowed if it is bound to some material that increases the size of the molecules.

Lipid solubility. Lipid-soluble compounds cross cell membranes easily and therefore are absorbed more rapidly than are water-soluble drugs.

Ionization. Ionized drugs are absorbed more slowly than those that are not ionized. For example, many drugs are weak acids or weak bases and are absorbed in the stomach or small intestine. Drugs that are either strongly acidic or basic are more ionized and cross lipid membranes poorly. Thus, they are poorly absorbed.

Effect of Gastric Emptying. Drugs that retard gastric emptying, such as chloroquine (an amebicide), will have decreased rates of absorption from the intestine.

Blood Supply at Injection Site. The rate of absorption from an injection site will vary with the blood supply at that site. Absorption from muscle is more rapid than absorption from subcutaneous fat.

Distribution

The term *distribution* includes the processes by which a drug, given for its systemic effect, is distributed in the body from the site at which it enters the circulatory system. The distribution of a drug influences its concentration and thus the rate and magnitude of its effects. When the drug is absorbed from the gastrointestinal tract or another site, it is distributed by the bloodstream or lymph. When it reaches the area of its target cell, the drug again must cross membranes to make contact with its receptor. These membranes usually are capillary cells but sometimes include the membranes of the target cells themselves. Those factors, previously listed, that affect absorption by their effect on the ability of the drug to cross cell membranes also influence the distribution of drugs by their effect on the drug's ability to cross membranes at the target cell.

There are additional factors that must be considered in drug distribution.

Volume of Distribution. When a specified dose of a drug is given and absorbed into the circulatory system, it becomes diluted by the blood, and its concentration decreases. If a drug could not be transferred out of the circulatory system, it would be diluted by the fluid of the blood plasma, approximately 3 liters in an average adult. This 3 liters is its volume of distribution. If the drug diffuses throughout the extracellular fluid, its volume of distribution could be approximately 12 liters in the same adult. If the drug can diffuse across all membranes and is evenly distributed within the cells as well, its volume of distribution might be approximately 40 liters, and its concentration in that fluid would be correspondingly reduced if the dose were the same.

Blood Supply to Target Organ. Many drugs are used for their effect on a specific organ. If the target organ has a large blood supply, such as the liver or kidneys, it will receive a larger proportion of the drug. In the liver and kidneys, endothelial linings of the liver sinusoids and renal glomerular capillaries permit faster transport of drugs; therefore, the liver and kidneys are associated with faster drug distribution than are other organs.

Plasma Protein Binding. Drugs bind to plasma protein and protein other than their specific receptors. The binding to plasma albumin is quantitatively the most important of these, although some binding to globulin does occur. When a drug is bound to such a protein, it does not cross membranes and may not reach its active site. Alternatively, some drugs have an affinity for a cellular constituent, such as certain nucleoproteins in cells that are not necessarily target cells. The net effect of protein binding is to reduce the concentration of free, or active, drug produced by a given dose. However, the bound and free drug forms are in equilibrium. As the free drug is absorbed from the circulatory system, the drug–plasma protein complex dissociates to restore the equilibrium and provide free drug. Therefore, protein binding tends to prolong the action of a drug. There are, however, limits to the capacity for protein binding. Once the system becomes saturated, additional drug may reach toxic levels quickly.

There are many factors affecting plasma protein concentration; these are discussed in later chapters. It is important to realize that a patient with decreased levels of plasma proteins—as a result of malnutrition, for example—may require smaller doses of drugs, since smaller amounts will be bound. Toxic levels will also be more easily reached in these patients.

Concentration in Adipose and Other Tissues. Lipid-soluble drugs may concentrate in adipose tissue but will be in equilibrium with the drug concentration in the plasma. This may increase the length of time a drug is active, a factor that may be important in patients who are severely under or over normal weight.

Some drugs, such as quinacrine hydrochloride, localize in the liver and are protected against degradation. Thus, their half-lives are prolonged. A drug that precipitates in the gastrointestinal tract is distributed more slowly and so its action may be prolonged.

Blood-Brain Barrier. The capillaries in the brain are more tightly bound to each other and are surrounded by a thicker basement membrane than are the capillaries in other organs. They are enveloped by *glial cells,* which act as a barrier to many water-soluble compounds. These factors are referred to collectively as the *blood-brain barrier.* They form a barrier to absorption by passive diffusion of water-soluble or ionized drugs. The blood-brain barrier interferes with drug transfer to the central nervous system, cerebrospinal fluid, and the aqueous humor of the eye.

Placental Barrier. The placenta serves as a barrier to some drugs. In general, the placenta presents a greater barrier to large molecules and a lesser barrier to drugs composed of small molecules.

Inflammation. The permeability of some membranes to drugs changes in the presence of inflammation. Penicillin, for example, will penetrate into the cerebrospinal fluid of a patient with meningitis more easily than in a person without infection.

Drug Metabolism and Excretion

The discussion thus far has been based on an idealized model in which termination of drug activity, which begins almost immediately following its administration, has not been considered. A drug must be either excreted or inactivated to stop its activity. A common unit of measure for a drug's activity is *half-life,* the time in which the concentration of a drug in the plasma is reduced to half its original concentration.

Excretion

Most drugs or their metabolites are in solution and are excreted in the urine. Some are excreted into the bile and thence into the intestine to be excreted in the feces; however, many of these are reabsorbed from the intestine and recycled so that urinary excretion remains the primary excretory pathway. Some other, usually minor, excretory pathways include the lungs for volatile compounds, and other body fluids such as sweat, tears, saliva, and milk. Excretion in milk may be an important consideration for the infants of nursing mothers but is not usually a major excretory pathway for the mother herself.

Various methods may be used to alter the rate of excretion of a drug, including changing the pH of the urine and decreasing renal tubular secretion of the drug. These methods may be used to decrease the excretion rate and prolong drug action or to increase the excretion rate to eliminate toxic materials.

Drug Biotransformations

Many drugs undergo one or more molecular changes while they are in the body. These changes are referred to as *biotransformations* or *metabolism* and often involve specific nutrients (Table 3-1). Some of these reactions are therefore influenced by nutritional status. The effects of some drugs are produced before or during such transformations. Other drugs undergo a biotransformation to produce a metabolic product which is the active compound. Many drugs undergo a biotransformation for purposes of *detoxification* — that is, altering the drug so as to stop its action. Many of these reactions also convert lipid-soluble drugs into more polar and

Table 3-1. Nutrients Used in Drug Oxidation and Conjugation

Nutrient	Oxidation	Conjugation
Carbohydrate		Glucose
Lipid	Lecithin	Acetyl (also from protein and carbohydrate)
Amino acids and derivatives	Glycine Protein	Glycine Glutamic acid, glutamine Cysteine, cystine Methionine Serine Arginine Alanine Some peptides
Minerals	Iron, copper, calcium, zinc, magnesium	
Vitamins	Pantothenate Niacin Riboflavin Ascorbic acid(?)	Pantothenate Niacin Folate Vitamin B_{12}

more water-soluble drugs that can be excreted in the urine. Otherwise, lipid-soluble drugs might remain in the body almost indefinitely.

The reactions that occur in biotransformations commonly are classified into two categories, *nonsynthetic* and *synthetic* reactions.

Nonsynthetic Reactions. Nonsynthetic reactions, including oxidation, reduction, and hydrolysis, may make the drug more active or less active or may increase its toxicity. The reactions are catalyzed by specific enzymes, such as esterases, or by nonspecific enzymes. The latter are the microsomal enzymes, found mostly in the liver in the smooth endoplasmic reticulum of the hepatocytes.

Most oxidations are accomplished by the *mixed-function oxidizing* (MFO) *system* (Fig. 3-2), which requires (1) cytochrome P-450, (2) NADPH-cytochrome c reductase (a flavoprotein), (3) lecithin, (4) NADPH, and (5) oxygen. Some reduction reactions occur in the microsomal fraction of cells and others in the cytosol. Hydrolysis reactions occur in the blood plasma and in the soluble fraction of cells. The nutrients needed for oxidation reactions are shown in Table 3-1; those required for reduction or hydrolysis are less well understood but seem to be similar.

Synthetic Reactions. Synthetic reactions, including acetylation, sulfation, methylation, or combination with glycine, glutamine, or glucuronic acid, are called *conjugations* and consist of the combination of two materials in the body to form a new compound. In drug metabolism, one of the components involved in a conjugation reaction is the drug or a metabolite produced by one of the

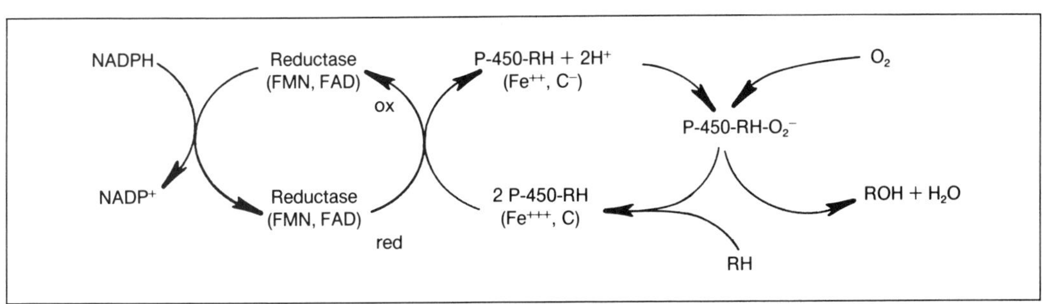

Figure 3-2. Mixed function oxidizing (MFO) system. RH = a substrate; C = an unidentified electron acceptor; ROH = the oxidized RH substrate. (Adapted with permission from Williams, R.T., Nutrients in drug detoxication reactions. In J.N. Hathcock and J. Coon, Eds., Nutrition and Drug Interrelations. *New York: Academic, 1978, p. 306.)*

nonsynthetic reactions. The other component, the *conjugating agent,* is provided by the body.

One of the most important of the conjugating agents is glucuronic acid, which is derived from carbohydrate. Protein provides glycine, glutamine, cysteine, glutathione, and methionine as sources of conjugating agents and also serves as a source of sulfate. Acetyl groups can be derived from protein, fat, or carbohydrates. Other nutrients necessary for some of the common conjugations are shown in Table 3-1.

Factors Influencing Rate of Metabolism. Drugs usually are metabolized at rates dependent on their concentration, but there are several factors that influence and alter this generalization. First, decreased concentration of the circulating free drug, such as that resulting from protein binding or concentration in adipose tissue, will reduce the rate of drug biotransformation. Second, the metabolism of drugs is dependent on the nutrient supply, and so clinical conditions that compromise the supply of these nutrients may affect the biotransformations of drugs. Third, depressed levels of drug-metabolizing enzymes resulting, for example, from liver disease, or occurring in a newborn infant will lower the rate of drug metabolism. Finally, one drug may alter the metabolism of another. Drug interactions with nutrients will be discussed in more detail in the next section.

Drug Safety and Effectiveness in Individuals

Factors Modifying Drug Effects in Individuals

A number of factors modify the effect of drugs in individuals. Some of these apply to all persons, and some only to selected individuals.

Body weight: In individuals of normal weight, a larger person will require a larger dose of a given drug than will the smaller person to maintain an equal concentration of the drug.

Body composition: If a person is seriously overweight or underweight, efficacy of drugs may be altered because of the differences in proportions of body fat and body water.

Age: In addition to its obvious effect on body size, in the early years age has a significant effect on drug metabolism. Some enzyme systems for drug metabolism are underdeveloped in infants, resulting in increased and prolonged drug action. The elderly may also have altered absorption or metabolism of drugs.

Gender: Women normally have more fat and less water than do men of equal weight and usually will require less drug. In addition, if the woman is pregnant or lactating, the effect of the drug on the fetus or on the nursing infant is an important consideration.

General physical condition: Severe renal or liver disease decreases the ability to excrete many drugs and thus will prolong their effect. Diseases that reduce the hydration of the body may affect drug action as a result of the change in the volume of distribution. For example, as the water content of the body is decreased, the volume of distribution also decreases with a consequent increase in drug concentration. Conversely, if the patient is edematous, the volume of distribution may be expanded.

Individual Variations in Drug Response

Some patients may develop an allergy to a drug. The allergic reaction is an unusual response of the immune system, the mechanism of which is described in Chapter 4. The magnitude of the response is not related to the size of the dose but, in order for an allergic response to occur, the patient must have had a previous exposure to the drug or a molecule of similar structure.

Some individuals react to a drug in a manner that is different from the usual but is not an allergy. This is called an *idiosyncrasy* and is believed to be the result of a mutation. It differs from a *toxicity* in that a toxicity will occur in all persons. In both an idiosyncrasy and a toxicity, unlike allergy, the magnitude of the response is related to the size of the dose, and the first dose can elicit the abnormal response.

After repeated exposure to some drugs, a patient may develop a drug *tolerance;* that is, an increasing amount is needed to cause the same response. This occurs especially with those drugs acting on the central nervous system. The mechanisms by which drug tolerances develop are not understood completely. It has been suggested that there may be a decrease in the rate of absorption, in the rate of transfer to the active site, or in the response of the receptor cells, resulting in diminished or slower reaction, or a drug may induce the enzymes of the MFO system. The phenomenon of drug tolerance is relevant to the abuse of "hard" drugs.

Drug Interactions

Patients frequently receive more than one drug at a time. There are several types of drug interactions which may be important. *Summation* occurs when two or more drugs elicit the same response, and the combined response is the sum of the effect of each. If each of these drugs elicits the response by acting via the same mechanism, the effect is *additive.* An additive response is, therefore, a form of summation.

Sometimes, two or more drugs that elicit the same response, such as raising blood glucose, have a greater effect together than the sum of each separately. This is called *synergism.* If, on the other hand, the effect of two or more drugs is less than the sum of each separately, the effect is referred to as an *antagonism.* Antagonistic reactions may be (1) pharmacologic (the drugs compete for the same receptor); (2) physiologic (the drugs have opposing actions at different receptors); or (3) chemical (the drugs react with each other to produce an inactive substance).

Classification and Terminology

Drugs may be classified in several ways. One of the simplest systems is a grouping into three categories:

1. *Drugs that fight infection:* These are the only drugs that actually cure a disease. They are toxic to the infecting organism, with little or no toxicity to the host.
2. *Drugs that replace inadequate materials:* Hormones, for example, sometimes are administered in amounts to replace inadequate levels in the body. When a drug is given at a dose level to provide replacement only, the amount is called a *physiologic dose.* A much larger *pharmacologic dose* is used for some purposes, but side effects will be more severe.
3. *Drugs that affect regulation:* Most drugs fall into this category. Examples include drugs that control blood pressure and those that control water and electrolyte balance.

Drugs may also be classified on the basis of the organ or tissue affected or on the basis of their type of action. The latter includes categories such as antiinfectives, anticonvulsants, hypotensive drugs, and anesthetics.

The naming of specific drugs within these categories has presented some problems. Drugs, as chemical compounds, have names that indicate their structure, but these names often are long and too difficult to pronounce or remember for common use. Therefore, when a drug is accepted for therapeutic use, it is assigned a name that is shorter and usually more pronounceable but still gives some indication of its chemical structure. This *generic* name is available for use in referring to the drug regardless of the manufacturer. In addition, manufacturers give their particular products names which only that manufacturer can use. Usually these names, the *proprietary* (or brand or trade) names, are the easiest to pronounce. In this book, the generic names of drugs are used, and an indication of the type of action of the drug is provided whenever possible. The professional in nutritional care may need to know the proprietary names that are equivalent to the various generic drug names. This information is contained in recent issues of one or more of various pharmaceutical indexes, some of which are listed in the Bibliography of this chapter.

NUTRITION-DRUG INTERRELATIONSHIPS

The interrelationships between nutrition and drugs may be examined broadly from two perspectives. One of these is the effects of drugs on the nutrition of the patient. The other is the influence of nutrition on drug action. Either or both of these may be important in a given patient.

Effects of Drugs on Nutrition

The specialist in nutritional care must be alert to medications that may contribute, either directly or indirectly, to malnutrition. This is true, of course, primarily when the drug is given over a long period of time.

Drug Effects on Taste, Appetite, and Food Intake

Some drugs are used specifically for the purpose of increasing or decreasing the food intake of the patient (see Chapter 15). Other drugs, used for purposes unrelated to food intake regulation, affect food intake as a side effect of their primary function. It is these drugs that will be discussed in this chapter.

Anatomy of Taste and Odor. The *flavor* of food is a sensation that is thought to combine the effects of stimulation of sensory receptors in the tongue, palate, and pharynx, providing a sense of taste (*gustation*), stimulation of receptors for *odor* in the nose, providing the sense of smell (*olfaction*), and also temperature, texture and color. The relative importance of the perception of taste and odor are not understood completely.

The sensory structures of the tongue and their innervation are depicted in Fig. 3-3. Taste perception results from combinations of varying amounts of the sensations traditionally called *sweet, salty, sour,* and *bitter* and probably others. The ability to detect and recognize the "traditional" tastes are measured using pure chemicals—sugar, sodium chloride, citric acid, or caffeine—in solution, for convenience and to make comparisons possible. However, chemosensory scientists generally believe there are other tastes but have not agreed on terminology.

Taste buds located in the back of the tongue innervated by the ninth cranial (glossopharyngeal) nerve are more sensitive to bitter compounds and generally less sensitive to those classified as sweet, salty, or sour, in comparison to taste buds located on the anterior portion of the tongue. These anteriorly located taste buds are innervated by the *chorda tympani* (a branch of the facial or seventh cranial nerve). Within the individual taste buds, there are approximately sixty individual taste bud cells. Most of these respond to many stimuli but to varying degrees. The final taste perceived is the result of a complicated pattern of individual nerve fiber responses to stimuli.

Basic odors are much less precisely defined. It has been suggested that some of these may be *putrid, ethereal, musky,* and *camphoric.*[1] Detection and recognition of these odors are tested using butylmercaptan, diethyl ether, butylbenzene, or camphor in an odorless solvent. In addition, modern researchers classify odors on the basis of the molecular structure of the compounds and on the basis of portions of the molecule. Receptors are located in the mucosa high in the nose and are innervated by the olfactory

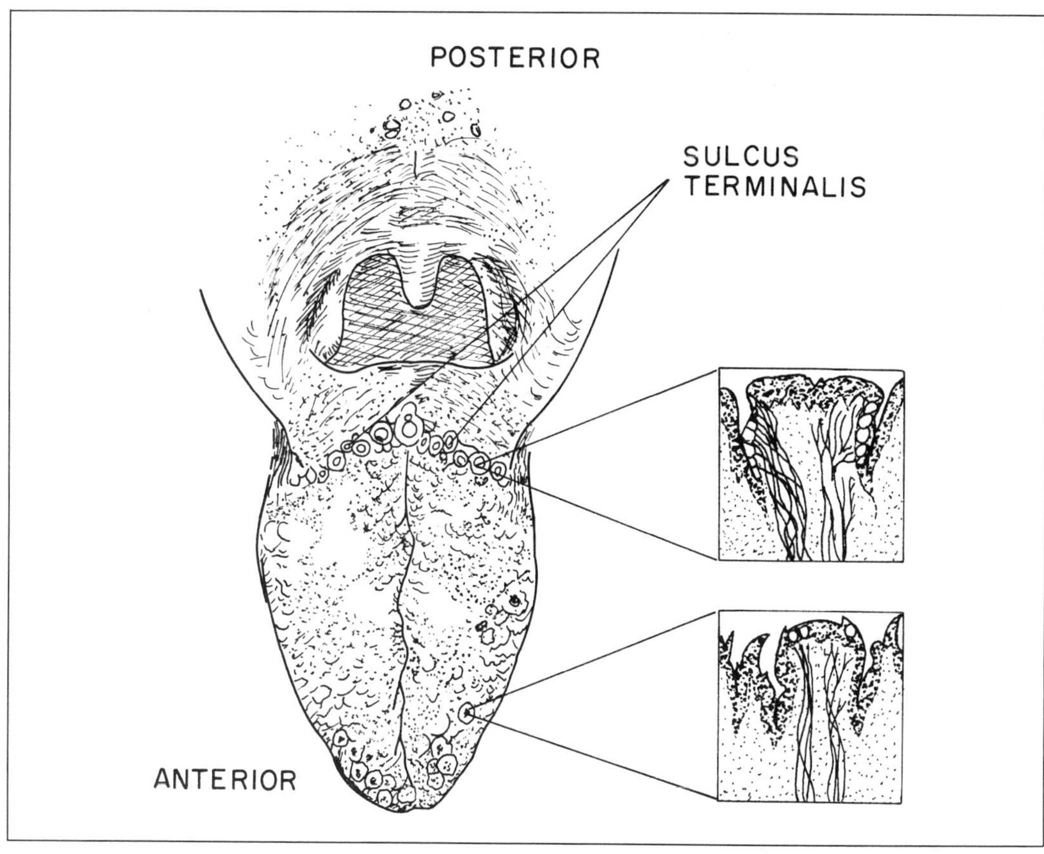

Figure 3-3. The surface of a normal tongue and palate. Filiform papillae may be seen covering the entire lingual surface. Fungiform papillae, somewhat larger and raised, may be seen covering the anterior two-thirds of the surface; they terminate at a V-shaped groove, the sulcus terminalis. Circumvallate papillae are seen over the posterior one-third of the lingual surface. Papillae may also be seen covering the area of the palate near the junction of the hard and soft palates. Lower insert: *Light microscopic appearance of a fungiform papilla. The taste buds, innervated by the chorda tympani branch of the facial nerve, are located at the top of the papilla only; free nerve endings may also be seen.* Upper insert: *Light microscopic appearance of a circumvallate papilla. The number of taste buds, innervated by a branch of the glossopharyngeal nerve, is much greater than in a fungiform papilla. These taste buds usually are located along the sides of the papilla. Free nerve endings may also be seen and are greater in number than in a fungiform papilla. (Adapted from Henkin, R.I., The role of taste in disease and nutrition.* Borden's Rev. Nutr. Res. *28:71, 1967, pp. 72–73.)*

nerve. Oral and nasal cavities are richly innervated also with free nerve endings (pain receptors), which respond to noxious stimuli from materials such as pepper, chili, and ammonia.

Effect of Disease on Taste and Odor Perception. Even before a diagnosis is made and before any drugs are prescribed, the disease process itself may affect the patient's sensitivity to taste. If the membrane characteristics of the taste bud cells or olfactory receptors are altered or if electrical activity of the nerve cells involved in sensations of taste or smell is distorted, the message may be misinterpreted by the brain. "Salty" may be interpreted as "bitter," for example. If the electrical activity is blocked, reduced, or increased in intensity, the perception of the taste or

Table 3-2. Alterations in Senses of Taste and Smell

Term		
Taste	Odor	Definition
Ageusia	Anosmia	Total loss of the perception
Hypogeusia	Hyposmia	Decreased ability to detect or identify a taste or odor
Hypergeusia	Hyperosmia	Increased sensitivity in detecting or recognizing a taste or odor
Dysgeusia	Dysosmia	Distortion (usually unpleasant) in the perception

odor would be absent, decreased, or increased accordingly. The descriptive terms used to define alterations in these senses are listed in Table 3-2.

Table 3-3 lists various conditions that may cause alterations in taste or odor sensitivity. It is important to recognize that the symptoms may or may not be seen in an individual patient. In addition, these data are obtained from studies of responses to threshold levels of the stimulant. In a practical situation, stimuli are well above threshold concentrations and so data on threshold responses may not be meaningful.

Drug Effects on Taste and Odor Perception. In addition to patients with the conditions listed in Table 3-3, patients who are receiving any of a wide variety of drugs may suffer from similar alterations in taste or odor perceptions. Table 3-4 lists a number of these drugs.

Some drugs, such as potassium iodide and those containing bromides, are secreted into the saliva and thereby produce an unpleasant taste in the mouth. Others produce an unpleasant aftertaste or are themselves simply unpleasant tasting. These include penicillin, clofibrate, chloral hydrate, paraldehyde, and B-complex vitamins.

Table 3-3. Conditions That Might Alter Taste or Odor Sensitivities

Increased Detection Threshold[a]
Advanced age
Congenital defect
Copper deficiency
Zinc deficiency
Familial dysautonomia
Facial paralysis
Trauma (head injuries, gunshots, burns)
Sjögren's syndrome
Hypothyroidism
Mental depression
Chronic renal insufficiency
Cystic fibrosis of the pancreas (↓odor; normal taste?)

Decreased Detection Threshold
Adrenocortical insufficiency
Panhypopituitarism
Congenital adrenal hyperplasia
Cystic fibrosis of the pancreas (↑odor and taste?)
Congenital defect
Epileptic syndromes

Specific Alterations in Sensitivity
Turner's syndrome (↓sour, ↓bitter)
Gonadal dysgenesis
Pseudohypoparathyroidism (↓sour, ↓bitter)
Congenital cretinism
Congenital taste blindness
Drug-induced
Lesions of tongue or palate (tumor, infection, trauma, granuloma, irradiation, postsurgery) (↓salt, ↓sweet)
Maxillary dentures (↓sour, ↓bitter)
Menses
Pregnancy
Diabetes mellitus (↓sweet if ↑blood sugar)
Cancer (↓sweet, ↓salt, altered bitter)
Renal failure (↓sweet, ↓salt, ↓sour)
Sjögren's syndrome (↓bitter, ↓sour, ↓salt)
Schizophrenia

Compiled from Campanella, G., Filla, A., and DeMichele, G., Smell and taste acuity in epileptic syndromes. *Eur. Neurol.* 17:136, 1978; Henkin, R.I., The role of taste in disease and nutrition. *Borden's Rev. Nutr. Res.* 28:71, 1967; Henkin, R.I., and Christiansen, R.L., Taste thresholds in patients with dentures. *J. Am. Diet. Assoc.* 75:118, 1967; and Hertz, J., Cain, W.S., Bartoshuk, L.M., and Dolan, T.F., Jr., Olfactory and taste sensitivity in children with cystic fibrosis. *Physiol. Behav.* 14:89, 1975.

[a] Detection threshold is the lowest concentration of a substance that a person can discriminate as being different from water. Increased threshold indicates decreased sensitivity.

Table 3-4. Drugs That May Alter Taste Sensation

Decreased Taste Acuity		Specific Alterations in Sensation	
Drug	Function	Drug	Function
Amydricaine	Anesthetic	Allopurinol[a]	
Anisotropine methylbromide	Cholinergic-blocking	Amphetamines (↓sweet, ↑bitter)	Stimulant
Azathioprine	Immunosuppressant	Amydricaine (↓bitter, ↓salt)	Anesthetic
Baclofen	Skeletal muscle relaxant	Benzocaine (↑sour)	Anesthetic
Carbamazepine	Anticonvulsant	Bromocriptine mesylate[a]	
Cholestyramine	Antihyperlipemic	Captopril[a] (sweet tastes salty)	
Clofibrate	Antihyperlipemic	Chloral hydrate[a]	
Cocaine	Anesthetic	Chlorpromazine[a] (metallic taste)	Tranquilizer; antipsychotic
Eucaine	Anesthetic	Clindamycin	Antibiotic
Griseofulvin	Antifungal	Clofibrate (unpleasant aftertaste)	Antihyperlipemic
Levodopa	Antiparkinsonism agent	Cocaine (↓bitter, ↓sweet)	Anesthetic
Lidocaine	Anesthetic	Ethambutol hydrochloride[a]	
Lincomycin hydrochloride monohydrate	Antibiotic	Ethionamide (metallic taste)	Antituberculotic
Methimazole	Antithyroid	Eucaine (↓bitter, ↓sweet)	Anesthetic
Methylthiouracil	Antithyroid	Fluorouracil (altered bitter and sour, ↓sweet)	Antineoplastic
Metronidazole	Amebicide and trichomonacide	Furosemide (↓sweet)	Diuretic
Oxyphencyclimine hydrochloride	Cholinergic-blocking	Gold compounds[a]	
Penicillamine	Chelating agent	Griseofulvin	Antifungal
Phenindione	Anticoagulant	Histidine[a]	Amino acid
Phenylbutazone	Antiarthritic, antiinflammatory	Insulin (↓salt, ↓sweet with prolonged use)	Hormone
Phenytoin sodium	Anticonvulsant	Levodopa	Antiparkinsonism agent
Procaine hydrochloride	Anesthetic	Lidocaine (↓sweet, ↓salt)	Anesthetic
Rifampin	Antituberculotic	Lincomycin hydrochloride monohydrate (↓sweet)	Antibiotic
Sulfasalazine		Lithium carbonate (unpleasant metallic, dairy products taste spoiled)	Psychotherapeutic
Tetracaine hydrochloride	Anesthetic	Metronidazole[a] (metallic, sharp taste)	Amebicide and trichomonacide
		Nortriptyline hydrochloride (unspecified, unpleasant taste)	Antidepressant
		Penicillamine (↓sweet, ↓salt)	Chelating agent
		Penicillin[a]	Antibiotic
		Procaine hydrochloride (↑sweet)	Anesthetic
		Quinidine[a]	
		Streptomycin sulfate	Antibiotic

(*continued*)

Table 3-4. Drugs That May Alter Taste Sensation (continued)

Decreased Taste Acuity		Specific Alterations in Sensation	
Drug	Function	Drug	Function
		Tetracaine hydrochloride (↓bitter, ↑sweet)	Anesthetic
		Thioridazine[a]	
		Triclofos sodium (↑bitter)	Sedative

Compiled from Carson, J.S., and Gormican, A., Disease-medication relationships in altered taste sensitivity. *J. Am. Diet. Assoc.* 68:550, 1976; March, D.C., *Handbook: Interaction of Selected Drugs with Nutritional Status in Man,* 2nd ed. Chicago: American Dietetic Association, 1978; and Maslakowski, C.J., Drug-nutrient interactions/interrelationships. *Nutr. Supp. Serv.* 1:14, 1981.

[a] Induces a bad taste.

Drug Effects on Appetite and Food Intake. Some drugs tend to decrease appetite as a side effect. Included among these are the drugs previously listed that have an unpleasant taste in the mouth. Additionally, drugs and other compounds can be borne to the taste receptors intravascularly via the capillaries supplying the receptors. As a consequence, there may be a lingering sensation after the stimulation from the inhaled or ingested substance is over. Other drugs depress food intake because they cause nausea, and some produce *anorexia* (abnormal absence of the desire for food) by mechanisms that are not understood. March[2] notes that an extensive number of drugs can cause nausea, vomiting, and anorexia. Table 3-5 lists those in which the action is frequent or more severe. Many antineoplastic agents cause severe nausea and vomiting as well as other symptoms that tend to decrease nutrient intake. They are discussed in greater detail in Chapter 13.

Some drugs tend to increase appetite as a side effect, but there are no safe and effective drugs whose primary function in humans is to increase food intake.[3] Those that have some appetite-stimulating side effects are listed in Table 3-6.

Drug Effects on Nutrient Absorption

Some drugs adversely affect the absorption of nutrients and thereby influence the nutritional status of the patient. The resulting malabsorption defects have been classified as *primary* or *secondary.*[4]

Primary malabsorption is caused by action in the lumen or on the intestinal mucosa. The most severe primary malabsorption results from actions of drugs that damage the absorptive cells of the small intestine. Other mechanisms of action include (1) altering transit time, (2) binding bile acids and decreasing micelle formation, (3) acting as a physical barrier, and (4) altering the pH in the lumen of the gastrointestinal tract. Table 3-7 contains a list of drugs that cause primary malabsorption of various nutrients.

Secondary malabsorption of a nutrient is due to the interference of a drug with the absorption or metabolism of another nutrient. The primary example involves the interrelationship of drugs and vitamin D metabolism, which results in calcium malabsorption.[5]

Some drugs cause gastrointestinal upsets and diarrhea by causing changes in the intestinal flora.

Drug Effects on Nutrient Metabolism

The desirable effects of some drugs are based on their action of interfering with the activity of a nutrient. Anticoagulant drugs, for example, are antagonists to vitamin K action. Other drugs affect nutrient metabolism as a side effect.

Table 3-5. Drugs That Cause Frequent or Severe Nausea, Vomiting, or Anorexia as a Side Effect

Drug	Function	Notes
Amphetamine	Cerebral stimulant	Frequent
p-Aminosalicylic acid	Antituberculotic	Frequent
β-Sitosterol	Antihyperlipemic	Common
Cancer therapy drugs[a]	Antineoplastic	Severe
Digitalis	Antiarrhythmic	Frequent
Estrogen	Hormone	
Ethosuximide	Anticonvulsant	Frequent
Griseofulvin	Antifungal	
Levodopa	Antiparkinsonism agent	Occasional
Nitrofurantoin	Urinary germicide	Frequent
Penicillamine	Chelating agent	In initial doses
Penicillins	Antibiotic	
Phensuximide	Anticonvulsant	Frequent
Procainamide	Antiarrhythmic	
Propoxyphene	Analgesic	Undetermined mechanism
Reserpine	Hypotensive agent	Undetermined mechanism
Sulfonamides	Antiinfective	
Tetracycline	Antibiotic	Can be severe

[a] See Chapter 13 for more information.

Table 3-6. Drugs That Tend to Increase Appetite

Drug	Function	Suggested Mechanism
Alcohol	Social beverage	Stimulate sense of taste; increase flow of secretions in digestive system; promote relaxation
Androgens	Hormone	
Benzodiazepines	Antidepressant; tranquilizer	Promote relaxation
Corticosteroids	Hormone	
Cyproheptadine hydrochloride	Antihistamine	Direct effect on hypothalamus or hypoglycemic effect
Insulin	Hormone	Hypoglycemic effect
Phenothiazines	Antipsychotic; tranquilizer	Promote relaxation; antiemetic
Sulfonylureas (e.g., tolbutamide,chlorpropamide)	Hypoglycemic agents	Stimulate insulin release

Table 3-7. Primary Intestinal Absorptive Defects Induced by Drugs

Drug	Function	Malabsorptive or Fecal Nutrient Loss	Mechanisms	Nutritional Care Recommendations
Mineral oil	Laxative	Carotene, vitamins A, D, K	Physical barrier; nutrients dissolve in mineral oil and are lost; micelle formation	Mineral oil not given at or close to meal times if used for extended time
Castor oil, milk of magnesia	Cathartic	Calcium and potassium loss		Calcium and potassium supplements if used for extended time
Phenolphthalein	Laxative	Vitamin D, calcium	Intestinal "hurry"; potassium depletion; loss of structural integrity	Monitor serum potassium and calcium status; supplement if used for extended time
Neomycin, cycloserine, erythromycin, tetracyclines	Antibiotic	Fat, nitrogen, sodium, potassium, calcium, magnesium, iron, lactose, sucrose, vitamin B_{12}, folate	Structural defect; pancreatic lipase; binding of bile acids (salts)	Vitamin and mineral supplements if used for extended time
Cholestyramine	Hypocholesterolemic agent; binds bile acid	Fat, fat-soluble vitamins, carotene, vitamin B_{12}, iron	Binding of bile acids (salts and nutrients—e.g., iron)	Monitor vitamins B_{12} and A and iron status
Potassium chloride	Potassium repletion	Vitamin B_{12}	Change in ileal pH	Monitor vitamin B_{12} status
Colchicine	Antiinflammatory agent in gout	Fat, carotene, sodium, potassium, vitamin B_{12}, lactose	Mitotic arrest; structural defect; enzyme damage	Monitor vitamins B_{12} and A and electrolyte status
Para-aminosalicylic acid	Antituberculotic	Fat, folate, vitamin B_{12}, calcium, magnesium, iron	Mucosal block in B_{12} uptake	Monitor vitamin B_{12} and folate status
Phenytoin sodium	Anticonvulsant	Folate, vitamin B_{12}		Monitor vitamin B_{12} and folate status
Methotrexate	Antineoplastic	Folate, vitamin B_{12}		Monitor vitamin B_{12} and folate status

Compiled from Roe, D.A., *Drug-Induced Nutritional Deficiencies*. Westport, Conn.: AVI, 1976; and Utah Dietetic Association, *Handbook of Clinical Dietetics*, 1977.

Alcohol, in particular, has a wide range of effects on nutrient metabolism. However, in view of its wide use as a social beverage and its association with liver disease, the nutritional effects of chronic alcoholism will be discussed in Chapter 11.

Protein. A number of drugs affect the metabolism of proteins and amino acids (Table 3-8). A few stimulate protein synthesis, but the majority have the opposite effect. The mode of action of many of these drugs is unknown. For patients receiving long-term therapy, it is important that their protein status be monitored frequently.

Lipids. Drugs that influence lipid metabolism may be divided roughly into those that raise plasma triglyceride or cholesterol levels and those that lower them. Some drugs are used for the primary purpose of lowering blood lipid levels. These will be discussed in Chapter 11. Others affect lipid metabolism as a side effect. These are listed in Table 3-9 and are categorized according to the direction of their effects.

Carbohydrates. Drugs that affect carbohydrate metabolism may be divided into those that increase blood glucose levels and those that lower them. Some affect blood glucose levels as side effects of their intended actions (Table 3-10), whereas it is the primary purpose of others, such as insulin and the oral hypoglycemic agents, to alter blood glucose levels.

Vitamins and Minerals. Some drugs are useful primarily as a result of their relationship to minerals or vitamins in the body. As previously mentioned, penicillamine is a chelating agent used in the treatment of Wilson's disease to remove excess copper. There

Table 3-8. Drugs That Affect Protein Metabolism

Drug	Function	Action
Amphotericin B	Antifungal	Accelerates protein catabolism
Anabolic steroids	Hormone	Stimulate protein synthesis
Azathioprine	Antineoplastic	Undefined
Chloramphenicol	Antibiotic	
Corticosteroids	Hormone	Increases gluconeogenesis; increases urinary nitrogen excretion
Dactinomycin	Antineoplastic	Inhibits protein synthesis
Estrogen/progesterone combination	Hormone (contraceptive)	Changes in plasma amino acid pattern; questionable significance
Indomethacin	Analgesic, antipyretic, antiinflammatory	Promotes gastric emptying; decreases amino acid absorption
Insulin	Hormone	Stimulates protein synthesis
Kanamycin sulfate	Antibiotic	Decreases absorption
Methotrexate	Antineoplastic	Folic acid antagonist; interferes with phenylalanine metabolism
Neomycin	Antibiotic	Decreases absorption
Salicylates	Analgesic	Produces aminoaciduria
Tetracyclines	Antibiotic	Increases urinary nitrogen excretion
Thyroid	Hormone	Increases urinary nitrogen excretion

Table 3-9. Drugs with Side Effects That Result in Alteration of Serum Lipid Levels

Drug	Function
Increased serum lipid	
Alcohol	Social beverage
Chlorpromazine	Tranquilizer; antipsychotic
Corticosteroids	Hormone
Estrogen/progesterone	Oral contraceptives
Growth hormone	Hormone
Thiouracil	Hormone antagonist
Vitamin D	Hormone
Decreased serum lipid	
p-Aminosalicylic acid	Anti-tuberculotic
Aspirin	Analgesic
Chlortetracycline hydrochloride	Antibiotic
Colchicine	Antiinflammatory
Fenfluramine hydrochloride	Antiobesity agent
Glucagon	Hormone
Phenindione	Anticoagulant
Sulfinpyrazone	Uricosuric

Table 3-10. Drugs That Alter Blood Glucose Levels as a Side Effect

Drug	Function
Increased blood glucose (hyperglycemia)	
Corticosteroids	Hormones
Coumarin derivatives	Anticoagulant
Diazoxide	Antihypertensive
Estrogen	Hormone
Morphine	Analgesic
Phenothiazines	Tranquilizer
Phenytoin sodium	Anticonvulsants
Probenecid	Uricosuric
Thiazides	Diuretic
Decreased blood glucose (hypoglycemia)	
Aspirin	Analgesic
Barbiturates	Sedatives
Monoamine oxidase inhibitors	Antihypotensive; antidepressant
Phenacetin	Analgesic
Phenylbutazone	Analgesic; antiinflammatory
Propranolol hydrochloride	Cardiovascular drug (beta-adrenergic blocker)
Sulfonamides	Antiinfective

are diuretics that function primarily because of their effects on sodium excretion.

However, drugs may have important side effects as a result of their actions on mineral or vitamin metabolism. When these alterations result in increased nutrient requirements, the possibility of deficiency results, particularly in patients who have had marginal diets over extended periods or in those whose nutritional status has been damaged by the disease process. The nutritional care specialist should be alert to the increased needs of such patients, particularly when treatments involve long-term, high dosages of the drugs listed in Table 3-11. Detailed information on the interactions of vitamins or minerals and drugs is contained in the handbook by March.[2]

Effects of Food and Nutrients on Drugs

Effects of Food on Drug Absorption

Food in the Digestive Tract. Many drugs act as gastric irritants when taken orally (Table 3-12). It is recommended that these drugs be taken with food.[6] The presence of food may change the pH, osmolality, amount of various secretions, or motility of the gastrointestinal tract. Any of these changes can, in turn, alter the absorption of drugs by causing alterations in their ionization, stability, solubility, or transit time. There is no constant effect of food on drug absorption. It may be decreased, delayed, or increased (Table 3-13), depending on the drug involved. As Table 3-13 suggests, the more frequent effect is a reduction in the amount or rate of drug absorption. Such changes reduce the blood level of the drug, thus reducing its effectiveness. When the rate of absorption is reduced, the action of the drug is prolonged. Conversely, when absorption is increased, the blood level may be increased, perhaps to toxic levels. These effects are of clinical importance when fast action of the drug is needed.

Specific Nutrients. Individual nutrients also affect the absorption of some drugs. The interactions of certain nutrients with tetracycline, griseofulvin, or tetrachloroethylene may be of particular clinical importance.

Tetracycline forms an insoluble complex with calcium, magnesium, iron, or aluminum, which inhibits tetracycline absorption; therefore, it usually is recommended that tetracycline or its derivatives be taken without milk or milk products. In addition, the drug should be taken more than 1 hour before or 2 hours after a meal. Tetracycline can cause serious nausea and vomiting, and sodium bicarbonate, which some patients may take for their gastrointestinal symptoms, seems to reduce tetracycline absorption. Possibly, the mechanism of action involves the change in pH of the gastric contents. In any case, there is danger that the drug will be rendered ineffective, with potentially serious consequences.

Griseofulvin (an antifungal agent) and tetrachloroethylene (an anthelmintic) are absorbed more rapidly if taken with a high-fat meal.

Effects of Nutritional Status on Drug Metabolism and Excretion

The malnutrition that often can occur in hospitalized patients may have a detrimental effect on the metabolism of many drugs.[7–9] Many nutrients can be involved.

Protein. Protein deprivation can affect drug binding in two ways. First, it reduces the amount of plasma albumin available for binding. Since the unbound, or free, drug is the active component, a decrease in plasma albumin results in an increase in the amount of drug available to react with binding sites, to be metabolized, and to be excreted. The net effect is an increase in drug potency in a shorter time. Second, other substances such as nonpolar amino acids and free fatty acids

Table 3-11. Drugs That Affect Vitamin Requirements

Drug	Vitamin with Which Drug Interacts	Possible Mechanisms	Possible Symptoms
p-Aminosalicylic acid	Vitamin B_{12}	Decreased absorption	Megaloblastic anemia
Antacid	Thiamine	Decreased absorption	Thiamine deficiency
Anticonvulsants	Folate	Decreased absorption; competitive inhibition of vitamin coenzymes; enzyme induction	Megaloblastic anemia
	Vitamin D	Enzyme induction	Rickets, osteomalacia
	Vitamin K	Enzyme induction	Neonatal hemorrhage
Cathartics (irritant)	Vitamin D	Increased peristalsis; damage to the intestinal wall	Osteomalacia
Cholestyramine	Folate	Complexation of the vitamin	
	Vitamin B_{12}	Inhibition of intrinsic factor function	
	Vitamin A		
	Vitamin D	Binding of bile salts	Osteomalacia
	Vitamin K		
Cinchona alkaloids	Vitamin K		
Colchicine	Vitamin B_{12}	Absorptive enzyme damage; damage to the intestinal wall	
Coumarin anticoagulants	Vitamin K		Hemorrhage
Estrogen-containing hormonal contraceptives	Folate	Inhibition of absorptive enzymes; increased synthesis of folate-binding macroglobulin; enzyme induction	Megaloblastic anemia
	Vitamin B_{12}	Changes in tissue distribution	
	Vitamin B_6	Induction of tryptophan oxygenase enzyme; competition for vitamin-binding sites on apoenzyme	Depression
	Riboflavin		
	Thiamine		
	Vitamin C	Decreased absorption; increased ceruloplasmin concentration; increased concentration of reducing compounds; changes in tissue distribution	

Glutethimide	Vitamin D	Enzyme induction	Osteomalacia
Hydralazine	Vitamin B_6	Increased excretion of vitamin-drug complex	Peripheral neuropathy
Isoniazid	Vitamin B_6	Increased excretion of vitamin-drug complex	Peripheral neuropathy; generalized convulsions (infants); anemia
	Niacin	Competitive inhibition of vitamin coenzymes; secondary to vitamin B_6 deficiency	Pellagra
Levodopa	Vitamin B_6	Increased excretion of vitamin-drug complex	Peripheral neuropathy
Methotrexate	Folate	Inhibition of dihydrofolate reductase enzyme	Megaloblastic anemia
Mineral oil	Vitamin A	Lipid solvent	
	Vitamin D		Rickets
	Vitamin K		
Neomycin	Vitamin B_{12}	Damage to the intestinal wall; inhibition of intrinsic factor function	
	Vitamin A	Damage to the intestinal wall; inhibition of pancreatic lipase; binding of bile salts	
Penicillamine	Vitamin B_6	Increased excretion of vitamin-drug complex	Peripheral neuropathy
Potassium chloride	Vitamin B_{12}	Decreased ileal pH	
Pyrimethamine	Folate	Inhibition of dihydrofolate reductase enzyme	Megaloblastic anemia
Salicylates	Folate	Decreased protein binding	
	Vitamin C	Decreased uptake in thrombocytes and leukocytes	
	Vitamin K		
Sulfasalazine	Folate	Decreased absorption	
Tetracycline	Vitamin C	Increased excretion	
Triamterene	Folate	Inhibition of dihydrofolate reductase enzyme	Megaloblastic anemia
Trimethoprim	Folate	Inhibition of dihydrofolate reductase enzyme	Megaloblastic anemia

Adapted with permission from Ovesen, L., Drugs and vitamin deficiency. *Drugs* 18:293, 1979.

Table 3-12. Drugs Reported to Irritate the Gastrointestinal Tract

Drug	Function
Aminophylline	Bronchodilator
Aminosalicylic acid	Antituberculotic
Aspirin	Analgesic
Aspirin-phenacetin-caffeine (APC)	Analgesic
Chlorpromazine	Major tranquilizer
Chlorpropamide	Oral hypoglycemic
Ferrous fumarate	Iron replacement
Ferrous gluconate	Iron replacement
Ferrous lactate	Iron replacement
Ferrous sulfate	Iron replacement
Hydrochlorothiazide	Diuretic
Hydrocortisone	Antiinflammatory
Indomethacin	Nonsteroidal antiinflammatory
Isoniazid	Antituberculotic
Metronidazole	Antifungal
Nalidixic acid	Urinary tract antiinfective
Potassium salts (bicarbonate, chloride, gluconate, etc.)	Potassium replacement
Prednisolone	Antiinflammatory
Prednisone	Antiinflammatory
Procyclidine hydrochloride	Antiparkinsonism agent
Reserpine	Antihypertensive
Sulfinpyrazone	Uricosuric
Tolbutamide	Hypoglycemic
Triamterene	Potassium-sparing diuretic
Trihexyphenidyl preparations	Antiparkinsonism agent
Trimeprazine tartrate	Antihistamine

Reprinted with permission from Visconti, J.A., *Drug-Food Interaction.* Nutrition and Disease series. Columbus, Ohio: Ross Laboratories, 1977, p. 16.

Table 3-13. Effects of Food on Drug Absorption

Drugs with which food reduces absorption
Ampicillin
Aspirin
Demeclocycline
Erythromycin
Erythromycin stearate
Levodopa
Methacycline hydrochloride
Oxytetracycline
Penicillin V
Phenethicillin
Pivampicillin hydrochloride
Propantheline bromide
Rifampin
Sulfadiazine sodium
Tetracycline

Drugs with which food delays absorption
Acetaminophen
Amoxicillin
Aspirin
Cephalexin
Cephradine
Digoxin
Furosemide
Nitrofurantoin
Potassium ion
Sulfadiazine
Sulfadimethoxine
Sulfanilamide
Sulfisoxazole

Drugs with which food increases absorption
Erythromycin ethylsuccinate
Griseofulvin
Lithium ion
Nitrofurantoin
Riboflavin

carried by albumin may affect drug binding.[10] The clinical significance of altered levels of these substances is unknown.

In addition to the effects on drug binding, protein deficiency depresses both the cytochrome P-450 content and P-450 reductase activity in the MFO system.[11] The consequences of these actions vary. If the MFO system detoxifies a drug, the protein deficiency would have the effect of making the drug more toxic. If, however, the MFO system metabolizes a drug to a more toxic compound, protein deficiency would decrease the toxicity of the drug. These statements, however, assume a simple one-step metabolic pathway. The effects of protein deficiency in more complex systems needs additional study.

Lipids. Lipids have been reported to be essential for normal functioning of the MFO system,[12] although their precise function is not understood entirely.[13] A fat-free diet has been shown to decrease the activity of the drug-metabolizing enzyme system in the rat, and drug-metabolizing enzymes are induced in rats fed diets with added polyunsaturated fatty acids.[14-16]

Minerals. There is a paucity of information concerning the effects of mineral nutrition on drug metabolism in humans. Experiments with animals have indicated that dietary deficiencies of calcium, magnesium, and zinc alter the rate of metabolism of a variety of drugs, and iron deficiency stimulates hepatic drug metabolism.[17] Hypokalemia alters the plasma half-life of some drugs. The significance of these changes in human patients is unknown, and the effects of multiple deficiencies also need investigation.

Vitamins. There is evidence that several vitamins affect the drug-metabolizing enzyme system. These include ascorbic acid (vitamin C), riboflavin, and alpha-tocopherol (vitamin E).[18] Niacin deficiency may also be included, possibly in relation to NADPH levels. Further investigation is needed on (1) the function of these vitamins in the drug-metabolizing enzyme system, (2) the possible involvement of other vitamins, and (3) the effects of multivitamin deficiencies and of combined mineral-vitamin deficiencies.

Two more specific reactions may be of clinical importance. Pyridoxine blocks the effects of the drug levodopa, used in the treatment of Parkinson's disease. Foods do

Table 3-14. Drug-Food and Drug-Alcohol Incompatibilities

	Reactants		
Reaction Classification	1	2	Effect
Tyramine reactions	Monoamine oxidase inhibitors; antidepressants (e.g., phenelzine sulfate); procarbazine hydrochloride; isoniazid (INH)	Foods rich in tyramine or dopamine Cheese; red wines; chicken liver; broad beans; yeast extracts	Flushing; hypertension; cerebrovascular accidents
Disulfiram reactions	Aldehyde dehydrogenase inhibitors Disulfiram (Antabuse); calcium cyanamide; metronidazole; nitrofurantoin; *Coprinus atramentarius* (inky cap mushroom); sulfonylureas; furazolidone; quinacrine hydrochloride; chloramphenicol	Alcohol Beer; wine; liquor; foods containing alcohol	Flushing, headache; nausea, vomiting; chest and abdominal pain
Hypoglycemic reactions	Insulin releasers Oral hypoglycemic agents; sugar (as in sweet mixes)	Alcohol	Weakness; mental confusion; irrational behavior; loss of consciousness
Flush reactions (see disulfiram reactions)	Miscellaneous Chlorpropamide (diabetes); griseofulvin; tetrachlorethylene	Alcohol	Flush; dyspnea; headache

Adapted from Roe, D.A., Interactions between drugs and nutrients. *Med. Clin. North Am.* 63:988, 1979.

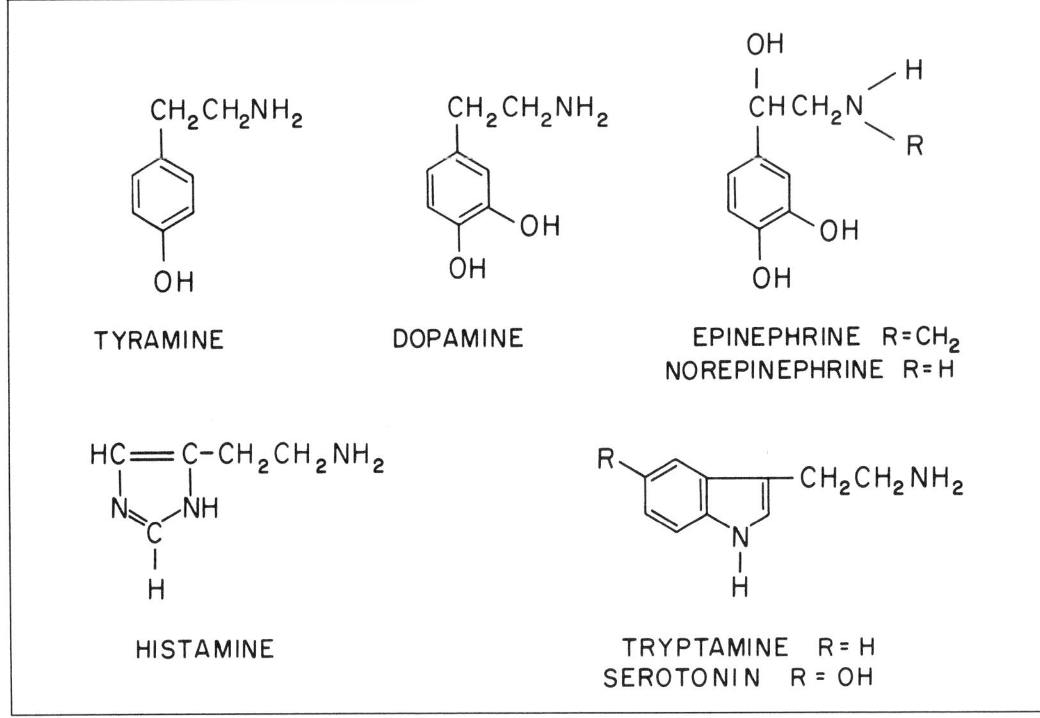

Figure 3-4. Vasoactive amines in food.

not contain enough pyridoxine to inhibit levodopa, but supplementation with 1.0 mg or more of pyridoxine should be avoided. Vitamin K interacts with and decreases the effect of warfarin sodium (an anticoagulant). Vitamin K supplementation or excessive intake should be avoided.

Detrimental Systemic Food-Drug Interactions

Some interactions between drugs and certain foods or alcohol result in systemic reactions that may be unpleasant or even life-threatening. Four types of these reactions are listed in Table 3-14.

Vasoactive Compounds and Monoamine Oxidase Inhibitors. There are a number of compounds, found naturally in food, that can cause a marked increase in blood pressure if they appear in the circulation. They include tyramine, dopamine, and norepinephrine, which are phenethylamine derivatives, and, in addition, histamine and serotonin (5-HT) (Fig. 3-4). These amines can be synthesized by some plants and also appear in animal products in which there is some fermentation or microbial contamination. Of these compounds, tyramine has been found to be the most clinically significant. As a result of sympathetic overstimulation, *tyramine* produces a marked elevation in blood pressure along with occipital headache, nausea, and vomiting. If severe, the effects cause a hypertensive crisis which can be life-threatening.

Monoamine oxidase (MAO) is found in the liver, gastrointestinal tract, and adrenergic nerve endings where it metabolizes norepinephrine, tyramine, and other pressor amines. Normally, MAO metabolizes the tyramine in food before it reaches the systemic circulation. The action of MAO is inhibited by a number of drugs known as *monoamine oxidase inhibitors* (MAOIs). This category of drugs includes isocarboxazid, nialamide, phenelzine sulfate, and tranylcypromine sulfate. They sometimes are used in the treatment of severe depression in patients who do not respond to the tricyclic antidepressants. They also are used occasionally in the treatment of postural hypotension. There are other drugs that inhibit MAO. These include procarbazine hydrochloride (an antineoplastic), pargyline hydrochloride (an antihypertensive), and furazolidone (an antibiotic). If a patient is taking any of these drugs and eats food containing tyramine, the tyramine is not metabolized, reaches the systemic circulation, and causes the symptoms described previously.

Because of the hazards of the reaction, the patient should avoid foods that contain tyramine and other foods with which MAOIs are thought to react, such as raisins. Similar reactions have been reported in patients who have eaten broad beans (*Vicia fava*), presumably due to the presence in the beans of dopa which is metabolized to dopamine. As a result, it also is recommended that these be avoided. Table 3-15 lists foods that contain tyramine or dopamine and that should be avoided by patients taking MAOIs. Blood pressure can be increased by 6 mg tyramine, and 25 mg produces severe hypertension.[19]

There is uncertainty concerning some other food items. Studies on rats indicate that methylxanthines found in coffee, tea, cocoa, and cola drinks react with MAOIs. The patient's physician may decide that it is necessary to eliminate these beverages from the diet.

Little is known about the metabolism of other amines, such as histamine, serotonin, and norepinephrine. It may become necessary to restrict other foods as the interactions between these substances and drugs become known. If a drug acted as a histaminase inhibitor, for example, a diet restricted in histamine might be necessary. The diet would require the elimination of fermented foods such as chocolate and sauerkraut.

Table 3-15. Foods Reported to Contain Tyramine or Dopamine

- Cheeses
  - Cheddar
  - Camembert
  - Emmenthaler
  - Brie
  - Stilton blue
  - Processed
  - Gruyère
  - Gouda
  - Brick, natural
  - Mozzarella
  - Bleu
  - Roquefort
  - Boursault
  - Parmesan
  - Romano
  - Provolone
- Beer and ale
- Wines
  - Chianti
  - Riesling
  - Sauterne
  - Sherry
- Marmite yeast and yeast extract
  - Products made with large amounts of yeast (e.g., homemade bread)
- Fish
  - Salted dried fish
  - Pickled herring
- Meat
  - Meat extracts
  - Beef liver (stored)
  - Chicken liver (stored)
  - Aged game
  - Salami, sausage, bologna
  - Pepperoni
- Vegetables
  - Avocado
  - Tomato
  - Green bean pods
  - Eggplant
  - Italian broad beans
- Fruit
  - Banana
  - Red plums
  - Orange (limit to 1 small orange per day)
  - Figs
  - Raisins
- Miscellaneous
  - Soya and soy sauce
  - Bouillon cubes

Compiled from Lovenberg, W., Some vasoactive and psychoactive substances in food: Amines, stimulants, depressants and hallucinogens. In *Toxicants Occurring Naturally in Foods.* Washington, D.C.: National Academy of Sciences, 1973, pp. 172–174; and Horwitz, O., Lovenberg, W., Engelman, K., and Sjoerdsma, A., Monoamine oxidase inhibitors, tyramine and cheese. *J.A.M.A.* 188:1108, 1964.

Table 3-16. Drugs Reported to Interact with Alcohol

Anticoagulants, oral
Antidepressants, tricyclic
Antihistamines
CNS depressants
Chloramphenicol
Disulfiram
Ethionamide
Furazolidone
Griseofulvin
Guanethidine
Isoniazid
Methotrexate
Methotrimeprazine
Metronidazole
Monoamine oxidase inhibitors
Narcotic analgesics
Nitroglycerin
Phenothiazines
Phenytoin sodium
Procarbazine hydrochloride
Quinacrine hydrochloride
Salicylates
Sulfonamides
Tetrachlorethylene
Tolazoline hydrochloride
Tolbutamide

Reprinted with permission from Visconti, J.A., *Drug-Food Interaction.* Nutrition in Disease series. Columbus, Ohio: Ross Laboratories, 1977, p. 20.

Alcohol-Drug Interactions. Although alcohol has been considered both a drug and a nutrient, it will be considered here as a beverage which can interact with various drugs (Table 3-16). It has been shown to decrease the absorption of many nutrients and to alter the metabolism of drugs. Some of the types of reactions are described in Table 3-14. The reactions with alcohol of disulfiram and of hypoglycemic drugs are particularly important. Patients taking these drugs may need to be counseled concerning alcohol intake.

References

1. Maller, O., and Cardello, A. The sick senses. Functions of taste and smell. *The Professional Nutritionist* 10:1, 1978.
2. March, D.C. *Handbook: Interactions of Selected Drugs with Nutritional Status in Man,* 2nd ed. Chicago: American Dietetic Association, 1978.
3. Pawan, G.L.S. Drugs and appetite. *Proc. Nutr. Soc.* 33:239, 1974.
4. Roe, D.A. Interactions between drugs and nutrients. *Med. Clin. North Am.* 63:985, 1979.
5. Roe, D.A. Effects of drugs on nutrition. *Life Sci.* 15:1219, 1974.
6. Visconti, J.A. Drug-food interaction. In *Nutrition in Disease.* Columbus, Ohio: Ross Laboratories, 1977.
7. Bistrian, B.R., Blackburn, G.L., Hallowell, E., and Heddle, R. Protein status of general surgical patients. *J.A.M.A.* 230:858, 1974.
8. Bistrian, B.R., Blackburn, G.L., Vitale, J., et al. Nutritional status of general medical patients. *Clin. Res.* 22:692A, 1974.
9. Bistrian, B.R., Blackburn, G.L., and Sherman, M. Therapeutic index of nutritional depletion in surgical patients. *Surg. Gynecol. Obstet.* 141:512, 1975.
10. Spector, A.A., and Fletcher, J.E. Nutritional effects on drug-protein binding. In J.N. Hathcock and J. Coon, Eds., *Nutrition and Drug Interrelations.* New York: Academic, 1978.
11. Campbell, T.C. Effect of dietary protein on drug metabolism. In J.N. Hathcock and J. Coon, Eds., *Nutrition and Drug Interrelations.* New York: Academic, 1978.
12. Wade, A.E., and Norred, W.P. Effect of dietary lipid on drug-metabolizing enzymes. *Fed. Proc.* 35:2475, 1976.
13. Wade, A.E., Norred, W.P., and Evans, J.S. Lipids in drug detoxication. In J.N. Hathcock and J. Coon, Eds., *Nutrition and Drug Interrelations.* New York: Academic, 1978. P. 476.
14. Norred, W.P., and Wade, A.E. Dietary fatty acid-induced alterations of hepatic microsomal drug-metabolizing enzymes. *Biochem. Pharmacol.* 21:2887, 1972.
15. Century, B., and Horwitt, M.K. A role of dietary lipid in the ability of phenobarbital to stimulate hexobarbital and aminopyrine metabolism. *Fed. Proc.* 27:349, 1968.
16. Marshall, W.J., and McLean, A.E.M. A requirement for dietary lipids for induction of cytochrome P-450 by phenobarbitone in rat liver microsomal fraction. *Biochem. J.* 122: 569, 1971.
17. Becking, G.C. Hepatic drug metabolism in iron-, magnesium-, and potassium-deficient rats. *Fed. Proc.* 35:2480, 1974.
18. Zannoni, V.G., and Sato, P.H. The effect of certain vitamin deficiencies on hepatic drug metabolism. *Fed. Proc.* 35:2464, 1974.

19. Blackwell, B. Hypertensive interactions between monoamine oxidase inhibitors and foodstuffs. *Br. J. Psychiatry* 113:349, 1967.

Bibliography

AMA Department of Drugs. *AMA Drug Evaluations,* 4th ed. Chicago: American Medical Association, 1980.

Csaky, T.Z. *Introduction to General Pharmacology,* 2nd ed. New York: Appleton-Century-Crofts, 1979.

Dukes, M.N.G. *Meyler's Side Effects of Drugs Annual,* No. 5. Amsterdam: Excerpta Medica, 1981.

Food and Nutrition Board. *Toxicants Occurring Naturally in Foods,* 2nd ed. Washington, D.C.: National Academy of Sciences, 1973.

Gilman, A.G., Goodman, L.S., and Gilman, A. *The Pharmacological Basis of Therapeutics,* 6th ed. New York: Macmillan, 1980.

Goth, A. *Medical Pharmacology,* 10th ed. St. Louis: C.V. Mosby, 1981.

Grollman, A., and Grollman, E.F. *Pharmacology and Therapeutics,* 7th ed. Philadelphia: Lea and Febiger, 1970.

Hartshorn, E.A. Food and drug interactions. *J. Am. Diet. Assoc.* 70:15, 1977.

Hathcock, J.N., and Coon, J., Eds. *Nutrition and Drug Interrelations.* New York: Academic, 1978.

Levine, R.R. *Pharmacology: Drug Actions and Reactions,* 2nd ed. Boston: Little, Brown, 1978.

Long, J.W. *The Essential Guide to Prescription Drugs,* 3rd ed. New York: Harper and Row, 1982.

March, D.C. *Handbook: Interactions of Selected Drugs with Vitamin Status in Man,* 2nd ed. Chicago: American Dietetic Association, 1978.

Miller, O.N. Symposium: Nutrition and drug metabolism. *Fed. Proc.* 35:2459, 1976.

Moore, A.O., and Powers, D.E. *Food-Medication Interactions.* Tempe, Ariz.: Food-Medication Interactions, 1981.

Parke, D.V. Symposium: Interaction of drugs and nutrients. *Proc. Nutr. Soc.* 33:191, 1974.

Physicians' Desk Reference. Oradell, N.J.: Medical Economics, 1982.

Roe, D.A. *Drug-Induced Nutritional Deficiencies.* Westport, Conn.: AVI, 1976.

The United States Pharmacopeia, 20th ed. Rockwell, Md.: United States Pharmacopeia Convention, 1980.

II. Diseases of the Immune System

4. Nutrition in Diseases of the Immune System

- I. The Normal Immune System
  - A. Components of the systemic immune system
    - 1. Mobile cells
      - a. neutrophils
      - b. eosinophils
      - c. basophils
      - d. lymphocytes
      - e. monocytes
    - 2. Fixed organs and tissues
      - a. thymus
      - b. lymph nodes
      - c. spleen
      - d. unencapsulated lymphoid tissue
  - B. The immune response
    - 1. Antigens
    - 2. The humoral response
      - a. immunoglobulins
      - b. mediators
    - 3. Cell-mediated response
    - 4. Genetic regulation
  - C. Local immunity
- II. Disorders of the Immune System
  - A. Immunoproliferative disease
  - B. Immunologic deficiency
    - 1. causes
    - 2. tests for immunocompetency
  - C. Hypersensitivity
    - 1. Types
      - a. immediate (type I)
      - b. cytotoxic antibody (type II)
      - c. immune complex disease (type III)
      - d. delayed (type IV)
    - 2. Food allergy
      - a. allergens
      - b. mode of contact
      - c. clinical manifestations
      - d. prevention
      - e. diagnosis
      - f. treatment
        - (1) avoidance of allergen
        - (2) other considerations
        - (3) drugs
        - (4) hyposensitization
    - 3. Autoimmune diseases
    - 4. Graft rejection

An appreciation of the interrelationships of nutrition and immune responses is fairly new and there is much information yet to be obtained. It is already clear that malnutrition depresses some aspects of immune function. In addition, it has become evident that the immune responses that have beneficial effects by providing resistance to infection also are capable of causing serious disease. Since nutritional care is important in the treatment of some of these disease states, it is desirable for nutritional care specialists to have an understanding of the principles of immunology.

The objects of this chapter are threefold: (1) to provide the basis for an understanding of normal immune responses and, from that perspective, an understanding of the mechanisms of immune disease; (2) to promote understanding of the relationship of immune function, or malfunction, to the diseases described in succeeding chapters; and (3) to provide the information fundamental to nutritional care for patients with abnormal immune responses to common foods.

THE NORMAL IMMUNE SYSTEM

The immune system protects the body against "foreign" materials called *immunogens* or *antigens.* These terms are not precisely equivalent in meaning but can be used interchangeably for our purposes in this chapter. The immune system, in protecting the body from foreign materials, recognizes materials that are part of "self" and protects us against those materials that are *not* self. The process by which the immune system learns to recognize self is not understood precisely, but recognition apparently develops during gestation and the newborn period.

The mechanisms mediating resistance to disease can be divided into two categories. *Natural, constitutive,* or *nonspecific immunity* consists largely of mechanisms responsible for somewhat nonspecific inflammatory response to tissue damage described in Chapter 1. *Adaptive immunity* is based on the properties of lymphocytes to respond to, or adapt to, specific antigens to produce a permanently altered response. The mechanisms are also classified as *systemic* or *localized,* and some aspects of their interrelationship will now be described.

Components of the Systemic Immune System

The immune system comprises a widely scattered group of organs, tissues, and cells known as the *lymphoreticular system.* It includes some tissues that are fixed in place. These are the thymus, lymph nodes, spleen, bone marrow, Kupffer cells in the liver, tonsils, the lymphoid tissue of the respiratory and genitourinary systems, Peyer's patches of the small intestine, and probably the appendix. The other component of the immune system consists of mobile cells and soluble components that the mobile cells synthesize. The mobile cells have their origin in various of the fixed tissues and are carried in the blood to the site of their function. The action of cells of adaptive immunity often is integrated with the action of phagocytic cells. These cells—monocytes, macrophages, and neutrophils—often called *accessory cells,* are part of the nonspecific immunity mechanism.

Mobile Cells

The *leukocytes* (white blood cells) are derived from *hematopoietic stem cells,* which are also the source of red blood cells and platelets. Stem cells reside in the bone marrow in adults but are more widely distributed in infants. The mature forms of leukocytes are normal components of the blood and are classified into five groups. Three types of cells, known collectively as *granulocytes* because they contain visible granules when seen under the microscope, are *neutrophils* (or polymorphonuclear leukocytes; PMNs), *eosinophils,* and *basophils.* The other two groups of leukocytes, categorized together as *mononuclear cells,* are known individually as *lymphocytes* and *monocytes.* Cells in all five groups can migrate from blood and lymph into the tissues.

The lymphocytes are the principal mediators of the adaptive immune response and are distributed throughout the tissues and fluids of the body. There are two subtypes of lymphocytes. They cannot be distinguished by their appearance under a microscope, but they react differently. One type, the *T-lymphocyte,* reacts directly with a foreign substance or antigen to produce the *cell-mediated response.* In the formation of T-lymphocytes, hematopoietic stem cells mature in the thymus gland and then migrate to other tissues (Fig. 4-1). The cell thus is called *thymus-dependent* or *T cell.* The second type, the *B-lymphocyte,* produces an antibody that interacts with the antigen. This is called the *humoral response* since antibodies are carried in the body fluids. The site of transformation of the stem cell to the B cell in humans is not known. In birds, it occurs in the *bursa of Fabricius*—hence, *bursa-dependent* or *B cell* (see Fig. 4-1). It has frequently been suggested that, in humans, the equivalents to the bursa are located in the appendix and Peyer's patches of the intestine or in the bone marrow. Of the circulating lymphocytes, 70 to 80 percent are T cells and the remainder are B cells.

Macrophages are derived from monocytes, both of which function as phagocytic cells. Macrophages are activated by T cells and then present the phagocytized antigen to the B cell. Macrophage plus antigen is a particularly potent immunogen.

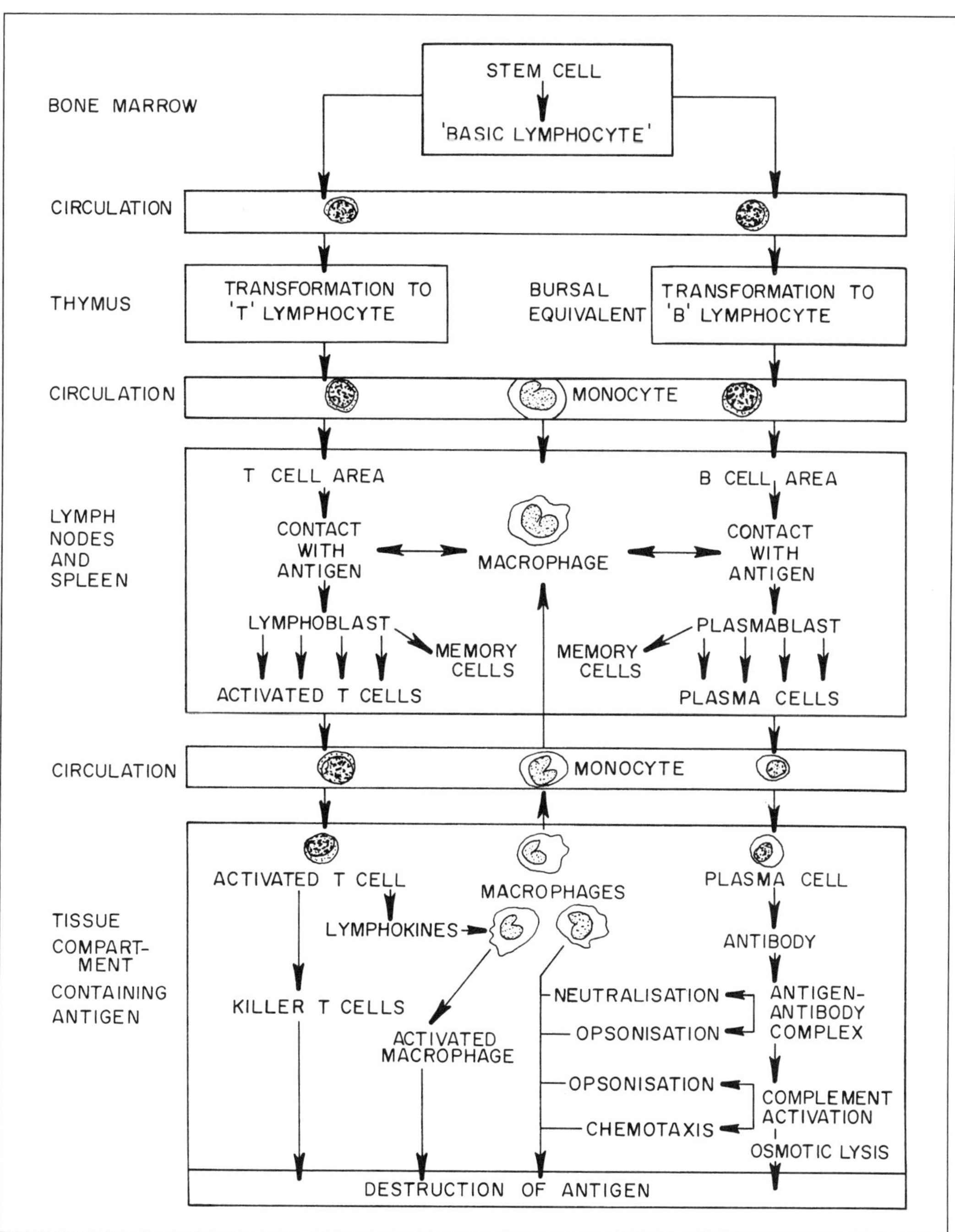

Figure 4-1. The role of lymphocytes in the adaptive immune response. T-lymphocytes activate the cell-mediated response, whereas B-lymphocytes are responsible for the humoral response. (Reprinted with permission from Wheater, P.R., Burkitt, H.G., and Daniels, V.G., Functional Histology. *Edinburgh: Churchill Livingstone, 1979, p. 146.)*

Neutrophils are the predominant phagocytic cells found in localized infections and are part of the constitutive mechanism. They engulf bacteria and cellular debris and digest them by means of lysosomal enzymes. The other two granulocytes, the eosinophils and basophils, play a role in a particular type of immune response classified as hypersensitivities, discussed later in this chapter. Basophils are the source of *mast cells* (connective tissue cells containing histamine granules). The function of eosinophils is unknown. It has been suggested that they reduce the severity of some types of immune response, but the mode of action is unknown.[1]

Fixed Organs and Tissues

In the lymphoreticular system, certain organs consist of a web of extremely fine (*reticular*) fibers, the meshwork of which supports the *reticuloendothelial cells.* These are fixed phagocytic cells, part of the constitutive mechanism, which form a portion of the walls of the channels of the thymus, spleen, lymph nodes, and liver. Lymphocytes are scattered between the sinusoidal spaces.

The *thymus,* lying high in the chest between the aorta and sternum, is considered to be the "master gland" of the immune system. It is essential for differentiation of the T cells and also produces humoral factors essential for normal immune function. It has an outer cortex and a central medulla, each with a reticular network. The cortex contains a large number of lymphocytes. Other lymphocytes migrate to the medulla, differentiate further, and then migrate to the peripheral lymphoid tissue. Although the thymus has the highest cell production rate in the body and produces many lymphocytes, it does not participate directly in immune reactions.

The *lymph nodes* are situated at intervals along the course of the large lymph vessels. They occur mainly at the junctions of major vessels. Each node is associated with *afferent* lymph vessels carrying lymph into the node and *efferent* vessels carrying lymph away. The node itself consists of a cortex, a medulla, and a paracortical area between the two. T cells are present mainly in the medulla and paracortical area, whereas B cells occur primarily in follicles in the cortex. The lymph node also consists of a network of interlacing fibers that act as a filter for the lymph.

The *spleen* contains follicles with B cells as well as areas of T cell concentration. Its reticular network acts as a filter for the blood. Thus, the functional structure of the spleen is similar to that of the lymph node. Both organs create an opportunity for interaction between antigen and lymphocyte by filtering antigens from their respective fluids.

Unencapsulated lymphoid tissue occurs in the alimentary, respiratory, and genitourinary tracts. Some of the tissue cells are widely scattered while others form dense collections. The latter occur in the appendix, the tonsils, and Peyer's patches of the small intestine.

The Immune Response

As previously noted, adaptive immune responses are conventionally divided into two categories known as *cell-mediated* and *humoral* (or *antibody-mediated*) responses. These can be described separately, but it is important to keep in mind that they frequently interact and function simultaneously.

Antigens

An *antigen* or *immunogen* is a substance perceived as foreign to the body which stimulates the immune system to respond specifically to the antigen and not to unrelated substances. The most potent antigens are proteins, but polysaccharides and synthetic polymers also can act as antigens, Lipids, with the exception of phospholipids, are poor immunogens.

The immune response is elicited by a specific chemical configuration of the molecule or one very similar to it called the *antigenic determinant.* The ability of the immune system to react with similar, but not identical, structures of antigens accounts for cross-reactivity.

In general, larger and more complex molecules tend to be more antigenic. Proteins with molecular weights of less than 10,000 and carbohydrates with molecular weights of less than 100,000 are only weakly antigenic. A polymer with a single repeating unit is much less antigenic than is a more complex one with many different units. Aromatic amino acids increase antigenicity much more than do aliphatic amino acids. The immune response may vary also with the dose and the route of administration, but this is not always the case.

It is not clear why some antigens elicit a humoral response and others, a cell-mediated response. As a general rule, cellular and particulate antigens stimulate a cell-mediated response. Humoral immunity is particularly associated with soluble antigens[2] but also is associated with cellular antigens.

A wide variety of materials can be recognized as antigens. These may include infectious organisms, venoms, and tumor cells. Some foods, some pollens, dusts, danders, and molds that a person inhales, plant, animal, or other materials that come in contact with the skin, cells from other humans as in blood transfusions, skin grafts, and organ transplants may be antigenic in the appropriate circumstances. It is even possible for a person's own tissue to be immunologically recognized as foreign. The antisera, hormones, enzymes, diagnostic agents, antibiotics, vitamins, and a variety of drugs used to treat disease may act as antigens. Some antigens are recognized as foreign by everyone. Others are foreign only in certain circumstances categorized as hypersensitivity.

Some special categories of antigens include *alloantigens,* present in certain individuals in a species, but not all. An example is the blood group antigens. *Heteroantigens* are from species different from the host. In humans, heteroantigens include bacteria, viruses, and materials from plants and other animals, including foods in some circumstances. *Haptens* are not antigenic alone but become antigenic when they complex with another substance. Drug allergies often occur by this means when a drug of low molecular weight complexes with a plasma protein to form a molecule with a sufficiently large molecular weight and foreign structure so that the complex is antigenic.

The Humoral Response

The membranes of B cells contain receptors for specific antigen binding. A simple model, sufficient for our purposes here, states that recognition of a specific antigen by a B cell consists of binding of the antigen to the membrane receptor. The sequence of events thereafter is not entirely clear. It is known that the B cell is stimulated to divide by a special type of cell division called *cloning.* The cells produced by cloning mature to form *plasma cells,* which then synthesize and release the *antibodies* or *immunoglobulins.*

Immunoglobulins. The antibody synthesized by each plasma cell is specific for the antigen that was initially recognized, bound, and programmed by the parent B cell. The antibody produced by the plasma cell then binds specifically to the antigen for which it was designed, thus inactivating and neutralizing it. When a virus is bound to an antibody, for example, its virulence and ability to cause disease is decreased. Antibodies also bind to foreign cells such as bacteria, tumor cells, or grafts and induce lysis of the cells. Some examples of the types of action of antibodies include *precipitation, agglutination,* and *opsonization,* the last of these a process by which the cell is made more vulnerable to phagocytosis. In addition, antibodies, by attachment to the antigenic cell surface, may damage it by altering its mobility, metabolism, or physical behavior in fluids. In some cases, the antibody functions via complement activation. *Complement* is a series of serum proteins of the constitutive system which often is called the *complement cascade.* The proteins in the series react with each other in a sequence so that one activates the next. Some of the effects of this action include cell lysis, altered vascular permeability to allow lymphocytes to move to the site of the antigen, increased phagocytosis, and degranulation of mast cells.

Most of these actions of antibodies facilitate clearance of the antigen by the reticuloendothelial system. Antibody-coated foreign cells are attacked by neutrophils or monocytes. The antigen-antibody (Ag/Ab) complex is phagocytized by neutrophils, macrophages, and monocytes.

When an antigen is first introduced, the response is relatively slow. One of the results of this primary response is the production of a special group of cells called *memory B cells* in addition to the plasma cells. When cells are exposed to the antigen again, these memory B cells "remember" that antigen. Their *secondary* or *anamnestic response* is greater than the primary response.

There are five classes of immunoglobulins—G, M, A, D, and E, abbreviated as IgG, IgM, IgA, IgD, and IgE, respectively. Each antibody molecule is made up of a basic unit of two long (*heavy* or *H*) chains and two short (*light* or *L*) chains. These are bound to each other by disulfide bonds in a symmetric structure, as shown in Fig. 4-2. Each of these units is made up of an *Fc portion* (Fragment, crystallizable), consisting of portions of the two H chains, and an *Fab portion* (Fragment, *a*ntigen-*b*inding), made up of the two L chains and the remainder of the H chains (see Fig. 4-2). The Fc portion binds to the macrophages, lymphocytes, or neutrophils. It also activates complement and releases soluble substances from mast

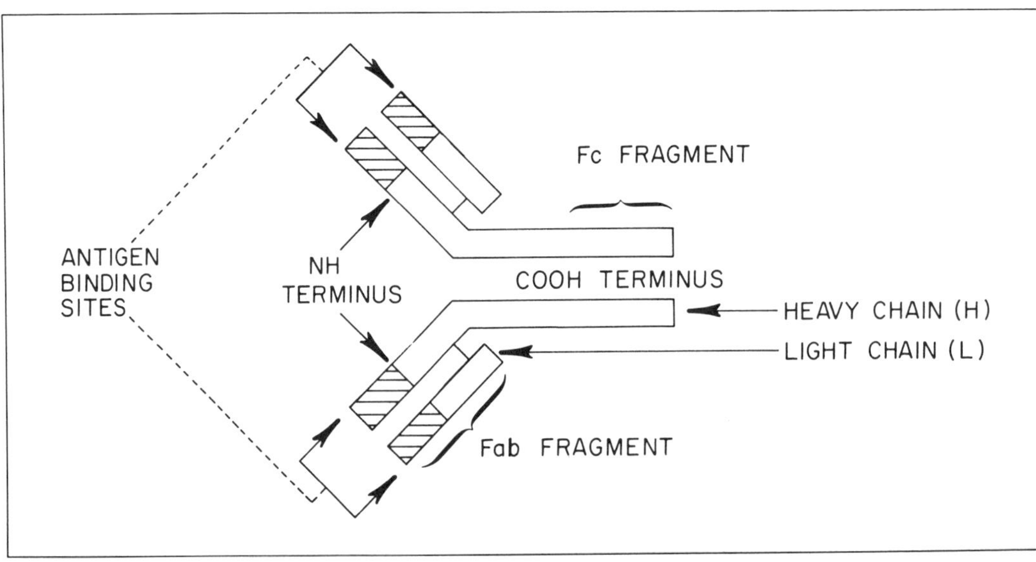

Figure 4-2. An immunoglobulin molecule. Basic units of all immunoglobulin molecules are two pairs of polypeptide chains joined by disulfide bonds. All immunoglobulins have the same light chain component, identifiable antigenically as kappa or lambda, with any given immunoglobulin having two kappa or two lambda chains. Heavy chains of each immunoglobulin class are unique for that class and determine its biologic properties. The Fc fragment is responsible for complement fixation, placental transfer, and skin fixation. Shading indicates the section of the Fab fragment where the amino acid sequence is variable; these are the antigen-binding sites. (Reprinted with permission from Barber, H.R.K., Immunobiology for the Clinician. *New York: John Wiley and Sons, 1977, p. 27.)*

cells. The Fc portion is much the same within a class of immunoglobulins, but varies from one class to another.[2]

The Fab portion has a section (shown by the shaded section in Fig. 4-2) in which the amino acid sequence is variable. These are the antigen-binding sites and are the source of the specificity of the antibody for its antigen. This region is identical in all cells of a single clone. Each basic antibody unit can bind with two antigenic sites and therefore has a valence of 2.

Immunoglobulin G (IgG) consists of a single unit, as previously described, with a valence of 2. It comprises approximately 75 percent of all immunoglobulin and is the major antibody of the anamnestic response. Immunoglobulin G is involved in opsonization and complement fixation. It is found in large quantities in the circulatory system and peripheral lymphoid tissue and is the only immunoglobulin capable of crossing the placenta.

Immunoglobulin A (IgA) has two subclasses, *serum IgA* and *secretory IgA*. Secretory IgA (sIgA) is synthesized by plasma cells in secretory glands of mucous membranes of the alimentary, respiratory, and genitourinary tracts, and the salivary, lacrimal, and mammary glands.[3-6] It occurs mostly in secretions of the mucous membranes and serves as a barrier against environmental pathogens.

The function of serum IgA is unknown. It is found in small but significant amounts in the blood and occurs as a *monomer*—that is, with one of the basic units described previously. However, secretory IgA is a *dimer:* Its two basic units are linked by a structure known as a *J* (joining) *chain,* originating in the plasma cell. These then are attached to a glycoprotein known as *secretory piece,* which is synthesized in the epithelial cells.[7-10] Its function may be to facilitate transport of sIgA through the mucosa[2] or to render the IgA resistant to proteolytic enzymes.[11]

Immunoglobulin M (IgM) also occurs as a *polymer,* usually as a *pentamer,* so it has a valence of 10. The units are linked by a J chain and the molecule also contains secretory piece. Approximately 10 percent of the immunoglobulins are IgM. It is the major mediator of the primary immune response. Other actions include formation of blood group antibodies, activation of complement, and destruction of antigens on initial exposure. Immunoglobulin M is very effective in opsonization. It forms antibodies to gram-negative bacteria and also is antiviral. Immunoglobulin M is found in all body fluids.

Immunoglobulin D (IgD) is found in small amounts in serum and also is associated with IgM on most B cells. Its function is unknown, but it may act as an antigen receptor on the cell surface, and it may be involved in B cell differentiation and memory cells.

Immunoglobulin E (IgE) is found in low concentration in normal serum but in high concentration in the serum of many patients with allergies. Immunoglobulin E can attach to cells of the skin, mast cells, basophils, or neutrophils. Since it can attach to self cells, it is termed *homocytotropic.* When IgE attaches, these cells become sensitized to the antigen. The binding of some sensitized cells (usually basophils and mast cells) to the antigen causes the release of pharmacologically active amines known as *mediators.*

Mediators. There are several mediators known to participate in the humoral response. Of these, *histamine* is the most important. It occurs in mast cells, basophils, platelets, and perhaps in other cells. It is released when an antigen–IgE antibody complex binds to a histamine-containing cell. It causes vasodilation and increased capillary permeability leading to erythema (redness) and edema in the mucous membranes of the skin. Antihistamine drugs inhibit its actions. *Slow-reacting substance of anaphylaxis* (SRS-A), released from mast cells, is a mediator that causes increased vascular permeability and contraction of smooth muscle. Antihistamines do not inhibit SRS-A. *Eosinophil chemotactic factor of anaphylaxis* (ECF-A) is found in mast cells. It increases the movement of eosinophils to areas of Ag/Ab reactions. *Serotonin* (5-hydroxytryptamine or 5-HT) is found in mast cells, platelets, and enterochromaffin cells. It causes capillary dilation and increased permeability. It is discussed further in Chapter 6 in relation to tumors involving enterochromaffin cells. *Prostaglandins* have various activities. They increase the dilation and permeability of capillaries, increase smooth muscle contraction, and alter the pain threshold. *Bradykinin* is produced by the *kallikrein* or *kinin* system and is released from mast cells. It produces prolonged, slow contractions of smooth muscle. There are other substances in this group having similar effects.

The consequences of the actions of these mediators are described in relation to allergies later in this chapter.

Cell-Mediated Response

The *cell-mediated immune response* involves primarily the T-lymphocytes and operates against bacteria, some viruses and fungi, tumor cells, and foreign tissue such as transplants. T-lymphocytes are responsible for the delayed allergic reactions described later in this chapter. There are a number of subpopulations of T cells that have specialized functions and are known as *memory* T cells, *suppressor* T cells, *helper* cells, and *killer* cells. Many of these function in the interactions between B cells and T cells.

T cells produce mediators known as *lymphokines,* a group of substances that can cause the death of antigenic cells and a variety of other activities. Lymphokines are currently being studied actively, and much more information on these substances will be forthcoming.

When T-lymphocytes are activated by an antigen, usually on the surface of a macrophage, they are transformed to large *immunoblasts* (*lymphoblasts*). These cells divide by mitosis. The daughter cells already are activated and have the same immunologic specificity as the parent cell. As in the case with B cells, the secondary response is stronger and faster than the primary response. The sensitized T cells kill viable antigenic cells by direct attachment. The antigenic cells are lysed and then phagocytized by activated macrophages.

Genetic Regulation of the Immune Response

The cells of each person's body have protein molecules called *histocompatibility antigens* on their cell membranes, which provide the identity of self. These are called *human leukocyte antigens* (*HLA*) because they were first discovered on the surface of human leukocytes, but it now is known that they are present on almost all body cells. The specific nature of these antigens in each individual is determined by a cluster of genes on the sixth chromosome pair in an area called the *major histocompatibility complex.* Four loci within this complex have been identified and have been labeled *HLA-A, HLA-B, HLA-C,* and *HLA-D.* It is thought that there are others, but they have not been identified.

Each locus in an individual has two alleles. A person inherits one of each pair of alleles in each locus from each parent. A large number of alleles occur in the population for each gene. At present, there are seven known alleles for HLA-C and more than thirty for HLA-B, each identified by a letter and a number, such as HLA-B26. The number of known HLA-A and HLA-D alleles lie between these two extremes. The number of possible combinations in the general population is at least several thousand, but the number in the offspring of a single pair of parents is much smaller.

Near the HLA-D locus, there are *immune response* (Ir) genes believed to have some control over the immune response and the degree of responsiveness in T cells. Other genes appear to control antibody production and macrophage function.

Some HLA antigens have been associated with specific diseases. For example, juvenile diabetes mellitus is associated with persons with HLA-B8. When the persons suffering from a given disease have the same antigen, that antigen is a *marker.* It indicates that those carrying that antigen have an increased susceptibility to the disease in question, but they may not actually have the disease unless the necessary environmental conditions also exist. The mechanism of the association of HLA antigens with the occurrence of certain diseases is unknown.

Local Immunity

Nonspecific local defenses exist at surface areas that are exposed to antigens. These barriers to environmental antigens include the skin, respiratory tract, genitourinary tract, eyes, and ears. Some of the mechanisms involved include trapping in mucus, clearance by the cilia, and action of digestive enzymes, acids, and alkalies, and a washout action by intestinal motility. Specific local defenses include IgA antibody and the large population of lymphocytes in the respiratory and gastrointestinal tracts.

DISORDERS OF THE IMMUNE SYSTEM

Although the purpose of the immune system is protection of the body's cells from foreign materials (*immunity*), it sometimes malfunctions and may actually cause disease. These diseases are the subject of *clinical immunology.* Diseases of the immune system can conveniently be divided into three categories: (1) excess proliferation of immune cells or their products, (2) deficiency of function, and (3) inappropriate immune response (hypersensitivity). Within each category, there are some conditions in which nutritional care is important. Each category will be briefly described in turn, and those conditions in which nutritional care is of special importance will be described in more detail.

Immunoproliferative Disease

Immunoproliferative disease (excess production of one or more components of the immune system) can affect either the humoral or cellular system. There is a wide spectrum of these diseases, and they are referred to as *gammopathies.* Gammopathies may be produced by one clone only (*monoclonal*) or by more than one (*polyclonal*). There may be high concentrations of the whole antibody or of only the H chain or the L chain. Gammopathies of the latter types are referred to as *heavy chain disease* or *light chain disease.* Monoclonal gammopathy may be benign or malignant, the most common malignant form being multiple myeloma.

One group of immunoproliferative diseases is categorized as *plasma cell dyscrasia,* in which abnormally large quantities of antibodies, especially IgG, are produced. Other categories of immunoproliferative disease are the *leukemias* (abnormal proliferation and accumulation of leukocytes) and the *lymphomas* (solid tumors of stem cells).

Nutritional care is directed primarily toward alleviation of the symptoms produced as a result of the effect of the immune system disease on other organ systems or as a result of the side effects of treatment. The consequences of some of these conditions include renal disease and require some of the nutritional manipulations indicated in other renal diseases (see Chapter 7). Other conditions cause diarrhea, the nutritional implications of which are described in Chapter 6. Leukemia and the nutritional care of leukemia patients is described, along with other forms of cancer, in Chapter 13, where the nutritional implications of some cancer treatments also are discussed.

Immunologic Deficiency

Causes

Another group of immune diseases consists of those in which the *immune function is deficient.* The cause may be congenital or secondary to other conditions (Table 4-1). Congenital absence or deficiency of humoral or cellular immunity, or both, is seen occasionally in newborns as the results of failure

Table 4-1. Some Drugs and Conditions Associated with Depressed Delayed Hypersensitivity

Drugs
Glucocorticoids
Cancer chemotherapeutic agents (e.g., cyclophosphamide, methotrexate)
Rifampin
Niridazole
Congenital defects
Thymic-parathyroid aplasia (DiGeorge's syndrome)
Autosomal recessive lymphopenia (Nezelof's syndrome)
Combined deficiency disease
Cancer
Hodgkin's disease
Other lymphomas
Advanced carcinoma
Infection and Vaccination
Viral
Measles (and vaccine)
Mumps
Chickenpox
Influenza
Infectious mononucleosis
Measles-mumps-rubella vaccine
Bacterial
Tuberculosis
Leprosy
Streptococcal infection
Brucellosis
Bacterial pneumonia
Fungal
Coccidioidomycosis
Histoplasmosis
Blastomycosis
Age
Malnutrition and low birth weight in children
Diabetes mellitus
Uremia
Surgical operations and anesthesia
Sarcoidosis
Burns

Reprinted with permission from Wing, E.J., and Remington, J.S., Delayed hypersensitivity and macrophage functions. In H.H. Fudenberg, D.P. Stites, J.L. Caldwell, and J.V. Wells, Eds., *Basic and Clinical Immunology*, 3rd ed. Los Altos, Calif.: Lange Medical, 1980, p. 132.

of proper development, but these conditions are rare. It is more common to find immunologic deficiencies secondary to physical or emotional stress. This condition is called *anergy* and is the opposite of the anamnestic response.

The means by which emotional disturbance affects immunity are not clear, but the effect may be mediated via the hypothalamus and, thence, to the pituitary and adrenal glands. Glucocorticoids, produced by the adrenals, are lympholytic and thus might reduce the number of functioning lymphocytes. Increased incidence of infections, increased incidence of cancer, and delayed recovery, all of which are possible consequences of immunodeficiency, have been seen in emotionally disturbed patients.

Physical stresses, including surgery and anesthesia, major burns, neoplasms, and virus infections, also depress immune function. These stresses may function by stimulating the adrenals to produce glucocorticoids. Diabetes mellitus and uremia in chronic renal failure also have a depressive effect.

Studies of malnutrition and immune function have shown numerous interrelationships.[12,13] For many years, malnutrition has been associated with increased susceptibility to infection in underdeveloped countries. It is now recognized that the mechanisms involved are not fundamentally different from those seen in malnourished hospitalized patients in developed countries.[14,15] Immune function has been shown to be adversely affected by every nutritional deficiency that has been investigated. Malnutrition decreases the thickness of the skin and connective tissue and reduces their ability to act as barriers to infection.[16] Protein-energy malnutrition appears to affect cell-mediated and humoral immunity in different ways. The number of T cells, levels of thymic hormones, and production of some mediators are decreased.[17–19] In contrast, the numbers of B cells and plasma cells remain normal and sometimes are increased, but the effects on subclasses of B cells are unknown.[14,20,21] Serum IgE and IgA levels are high, possibly reflecting an increase in the incidence of parasites or a decrease in T cell control.[14,22] Secretory IgA and complement usually are decreased.[21,23–25] Phagocytic cell function has been shown to be significantly abnormal in protein-energy malnutrition.[14,26,27] Other indications of effects of protein malnutrition on immune function include thymus atrophy,[28–30] inability to respond to some antigens with antibody production,[31] and decreased production of some mediators.[32] On the other hand, experiments with animals have shown that moderate calorie restriction may be beneficial, provided the intake of nutrients is adequate.[33,34]

Lipids also are involved in the immune response. Polyunsaturated fatty acids have been shown to depress T cell function. The mechanism is unknown, but it has been suggested that these fatty acids be used in increased quantities in the diet as an adjuvant to immunosuppressive drugs given to transplant patients.[35–37] In contrast, esterified fatty acids increase the *mitogenic* (promoting mitosis) response of the T cells. Therefore, it has been suggested that lipids be included in parenteral feeding to improve the immune response in malnourished patients.[38]

Vitamin A, pyridoxine, zinc, and iron deficiencies impair cell-mediated immunity.[19,39] Vitamin A deficiency has been associated with reduced antibody formation in animals.[40] Relationships to deficiencies of vitamin B_{12}, folate, pantothenate, thiamin, riboflavin, and ascorbic acid have also been noted, but much more information is needed.[39]

In malnourished hospitalized patients, the malnutrition often is secondary to other conditions. For example, immunoglobulin deficiency may result from excess protein loss from a diseased intestine or kidneys. Nutritional care is important in maintaining adequate nutritional status and preventing anergy in this type of patient, particularly the patient whose disease depresses immune function in addition to causing malnutrition.

The number of T cells declines with age. Although this decrease is apparently inevitable and normal, it may be considered a deficiency since it is associated with an increase in the occurrence of some diseases.

Sometimes, the immune deficiency is *iatrogenic*—that is, the result of therapy. In organ transplants, for example, the immune response is deliberately suppressed in order to prevent rejection of the graft. The immune response is often depressed also in the treatment of cancer, either deliberately or as a side effect of treatment.

It is clear that malnutrition can occur as a significant side effect of other diseases and markedly affects immune function. For those patients, and also for patients who have primary immunodeficiency disease, for the elderly, and for those with iatrogenic immune deficits, it is important to provide an adequate diet to support maximum immune function. In the chapters that follow, nutritional needs in these conditions and procedures for meeting these needs are discussed.

Tests for Immunocompetency

The complexity of the immune system prevents the development of a single test to measure the adequacy of the immune response. The available tests vary from those that are very simple to those that are extremely sophisticated. The most sophisticated tests are used in the diagnosis of various immune disorders and are not within the scope of this text. They are described in other texts and monographs for those who are interested in further information.[41,42]

Some simple tests of immunocompetency are of interest to nutritional care specialists, since they are used in some institutions as an indicator of nutritional status and to identify patients in particular need of nutritional support. There are two procedures in common use in the nutritional assessment procedures described in Chapter 2.

Enumeration of *lymphocytes in the peripheral circulation,* a measurement that is affected by many variables, is easily obtained since it is done routinely on almost all patients. *Delayed cutaneous hypersensitivity* (DCH) *skin tests* often are used to indicate the presence of protein-energy malnutrition in hospital patients. The antigens commonly used are purified protein derivative of tuberculin (PPD), histoplasmin, *Candida,* streptokinase-streptodornase (SK/SD), and mumps. The use of these antigens is based on the assumption that DCH is a good indicator of nutritional status. There is evidence that the severity of defective T cell function correlates to some degree with the severity of malnutrition,[17,43,44] but serious questions exist concerning the validity and reliability of these procedures.[45]

Another test of immune function somewhat less frequently used is the determination of T cell blast formation. The uptake by lymphocytes of tritiated thymidine (labeled with ^3H) is used as a measure of the response to *mitogens* (substances that cause cell mitosis). The amount taken up provides some evaluation of the immune system.

The response of an individual to active sensitization can be measured by application of dinitrochlorobenzene to the skin. The procedure is repeated in 2 to 3 weeks. If the cellular immunity is intact, the patient develops a lesion at the site.

A great deal more research is needed before the best procedures for evaluating nutritional status with tests of immune function are determined.

Hypersensitivity

Hypersensitivity is a harmful response and is defined as an adverse immunologic reaction to a substance that is harmless to most people. The term *allergy* is used to refer to a hypersensitivity to a foreign antigen that does not have a beneficial effect such as does immunity to infection. It is important to remember that allergy is an *immune* response and, when the term is applied to foods, must not be confused with food poisoning or with a food intolerance resulting from an enzyme deficiency. In hypersensitivity, the antigen often is called an *allergen.*

Types of Hypersensitivity

The most common classification of hypersensitivity reactions is that of Gell and Coombs,[46] who listed four types. Their essential features are compared in Table 4-2. Some diseases may be expressions of two or more types or are variants of these classifications.

Type I. In type I (immediate, anaphylactic, or reagin-dependent) hypersensitivity (Fig. 4-3), a sensitizing dose is necessary first (Fig. 4-4). Then a specific antibody, usually IgE, is bound to and sensitizes tissue cells such as mast cells and basophils. In following exposures, the antigen seeks out and reacts with the specific antibody at the cell surface. The sensitized cell releases histamine and other mediators (Fig. 4-5). This response is considered immediate, usually occurring in less than 60 minutes. The results of this sequence of events, called *anaphylaxis,* affect organs in which mast cells are fixed. These "shock organs" are smooth muscle in lung and bronchi, endothelial cells of the blood vessels, and associated secretory glands which contain mast cells in large numbers. The response occurs in genetically susceptible individuals who produce IgE antibodies to allergens to which most of the population does not respond.

Some anaphylactic responses are normal in the sense that all individuals will react similarly. Individuals who have abnormal responses, or hypersensitivity, have a genetically based susceptibility. The term *atopy* has been coined to indicate these abnormal responses.

The response may be local or systemic.

Table 4-2. Four Types of Hypersensitivity Reactions

	Anaphylactic (Type I)	Cytotoxic (Type II)	Immune Complex Disease (Type III)	Cell-Mediated (Type IV)
Antibody-mediating reaction	IgE, mast-cell binding	IgG or IgM	IgG	Receptor on T-lymphocyte
Antigen	Usually exogenous	Cell surface	Extracellular	Extracellular or cell surface
Response to intradermal antigen				
Maximum reaction	30 min.		3–8 hr	24–48 hr
Appearance	Wheal and flare		Erythema and edema	Erythema and induration
Histology	Degranulated mast cells, edema, eosinophils		Acute inflammatory reaction; predominant neutrophils	Perivascular inflammation; neutrophils migrate out leaving predominantly mononuclear cells
Damaging agent	Biochemical mediators from IgE-sensitized cells produce tissue response	Complement may or may not be involved	Complement and neutrophils produce tissue damage	Lymphokines released from antigen-sensitized lymphocyte; reactions produce tissue damage
Transfer sensitivity to normal subject	Serum antibody	Serum antibody	Serum antibody	Lymphoid cells, transfer factor
Examples	Atopic allergy (e.g., hay fever)	Hemolytic disease of newborn (Rh factor)	Serum sickness; complex glomerulonephritis	Tuberculin skin reaction; contact dermatitis

Reprinted with permission from Boyd, W., and Sheldon, H., *Introduction to the Study of Disease,* 8th ed. Philadelphia: Lea and Febiger, 1980, p. 155.

IMMEDIATE TYPE

(Antibody-mediated, types I–III)

Type I: Anaphylactic

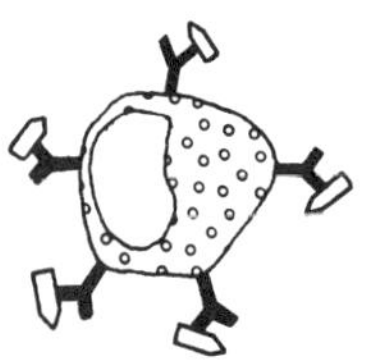

Antibody IgE bound to cell causes release of vasoactive substance on contact with antigen (e.g., asthma, hay fever).

Y = IgE   ▭ = Antigen

Type II: Cytotoxic

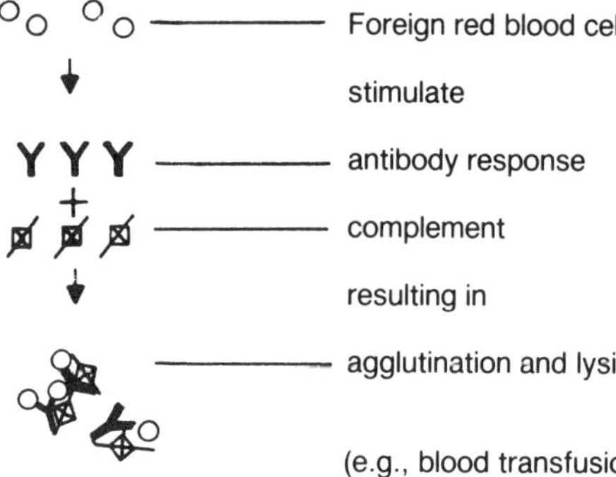

(e.g., blood transfusion reaction, hemolytic disease of newborns)

Type III: Immune complex disease

Antigen and antibody combine in the presence of complement to damage small blood vessels (e.g., serum sickness).

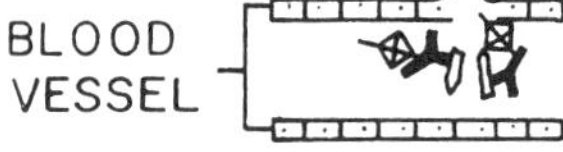

DELAYED TYPE

Type IV: Cell-Mediated

Sensitized lymphocytes react with specific antigens to release lymphokines (e.g., contact dermatitis, tuberculin reaction, skin reaction to dinitrochlorobenzene, homograft rejection).

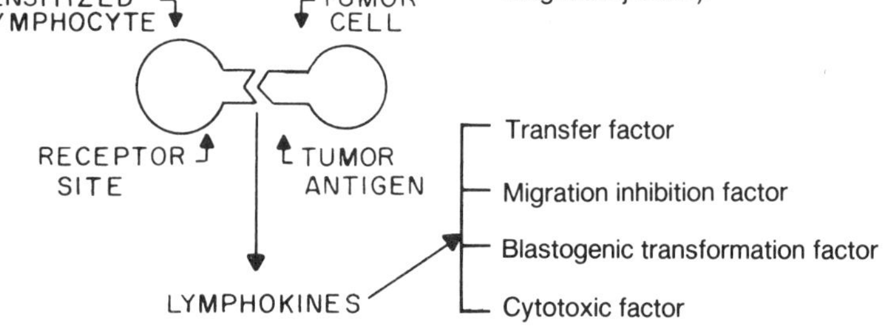

Figure 4-3. Types I through IV hypersensitivity reactions. (Reprinted with permission from Barber, H.R.K., Immunobiology for the Clinician. *New York: John Wiley and Sons, 1977, pp. 76–77.)*

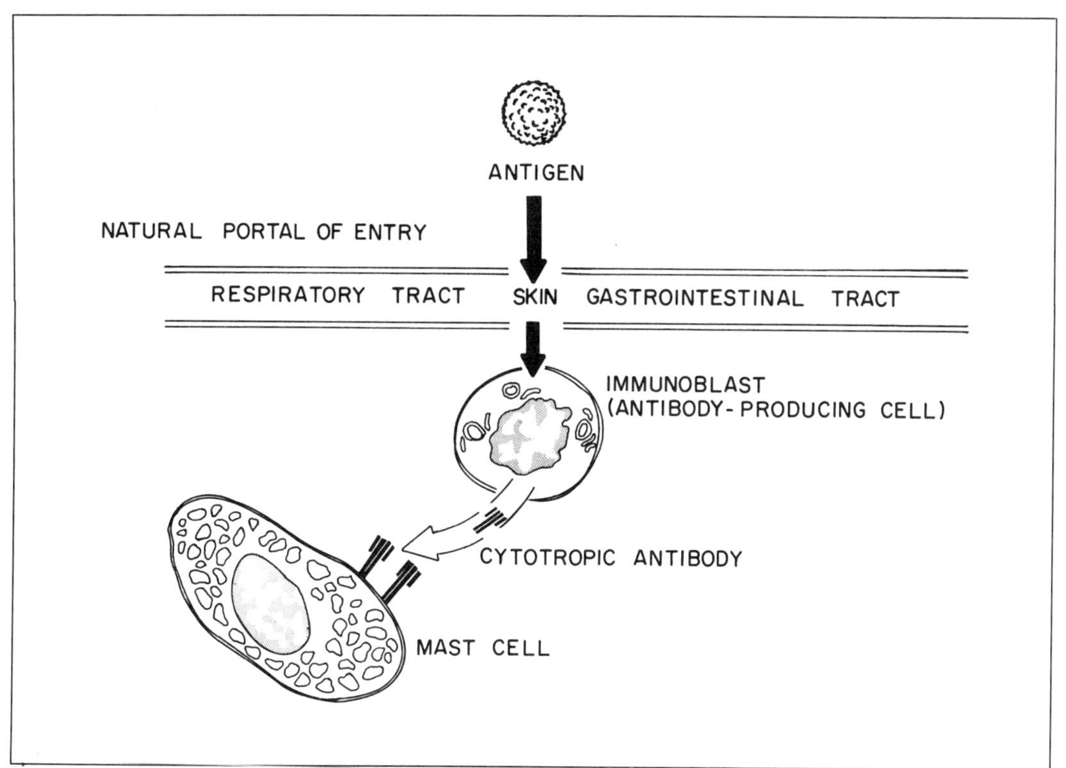

Figure 4-4. Atopic sensitization in type I hypersensitivity. (Reprinted with permission from Frick, O.L., Immediate hypersensitivity. In H.H. Fudenberg, D.P. Stites, J.L. Caldwell, and J.V. Wells, Eds., Basic and Clinical Immunology, *3rd ed. Los Altos, Calif.: Lange Medical, 1980, p. 275.)*

When the Ag/Ab response is on a mucosal surface, the consequences are fairly mild. This type of response occurs most often to airborne allergens (inhalants) such as pollens, molds, fungal spores, dusts, animal danders, and various substances with volatile components and strong odors. In atopy, allergic rhinitis (hay fever) is, by far, the most common manifestation, usually as a response to seasonal pollens. Bronchial asthma, atopic dermatitis, and gastrointestinal allergy occur less often. Some patients have more than one manifestation of atopy, but not usually at the same time.

The shock organ in atopic individuals varies, but there usually is only one in a given individual. The means by which the symptoms are produced in the shock organ are based on the actions of the mediators. For example, when the allergen-IgE reaction occurs in the nose, release of histamine causes vasodilation and increased capillary permeability. These effects cause leakage of nasal fluid (rhinorrhea). Other factors cause sneezing and nasal itching. The total syndrome is allergic rhinitis or hay fever. In urticaria (hives), which involve superficial capillaries, histamine is released locally, causing vasodilation and producing a red flare. The increased permeability of the capillaries allows movement of plasma into the

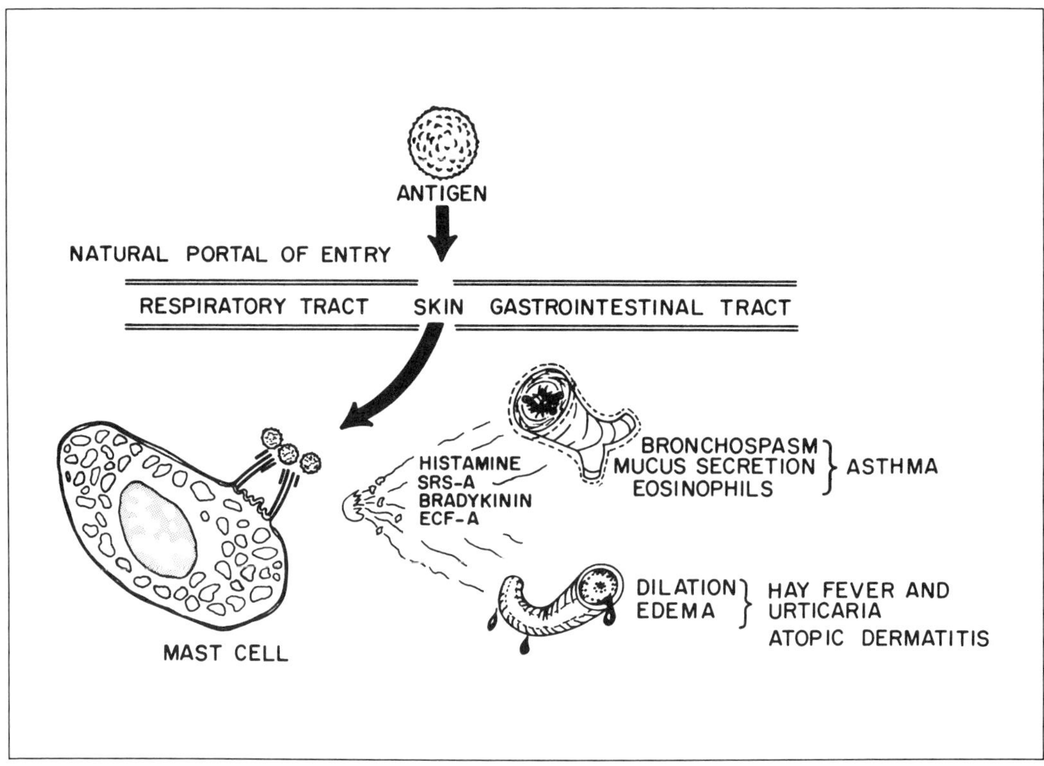

Figure 4-5. Atopic reaction in type I hypersensitivity. The sensitized cell releases histamine and other mediators. SRS-A = slow-reacting substance of anaphylaxis; ECF-A = eosinophil chemotactic factor of anaphylaxis. (Reprinted with permission from Frick, O.L., Immediate hypersensitivity. In H.H. Fudenberg, D.P. Stites, J.L. Caldwell, and J.V. Wells, Eds., Basic and Clinical Immunology, *3rd ed. Los Altos, Calif.: Lange Medical, 1980; p. 276.)*

tissue, leading to swelling and formation of a wheal. The raised area plus red flare of hives is referred to as a *wheal-flare* reaction. In asthma, the allergen-IgE reaction releases SRS-A and causes a spasm in the bronchioles of the lung. As a result, the patient has difficulty in breathing.

The systemic response may be more severe. It can occur very rapidly following injection of a drug, insect venom, or foreign serum. The antigen can also be absorbed through the intestinal tract. The possible consequences of systemic anaphylaxis can include bronchospasm and edema of the larynx, sometimes leading to dyspnea, cyanosis, and severe hypotension. If interference with respiration is very severe, it can be life-threatening. This severe form is called *anaphylactic shock.*

Table 4-3 provides a summary of atopic conditions.

Type II. In type II (*cytotoxic or cytolytic antibody*) hypersensitivity (see Table 4-2), IgG or IgM binds to an antigen on a cell membrane and activates complement, resulting in a toxic effect on the cell or cell lysis (see Fig. 4-3). Among the conditions resulting from this type of immune disorder are renal diseases including renal complications of systemic lupus erythematosus and scleroderma. Information on their nutritional care is

Table 4-3. Atopic Conditions

Condition	Commonly Associated Allergens
Allergic rhinitis	Inhalants (spores, pollens, animal dander)
Extrinsic asthma	Mold spores
Atopic conjunctivitis	Inhalants (spores, pollens, animal dander)
Atopic dermatitis	Various food allergies; drug hypersensitivities (especially penicillins, sulfonamides, streptomycin); local anesthetics; heavy metals; reactive chemicals
Urticaria-angioedema	Insect bites; food allergies
Gastrointestinal allergy	Food allergies (cereals, milk, eggs, shellfish, fruit); drug hypersensitivities
Serum sickness	Drugs, especially penicillin
Anaphylaxis	Heterologous antisera; vaccines; iodinated radiographic material

Adapted from Bach, M.K., Reagin allergy. In B.A. Thomas, Ed., *Immunology.* Scope Monograph Series. Kalamazoo, Mich.: Upjohn, 1975.

Reprinted with permission from Boyd, W., and Sheldon, H., *Introduction to the Study of Disease,* 8th ed. Philadelphia: Lea and Febiger, 1980, p. 154.

found in later chapters. Some antibodies stimulate their target cells instead of inhibiting or killing them.[1] This is thought to be the mechanism for thyrotoxicosis.

Type III. In type III hypersensitivity (immune complex disease) (see Table 4-2), Ag/Ab complexes deposit in tissues and activate complement, with consequent release of chemotactic factors, cell infiltration, and release of lysosomal enzymes. A chronic inflammatory response follows. When the immune complexes are not cleared in the usual way by the reticuloendothelial system, they continue to circulate and deposit in small blood vessels, producing vasculitis and interfering with blood supply to the tissues (see Fig. 4-3). The ability to remove the immune complex depends on the solubility and size of the Ag/Ab particle. When antigen is present in excess, particles are larger and more difficult to remove. The consequences may be systemic (serum sickness) or local (Arthus reaction), occurring at the site of the injection.

The consequences of the disorder vary with the specific organs involved. In some diseases, the association with immune complex disease is suspected but not proved. Some of the disorders of interest to the nutritional care specialist which possibly are included in this category are:

In the digestive system, Crohn's disease and chronic ulcerative colitis
In the kidney, glomerulonephritis and some cases of systemic lupus erythematosus
In the liver, some cases of hepatitis with cirrhosis

These conditions are discussed in later chapters.

Type IV. In type IV (delayed or cell-mediated) hypersensitivity (see Table 4-2), the condition results from the stimulation of lymphocytes specifically sensitized to the antigen. In some cases, it does not involve production of antibodies or complement activation. There is, instead, cytotoxicity from the release of lymphokines, direct attachment to the sensitized lymphocyte with lysis of the antigen cell, or both (see Fig. 4-3). The cells responsible for this type of toxicity are not known. They do not seem to be either typical B or T cells and have therefore been called *K* (killer) *cells.*

The response is slower than is the response to type I hypersensitivity. It may occur hours to days following exposure to the antigen. The symptoms are extremely variable and often mimic other disorders. The severity of the symptoms usually is dose-related. Conditions in this category include contact dermatitis, graft rejection,

Table 4-4. Comparison of Types I and IV Food Allergy Reactions

Immediate (Type I)	Delayed (Type IV)
Not quantitative; all-or-none reaction	Usually dose-related
Immediate, within 1–60 min.	Delayed up to 5 days
IgE-mediated	May be due in part to faulty and deficient digestive or absorptive processes
Less common and at times dangerous	Very prevalent
Skin test usually positive	Skin test negative or unreliable
Mortality possible	Morbidity great, but no mortality
Severity predictable; shock-type reaction	Severity cyclic, but morbidity prevalent and chronic
Usually involving one shock organ	Systemic malaise
Often permanent	Usually diminishes with prolonged avoidance
May result from prolonged delayed sensitivity	May be converted to immediate-type sensitivity

Reprinted with permission from Breneman, J.C., *Basics of Food Allergy,* 1978, p. 15. Courtesy of Charles C Thomas, Publisher, Springfield, Illinois.

some autoimmune diseases, and some food allergies.

Food Allergy

Hypersensitivity reactions to food usually are type I (about 5 percent) or type IV (about 95 percent). Type III has been reported to occur in addition, but the relationship is controversial. The essential features of types I and IV food allergies are compared in Table 4-4.

Allergens. It is believed that food allergens gain access to the body by absorption from the digestive tract. The majority are plants, and an allergic patient often is sensitive to foods in the same botanical family. Few animal foods are allergens, but they can be important. The most common food allergens are listed in Table 4-5. Allergies to wheat, cow's milk, and chicken eggs, especially if all three are present in the same person, can be particularly troublesome in meal planning.

There is very little cross-reactivity in allergies to animal foods. Patients allergic to eggs are not usually allergic to chicken. Allergies to milk and beef only occasionally occur in the same patient. Of the two, milk allergy is much more common.

Some chemicals used in food processing may be allergens. In some cases, they are haptens. An important group of additives which are considered by some to be causes of atopic reactions are the artificial food colors, but this is very controversial. If a diet free of these products is prescribed, certain facts should be kept in mind. Most are petroleum products and are used in very small amounts. Some color is imparted by concentrations of 0.001 percent. At the other extreme, objectionable overcoloring occurs at

Table 4-5. Common Food Allergens

Immediate hypersensitivity
Fish
Seafood
Nuts
Legumes (especially peanuts)
Eggs
Salicylates

Delayed hypersensitivity
Milk
Wheat
Chocolate
Cola
Corn
Citrus fruit
Eggs
Beef
White potatoes
Pork
Legumes
Chicken
Oatmeal
Rye
Oranges
Cottonseed
Mustard
Tomatoes
Cucumbers
Garlic

Table 4-6. Food Sources of Substantial Amounts of Artificial Colors

Baked goods
Breakfast cereals
Cake mixes
Candies
Carbonated drinks
Cherry pie mix
Colored sugar
Drug syrups (e.g., cough syrup)
Frankfurters
Fruit cocktail, canned
Fruit drinks, artificial
Fruit salad, canned
Gelatin desserts
Gum, bubble
Gum, chewing
Ice creams and cones
Maraschino cherries
Mint jelly
Popsicles

approximately 0.008 percent. Some colors used in foods are Blue No. 1 (brilliant blue), Green No. 3, Red No. 3 (erythrosine), Yellow No. 5 (tartrazine), and Yellow No. 6. Orange color is made by mixing red and yellow, and green sometimes is achieved by mixing blue and yellow. Purple is a combination of red and blue. The red, blue, and yellow colors and their derivatives, orange, green, and purple, are found in large quantities in the foods listed in Table 4-6. Brown products, such as root beer and colas, are colored with caramel.

Mode of Contact. Allergens in type I and type IV hypersensitivities often are classified according to their mode of contact. The most common allergens in type I atopy are the inhalants. This group comprises pollens, dusts, molds, fungal spores, and other airborne materials. Their primary area of contact is the respiratory tract. Few of these are food-related, but some patients find that strong odors from some foods are antigenic.

Ingestants are substances taken internally as food or drink. Some drugs may be included here, as well as chemical additives and unintentional ingestants such as mouthwashes and toothpastes. The ingestants obviously are of primary interest to the nutritional care specialist.

Contactants are allergenic on direct skin or mucous membrane contact. They may include pollens and food as well as other substances in the environment. Contact allergies are type IV hypersensitivities. When a patient is highly sensitive to a specific ingested food, he or she sometimes also develops a contact dermatitis when handling that food. This reaction is not invariable, but the possibility does exist.

Injectants are those substances that cause reactions when injected into the body. Injected drugs and sera used in medical treatment as well as insect venoms are in this group.

Clinical Manifestations. With food allergies, the allergen may react with the IgE antibodies locally and produce symptoms in the gastrointestinal tract itself or may affect organs elsewhere in the body. Only when the symptoms occur in the gastrointestinal tract is the condition known as *gastrointestinal allergy.* When organs elsewhere in the body are affected, two possible mechanisms are theoretically possible: (1) the mediators are transmitted systemically and affect the susceptible shock organ or (2) the antigen itself is absorbed into the systemic circulation and has a direct effect on the shock organ. At the present time, the first of these is more commonly accepted.[47]

Table 4-7 gives a comprehensive list of clinical manifestations that have been suspected to result from allergies to ingested foods. Some of the symptoms in the gastrointestinal tract itself—vomiting, diarrhea, malabsorption, and constipation—are common to many other disorders and therefore are discussed in detail in Chapters 5 and 6.

Anaphylaxis usually occurs promptly after the allergenic food is eaten. Typically, offending foods are legumes, especially peanuts, and also berries, nuts, and seafoods, particularly shellfish. Urticaria and angioedema are common allergic symptoms to a

Table 4-7. Possible Clinical Manifestations of Food Allergy

Gastrointestinal
Nausea
Vomiting
Diarrhea
Abdominal pain and colic
Loss of appetite
Intestinal hemorrhage
Hepatosplenomegaly
Constipation
Malabsorption
Functional intestinal obstruction
Cheilitis
Stomatitis

Dermatologic
Urticaria
Angioedema
Circumoral rashes
Eczema
Perianal dermatitis
Aphthous ulcers

Respiratory system
Chronic rhinitis
Asthma
Recurrent bronchitis
Recurrent croup
Recurrent otitis media
Chronic coughing
Hemoptysis

Central nervous system
Headache
Insomnia
Irritability
Listlessness
Drowsiness

Hematologic
Anemia
Eosinophilia

Systemic
Anaphylaxis
Failure to thrive
Malnutrition

Other (controversial)
Crib death
Celiac disease
Ulcerative colitis
Tension fatigue syndrome
Hyperkinesia
Migraine
Peptic ulcer
Irritable colon

variety of foods. Atopic dermatitis (*eczema*) occurs frequently from milk, wheat, corn, fish, and legume allergies, but may result from a wide variety of others.[47] Asthma is most often associated with inhalants, but approximately 10 percent of asthma patients have a sensitivity to aspirin. Cross-reactivity in some of these patients make them sensitive to some foods and food additives, especially tartrazine yellow.

There are two behavioral alterations that possibly are related to allergic reactions. Children with *tension fatigue syndrome* are described as having a variety of symptoms, some of which are contradictory. They are listed in Table 4-8. Feingold[48] has suggested that food additives and *hyperactivity* are related. In particular, he points to tartrazine and salicylates as offenders. His reports have been based on clinical experience and the concept has not been universally accepted. Controlled studies have not been conclusive.[49]

The immune responses to ingestants obviously are of primary interest to the nutritional care specialist; however, it is important to recognize that individual patients may simultaneously be allergic to inhalants and contactants. Under these circumstances,

Table 4-8. Symptoms and Signs Associated with the Tension Fatigue Syndrome

	Clinical Features
Behavior	Wild, maniacal, impulsive, tired, lethargic, lacking energy
Disposition	Talkative, restless, inattentive, aggressive, listless, depressed
Sleep habits	Inability to sleep, nightmares, always sleepy
Symptoms	Headaches, abdominal pains, leg aches, jitteriness, restless legs, enuresis, nausea, bloating, abdominal pains, diarrhea and constipation, halitosis, excessive perspiration
Signs	Pallor, circles under eyes, Dennie's sign, nasal stuffiness, aphthous ulcers

Reprinted with permission from Rapp, D.J., The management of food allergy. In J.W. Gerrard, Ed., *Food Allergy: New Perspectives,* 1980, p. 188. Courtesy of Charles C Thomas, Publisher, Springfield, Illinois.

these allergies have some effect on each other. It has been suggested that each patient has a limit of tolerance or threshold for the appearance of symptoms.[50] Thus, some food allergies cause obvious symptoms in the ragweed-sensitive patient only in the season when ragweed is in bloom.

The severity of the clinical manifestations of atopy or delayed hypersensitivity is affected by a number of other factors which add to the patient's *total allergic load.* One of these is the patient's genetic constitution. A tendency to hypersensitivity seems to recur in certain families; however, the specific clinical manifestations may vary within that family. One person might have hay fever, another hives, and so on. An individual's reaction to a given allergen is consistent, though. For example, a person who develops hives from eating strawberries will continue to have hives and will not develop hay fever on the next exposure to strawberries.

In addition to the genetic predisposition, symptoms also tend to be more severe when the patient is physically less well than normal, during emotional stress, and during inclement weather. The question of emotional involvement in allergic patients is a complicated one. The nutritional care specialist should keep in mind that not only does emotional stress exacerbate the symptoms, but also the disease itself may cause emotional problems which must be considered in treatment.

Another important point is that sensitization by one mode of contact may lead to allergic reactions when other means of contact occur. If a patient becomes sensitized to an injected drug, for example, the sensitivity can result in an allergic reaction if that substance or a closely related material is contained in an ingested food. Penicillin sensitivity is an example which will be discussed in more detail.

Prevention. Although most foods are digested prior to absorption, trace amounts can be absorbed in the form of molecules sufficiently large to be antigenic.[51] The prevalence of food allergy is inversely proportionate to age. It is not known whether this results from maturation of the gastrointestinal tract, thus reducing absorption of antigen, or whether an acquired immunity develops.[47] Antigen absorption occurs more commonly in early infancy than in adults, possibly because of low levels of sIgA in the intestine.[52–55]

The infant may also become sensitized to foods that the mother eats in large quantities during pregnancy.[56] Immunoglobulin E does not cross the placenta; therefore, type I allergies are not acquired passively, but foods eaten and absorbed as antigen by a pregnant woman are believed to be capable of crossing the placenta. Antibodies can then be made by the fetus.[57,58] A mixed diet without emphasis on any one food in pregnancy is recommended in families with a genetic predisposition to allergy.

Breast feeding may prevent sensitization in atopic families, since the milk contains less foreign protein.[59] However, some antigens in the mother's diet have been found in the milk.[60] For protection against allergies, long-term breast feeding of the atopic infant and a varied diet for the mother, avoiding large quantities of foods that are common allergens, are recommended.[61] The introduction of new foods to the infant should be delayed as long as possible.

Diagnosis of Food Allergy. The occurrence of clinical manifestations of food allergy does not require the presence of antibodies.[62] In addition to the occurrence of delayed sensitivity which is not antibody-dependent, antibodies can be found before allergic symptoms begin to occur. As a consequence, measurement of total IgE level in the serum is inadequate for diagnosis. The problem often is approached more indirectly.

The physician is faced with several problems in the diagnosis of food hypersensitivity. One of these is differential diagnosis. For example, some allergic reactions mimic other gastrointestinal diseases such as gluten intolerance and lactose intolerance. It also is important to distinguish hypersensitivity reactions from infections. The problem may be complex, and the diagnosis of hypersensitivity sometimes is made by a process of elimination.

A second problem in diagnosis is the identification of the offending food or other allergens. It is in this process that the skillful nutritional care specialist can be invaluable. The available procedures vary greatly in their innate dependability, and some are more than usually dependent on the skills of the health care professional.

The *diet history* can be important and should be the first procedure used. When allergy is of the immediate reaction type and the response is severe to an obviously present allergen, the patient, or the parent of a child patient, will usually be aware of the identity of the allergen. However, when allergic responses are delayed, are nonspecific in nature, moderate in severity, or result from hidden allergens, skillful and thorough questioning is required. In addition, detailed knowledge of food composition, botanical relationships, and food preparation methods are essential. It is insufficient to ask the patient simply to describe his or her diet. Some useful general lines of questioning are listed here. Judgment must be exercised in choosing which to use in specific cases.

What foods were eaten, how often, and in what amounts?

What are the sources of these foods: Home-prepared? Away from home? If away from home, where? Brands? Specific content of mixed dishes? Is the food eaten cooked or raw?

Is chewing gum used? If so, what brand? How often? When?

What is the patient's meal pattern? Time? Amount? Frequency?

Which foods were eaten in especially large quantities compared to normal?

Are there foods eaten to which other members of the family are known to be allergic, particularly parents, grandparents or siblings?

Do symptoms develop as the result of smelling or handling certain foods?

Do symptoms develop only when exposure occurs in only certain locations? Only after certain activities?

Is the patient under emotional stress? Constantly? At recurring intervals?

What cleaning compounds are used? Dishwashing methods?

What drugs, cosmetics, and personal hygiene products are used? Brands? Time and frequency of use? Inquire about aspirin, toothpastes, mouthwashes, throat lozenges, laxatives, and other products in or around the mouth, even if the patient is not conscious of swallowing them.

The answers to these questions may well lead to others.

Another diagnostic method is the *food diary.* Total recall of the diet information in the diet history interview is difficult, if not impossible. Therefore, the patient may be asked to keep a diary for a period of a week or several weeks. The patient will require careful instruction on the information to be entered in this diary and will need encouragement to complete the record carefully and accurately in order for the diary to be useful. The patient should record all food, drink, and other ingestants, along with the time of intake or use, amounts, and preparation methods. Ingredients for all mixtures, as well as the brand names of prepared or packaged items, should be listed. At the same time, the nature, time of onset, and severity of symptoms must be recorded. This information then is examined to detect a relationship between the ingestion of a specific item and the onset of symptoms within approximately 3 days. A food should be suspected particularly if the interval between ingestion and onset of symptoms is relatively constant.

Cutaneous testing sometimes is used in addition to the history and diary. Specific items that precipitate severe responses may be identified by the history or diary; these should not be the subject for cutaneous testing because the process can be hazardous. However, a list of suspected foods in which the relationship to symptoms is less clear sometimes is also obtained. Cutaneous testing (skin tests) may be used in investigating these suspected allergens. Extracts of suspected offenders are applied to a "scratched" area of the skin or put into areas where the skin is pricked. These epicutaneous tests are known as *scratch* (cutireaction) or *prick tests.* Alternatively, the extract sometimes is injected intracutaneously. Results are interpreted in terms of the size of the wheal-flare reactions elicited at each site compared to that produced by administration of the solvent alone. Theoretically, a large wheal and flare indicates greater sensitivity. A reaction in 15 to 20 minutes suggests an IgE-mediated reaction. An Arthus-like (type III) reaction is suggested with a reaction in 4 to 8 hours, and a type IV cell-mediated response is probable if the wheal-flare reaction appears in 24 to 72 hours.

The *skin-window test* is also a form of cutaneous testing.[63,64] The surface of the skin is scraped with a blade, a drop of antigen extract is applied, and a microscope slide is taped over the area. The slide is stained and examined for eosinophils and other cells in 24 hours. The test is positive if eosinophils are three times more numerous than in a control area.

Unfortunately, cutaneous testing is not especially reliable in diagnosis of food allergies. Prick or scratch tests often are positive in type I hypersensitivity[65,66] and negative in type IV,[67,68] but there are many false-positive responses, some resulting from nonspecific skin irritation. False-negative responses also are common.[64,69] Intradermal tests are more dependable in type IV sensitivities. One reason for the unreliability of skin tests may be that extracts are made from raw materials and so may not sufficiently closely resemble the cooked items that the patient normally eats. In addition, the allergen may be altered chemically when the extracts are prepared or during storage. An additional problem arises in that extracts are not available for every possible antigen. The patient may be allergic to substances not tested. Lastly, it is important to remember that the skin does not always respond in the same way as other shock organs.

Laboratory tests are of limited usefulness but may be used to suggest or confirm the diagnosis. They are not definitive. Increased eosinophil levels in the blood (eosinophilia) suggests allergy,[70] but it occasionally is present in other conditions.[71] Therefore, this test is not useful in differential diagnosis. Increased serum IgE often is seen in type I hypersensitivity, but it, too, is found in other conditions.[69,72] Low serum IgA usually is associated with sIgA deficiency. In the *radioallergosorbent test* (RAST), the amount of the patient's IgE antibody to specified antigens is measured. It therefore tends to be positive in type I sensitivities and negative in type IV.[67,68] The test is expensive, not all antigens are available for use with this method, and it is considered to be less sensitive than intradermal skin testing. Further developments may eventually make this technique more useful.[41]

Diet testing often is of great value, given the limitations of in vitro and skin tests. There are several procedures available for use under appropriate circumstances. One of these procedures is the *restriction of specific foods and diet challenge.* In this procedure, the foods on the suspect list are eliminated from the diet. The patient is given a list of those foods to be eliminated and also a list of foods that may be eaten. Usually, all commercially prepared foods are banned for the duration of the test. The patient should also be advised on meal planning for nutritional adequacy. If the list of foods to be eliminated is long or if many foods in a single group are restricted, the physician may prescribe vitamin and mineral supplementation. It must be remembered that these often contain artificial colors, binders, and other materials to which the patient may be sensitive.

The diet should be followed for 3 to 4 weeks. If the patient's symptoms subside, the restricted foods are added to the diet *one at a time.* This challenge test consists of adding the items to the diet in a large serving at each meal for 3 days. If the symptoms recur during that period, the food item is removed from the diet. The patient uses the previous diet until all symptoms subside and then proceeds to the next test item. A careful food diary is kept by the patient throughout. The procedure is repeated for each item on the suspect list.

Foods added first in the challenge test are those that occur most frequently in the diet and to which patients are most frequently sensitive. Most patients complete this procedure with a very short list of foods to which they are allergic. It may consist of only one or two items. Foods that are shown by this procedure to be allergens should be retested at a later date, perhaps at yearly intervals, since sensitivities sometimes change with time.

A more restrictive or *elimination diet* may be used if specific restriction and diet challenge does not render the patient symptom free. There are several versions of elimination diets available.[73] Some eliminate foods only in a specific category. Others are much more restrictive and consist only of a limited number of foods, those that past clinical experience has shown to be rarely, if ever, the cause of hypersensitivity responses. The chosen diet is used until all symptoms subside. Then foods are added one at a time as described previously. The time intervals are important. If the patient does not become symptom free on one of these diets, another with entirely different components can be tried.

If the symptoms do not subside on even the most restricted of the elimination diets, food allergy is an unlikely diagnosis. The patient may, instead, be allergic to an inhalant or other nonfood substances. In some cases, the problem is not an allergy, and the physician must seek the cause elsewhere. The use of elimination diets is hazardous for children if not carefully managed. Such diets may be inadequate for the growing child.

Treatment. Once the foods causing the symptoms are identified, the most effective treatment is complete avoidance of these foods. In immediate reactions (type I), the immune response is permanent and will recur on reexposure at any time. The avoidance of the allergen, therefore, is needed permanently. In delayed reactions (type IV), a tolerance sometimes develops during a period of abstinence. If, however, the period of abstinence is too short, the recurring symptoms may be more severe.[74]

Avoidance diets. Avoidance of allergens is a simple procedure when the offending foods are eaten only occasionally and if their presence is obvious, but it presents a great problem in sensitivities to foods such as milk, eggs, wheat, corn, and other very common items. Patients, or the parents, must be given lists of foods to be avoided and careful instruction on reading labels and detecting hidden sources of the allergen. Copies of diet lists are not always available in institutional diet manuals, since the patients are most often treated on an outpatient basis. Some books on allergy management give diet suggestions but must be modified to the individual needs of the patient.[75–81] The process requires that the nutritional care specialist be very knowledgeable of food composition and processing methods. In many circumstances, the patient is allergic to more than one item and several diets must be combined with great care. In view of the need for individualization, diet lists are not included in this book, but some examples will provide an appreciation of the knowledge required and the dimensions of the patient's problem.

The *milk-free diet* presents special problems when, as is often the case, the patient is an infant. Breast feeding is highly recommended for prevention of the sensitization of infants from families in which allergies are common. If the infant does not tolerate breast milk, the mother's diet should be examined for potential sources of allergens, since some allergens can be secreted into the breast milk. Elimination from her diet of some of the more common allergens, such as eggs, may solve the problem.

Patients who are only moderately reactive to cow's milk may tolerate "superheated" milk that has been boiled 15 to 30 minutes at 240°F. or powdered, evaporated, or lactic acid–treated milk.[82] Heating probably is most useful to those patients who are allergic to the heat-labile protein in milk, that is, to albumin and gamma globulin. It is not effective in sensitivity to casein.

Approximately 40 percent of patients sensitive to cow's milk are able to tolerate goat's milk.[50] These patients may be sensitive to lactalbumin, which is species specific. The other protein fractions in milk, such as lactoglobulin, are not species specific. Sensitivity to these fractions will occur with goat's milk as well as cow's milk.

Many milk-sensitive infants may be successfully fed formulas using soy protein as the protein source. Several of these are available commercially. Other nutrients are added to make them complete formulas for infant feeding (see Appendix L). These are less successful as milk substitutes for older children or adults, who may find the taste objectionable.

If an infant does not tolerate the soy protein well, other formulations that may be usable include Pregestimil and Nutramigen (Appendix L). The protein in these products is a hydrolysate of bovine casein and is filtered to remove large protein molecules. Both products contain corn oil. A meat-base formula, made from beef heart, also is available as a substitute for milk and is sometimes successful.

The nutritional care specialist must be prepared to help patients identify hidden sources of milk. In addition to warning against obvious forms of milk such as cream, cheese, butter, ice cream, sherbet, yogurt, and creamed foods, the patient needs to avoid such items as:

- Any foods that contain casein, caseinate, whey, or "milk solids" (see product labels), including nondairy items such as Coffee-mate, Imo, and Cool-Whip, which contain caseinate
- Most chocolate and many other candies
- Most breads except Kosher bread (*challah*) and some French, Italian, and Syrian breads
- Many cereals and most crackers, rolls, biscuits, and similar products
- Most frankfurters, sausages, and cold cuts
- Most margarines

The patient must also be given suggestions on items that are safe to use. Lists of commercial baked products that do not contain milk have been published.[4] Some margarines sold as Kosher products do not contain milk products but may be colored with tartrazine. Kosher foods in general can be relied on to be milk-free.

Patients must also be given guidance on meal planning for nutritional adequacy. The physician probably will prescribe vitamin and mineral supplements.

The *wheat-free diet* presents a difficult problem in the older child and the adult because of the wide variety of foods containing wheat products. All forms of wheat in cereals, flour, bread, and other baked goods must be avoided. Flour must be assumed to be wheat flour unless otherwise stated. The term *graham,* as in graham crackers, refers to wheat. Malt, used in malted products and beer, may be made from wheat or from other cereals such as barley or corn. The term *cereal extract* on a label is also a danger signal. Products such as rye bread almost always contain some wheat flour unless labeled "100 percent rye bread" and packaged in a can. If the product were not canned, it would dry out very rapidly and be inedible. Few breakfast cereals are wheat-free. Corn flakes, for example, almost invariably contain some wheat. Most creamed, thickened, or breaded foods contain wheat. Paste products, noodles, macaroni, spaghetti, and similar items are wheat products.

Patients should be given lists of usable commercial products and recipes using alternatives to wheat flour, particularly for baking. Some of these are available from commercial processors of other cereals. Rye, oats, rice, and barley flour may be used in home baking but cannot simply be substituted in recipes for products made with wheat flour. Special recipes are required, and the products still differ somewhat in texture and acceptability. There is often a cross-reactivity with buckwheat, so buckwheat flour should not be used in these recipes.

The *egg-free diet* is somewhat more easily managed than those without milk or wheat but still presents some problems. Although eggs in the obvious forms, such as fried or scrambled, are easy to avoid, the hidden forms are difficult to detect. The patient usually is sensitive to the egg white, not the yolk, but precise separation is very difficult.

Some hidden sources of eggs include coffee; wines; root beer; clear soups that have been clarified with egg white; any product labeled as containing albumin, vitellin, ovovitellin, livetin, ovomucin, or ovomucoid; breads, rolls, and pastries with a glazed crust and almost all other baked desserts; and waffles, pancakes, and similar products. Commercial mixtures such as salad dressings, puddings, custards, cookies, some ice cream, sherbet, cake flour, and some baking powders, many meat mixtures and prepared meats, many paste products, and some candies may contain egg white.

Patients must be given lists of commercial products known to be egg-free, useful recipes, especially for baking, and guidance in menu planning for good nutrition.

The *corn-free diet* is exceedingly difficult to manage since many foods contain corn products in hidden forms. Therefore, careful patient instruction is essential. The patient must avoid corn as a vegetable, hominy, grits, cereals containing corn, and popcorn. In addition, products containing corn oil and most cooking oils, cornstarch, corn syrup, corn sugar, dextrose or glucose, dexin, dextrin, dextrimaltose, commercial citric acid, and monosodium glutamate must be eliminated. Malt is often yeast-fermented corn. Commercial fructose may be made from corn. Many cardboard cartons, including milk cartons, are dusted with cornstarch. Many canned and frozen foods, especially fruits, are sweetened with corn syrup and must be avoided. The phrase "sugar added" on a label often refers to corn syrup, not sucrose. Cornstarch is a common thickener in a variety of products.

Corn is used in many products in processing or manufacturing and can occur in very unexpected places. Some examples are:

Carbonated beverages
Instant tea and coffee
Baked products baked on a hearth sprinkled with cornmeal
Frozen vegetables in waxed containers
Gelatin desserts
Salt
Peanut butter
Some brands of flour
Products containing baking powder or yeast
Cold cuts
Distilled vinegar
Beer, whiskey, gin, brandies, and wine

Many vitamin preparations and drugs in tablets, capsules, or liquids contain corn products. Sorbitol usually is made from corn. The patient may also need to be warned of other sources of corn such as breath sprays and drops, many dentifrices, gum on envelopes, labels, stickers, and tapes, chewing gum, and plastic food wrappers.

Some products containing corn are not intended to be ingested but may cause problems if inhaled. These include bath powders, hair sprays, talcum powder, and laundry starch. The cooking fumes from fresh corn are irritants in some patients.

The dimensions of the problem should now be obvious. A list of corn-free products should be given to the patient[4] along with careful counseling on meal planning for good nutrition. Some patients need a combined diet free of wheat, milk, egg, and corn and obviously will need a great deal of assistance.

Other avoidance diets that are encountered less frequently include those that require elimination of soy, cottonseed, linseed, or peanuts. In addition to use in a variety of manufactured foods, these items are found in many industrial products.

Sometimes food restrictions are necessary because the foods contain material not commonly considered to be a food, such as penicillin and salicylates. The sensitivity to the antibiotic *penicillin* most commonly develops in the course of drug therapy. It can be very severe, causing anaphylactic shock, and, as such, can be life-threatening. Penicillin once was used widely to treat infections in cows and then appeared in the milk.[83] Most states now require that milk be tested and found to be free of penicillin before it can be sold, but patients with severe penicillin allergies still are reported to have problems when drinking milk.[79]

Penicillium is a mold found in some cheeses. It is important to understand that it is unrelated to the antibiotic penicillin. Patients allergic to penicillin are not necessarily allergic to penicillium, but some patients are allergic to molds and can be expected to react to penicillium.

Salicylates are found in both food and drugs. Allergy to aspirin (acetylsalicylic acid) is fairly common. In addition to aspirin's presence in a long list of over-the-counter and prescription drugs, salicylates occur naturally in some foods, especially fruits.[84] Salicylates also are used in flavoring materials in processed foods and are found in beer, cider, wine, most distilled beverages, carbonated beverages, and tea. Aspirin sensitivity sometimes is accompanied by a sensitivity to benzoates and tartrazine.[85] The many foods containing these additives must then be eliminated, too. Salicylates also are used in suntan lotions, soaps, and in some other manufactured products. The patient may react to these products and needs careful instruction and a list of aspirin-free substitutes for aspirin.

The diet of the patient with many sensitivities may be very restricted in variety. Foods that the patient has not eaten before often are better tolerated and can provide interesting alternatives. Sometimes items new to the patient's diet may be obtained in the gourmet section of food stores, health food stores, and from shippers who specialize in special and exotic items. These foodstuffs may be more expensive but, if the patient can afford them, will provide variety in his or her meals.

The patient allergic to food is most frequently a child. The diet must then be adjusted for age and for the physiologic needs of growth. The nutritional consultant must have a knowledge of child development and be able to apply that knowledge in counseling.

Drug therapy. Although allergen avoidance is usually the mainstay of treatment, some drugs may be used. Antihistamines are used to prevent symptoms while aminophylline or epinephrine commonly are used to control symptoms once they occur. Cromolyn sodium is reported to prevent allergic reactions by preventing the release of mediators from mast cell granules. It probably stabilizes the lysosomal membranes. However, its use is still experimental in the United States.[47] Sometimes corticosteroids and other drugs are prescribed to reduce the response at the target cells. Corticosteroids may inhibit the histidine carboxylase that functions in the conversion of histidine to histamine.

Several variations of *immunotherapy* are available, but none is widely accepted. *Hyposensitization* consists of injection or oral administration of frequent small doses of antigen to induce the formation of IgG antibody. Theoretically, IgG, circulating in tissue fluids, combines with antigen before it can reach the tissue containing the IgE. The antigen-IgG complex then is removed by the reticuloendothelial system. This method is used to treat systemic forms of anaphylaxis.[86] Although it is useful in sensitivity to inhalant, it is not widely regarded as being effective in food allergy.[41]

Neutralization is a variant form of hyposensitization. It is a controversial procedure, the mechanism of which has not been determined, but the technique sometimes is used in an attempt to relieve the symptoms of allergy. It involves intradermal injection of extracts of antigens in graduated concentrations. Injections of concentrated extracts often are associated with onset of the same symptoms seen when the food is eaten. The strongest dilution that produces a negative wheal has been associated with relief of symptoms. Regular injections of this dose are given. Some allergists have reported that they used this technique successfully so that, after a course of injections, eating the offending food no longer precipitated symptoms,[87] but the method is not generally accepted.[41,88] The use of drops of the extract under the tongue, as an alternative to intradermal testing, is similarly rejected as being too insensitive.[89]

Autoimmune Diseases

When the immune system damages cells of disease-producing organisms, the effect is beneficial, but it is now recognized that the immune system can cause disease by damaging the body's own cells. Conditions known as *autoimmune diseases* are believed to result from the development of an immune reaction to a person's own tissue and involve either the humoral or cellular systems. These diseases are particularly difficult because of the constant exposure of the antigen to the antibody or sensitized lymphocyte. Diseases included in this category that have nutritional significance are listed in Table 4-9.

Table 4-9. Some Autoimmune Diseases with Possible Nutritional Care Implications

Active chronic hepatitis
Dermatomyositis
Goodpasture's syndrome
Primary atrophic hypothyroidism
Sjögren's syndrome
Systemic lupus erythematosus
Thyrotoxicosis
Type 1 diabetes mellitus
Ulcerative colitis

Autoimmune diseases presently are classified as type II, III, or IV hypersensitivities, but there also may be other types. In addition, elevated antibody levels have been found in other diseases not currently classified as being of autoimmune origin. Their relationship to autoimmunity is not clear; it is possible that, in some cases, the antibody develops as a consequence, not a cause, of the tissue damage.

There are a number of theories to explain the means by which autoimmunity develops. Three major theories regarding the production of *humoral autoimmunity* have been proposed and are presented here.

1. An agent of some type affects a tissue and alters it sufficiently that it is perceived by the immune system as foreign. The types of agents possibly involved are infectious, physical, or chemical, including some drugs. The change is presumed not to be so great that the antibodies produced will not attack normal cells.

2. Some constituents of the body usually are isolated from the immune system. Thus during normal development, at the time that the immune system learns to recognize self, recognition is not established. The autoimmune disease process is initiated when one of these "hidden" antigens escapes into an area in which it is not normally found; that is, it is ectopic. It comes in contact with the

immune system and is perceived as foreign. The consequent immune response to the ectopic antigen causes the disease.

Low concentrations of antibodies to these ectopic materials probably are present normally as a response to the normal turnover of body protein. When large concentrations of tissue debris appear, the formation of antibodies is stimulated. A large number of Ag/Ab complexes are formed, sometimes accompanied by complement fixation. These reactions may lead to further injury of tissue. Immunoglobulin G is believed to be the primary offender in immune complex injury.

Materials that have been proposed as candidates for ectopic antigen status include the protein in the lens of the eye, sperm, thyroglobulin from the thyroid follicle, mitochondria from the inside of cells, and molecular DNA and those forms of RNA normally sequestered within the nucleus. An immune response to one of these substances is thought to cause conditions such as Hashimoto's disease. Immune complex injury also is proposed as the cause of the damage to the kidney in systemic lupus erythematosus.

3. Some cells may be genetically programmed to produce an antibody to self, possibly as the result of a mutation. Normally, these cells would be suppressed. If a disease process interferes with the suppressive mechanism, an autoimmune disease theoretically could result.

Autoimmune disease involving the *cell-mediated system* might be produced by some of the same general mechanisms. In addition, it has been proposed that there are parasites that can live in a cell and alter its surface sufficiently that the cell becomes perceived as foreign. It has been suggested that this mechanism may be responsible for the primary damage in systemic lupus erythematosus, scleroderma, and, possibly, rheumatoid arthritis.

Recent studies in inbred strains of mice have suggested that diet may alter the course of autoimmune disease. New Zealand black mice are prone to reduced immune competency and tend to develop an autoimmune hemolytic anemia. This anemia develops earlier in mice fed a low-protein, high-fat diet than in those fed a high-protein, low-fat diet.[90] Also, if these mice are mated with New Zealand white mice, the pups produced tend to develop an autoimmune damage to the kidneys. Caloric restriction prolonged their life span.[91,92] It is not known if such diet alterations would be effective in human patients with autoimmune disease.

Procedures in nutritional care of patients with autoimmune disease are determined by the effects of the disease on damaged organs rather than the effects on the immune system and will be discussed in the chapters on the relevant organ systems.

Graft Rejection

Graft rejection and its nutritional care is of interest in patients with kidney transplants (Chapter 7) and in the treatment of some cancer patients (Chapter 13). Given current trends, transplants of other organs can probably be anticipated to become accepted procedures in the future.

Currently, almost all grafts are *allografts* (*homografts*)—that is, grafts between two persons of the same species but differing in genetic constitution. Their differing HLA antigens are called *alloantigens.* When an organ—a kidney, for example—is transplanted from the donor to the host (recipient), some degree of immune response is to be expected, since the kidney consists of a large number of foreign proteins which are the antigens. Specifically, the host reacts immunologically to the histocompatibility antigens on the cells of the donor tissue. This process is called *rejection* and can occur in one of three forms.

1. *Immediate rejection* occurs when the recipient already has antibodies to the donor tissue. The antibodies may have developed as the result of a blood transfusion from the same donor, for example. In these circumstances, the rejection may begin in minutes

or a few hours with deposition of Ag/Ab complex in the blood vessels, activation of the complement cascade, and the usual subsequent events. This is a *hyperacute rejection.* An *accelerated rejection* is similar, but the response is somewhat slower because the number of antibodies is lower.

2. *Acute rejection* occurs in a few weeks. It is theorized that donor HLA circulates to lymph nodes and spleen and induces sensitization. Host lymphocytes become sensitized as they circulate to the graft. The cell-mediated response destroys the blood vessels and the kidney tubules by creating an ischemic necrosis. Humoral immunity probably also is involved in acute rejection.

3. *Chronic rejection* may follow in months or years. It appears to be the result of immunoproliferative lesions in the intrarenal arteries, leading to ischemia. The kidney is the only organ that has been transplanted successfully for a sufficiently long period that the mechanisms of chronic rejection are available for study.

Immunosuppressive drugs are used to prevent transplant rejection. Nutritional care in patients receiving these drugs is described in Chapter 7. Some investigation is beginning on the effects of deficiencies of specific nutrients or modified diets that have an immunosuppressive effect. These might then be used to increase the effects of immunosuppressive drugs.

It seems appropriate here to mention a condition in which, in effect, the graft rejects the host. The immune response is in the opposite direction from that seen in transplant rejection. It occurs in some patients if the host is immuno*in*competent but the donor is immunocompetent. The host may have become immunoincompetent as a consequence of drug treatment or irradiation, or the condition may be genetic. T-lymphocytes from the donor will recognize the host as foreign and will mount an immune response against the host. The result is termed *graft-versus-host* (GVH) *reaction.* Nutritional care in GVH disease is described in Chapter 13.

References

1. Irvine, W.J. *Medical Immunology.* Edinburgh: Teviot Scientific, 1979.
2. Dubiski, S. Diagnostic Immunology. In A.G. Gornall, Ed., *Applied Biochemistry of Clinical Disorders.* Hagerstown, Md.: Harper and Row, 1980.
3. Tomasi, T.B., and Bienenstock, J. Secretory immunoglobulin. *Adv. Immunol.* 9:1, 1968.
4. Heremanns, J.F. Immunoglobulin formation and function in different tissues. *Curr. Top. Microbiol. Immunol.* 45:131, 1968.
5. Crabbe, P.A., Carbonaru, A.O., and Heremanns, J.F. The normal human intestinal mucosa as a major source of plasma cells containing gamma A immunoglobulin. *Lab. Invest.* 14:235, 1965.
6. Bienenstock, J. The significance of secretory immunoglobulins. *Can. Med. Assoc. J.* 103:39, 1970.
7. Halpern, M.S., and Koshland, M.E. Novel subunit in secretory IgA. *Nature* 228:1276, 1970.
8. Mestecky, J., Zikan, J., and Butler, N.T. Immunoglobulin M and secretory immunoglobulin A: Presence of a common polypeptide chain different from light chain. *Science* 171:1163, 1971.
9. Morrison, S.L., and Koshland, M.E. Characterization of the J chain from polymeric immunoglobulins. *Proc. Natl. Acad. Sci. U.S.A.* 69:124, 1972.
10. Tomasi, T.B., Jr., Tan, E.M., Solomon, A., and Prendergast, R.A. Characteristics of an immune system common to certain external secretions. *J. Exp. Med.* 121:101, 1963.
11. Lindh, E. Increased resistance of immunoglobulin A dimers to proteolytic degradation after binding of secretory component. *J. Immunol.* 114:284, 1975.
12. Suskind, R.M., Ed. *Malnutrition and the Immune Response.* New York: Raven Press, 1977.
13. Beisel, W.R., Ed. Impact of infection on nutritional status of the host. *Am. J. Clin. Nutr.* 30:1206, 1977.
14. Keusch, G.T. The effects of malnutrition on host responses and the metabolic sequelae of infections. In M.H. Grieco, Ed., *Infections in the Abnormal Host.* New York: Yorke Medical, 1980.

15. Bistrian, B.R. Interaction of nutrition and infection in the hospital setting. *Am. J. Clin. Nutr.* 30:1228, 1977.
16. Schneider, R.E., and Viteri, F.E. Morphological aspects of the duodenojejunal mucosa in protein-calorie malnourished children and during recovery. *Am. J. Clin. Nutr.* 25:1092, 1972.
17. Ferguson, A.C., Lawlor, G.J., Jr., Neumann, C.G., et al. Decreased rosette-forming lymphocytes in malnutrition and intrauterine growth retardation. *J. Pediatr.* 85:717, 1974.
18. Chandra, R.K. T and B lymphocyte subpopulations and leukocyte terminal deoxynucleotidyl transferase in malnutrition. *Acta Paediatr. Scand.* 68:841, 1979.
19. Chandra, R.K. Cell-mediated immunity in nutritional imbalance. *Fed. Proc.* 39:3088, 1980.
20. Bang, B.G., Makalanabis, D., Mukherjee, K.L., and Bang, F.B. T and B lymphocyte rosetting in undernourished children. *Proc. Soc. Exp. Biol. Med.* 149:199, 1975.
21. Stiehm, E.R. Humoral immunity in malnutrition. *Fed. Proc.* 39:3093, 1980.
22. Johnson, S.G.O., Melbin, T., and Vahlquist, B. Immunoglobulin levels in Ethiopian preschool children with special reference to high concentrations of immunoglobulin E (IgE). *Lancet* 1:1118, 1968.
23. Chandra, R.K. Reduced secretory antibody response to live attenuated measles and poliovirus vaccines in malnourished children. *Br. Med. J.* 2:583, 1975.
24. Sirisinha, S., Suskind, R., Edelman, R., et al. Secretory and serum IgA in children with protein-calorie malnutrition. *Pediatrics* 55: 166, 1975.
25. Sirisinha, S., Suskind, R., Edelman, R., et al. Complement and C3-proactivator levels in children with protein-calorie malnutrition and effect of dietary treatment. *Lancet* 1:1016, 1973.
26. Douglas, S.D., and Schapfer, K. The phagocyte in protein-calorie malnutrition—a review. In R.M. Suskind, ed., *Malnutrition and the Immune Response.* New York: Raven Press, 1977.
27. Chandra, R.K., Seth, V., Chandra, S., et al. Polymorphonuclear leukocyte function in malnourished Indian children. In R.M. Suskind, Ed., *Malnutrition and the Immune Response.* New York: Raven Press, 1977, pp. 259–264.
28. Smythe, P.M., Brereton-Stiles, G.G., Coovadia, H.M., et al. Thymolymphatic deficiency and depression of cell-mediated immunity in protein-calorie malnutrition. *Lancet* 2:939, 1971.
29. Watts, T. Thymus weights in malnourished children. *J. Trop. Pediatr.* 15:155, 1969.
30. Mugerwa, J.W. The lymphoreticular system in kwashiorkor. *J. Pathol.* 105:105, 1971.
31. Law, D.K., Dudrick, S.J., and Abdou, N.I. Immunocompetence of patients with protein-calorie malnutrition. *Lancet* 2:939, 1971.
32. Hoffman-Goetz, L., and Kluger, M.J. Protein-deficiency: Its effects on body temperature in health and disease states. *Am. J. Clin. Nutr.* 32:1423, 1979.
33. McCay, C.M., Crowell, M.F., and Maynard, L.A. The effect of retarded growth upon the length of the life span and upon the ultimate body size. *J. Nutr.* 10:63, 1935.
34. Yunis, E.J., and Greenberg, L.J. Immunopathology of aging. *Hum. Pathol.* 5:122, 1974.
35. McHugh, M.I., Wilkinson, R., Elliott, R.W., et al. Immunosuppression with polyunsaturated fatty acids in renal transplantation. *Transplantation* 24:263, 1977.
36. Mertin, J., and Hunt, R. Influence of polyunsaturated fatty acids on survival of skin allografts and tumor incidence in mice. *Proc. Natl. Acad. Sci. U.S.A.* 73:928, 1976.
37. Broitman, S.A., Vitale, J.J., and Vavrousek-Jakuba, E. Polyunsaturated fat, cholesterol and large bowel tumorigenesis. *Cancer Res.* 40:2455, 1977.
38. Ota, D.M., Copeland, E.M., Corriere, J.N., Jr., et al. The effects of a 10% soybean oil emulsion on lymphocyte transformation. *J.P.E.N.* 2:112, 1978.
39. Gross, R.L., and Newberne, P.M. Role of nutrition in immunologic functions. *Physiol. Rev.* 60:188, 1980.
40. Rogers, A.E., Herndon, B.J., and Newberne, P.M. Induction by dimethylhydrazine of intestinal carcinoma in normal rats fed high or low levels of vitamin A. *Cancer Res.* 33:1003, 1973.
41. Bahna, S.L., and Heiner, D.C. *Allergies to Milk.* New York: Grune and Stratton, 1980.
42. Fudenberg, H.H., Stites, D.P., Caldwell, J.L., and Wells, J.V., Eds. *Basic and Clinical Immunology,* 4th ed. Los Altos, Calif.: Lange Medical, 1980.
43. Edelman, R., Suskind, R.M., Olsen, R.E., and Sirisinha, S. Mechanisms of defective delayed cutaneous hypersensitivity in children with protein-calorie malnutrition. *Lancet* 1:506, 1973.
44. Neumann, C.G., Lawlor, G.J., Jr., and Stiehm,

E.R. Immunologic responses in malnourished children. *Am. J. Clin. Nutr.* 28:89, 1975.
45. Miller, C.L. Immunological assays as measurements of nutritional status: A review. *J.P.E.N.* 2:554, 1978.
46. Coombs, R.R.A., and Gell, P.G.H. Classification of allergic reactions responsible for clinical hypersensitivity and disease. In P.G.H. Gell, R.R.A. Coombs, and P.J. Lachman, Eds., *Clinical Aspects of Immunology.* Oxford: Blackwell Scientific, 1975.
47. Terr, A.I. Allergic diseases. In H.H. Fudenberg, D.P. Stites, J.L. Caldwell, and J.V. Wells, Eds., *Basic and Clinical Immunology,* 3rd ed. Los Altos, Calif.: Lange Medical, 1980.
48. Feingold, B. Food additives and child development. *Hosp. Pract.* 8:11, 1973.
49. Palmer, S., Rapport, J.L., and Quinn, P. Food additives and hyperactivity. *Clin. Pediatr.* (Phila.) 14:956, 1975.
50. Breneman, J.C. *Basics of Food Allergy.* Springfield, Ill.: Charles C Thomas, 1978.
51. Walzer, M. Studies in absorption of undigested protein in human beings. *J. Immunol.* 14:143, 1927.
52. Walker, W.A., Isselbacher, K.J., and Block, K.J. Intestinal uptake of macromolecules: Effect of oral immunization. *Science* 177:608, 1972.
53. Walker, W.A., Wu, M., Isselbacher, K.J., and Bloch, K.J. Intestinal uptake of macromolecules: III. Studies of mechanisms by which immunization interferes with antigen uptake. *J. Immunol.* 115:854, 1975.
54. Walker, W.A. Host defense mechanisms in the gastrointestinal tract. *Pediatrics* 57:901, 1976.
55. Walker, W.A. Antigen absorption from the small intestine and gastrointestinal disease. *Pediatr. Clin. North Am.* 22:731, 1975.
56. Lyon, G.M. Allergy in an infant of three weeks. *Am. J. Dis. Child.* 36:1012, 1928.
57. Miller, D.L., Hirvonen, T., and Gitlin, D. Synthesis of IgE by the human conceptus. *J. Allergy Clin. Immunol.* 52:182, 1973.
58. Singer, A.D., Hobel, C.J., and Heiner, D.C. Evidence for secretory IgA and IgE in utero. *J. Allergy Clin. Immunol.* 53:94, 1974.
59. Matthew, D.J., Taylor, B., Norman, A.P., et al. Prevention of eczema. *Lancet* 1:321, 1977.
60. Donnally, H.H. The question of the elimination of foreign protein (egg white) in woman's milk. *J. Immunol.* 19:15, 1930.
61. Gerrard, J.W., Ed. *Food Allergy: New Perspectives.* Springfield, Ill.: Charles C Thomas, 1980.
62. Baldwin, J. Some observations of the skin and mucous membrane reactions in hay fever. *J. Immunol.* 13:345, 1917.
63. Galant, S.P., Bullock, J., and Frick, O.L. An immunological approach to the diagnosis of food sensitivity. *Clin. Allergy* 3:363, 1973.
64. Bullick, J.D., and Bodenbender, J.G. A simple laboratory aid in diagnosing food allergy. *Ann. Allergy* 28:127, 1970.
65. Chua, Y.Y., Bremner, K., Lakdawalla, N., et al. *In vivo* and *in vitro* correlates of food allergy. *J. Allergy Clin. Immunol.* 58:299, 1976.
66. Chua, Y.Y., Bremner, K., Llobet, J.L., and Collins-Williams, C. Diagnosis of food allergy by radioallergosorbent test. *J. Allergy Clin. Immunol.* 58:477, 1976.
67. Rowe, A.H. *Food Allergy, Its Manifestations and Control and the Elimination Diets.* Springfield, Ill.: Charles C Thomas, 1972.
68. Speer, F., and Dockhorn, R.J. *Allergy and Immunology in Childhood.* Springfield, Ill.: Charles C Thomas, 1973.
69. Bock, S.A., Lee, W.Y., Remigio, L.K., and May, C.D. Studies of hypersensitivity reactions to foods in infants and children. *J. Allergy Clin. Immunol.* 62:327, 1978.
70. Roth, A. Detection of food allergy. *Postgrad. Med.* 32:432, 1962.
71. Beeson, P.B., and Bass, D.A. *The Eosinophil.* Philadelphia: W.B. Saunders, 1977.
72. Bock, S.A., Buckley, J., Holst, A., and May, C.D. Proper use of skin tests with food extracts in diagnosis of hypersensitivity to food in children. *Clin. Allergy* 7:375, 1977.
73. Rowe, A.H. *Elimination Diets and the Patient's Allergies.* Philadelphia: Lea and Febiger, 1944.
74. Randolph, T.G. Adaptation to specific environmental exposures enhanced by individual susceptibility. In L.D. Dickey, Ed., *Clinical Ecology.* Springfield, Ill.: Charles C Thomas, 1976.
75. Conrad, M. *Allergy Cooking.* New York: Pyramid, 1960.
76. Wood, M. *Gourmet Food on a Wheat-Free Diet.* Springfield, Ill.: Charles C Thomas, 1967.
77. Larson, J., and Nugent, B. *Very Basically Yours.* Chicago: Human Ecology Study Group, 1967.
78. Sheedy, C.B., and Keifetz, M. *Cooking for Your Celiac Child.* New York: Dial Press, 1969.
79. Thomas, L.L. *Caring and Cooking for the Allergic Child.* New York: Drake, 1974.
80. Golos, N. *Management of Complex Allergies.* Norwalk, Conn.: New England Foundation

of Allergic and Environmental Diseases, 1975.
81. *Baking for People with Food Allergies.* U.S.D.A. Home and Garden Bull. No. 147. Washington, D.C.: U.S. Department of Agriculture, 1976.
82. Tuft, L. *Allergy Management in Clinical Practice.* St. Louis: C.V. Mosby, 1973.
83. Welch, H. Problems of antibiotics in foods as the Food and Drug Administration sees them. *Am. J. Public Health* 47:701–705, 1957.
84. Noid, H.E., Schulze, T.W., and Winkelmann, R.K. Diet plan for patients with salicylate-induced urticaria. *Arch. Dermatol.* 109:866, 1974.
85. Lockey, S.D. Hypersensitivity to tartrazine (FD&C Yellow No. 5) and other dyes and additives present in foods and pharmaceutical products. *Ann. Allergy* 38:206, 1977.
86. Weir, D.M. *Immunology for Undergraduates.* Edinburgh: E. and S. Livingstone, 1970.
87. Miller, J.B. The management of food allergy. In J.W. Gerrard, Ed., *Food Allergy: New Perspectives.* Springfield, Ill.: Charles C Thomas, 1980.
88. Caplin, I. Ad Hoc Committee Report to American College of Allergists Annual Meeting, Atlanta, Georgia, 1973. *Ann. Allergy* 31:375, 1975.
89. Breneman, J.C., Hurst, A., Heiner, D., et al. Final report of Food Allergy Committee—sublingual testing. *Ann. Allergy* 33:164, 1974.
90. Fernandes, G., Yunis, E.J., Smith, J., and Good, R.A. Dietary influence on breeding behavior, hemolytic anemia and longevity in NZB mice. *Proc. Soc. Exp. Biol. Med.* 139:1189, 1972.
91. Fernandes, G., Yunis, E.J., and Good, R.A. Diet and immunity of NZB mice. *J. Immunol.* 116:782, 1976.
92. Fernandes, G., Yunis, E.J., and Good, R.A. Influence of diet on survival of mice. *Proc. Natl. Acad. Sci. U.S.A.* 73:79, 1976.

Bibliography

Chandra, R.K. Immunodeficiency in undernutrition and overnutrition. *Nutr. Rev.* 39:225, 1981.

Chandra, R.K., and Newberne, P.M. *Nutrition, Immunity and Infection.* New York: Plenum Press, 1977.

Elwood, P.C. Nutrition and immunology (symposium). *Proc. Nutr. Soc.* 35:253, 1976.

Grieco, M.H., Ed. *Infections in the Abnormal Host.* New York: Yorke Medical, 1980.

Phillips, M., and Baetz, A. Diet and Resistance to Disease. *Adv. Exp. Med. Biol.* 135:1981.

Playfair, J.H.L. *Immunology at a Glance.* Oxford: Blackwell Scientific, 1979.

Speer, F. *Food Allergy.* Littleton, Mass.: PSG, 1978.

Sources of Current Information

American Journal of Clinical Nutrition
Annals of Allergy
Journal of Allergy and Clinical Immunology
Journal of Immunology
Journal of Pediatrics

III. Diseases of the Digestive System

5. The Oral Cavity, Esophagus, and Stomach

The alimentary tract obviously is of central importance to the maintenance of adequate nutrition. It follows that malfunctions of this system will affect the patient's nutritional status, and so nutritional care specialists have an important role in the management of these conditions.

THE ALIMENTARY TRACT DURING STRESS

Disorders of the digestive tract often appear first during periods of stress or emotional disturbance. These can frequently be related to alterations in the function of the system, but in only a minority of cases can a specific biochemical or morphological lesion be detected. Almy[1] suggests that the disorder results instead from a nonspecific reaction to *life stress,* defined as any situation regarded by an individual as a threat to his or her security.

A number of adaptive responses to stress are recognized. These include such phenomena as pallor, sweating, increase in blood pressure, and alterations in gastric secretions. It appears, therefore, that some symptoms of physiologic dysfunction, including digestive tract dysfunction, can result from stress. Some of the digestive responses to stress may be evolutionary in origin, having had survival value in earlier human forms. As such, the stress response would be expected to appear in all individuals, and there is some evidence that it does.[1]

The question remains, however, why the adaptive response becomes so severe and prolonged in some individuals that it develops into an incapacitating and clinically defined disorder. The difference may be attributable to factors in the genetic background, personality, and environment of the individual. Previous experience, family, and culture are among the suggested contributing factors. A second question involves the reason that the stress response affects different organs in different individuals. Why, for example, does stress affect the digestive system in one individual and the lungs in another, or why does it affect the stomach in one and the intestines in another?

The end-organ affected may be determined by genetic influences and also may be a conditioned response. In the case of digestive disorders, it frequently is suggested that early experiences in feeding and toilet training have prolonged effects. In addition, factors in the immediate environment, such as alcohol, coffee, spices, and laxatives, may be contributory.

It is believed that a stress response component is present in the etiology of many disorders of the digestive system. In general, stress responses of the digestive system are divided into two categories,[1] *psychophysiologic reactions,* in which there are alterations in function without change in structure, and *psychosomatic reactions,* in which there are morphological changes in the end-organ. Some of the conditions believed to fall into these categories, such as peptic ulcer, gastritis, irritable bowel syndrome, and constipation, will be discussed in more detail later.

In providing nutritional care, it is important to recognize the stress response component in the etiology of the disease. A nutritional care specialist who is able to provide reassurance and emotional support *in proper measure* to the patient will be much more effective than one who responds only to the physical needs of the patient. For those interested in further information on this subject, excellent reviews by Almy and colleagues are available.[1–3]

COMPONENTS OF THE ALIMENTARY TRACT

The components of the alimentary canal and the anatomic relationships to other organs important to digestion are shown in Fig. 5-1. Throughout much of its length, the digestive tract has a similar form, which is illustrated in Fig. 5-2. The innermost layer, the *mucosa,* consists of three parts, a layer of epithelium supported by an underlying, richly vascularized connective tissue and a thin smooth muscle layer, the *muscularis mucosa.* The

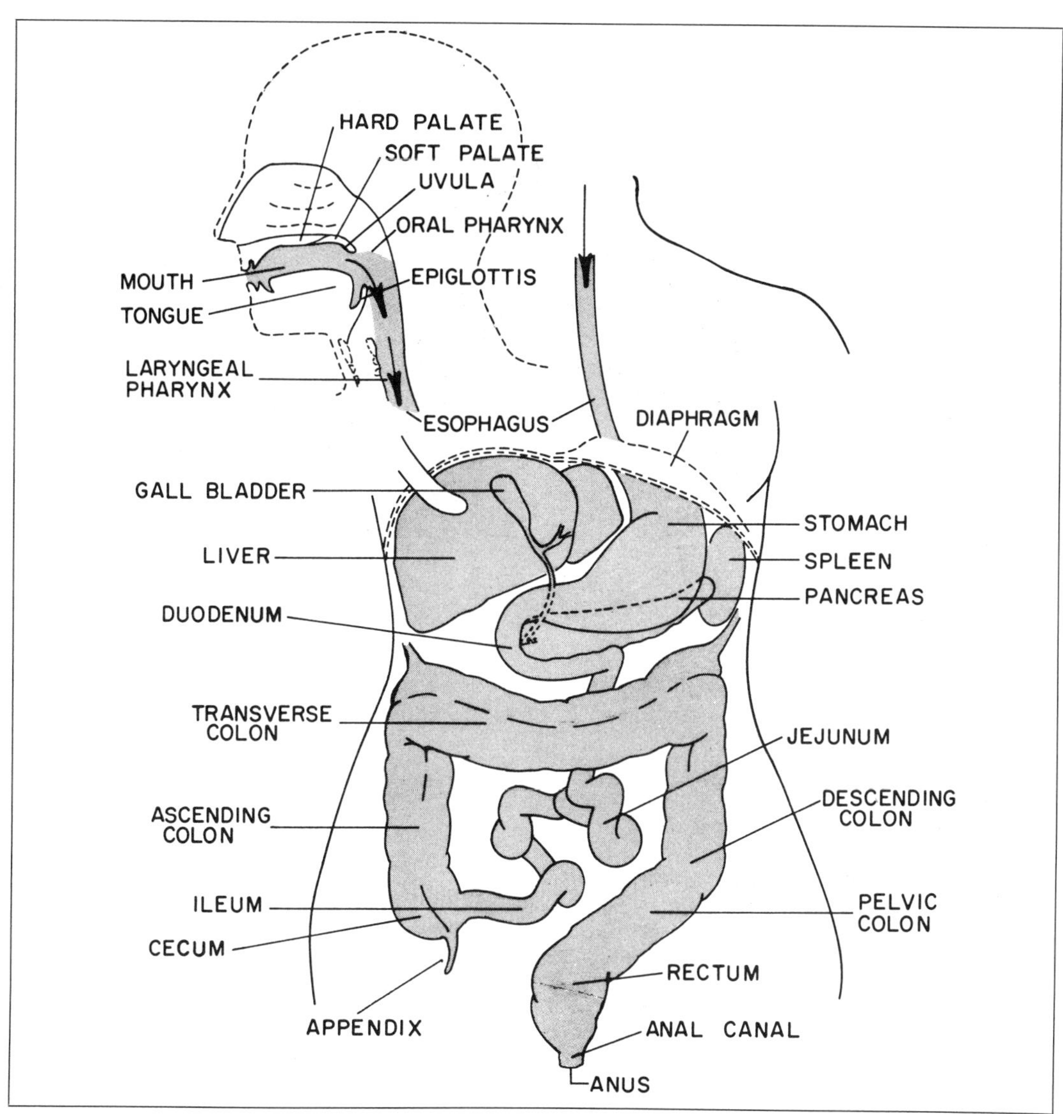

Figure 5-1. The parts of the digestive system. (Reprinted with permission from Ham, A.W., His*tology, 8th ed. Philadelphia: J.B. Lippincott, 1979, p. 645.)*

next layer, the *submucosa,* is composed of dense connective tissue containing larger blood vessels and a network of nerve cells and their processes called *Meissner's plexus.* The third layer, the *muscle layer,* consists of an inner circular muscle and an outer longitudinal muscle. Another network of nerves, the myenteric or Auerbach's plexus, lies between them. An outer *serosal layer,* primarily made of connective tissue, surrounds the gastrointestinal tract for most of its length.

THE ORAL CAVITY

Normal Anatomy and Physiology

The oral cavity consists of the *mouth* and the *pharynx,* a funnel-shaped organ which moves food from the mouth to the esophagus. It is obvious that the primary function of the oral cavity is to provide an opening for ingestion of food and access to the digestive and absorptive organs. Although

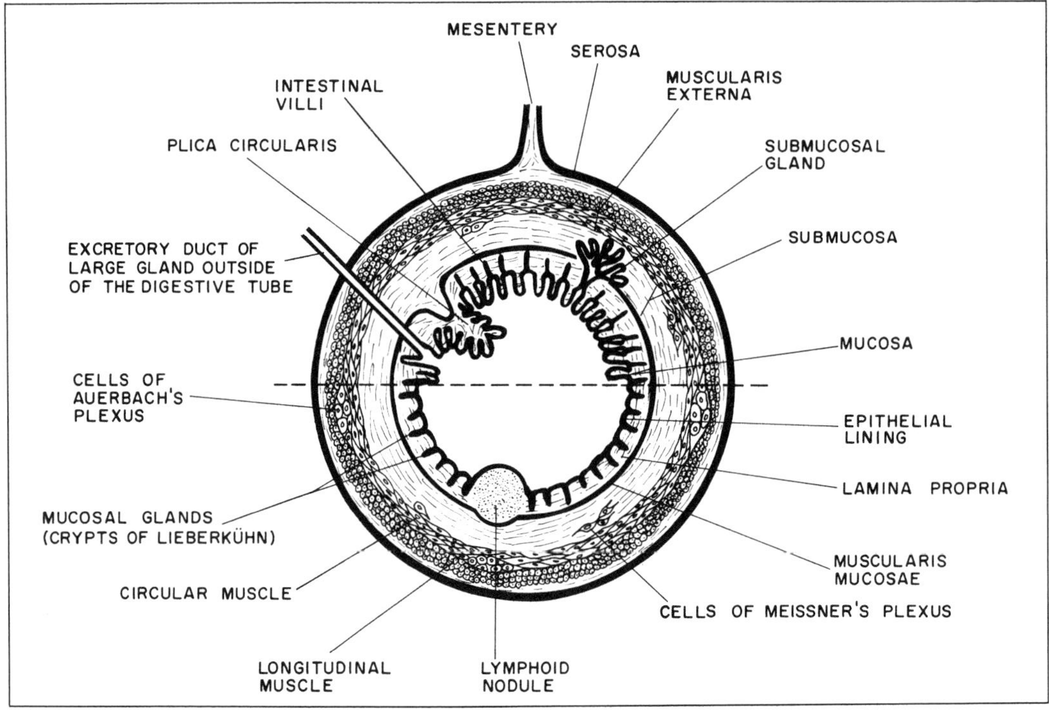

Figure 5-2. The general features of organization in the gastrointestinal tract. The concentric layers of serosa, muscularis, and mucosa are common to virtually all regions of the tract. In the upper half of the drawing, the mucosa is depicted with glands and villi as in the small intestine; in the lower half it is shown with glands only, as in the colon. (Adapted with permission from Bloom, W., and Fawcett, D.W., A Textbook of Histology, *10th ed. Philadelphia: W.B. Saunders, 1975, p. 599.)*

the oral cavity is simple in concept, it contains many tissues which exist in a complex relationship: teeth, gums (gingival tissue), tongue, taste buds, palate, salivary glands, mucous membranes, and alveolar (jaw) bones.

Salivary Glands and Salivation

The salivary glands consist of three pairs of major glands and numerous minor glands. Some glands secrete a *serous* (watery) saliva, and others, a more *mucous* material.

The functions of saliva are digestive or protective and include the following:

1. Moistening and lubricating food for easier swallowing
2. Holding particles together for easier swallowing
3. Acting as a buffer (salivary pH is approximately 6.8)
4. Beginning digestion of starch by action of salivary amylase (ptyalin), which continues until stopped by the low pH of the stomach
5. Promoting some remineralization of the teeth
6. Enhancing taste by dissolving and washing away food particles on taste buds so the person can taste the next food eaten
7. Dissolving and washing away food particles between the teeth
8. Facilitating speech

It should be obvious that malfunction can cause a variety of problems.

The main components of saliva are water, electrolytes, enzymes, and other proteins.

Potassium concentration is high, being almost equal to that in plasma. During sleep, saliva secretion is barely perceptible; maximum output may equal 4 ml/min. The usual daily secretion has been estimated to be between 0.5 and 1.5 liters, but others estimate 500 to 600 ml/day.[4] The high volume and high potassium content are important considerations in patients who have had head or neck surgery and whose saliva is draining externally. In these patients, careful replacement of fluid volume and of electrolytes is needed.

The volume of salivary secretion is controlled by the autonomic nervous system. As a consequence, surgery or trauma in which the nerves are severed has a severe effect on the amount of saliva produced. There is no known hormonal control of salivary volume, but its composition is under both nervous and hormonal control.[5]

Teeth and Mastication

The teeth are the major structures for *mastication* (chewing), which reduces food to a size appropriate for swallowing. The tongue also functions in dividing food, by mashing it against the palate and by moving food in place for chewing.

The teeth consist of four parts (Fig. 5-3). The *enamel, dentin,* and *cementum* are calcified tissues. The *pulp* is uncalcified connective tissue containing blood vessels, lymphatics, and nerves that transmit pain sensations only. The enamel, covering the *crown* or exposed portion of the teeth, is the hardest tissue in the body. It contains 96

Figure 5-3. Longitudinal section of a molar tooth in its alveolus. (Reprinted with permission from Crouch, J.E., Functional Human Anatomy, *3rd ed. Philadelphia: Lea and Febiger, 1978, p. 348.)*

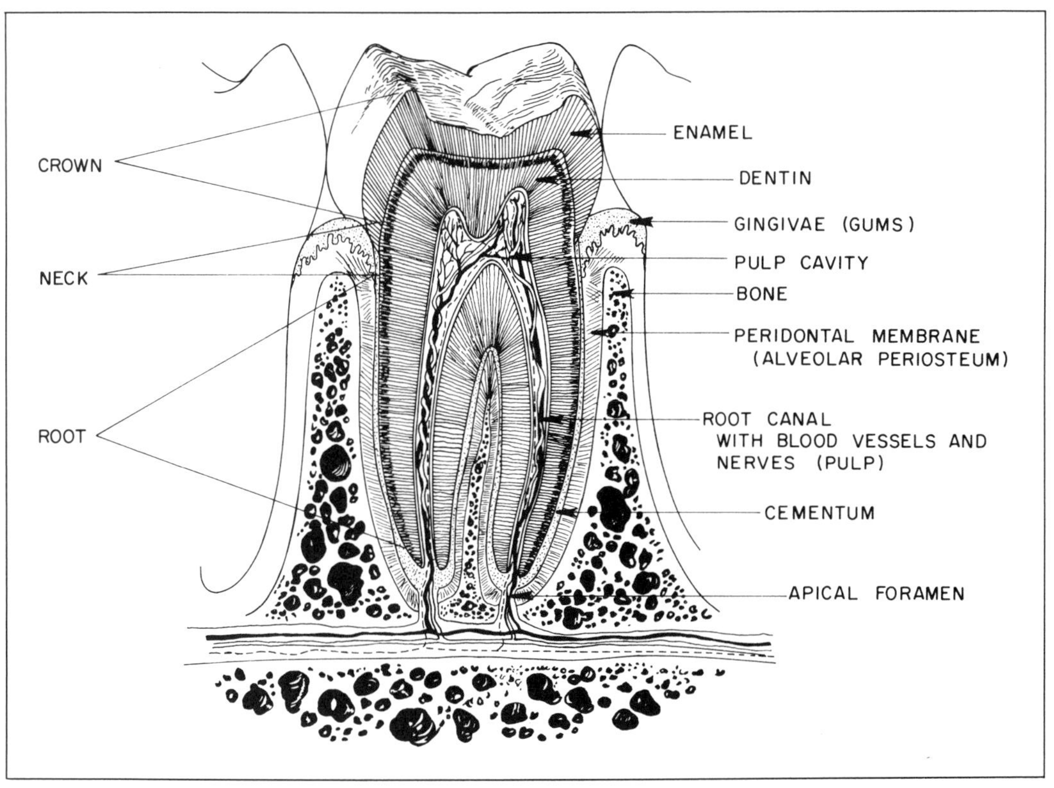

percent inorganic matter, mostly hydroxyapatite crystals, ($Ca_{10}[PO_4]_6[OH]_2$). Enamel is derived from ameloblasts which persist in the jaw only until the teeth erupt.

The dentin, lying immediately beneath the enamel, is the main component of the teeth. It is similar to bone in composition, containing 10 percent water, 20 percent organic matter, and 70 percent inorganic matter. The organic matter forms a matrix into which the hydroxyapatite is deposited. Dentin does not have a blood supply but is traversed by dentin tubules, a series of microscopic channels coursing through the dentin from the pulp to the enamel. These tubules may have a nutritional function. Dentin is formed by odontoblasts located at the periphery of the pulp. These cells continue to have the capacity to make dentin so that, in a protective response to damage, they form dentin on the border between the pulp cavity and root canal, narrowing the root canal.

Cementum is very much like bone in composition, with 45 percent inorganic matter. It is formed by cementoblasts and deposited in layers over the dentin of the *root* of the tooth. It is the site of the attachment of the *periodontal ligament* (or periodontal membrane) that anchors the tooth to the surrounding bone.

The maxilla (upper jaw bone) and the mandible (lower jaw bone) each have a thick projecting ridge called the *alveolar process,* containing sockets or alveoli, one for each tooth. The periodontal ligament extends from the alveolar process into the cementum to hold the tooth firmly in place. In addition to these supporting structures, the *gingiva* surrounds and is attached to the root of each tooth. Near the top of the gingiva, there is a gingival crevice or sulcus between it and the tooth. This is a matter of importance in dental disease. The supporting structures surrounding the teeth—the cementum, periodontal ligament, alveolar bone, and gingiva—are known collectively as the *periodontium.*

Swallowing

The act of swallowing or *deglutition* is a process in which related actions of the structures of the mouth, pharynx, and esophagus are carefully integrated (Fig. 5-4). The figure legend describes the sequence of events and should be studied carefully.

Abnormalities of the Oral Cavity

Effects of Malnutrition on Oral Tissues

The teeth initially form in the jaws by differentiation of specialized oral epithelial cells. These eventually form an organic matrix beginning at the top of the crown and proceeding toward the root. Calcification closely follows in similar fashion. The earliest differentiation of epithelium occurs in the 7-week embryo. Calcification in the primary teeth begins at 4 months' gestation and usually ends at 20 to 24 months of age postnatally. Eruption of primary teeth begins at 6 to 9 months and usually is complete at 3 years of age. The formation of the organic matrix and calcification of the permanent teeth are almost entirely postnatal, beginning at birth. The process extends to approximately age 25, when the third molar is complete.

From the fourth fetal month to 25 years of age, then, the forming teeth are vulnerable to various insults. The effect of nutrition during pregnancy on tooth development in the fetus has not been studied thoroughly. It appears that a nutritional deficiency must be severe before effects are obvious. The possibility remains, however, that milder deficiencies may cause subtle changes that alter the structure of the teeth and make them more vulnerable to decay.[6] Although the cause of many dental defects is unknown, there is some evidence that deficiencies of vitamins A or D, calcium, or phosphorus, or calcium-phosphorus ratio imbalance interfere with normal development of the teeth.[7] Research on animals has demonstrated that protein deprivation affects the development

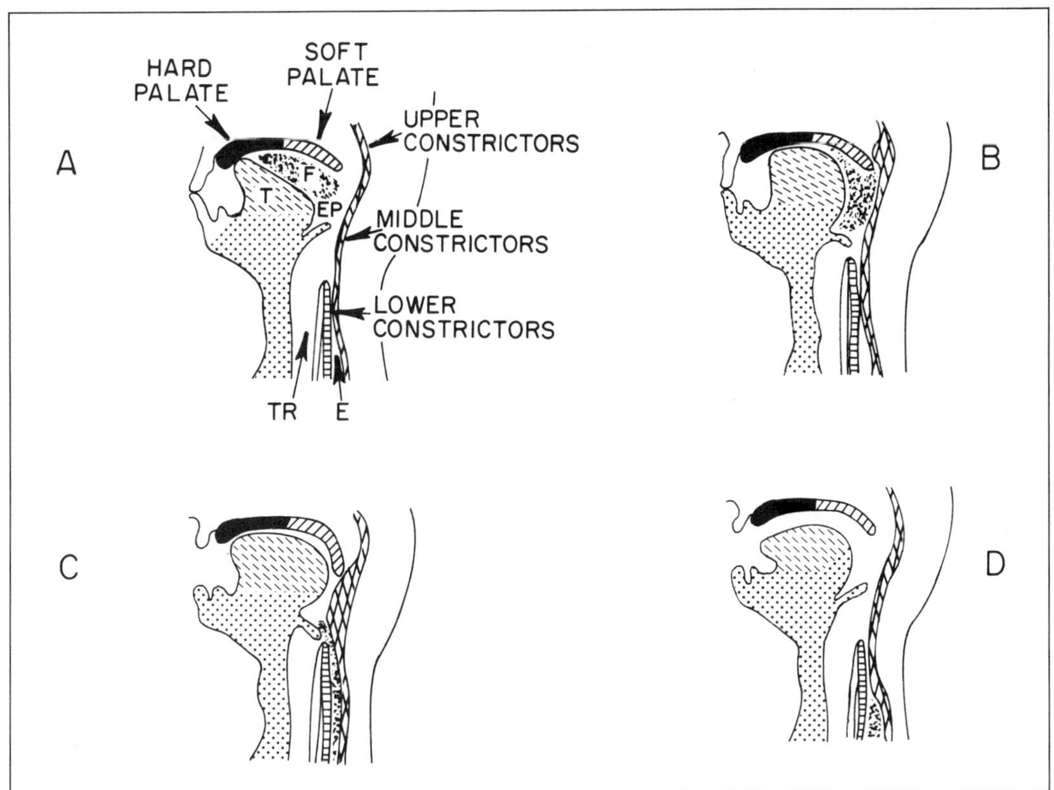

Figure 5-4. Oral and pharyngeal events during swallowing. **A.** *The bolus (F) to be swallowed is propelled into the pharynx by placement of the tongue (T) on the roof of the hard palate.* **B.** *Further propulsion is caused by movement of more distal regions of the tongue against the palate. Contraction of the upper constrictors of the pharynx and movement of the soft palate separate the oral pharynx from the nasopharynx.* **C.** *Propulsion through the upper esophageal sphincter is accomplished by contraction of the middle and lower constrictors of the pharynx and by relaxation of the cricopharyngeal muscle. Upward movement of the glottis and downward movement of the epiglottis (Ep) seals off the trachea (Tr)* **D.** *The bolus is now in the esophagus (E) and is propelled into the stomach by a peristaltic contraction. (Reprinted with permission from Weisbrodt, N.W., Esophageal motility. In L.R. Johnson, Ed.,* Gastrointestinal Physiology, *2nd ed. St. Louis: C.V. Mosby, 1981, p. 15.)*

of the teeth and their susceptibility to caries.[8–10]

In experimental animals, prenatal nutritional deficiencies contribute to the incidence of cleft lip, cleft palate, retarded development of salivary glands, and other congenital anomalies.[11] Of course, it is not possible to demonstrate this experimentally in human infants; therefore, the effects in humans are unknown.

After a tooth erupts, it apparently undergoes a maturation process during which its metabolism is different from that of a mature tooth. Studies with radioisotopes have shown that a recently erupted tooth can incorporate ions from its environment ten to twenty times faster than can a mature tooth.[12] Saliva may influence the maturation process, but the mechanism is unknown. We do not know whether malnutrition can cause changes in the amount or composition of saliva which could, in turn, affect maturation of the teeth. It does seem clear, however, that the erupted tooth is not so metabolically inert as was once believed.

Nutritional deficiencies are associated with several nonspecific conditions in the oral cavity. These include *gingivitis* (inflammation of the gingivae), *stomatitis* (inflammation of the oral mucosa), *glossitis* (inflammation of the tongue), and *cheilosis* (fissuring and scaling at the angle of the mouth). Their relationship to nutritional deficiency is described in many basic texts on normal nutrition. The nutritional care specialist should be alert to the possibility of oral disease in patients at risk of malnutrition, but it is equally important to realize that, since these conditions are nonspecific, they also occur as a result of nonnutritional factors. Their presence alone does not prove the existence of malnutrition.

Dental Diseases

The diseases described in this section can occur in people who are otherwise in good health. They also appear as a complication of existing illnesses and may seriously limit food intake, with a consequent detrimental effect on the patient's nutritional status. The nutritional care specialist must be alert to the possibility of dental disease in patients with unrelated diseases. A protocol for nutritional evaluation in relation to dental disease has been published and is useful in identifying patients in need of nutritional counseling.[13]

There are three types of materials that react with the teeth and supporting tissue and are particularly important in the etiology of dental disease. *Enamel pellicle* is a thin film that adheres to the teeth immediately after cleaning. It is believed to be formed by the conversion of glycoproteins in saliva into adhesive polymers by oral bacteria. *Dental plaque* is a sticky, gelatinous material that adheres to the pellicle. It consists of bacteria, epithelial cells, and leukocytes. The bacterial population varies with the location and age of the plaque, which must be removed mechanically. *Dental calculus* is believed to result from mineralization of plaque with minerals from saliva and from fluid in the gingival crevice.

Dental Caries. Dental caries or tooth decay refers to the destruction of the enamel, dentin and, sometimes, cementum. It has been reported to be present in 99 percent of adults by the age of 50. Because dental caries occurs so commonly, there is a tendency to treat it very casually, but it can be a serious problem. The term *rampant caries* refers to the condition of the patient who has extensive caries that worsen rapidly. Rampant caries occurs as a complication of other illnesses.

The patient requires nutritional management, since rampant caries causes pain and tooth loss. The patient may decrease chewing and swallowing as a result of the pain, thus contributing to nutritional deficiency. It sometimes is necessary to provide the patient with a soft diet to reduce discomfort during an extended period of dental repair. Patients should also be instructed in diet modifications for prevention of future caries.

Although the subject is controversial, it is commonly believed that the tooth decay process is related to sugar intake and plaque formation. However, the relationship is not a simple one, since some people with high sugar intake and extensive plaque do not have caries. In general, the simultaneous presence, over a period of time, of three factors — a susceptible tooth, cariogenic bacteria, and substrates for bacterial action — is considered to be necessary to the *cariogenic* (caries-forming) process.

Conditions in the host that produce susceptible teeth are not entirely understood. The effect of nutrition during gestation may be one of these factors. Diet also is believed to have an effect by local action on the tooth while eating. In addition, nutrients from absorbed food secreted into saliva or entering the tooth via its blood supply may affect resistance to decay. These factors need additional study before their role in increasing caries susceptibility can be understood completely.

Cariogenic bacteria, the second requirement for decay, act on monosaccharides or disaccharides, which are the third requirement. Several actions of bacteria may be involved in caries formation. The organism *Streptococcus mutans* is able to synthesize a polysaccharide of glucose, *dextran,* from dietary sucrose. This dextran serves as a matrix that enables the organism to colonize and form plaque on the tooth surface. Various organisms also act on monosaccharides and disaccharides, producing acids which can decalcify the teeth over a period of time. Following this demineralization, proteolytic bacteria attack the protein matrix of the dentin.

The saccharides, or substrates for bacterial action, have been rated as to their cariogenicity: In descending order, they are sucrose, glucose, maltose, lactose, fructose, and sorbitol. When bacteria have access to these materials over a period of time, caries formation is exacerbated by prolonged exposure of the teeth to bacterially produced acid in contact with the teeth, also for an extended time. The most cariogenic foods, therefore, are those that are sweet and sticky and tend to adhere to the teeth. Caries formation is influenced also by the frequency of eating. The intake of cariogenic foods at frequent intervals is thought to be more damaging than eating the same amount all at one time.

Caries prevention is an important objective in nutritional care. Some nutrients are thought to be *cariostatic*—that is, they tend to prevent or arrest the decay process. The phosphate content of the diet may be very important in this way.[6,14] Fat increases saliva flow, forms a protective film on the teeth,[15] and has some antimicrobial activity.[16] Protein also may be cariostatic.[17] For example, the casein of milk has been shown to reduce enamel solubility.[18] Saliva has a urea content equal to that in blood. With increased protein intake, urea concentration rises in both blood and saliva, and ureolytic microorganisms in plaque convert urea to ammonia, raising the pH and decreasing the demineralization of the teeth by acids. The possible toxic effect of the ammonia on surrounding cells has not been investigated. Salivary proteins, such as secretory immunoglobulin A, lactoferrin, lactoperoxidase, and lysozyme, are assumed to minimize the action of pathogenic organisms. It has been suggested that the availability of these proteins can be affected by nutritional status.[19]

Some diseases frequently are associated with caries formation, and good nutritional care for these patients includes procedures for caries prevention, combining diet, oral hygiene, and fluoridation. The diet should be adequate, with the preponderance of the carbohydrate in the form of starch rather than sugar. "Sticky" foods should be avoided. Repetitive snacking, especially of refined sugar, resulting in multiple exposures of the teeth to cariogenic foods, should be avoided. Noncariogenic sweeteners have been suggested, but their systemic effects are as yet unknown. The effects of xylitol, a potential sugar substitute, are currently being investigated. *Fluoridation* is of most benefit when the teeth are being calcified. It is provided in the drinking water in some communities, at a concentration of 1 mg/L, or 1 ppm. It sometimes is provided in tablets or drops at 0.5 to 1.0 mg/day, in topical gels "painted" on by dentists, or in fluoride-containing mouthwashes.

The *nursing bottle syndrome* or *bottle caries syndrome* is another severe problem requiring preventive action. It occurs in young children who habitually are allowed to fall asleep while sucking on a nursing bottle containing fruit juice or a milk formula sweetened with glucose or sucrose. Sucking, swallowing, and salivation decrease during sleep. The liquid then remains in the mouth, and lactic acid formed from the carbohydrate is increased. The result is extensive decay and loss of many of the primary teeth.

To prevent this syndrome, children should not be put to bed with a bottle. If this cannot be avoided, parents are advised that water may be used more safely. Plain milk or a formula sweetened with lactose, but not glucose or sucrose, may be usable. There is some evidence that the milk-saliva mixture from such a formula actually prevents decalcification of the teeth.[20]

Acute Gingivitis and Stomatitis. Gingivitis and *stomatitis* occur as side effects of many other diseases and also can be a consequence of emotional stress. The conditions are seen in mild form in many persons, but gingivitis occasionally occurs in a severe form called *acute necrotizing ulcerative gingivitis* (trench mouth, or Vincent's gingivitis). The direct cause is an infectious organism, but emotional stress, hormone changes, and abnormal diet habits have been implicated as contributing factors.

Early clinical manifestations of gingivitis include easily bleeding gums, a bad taste in the mouth, and fetid breath. The gingivae are red, swollen, and tender. In severe disease, the papillae become ulcerated and necrotic, and the patient suffers from malaise, fever, and serious loss of appetite. The condition makes the mouth susceptible to colonization by other bacteria and predisposes the patient to periodontitis.

Food intake in the patient with gingivitis may be decreased because of pain, presenting a problem in nutritional care. The patient is given a high-protein, high-calorie liquid diet until the condition of the tissues improves. Then the diet is progressed to a soft diet, taking care to avoid spicy or acidic foods, and later, to a relatively unrestricted diet as tolerated. Vitamin supplements sometimes are necessary. Some patients with severe disease need a pain-relieving mouthwash before eating.

Periodontal Disease. Periodontal disease has been estimated to occur in approximately 65 million adults in the United States and to cause loss of teeth in approximately 20 million. It occurs most often in the elderly but is not necessarily related to age; it has been known to begin in adolescence. Periodontal disease tends to occur especially often in patients who are mouth-breathers, or who have diabetes, leukemia, hyperparathyroidism, or hypoparathyroidism. Other factors that contribute to periodontal disease include faulty restorations, missing teeth, misalignment, malocclusion, and the use of tobacco.

It is an inflammatory process that results in a breakdown of the supporting structures of the teeth. The etiology usually is poor oral hygiene, resulting in accumulated plaque and calculus. The gingivae adhere less well to the teeth and pockets form in which debris collects, causing irritation. The inflammation then spreads into the supporting tissue.

The role of nutrition in the etiology of periodontal disease is complex and poorly understood. Squamous epithelium lining the gingival sulcus has a very high turnover rate, being renewed every 3 to 7 days.[21] This fact suggests that gingival tissue is very sensitive to malnutrition. Although periodontal disease is not a primary deficiency disease, the progress of the disease may be affected by the patient's nutritional status.[19] The amount and kind of dental plaque apparently is influenced by diet. It has been suggested that calcium deficiency or phosphorus excess accelerates bone resorption by causing secondary hyperparathyroidism.[22] This is still under investigation. The suggestion that calcium supplements are useful[23] is not commonly accepted.[24] The epithelium in the gingival crevice serves as a protective barrier which may be compromised in nutritional stress.

For periodontal disease, the primary preventive measure is removal of plaque, but diet may serve a supporting role. Patients often are advised to reduce their intake of sucrose and increase their use of firm fibrous foods, such as raw fruits and vegetables. Fibrous foods are believed to provide stimulation to soft tissue, cleanse the teeth, decrease calculus formation, reduce salivary atrophy, and increase salivary flow rates and protein content of saliva. However, the effectiveness of fibrous foods in prevention of periodontal disease has not been documented adequately.[19]

Good nutrition also contributes to the control of periodontal disease by maintaining normal immune function.[19] There is a constant migration of leukocytes through the gingival epithelium into the gingival crevice. Some of the products of their metabolism may be irritants or a source of nutrients to bacteria. On the other hand, leukocytes also provide antibacterial agents such as lysozyme, complement, and antibodies. Generally, it is believed that the gingival fluid is more protective than damaging, but the effect of nutrition on its composition is unknown.[19]

Nutritional care in the treatment of patients with existing periodontal disease consists primarily of the same procedures described for patients with severe gingivitis.

The Edentulous Patient. Several studies have shown a high incidence of nutritional deficiencies in patients who have no teeth or serviceable dentures or in whom the number and location of teeth are inadequate.[25,26] The condition has been called *masticatory insufficiency.*

Patients who have lost part or all of their teeth may have difficulties with closure of the jaw and with chewing and swallowing. As a result, they may choose soft, low-fiber foods of limited variety and amount. The danger of nutrient deficiency thereby is increased. Those who have dentures sometimes have problems adjusting to the dentures and may respond in similar fashion. Both groups should be monitored for vitamin and mineral status. Bran and wheat germ sometimes are added to the diet to provide fiber until the dental problems are corrected and the patient has adjusted to wearing dentures.

Hospitalized elderly patients sometimes have dentures that are ill-fitting secondary to weight loss. The nutritional care specialist should modify the diet as necessary and attempt to promote weight gain to achieve normal weight in such patients.

Other Problems in Chewing and Swallowing

Other conditions, such as fractured jaws and cancer of the jaw, affect the ability to chew or swallow. Chewing and swallowing can also be affected by surgical resection of the tongue, palate, or facial muscles, or by severing the nerves that control these structures. For these patients, it may be necessary to provide all nutrients in liquid form. The types of products and formulations that can be used for this purpose are described under Special Techniques for Nutritional Support (p. 148).

Some patients develop a fear of eating (*sitophobia*), because they have pain or discomfort when they eat. This can occur with inflammation, ulceration, or structural defects in the oral cavity or esophagus. Sometimes medication for pain is provided just before meals. In addition, the following procedures may be helpful to modify the diet to the tolerance of the patient:

1. Avoid foods with high acid, salt, or spice content.
2. Avoid very hot foods.
3. Use cold foods if well tolerated; (these may be irritating to some patients).
4. Use very moist, smooth foods; include liquids with meals.
5. Avoid very dry foods.

Abnormalities of Salivary Gland Function

The symptoms of salivary gland disease are limited in number: swelling, pain, dryness of the mouth (*xerostomia*), and taste abnormalities. Nutritional care is important, because these symptoms often cause a decrease in food intake.

A bad taste is most commonly the result of inflammatory conditions in which pus is produced in the mouth. Xerostomia may be the result of mouth-breathing or of a number of systemic conditions. A classification of causes of xerostomia is given in Table 5-1, and drugs that induce xerostomia as a side effect are listed in Table 5-2. Nutritional care of patients with xerostomia primarily involves procedures to maintain moisture in the mouth. A glycerin-and-lemon mouthwash often is provided to the patients, and they are advised to increase their fluid intake. In severe cases, an artificial saliva may be used to maintain comfort and promote remineralization of the teeth.[27] Carbohydrate solutions are useful to stimulate salivation but should be recommended only for patients who are edentulous. Xerostomia predisposes the individual to dental caries, since saliva, which has a protective effect on the teeth, is lacking. Therefore, sugar solutions should not be recommended for xerostomia patients who have their teeth.

Table 5-1. Etiology of Xerostomia—Classification and Examples

Factors affecting the salivary center
Emotions (fear, excitement, depression, etc.)
Neuroses (endogenous depression)
Organic disease (brain tumor)
Drugs (see Table 5-2)
Factors affecting the autonomic outflow pathway
Encephalitis
Brain tumors
Accidents
Neurosurgical operations
Drugs (see Table 5-2)
Factors affecting salivary gland function
Aplasia
Sjögren's syndrome
Obstruction
Infection
Irradiation
Excision
Factors producing changes in fluid or electrolyte balance
Dehydration
Diabetes insipidus
Cardiac failure
Uremia
Edema

Reprinted with permission from Mason, D.K., and Chisholm, D.M., *Salivary Glands in Health and Disease*. London: W.B. Saunders, 1973, p. 120.

Table 5-2. Classes of Drugs with Xerostomic Side Effects

Analgesic mixtures
Anticonvulsants
Antiemetics
Antihistamines
Antihypertensives
Antinauseants
Antiparkinsonism agents
Antipruritics
Antispasmodics
Appetite suppressants
Cold medications
Decongestants
Diuretics
Expectorants
Muscle relaxants
Psychotropic drugs
Central nervous system depressants
Benzodiazepine derivatives
Monoamine oxidase inhibitors
Phenothiazine derivatives
Tranquilizers—major and minor
Sedatives

Reprinted with permission from Bahn, S.L., Drug-related dental destruction. *Oral Surg.* 33:50, 1972.

It is important to provide adequate nutrition at all times in salivary gland disease. The patient's preferences should be catered to as much as possible.

Loss of Taste Sensation

A description of the anatomic basis for taste sensations and a list of drugs that alter taste sensations and the acceptability of foods are included in Chapter 3. Changes in metabolism and the anatomy in the head area may result in alteration in taste. The palate is most sensitive to bitter and sour. Flavors including these components are altered in patients with upper dentures that cover the palate, with tumors of the palate, or in whom the palate has been surgically removed. Patients with Turner's syndrome, a chromosomal disorder, have highly arched palates and diminished taste perception. Diseases of the tongue may also affect the sense of taste. Some examples are abnormalities affecting the nerves of the tongue, as in Bell's palsy and neuritis, surgical resection of the nerves, and tumors of the tongue. In addition, patients receiving irradiation treatment to the mouth have a decreased sense of taste. Some nervous system conditions, such as multiple sclerosis and head injuries, can have a similar effect. Various metabolic abnormalities altering the sense of taste are listed in Table 3-3.

Since smell and taste interact to a great extent in producing flavor sensations, injury to the olfactory nerve, as from whiplash injury or fracture of the nose, can cause temporary or permanent impairment of olfactory sensation. This may erroneously be perceived by the patient as "taste" impairment.

The nutritional care specialist must be understanding of the problems of lost taste sensation and provide individualized attention to these patients. The patient's preferences should be considered in planning meals. Seasonings may be increased or decreased to conform with the patient's preference in order to make foods more acceptable. Heat tends to increase the sensation of flavor, and cold, to decrease it; flavorings and seasonings should be added with these facts in mind. The sense of taste sometimes varies during the day. If so, the patient can be expected to prefer to eat larger meals when the sense of taste is impaired the least.

Effect of Aging on the Oral Cavity

In the aged, the tongue tends to lose its papillae and the number of taste bud cells declines, with a consequent decrease in the sense of taste.[28] Both taste bud cells and olfactory receptors are replaced frequently; they have average life spans of 10 days and 30 days, respectively. Structural changes in the taste system and olfactory system in the brain have been observed in the aged.[29] Detrimental alterations have been reported in the amygdala, hippocampus, and olfactory bulb of the brain.[30–33] The sense of smell declines, and it has been shown that the aged have a decreased ability to identify tastes.[29] As a result, contrary to common belief, many aging patients find that highly seasoned foods are more acceptable. Enhancement with artificial flavors has been recommended.[29]

Also in elderly patients, the mucous membrane becomes thinner and more susceptible to injury. Consequently, patients may choose soft, easily chewed foods which do not adequately stimulate gingival circulation or saliva flow. At the same time, the cells in the salivary glands atrophy, causing a decrease in salivation and a change in saliva composition. The deficiency of saliva contributes to a dry mucosa and difficulties in chewing and swallowing. Patients may be advised to chew moist foods and sugarless gum to stimulate saliva flow. Lemons also stimulate saliva flow. Patients should be counseled on food choices to meet nutritional needs within the limits of the textures that they can tolerate.

Aging patients sometimes have teeth that are worn and shortened, producing overclosure of the jaws with pain and limitation of jaw movement. For them, a reduction in the intake of very hard foods may be helpful.

THE ESOPHAGUS

Normal Anatomy and Physiology

The esophagus is a tube that carries foods from the pharynx to the stomach. Its structure is similar to that of the intestine, which is shown in Fig. 5-2, except that the esophagus has no mesentery or serosa. The mucosa does not absorb as it does in some parts of the alimentary tract.

The *upper esophageal sphincter* (UES) remains closed except during swallowing, preventing the flow of air into the esophagus and into the stomach. At the lower end of the esophagus, there is no obvious sphincter muscle present, but a few centimeters above the entrance of the esophagus into the stomach, the muscle structure functions as if it were a sphincter and therefore is referred to in the literature as the *lower esophageal sphincter* (LES). The LES normally remains contracted, closing the entrance to the stomach and preventing reflux of the stomach contents into the lower esophagus. It opens when swallowed material reaches the bottom of the esophagus, allowing the bolus of material to enter the stomach. Defects of function of the LES may arise from alterations in the smooth muscle, the innervations of the muscle, or in its hormonal control. The interrelationships of hormone action and sphincter pressure is controversial. Gastrin has a major effect in increasing LES pressure.[34–36] Hormones decreasing pressure include secretin,[37,38] cholecystokinin,[39,40] and glucagon.[41]

The LES contains many drug receptors.[42] Peppermint,[43] spearmint, chocolate,[44] alcohol,[45] and fats,[46] including fat in whole milk, reduce LES pressure. The methylxanthines caffeine and theophylline, contained in coffee and tea, have been reported to increase LES pressure by inhibiting phosphodiesterase and thus increasing intracellular concentrations of cyclic adenosine monophosphate in the LES,[47] whereas other reports state that theophylline decreases LES pressure and caffeine has no effect.[46] Coffee is reported to have an effect different from that of pure caffeine. Both caffeinated and decaffeinated coffees were found to cause increased LES pressure in one study.[48] Therefore, some unknown substance in coffee may cause the increase. The mode of action of the carminatives peppermint and spearmint is unknown but is thought to be a local effect.

Since the intake and action of caffeine and related compounds is of concern in several diseases, relevant facts on these substances are outlined in Appendix I.

Esophageal Disease

Disorders of the esophagus may be classified as obstructive, inflammatory, or nervous in origin. Since they compromise the ability to swallow, they affect the ability to consume food and so place the patient at nutritional risk.

Conditions Causing Dysphagia and Odynophagia

In many esophageal diseases, the patient has *dysphagia* (difficulty in swallowing). The term does *not* include pain. Dysphagia has been classified as preesophageal or esophageal, depending on the localization of its cause.

In *preesophageal dysphagia,* the patient has difficulty moving the bolus of food from the oral pharynx to the esophagus. This occurs in patients with central nervous system lesions and other neuromuscular disorders, including parkinsonism, dermatomyositis (an inflammation of the skin, subcutaneous tissue, and muscle), myotonic dystrophy (a disease marked by stiffening and atrophy of the muscles, especially in the head and neck), myasthenia gravis (a disease marked by progressive paralysis, affecting especially the head and neck), and bulbar poliomyelitis.

The underlying lesion of *esophageal dysphagia* may be of the obstructive or motor type. *Obstructive* disorders are caused by factors that reduce the size of the lumen of the esophagus. These factors include trauma with development of scar tissue, inelasticity resulting from repeated inflammation, development of an esophageal ring or web, or the presence of a tumor in the esophagus or adjacent tissue. In *motor* disorders, lesions occur in the nervous or muscular system, with consequent paralysis or disordered swallowing mechanisms. Transport of the bolus is interrupted, but the lumen is not obstructed. An example is diffuse esophageal spasm or curling, in which the esophagus has segmental spasms so that fluoroscopy shows a string-of-beads appearance.

Dysphagia may consist of an interference with the transport of solids or liquids or both. This is a matter of importance in diagnosis and in nutritional management. Dysphagia from obstructive lesions affects the ability to swallow solids. In the motor or nervous type of lesion, dysphagia affects passage of both solids and liquids.

Pain on swallowing (*odynophagia*) frequently, but not always, accompanies dysphagia. It can result from a motor or nervous disorder, a neoplasm, infection, ingestion of caustic chemicals, or from other causes of destruction of the mucosa. Odynophagia can seriously interfere with adequate nutrient intake.

Nutritional care of patients with dysphagia or odynophagia includes changes in the consistency of the diet and in feeding techniques. Extremes of temperature of foods should be avoided for patients who complain of dysphagia for very hot or very cold foods. The patient with dysphagia for solids often finds a soft or semisoft diet more easily tolerated. A liquid diet may be useful for the patient with dysphagia for both solids and liquids. Tube feedings or other special techniques sometimes are required. Pain can be reduced by limiting foods that are high in salt, spices, or acid, or are very dry or very hot. Care is needed to assure that food intake is sufficient to maintain adequate nutritional status.

Disorders of the Lower Esophageal Sphincter

Some special considerations apply for patients with disorders of the LES.

Achalasia. Achalasia, also known as *esophageal dyssynergia, aperistalsis, megaesophagus,* or *cardiospasm,* is a condition in which the lower esophageal sphincter maintains an excessively high tone while resting and fails to open properly when the patient swallows. In addition, peristalsis in the upper esophagus often is disordered. As a result, the esophagus becomes shaped like a funnel or bag. Symptoms include dysphagia, a feeling of fullness in the chest, and frequent vomiting. The patient loses weight and becomes seriously malnourished if the condition remains uncorrected. Aspiration during the night may lead to pulmonary infection.

At one time, the condition was considered to be emotional in origin. However, there is some evidence that achalasia patients have fewer ganglion cells than normal in the myenteric plexus.[49] In addition, these ganglion cells are surrounded by inflammatory cells, suggesting a physiologic basis for the condition.

Treatment consists of dilating the LES with an air-filled or water-filled bag or partially slitting the muscle surgically (*esophagomyotomy*). These treatments improve the symptoms of obstruction but do not correct the deficit in peristalsis.

Nutritional care is particularly important in the period prior to dilation or surgical treatment. The major change is usually in the consistency of the diet. Semisolid or liquid foods often are tolerated best, since peristalsis is not required for fluids to move through the esophagus. This and other alterations in the diet that may be helpful in achalasia are given in Table 5-3.

Table 5-3. Nutritional Care in Achalasia

Give semisolid or liquid foods as tolerated.

Provide small, frequent meals as tolerated.

Reduce protein and carbohydrate and increase fat in the diet to promote reduced gastric secretion and a decrease in lower esophageal sphincter pressure.

Avoid temperature extremes in foods.

Avoid foods such as citrus juices and highly spiced foods, which can injure the esophageal mucosa if retained.

Use a low-fiber diet if the patient finds it easier to swallow.

Encourage the patient to eat slowly.

After dilation, the patient is not allowed to eat or drink for at least an hour to avoid spasm of the esophagus. A light meal may be eaten in several hours, and solid foods, the next day.[50]

Postoperative management of the patient with esophagomyotomy often allows oral fluid intake the same day. A normal diet is reinstated as soon as the patient can tolerate it, usually in less than 5 days. Reflux of gastric contents and the development of esophagitis are possible side effects of the surgery.

Stricture of the Esophagus. A *stricture* is narrowing of the lumen of the esophagus, usually in the lower two-thirds. It most often is due to inflammation from reflux of gastric acid, ingestion of caustic chemicals, or from a hernia or a tumor in or adjacent to the esophagus. A stricture interferes with food intake in the same way as does achalasia. The general approach to nutritional care is similar to that described for achalasia.

Lower Esophageal Sphincter Incompetence. If the lower esophageal sphincter does not maintain a pressure that is higher than the pressure in the stomach, the contents of the stomach will back up into the esophagus, a condition known as *gastroesophageal reflux.* The wall of the esophagus is not protected from the acid of the stomach and, during reflux, the patient feels a burning sensation behind the sternum that radiates toward the mouth. This condition is known as *heartburn* or *pyrosis.* It is unrelated to disease of the heart.

The hormone gastrin has been shown to cause an increase in LES pressure; therefore, it has been suggested that decreased LES pressure is caused by a deficiency of gastrin. Investigation of gastrin levels in patients, however, show that there are also other factors in lowered LES pressure. One possibility is an abnormality in the sphincter muscle itself.

Another factor is the presence of a *hiatal hernia,* in which a portion of the stomach protrudes up into the chest cavity through the opening where the esophagus penetrates the diaphragm. At one time, it was thought that hiatal hernia was the cause of gastroesophageal reflux, but surgical repair of the hernia did not always correct the symptoms. Recent evidence suggests that a hiatal hernia is not the major mechanism but may contribute to the symptoms by interfering with the process of clearing acid from the esophagus following reflux, especially if the patient is lying down.

Scleroderma is a connective tissue disease which often involves the gastrointestinal tract. It results in decreased peristalsis and LES pressure, possibly as the result of a neural dysfunction and muscle atrophy.[51]

Estrogen and progesterone have been shown to reduce LES pressure, possibly by diminishing the response to gastrin. This offers an explanation for the increase in heartburn in pregnancy and in women taking contraceptive drugs.[52] Cigarette smoking has a similar effect.

A number of drugs also lower LES pressure. As a result, gastroesophageal reflux and heartburn may occur as a side effect of the drugs used in the treatment of other conditions. Some of these drugs and their

Table 5-4. Drugs That Decrease Lower Esophageal Sphincter Pressure

Drug	Use
Atropine	Anticholinergic; antispasmodic
Diazepam	Tranquilizer
Dopamine HCl	Antiparkinsonism agent
Isoproterenol	Beta-adrenergic agent
Morphine	Narcotic; analgesic
Nitroglycerine	Treatment of symptoms of angina
Nitroprusside	Vasodilator
Phentolamine	Alpha-adrenergic antagonist (shown in animals only)
Theophylline	Smooth muscle relaxant; phosphodiesterase inhibitor

uses are listed in Table 5-4. When patients are receiving these drugs, nutritional care specialists should be alert to the development of reduced LES pressure as a side effect, since it may affect food intake.

Drugs and nutritional care are both components of treatment. A mainstay of drug treatment for gastroesophageal reflux is the use of antacids. A mixture of aluminum hydroxide and alginic acid (Gaviscon) floats on top of the gastric contents and reduces the tendency to reflux. Bethanechol chloride may be used to increase LES pressure in patients who are resistant to antacid and diet treatment.

Nutritional care in gastroesophageal reflux includes procedures to (1) increase LES pressure, (2) lessen esophageal irritation, (3) improve clearing of materials from the esophagus, and (4) decrease the frequency and volume of reflux. The general nutritional status of the patient should be monitored. Specific procedures are listed in Table 5-5.

Table 5-5. Nutritional Care in Gastroesophageal Reflux

Increase lower esophageal sphincter pressure
- Increase protein in diet
- Decrease fat in diet to <45 g/day
- Avoid alcohol, peppermint, spearmint
- Avoid coffee, strong tea, and chocolate if not well tolerated
- Use *skim* milk

Decrease irritation in the esophagus
- Avoid irritants: citrus juices, tomato, coffee, spicy foods, carbonated beverages
- Avoid any other foods that regularly cause heartburn (*may* include rich pastry and frosted cakes)

Improve clearing of the esophagus
- Do not recline for >2 hr after eating
- Elevate head of bed

Decrease frequency and volume of reflux
- Elevate head of bed
- Do not recline for >2 hr after eating
- Eat small meals, more frequent meals if necessary
- Reduce weight if overweight
- Sip only small amounts of fluids with meals
- Drink most fluids between meals
- Include enough fiber to avoid constipation (straining increases intraabdominal pressure)

Nutritional and other considerations
- Monitor effect of citrus and tomato avoidance on ascorbic acid status; supplement as necessary
- Monitor effect of antacids on iron status; supplement if necessary
- Avoid chewing gum (causes air swallowing)
- Avoid smoking immediately following meals

Esophagitis

Chronic esophageal reflux and heartburn can result in esophagitis of the lower esophagus. *Plummer-Vinson syndrome,* inflammation in the upper part of the organ, may result from iron and vitamin B complex deficiency. The nutritional deficiency causes changes in the mucosa, making it more susceptible to damage. A variety of other agents—bacterial, chemical, physical, and traumatic—also cause chronic esophagitis. Nutritional care is generally the same as that for gastroesophageal reflux.

Replacement of the Esophagus

Conditions that may require the replacement of the esophagus include congenital atresia of the esophagus, trauma, stricture, and carcinoma. A portion of the stomach, colon, or jejunum is used as the replacement.

Problems with eating and slow weight gain are common postoperatively. The patient sometimes continues to complain of dysphagia. Solid foods are especially troublesome, but the symptom improves with time. In the interim, suggestions for high-calorie foods to maintain weight are helpful to the patient. Some patients complain that food is tasteless or that there is a constant salty taste in the mouth. This also improves with time. Patients should be encouraged to eat small, frequent meals and to avoid taking solid and liquid foods at the same meal.[53]

THE STOMACH

Normal Anatomy and Physiology

The major parts of the stomach are shown in Fig. 5-5. The stomach's functions are storage, mixing, propulsion of its contents into the intestine, and a small amount of digestion. In addition, the stomach secretes intrinsic factor and gastrin.

Secretion

Important constituents of gastric juice are hydrochloric acid, pepsin, mucus, and intrinsic factor. The usual volume of gastric juice is 1 to 2 liters, but it may reach 8 liters in disease.

Secretion of gastric juice is stimulated by a large number of factors which are classified as cephalic, gastric, or intestinal. In the *cephalic phase,* the pleasant smell or taste of food, chewing, and swallowing stimulate receptors in the mouth and nose. Impulses travel via the vagus nerves to the stomach, where the release of acetylcholine stimulates mucus, acid, and pepsinogen secretion in the body and gastrin release in the antrum. The response is greater to food the person likes and is less marked in response to bland food. These facts should be kept in mind in nutritional care of the anorexic patient. In the *gastric phase,* protein and amino acids in the stomach stimulate secretion by direct contact. Food causes a rise in pH, stimulating the vagus nerves, while distension of the stomach stimulates mechanoreceptors in the mucosa. Calcium and caffeine stimulate acid-secreting cells directly. In the *intestinal phase,* the products of protein digestion stimulate hydrogen ion secretion in the stomach.

Gastric secretion is inhibited by drugs such as atropine and by reflexes initiated by acid, fat, and solutions with high osmotic activity. The hormones cholecystokinin and secretin also inhibit secretion.

The mucosal surface of the stomach is perforated by *gastric pits.* In the proximal two-thirds of the stomach, three to seven gastric glands extend down from the bottom of the pits. These glands contain four types of secretory cells.

Figure 5-5. The parts of the stomach and duodenum. The border between the pyloric glandular mucosa and the oxyntic glandular mucosa does not exactly coincide with the border between antrum and body. (Borders are indicated by straight arrowless lines through figure.) (Reprinted with permission from Davenport, H.W., A Digest of Digestion, *2nd ed. Copyright © 1978 by Year Book Medical Publishers, Inc., Chicago. P. 46.)*

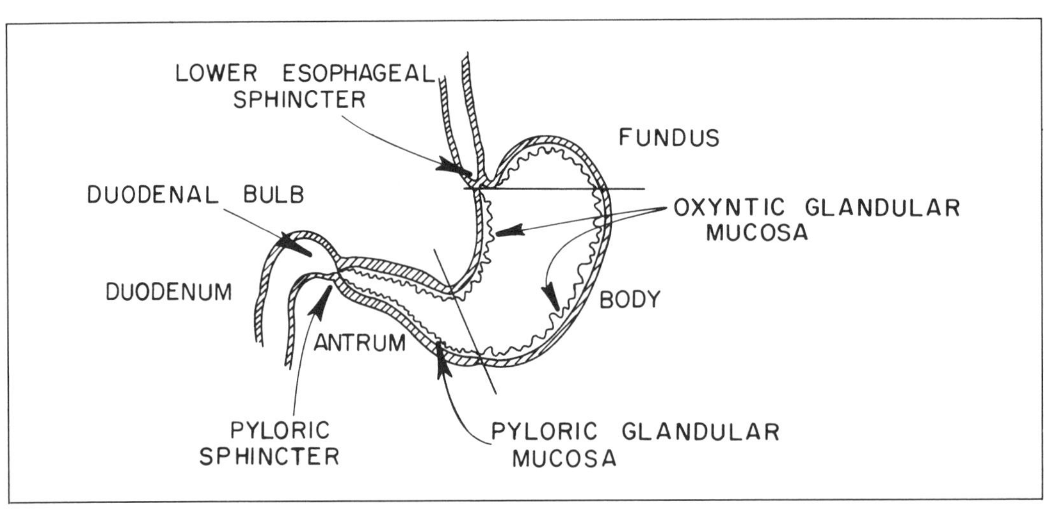

Chief or *peptic* or *zymogenic cells* line the walls of the base of the gland in a single layer and secrete pepsinogen into the lumen of the gland. The secretion of pepsinogen is strongly stimulated by acetylcholine, produced as a result of stimulation of the vagus nerves during the cephalic or gastric phase. The acid of the gastric juice also affects the production of pepsin by means of conversion of pepsinogen to pepsin at pH 2, stimulation of secretion of pepsinogen, and enhancement of other stimuli of chief cells.

Oxyntic or *parietal cells* lie between, and also peripheral to, the chief cells. They contain canaliculi (small channels) within the cell and extend between the chief cells to allow their secretions to be discharged into the lumen of the gland. Oxyntic cells secrete hydrochloric acid and intrinsic factor. The acid has many functions. It converts pepsinogen to pepsin, inhibits secretion of gastrin, stimulates secretion of secretin, and has a bacteriostatic effect, preventing infection in the gastrointestinal tract. The amount of acid produced normally and in some disease states is given in Appendix G. The amount that can be produced with maximum stimulation also is given. Histamine or pentagastrin are used as the stimulants. These values are important reference points when interpreting patients' charts.

Gastric juice also contains a large amount of water and sodium, potassium, and chloride ions. If a patient's gastric contents is being aspirated, the lost fluid and electrolytes must be carefully replaced.

Argentaffin cells also occur in the gastric glands and are responsible for the secretion of histamine, serotonin (5-hydroxytryptamine), and heparin. The cells occur singly between the chief cells and basement membrane.

The *mucous neck* or *mucous chief cells* line the neck of the gland. The neck is that area which extends from the gland to the epithelial cells lining the pit. They secrete mucus, as the name indicates, and are stimulated by the vagus nerves. They also provide replacement cells for surrounding areas.

The mucosal surface and pits in the stomach are covered with *surface mucous cells.* The mucus that they secrete stains differently in the laboratory from the mucus of the chief cells, indicating some difference in its composition. Secretion is stimulated by physical contact with stomach contents and by contact with certain specific materials in the stomach, such as alcohol. Mucus in the stomach protects the mucosal surface, particularly from autodigestion by gastric secretions.

Glands in other areas differ from those in the body of the stomach. In a band around the cardia, the glands are known as *cardiac glands* and contain some oxyntic cells. The *pyloric glands* occur in the distal one-ninth of the stomach. They contain mucous neck cells and a few oxyntic cells. *Surface mucous cells* occur throughout the stomach.

The mucosa of the antrum includes *G cells,* the source of gastrin, which stimulates acid and pepsinogen secretion. Gastrin also increases gastric blood flow, circular muscle contraction in the stomach, and growth of the mucosa of the stomach and small intestine. Alcohol or meat in the diet stimulates the release of gastrin.

Storage and Motility

The empty stomach has a volume of only 50 ml or so, but it relaxes and enlarges with each swallow. Its maximum capacity has been estimated to be approximately 1,600 ml. As the stomach empties, the *orad* half (closer to the mouth) contracts and maintains the pressure gradient toward the duodenum. There is little mixing of stomach contents in this area, since the fundus and body of the stomach have only weak contractions. Peristalsis begins in the middle of the stomach and progresses toward the duodenum, mixing ingested material and gastric secretions to produce *chyme.*

Peristalsis in the stomach also pushes some chyme into the duodenum. By this process, the stomach is emptied. The time required varies with the nature of the gastric contents and the degree of distension. Solids, lipids, and solutions of high osmotic pressure are emptied from the stomach more slowly than are isotonic solutions. Liquids are emptied more rapidly than solids. In the duodenum, receptors respond to the osmotic pressure, acidity, and lipid content of chyme. The means by which they control gastric emptying are incompletely understood, but some factors involved are gastrointestinal hormones and neurologic reflexes.

The *enterogastric reflex* inhibits peristalsis in the antrum. It is initiated when chyme in the stomach has high or low osmotic activity relative to plasma or when hydrogen ion concentration in the intestine is high. Particle size, viscosity of chyme, and volume of gastric contents also affect emptying time. Emotional stress affects motility by stimulation of the autonomic nervous system.

Digestion

Although some small molecules are absorbed from the stomach, only limited digestion occurs. Pepsin is specific for peptide bonds involving aromatic amino acids. The action of salivary amylase on starch continues when food reaches the stomach until terminated by the low pH of the gastric juice. The stomach produces some gastric lipase, which acts on short- and medium-chain triglycerides. None of these actions are extensive or essential for digestion.

Nausea and Vomiting

Nausea is a feeling of distress with the sensation of the need to vomit. The mechanism by which it is produced is unclear. The vestibules of the ears may be involved, as they are in motion sickness. The nauseated patient has a contraction of the duodenum along with decreased tone and motility in the stomach.

Vomiting or *emesis,* the forceful expulsion of gastrointestinal contents via the mouth, is distinct from *regurgitation,* the slow return of food to the mouth. Vomiting usually is accompanied by nausea but may occur independently. Vomiting usually is preceded by activity of the sympathetic nervous system, indicated by sweating, salivation, pallor, dilated pupils, and sometimes by retching (involuntary movements of vomiting without expulsion of vomitus). During vomiting, abdominal muscles and the diaphragm contract, increasing pressure in the stomach. The LES relaxes, allowing expulsion of the gastric contents.

Nausea and vomiting are manifestations of many diseases. They often occur in acute abdominal emergencies such as appendicitis, peritonitis, and intestinal obstruction. In addition, nausea and vomiting are symptoms of diseases of other organ systems. They occur in some cardiovascular diseases such as myocardial infarction and congestive heart failure. Central nervous system disorders, disorders of the labyrinths of the ear, and endocrine disorders, such as diabetic acidosis and adrenal insufficiency, also lead to vomiting. The morning sickness of early pregnancy probably is hormonal in origin. Drugs causing severe nausea and vomiting are listed in Chapter 3.

A brief episode of vomiting is not usually of consequence to the patient's nutrition, but prolonged vomiting may have many deleterious effects. The metabolic effects are diagrammed in Fig. 5-6. Patients also may have extreme weight loss with deficiencies of many nutrients. Severe vomiting sometimes tears the junction of the esophagus and stomach (Mallory-Weiss syndrome). Some patients—infants and those in a coma, for example—may aspirate vomitus, producing aspiration pneumonia.

Nutritional care of the patient with severe and prolonged vomiting is difficult. In many instances, no food intake is possible and the

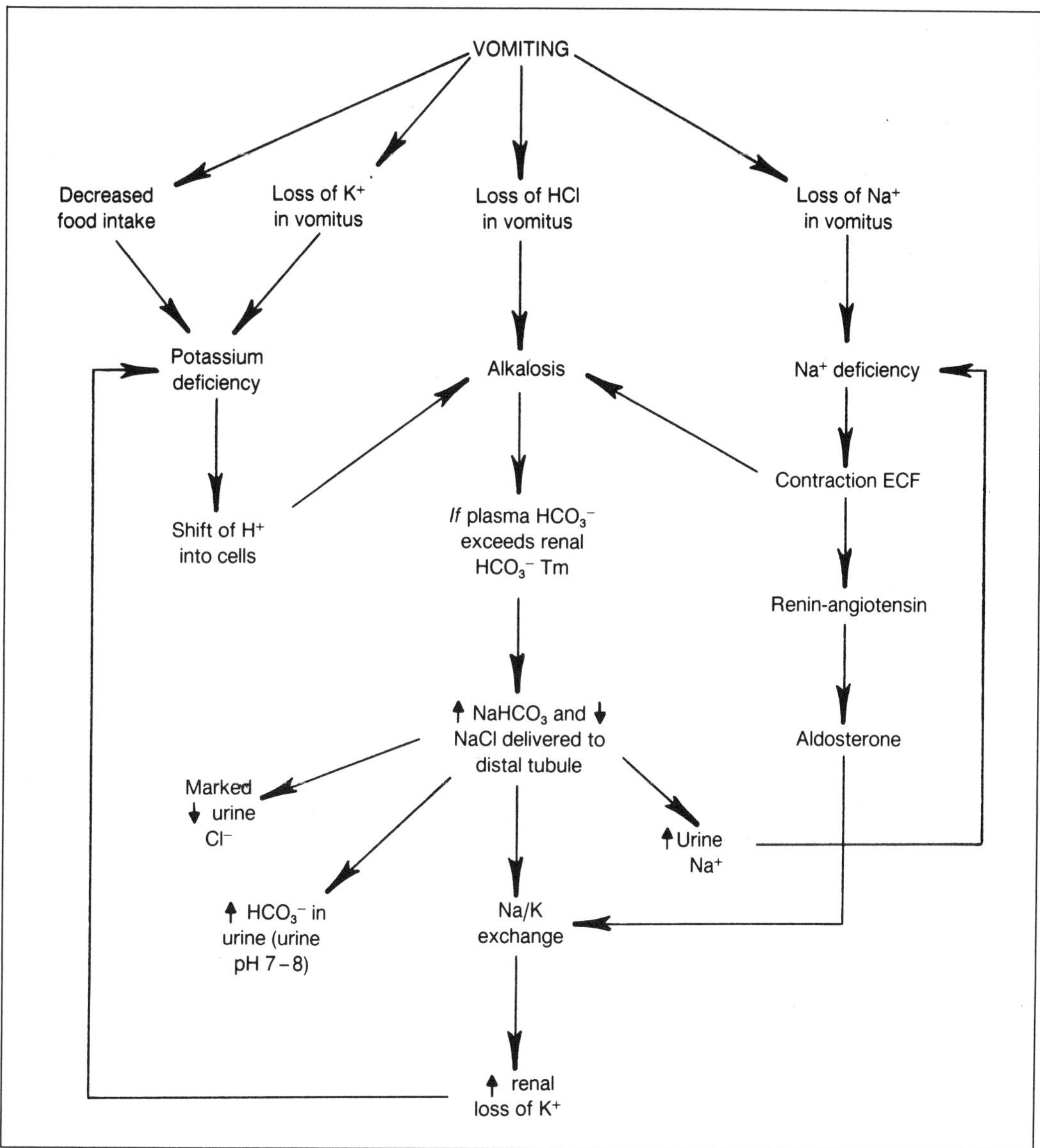

Figure 5-6. Metabolic consequences of vomiting. ECF = extracellular fluid; Tm = renal tubular maximum. (Reprinted with permission from Fordtran, J.S., Vomiting. In M.H. Sleisenger and J.S. Fordtran, Eds., Gastrointestinal Disease. *Philadelphia: W.B. Saunders, 1973, p. 140.)*

patient must be fed parenterally. The techniques in Table 5-6 may be useful if oral intake is possible.

Gastritis

Symptoms

Gastritis, an inflammation of the gastric mucosa, may be acute or chronic. The usual

Table 5-6. Suggestions for Nutritional Care in Prolonged Vomiting

Recommended foods and foods to avoid

Avoid intake of liquids with meals. Drink liquids between meals, at least 1 hr before or after meals.

Cold liquids may be tolerated better than those that are hot.

Carbonated beverages sometimes can reduce nausea. Popsicles and gelatin dishes are useful to increase fluid intake.

Eat dry toast, crackers, or dry cereal when feeling nauseated. These sometimes are helpful before arising if morning nausea occurs.

Avoid foods that many persons find difficult to tolerate, including strong-flavored vegetables such as those in the onion and cabbage family, coffee, highly spiced foods, and high-fat and fried foods. Try skim milk in place of whole milk.

Avoid highly acidic foods if they are troublesome; in some cases, tart foods may help to control nausea.

Use cold foods without aromas which may cause nausea. Try sandwiches, fruit plates, or cold meat plates.

Eat frequent small meals. This may be helpful to avoid overdistention of the abdomen and, at the same time, avoid having an empty stomach for a prolonged period.

Other recommendations

If vomiting is sporadic and predictable, eat rapidly digested and absorbed foods in the intervals between episodes of vomiting.

Relax, chew foods well, and breathe deeply and swallow when feeling nauseated. Eat and drink slowly.

Stay quiet 1 hr or more following meals.

Eat whatever will stay down. Cater to the patient's preferences.

symptoms of gastritis include a feeling of fullness, anorexia, nausea and vomiting, fever, and epigastric pain, but chronic gastritis sometimes is asymptomatic.

Acute Gastritis

Acute gastritis frequently is the result of alcoholic abuse or ingestion of corrosive chemicals. Other causes include overeating, eating too fast, and eating when emotionally upset. Gastritis may result from bacterial or viral infection, including food poisoning. The infection sometimes enters from the blood, and the condition then is called *hematogenous gastritis.* Diseased periodontal tissue, tonsils, or sinuses sometimes are the source of infection. Gastritis may be secondary to other conditions, including uremia (see Chapter 7), conditions causing shock, and allergies. Intake of drugs such as salicylates, some antibiotics, and ammonium chloride also may cause gastritis. Gastritis from all causes is much more common than are ulcers.

The patient with acute gastritis is not given any food for 1 to 2 days but may be given ice for comfort to reduce mouth dryness. Drinking water is avoided, since water stimulates gastric secretion. Liquids are added as tolerated as recovery progresses. When the patient is free of symptoms, the diet is progressed to a soft and then a house diet, similar to those described in Chapter 2 with omission of those food items that tend to cause gastric irritation. These are somewhat variable among individuals but usually include alcohol, black pepper, chili powder, and the sources of caffeine listed in Appendix I.

Chronic Gastritis

There are several forms of *chronic gastritis* which are distinguished by the appearance of the tissues—*superficial, atrophic,* or *hypertrophic. Menetrier's disease* is a hypertrophic type characterized by increased height and thickness of the gastric folds on the greater curvature of the stomach. There also are changes in the cell structure of the mucosa, which becomes very permeable to serum proteins. Proteins exude into the stomach and are digested. The condition may cause protein deficiency with hypoproteinemia and edema.

The cause of chronic gastritis is unknown. It precedes or occurs along with gastric ulcers, cancer of the stomach, pernicious anemia, diabetes, tuberculosis, heart failure, or nephritis. It also occurs in chronic iron deficiency. Patients who take aspirin frequently, such as those with arthritis, frequently develop chronic gastritis. It also is seen in patients of advanced age. An immune mechanism may be involved in gastric atrophy.[54]

The major objectives of nutritional care for chronic gastritis are the avoidance of irritants and promotion of patient comfort. Small, frequent feedings of soft foods are given. Excess amounts of liquid with meals, as well as the specific gastric irritants listed previously, should be avoided, and a bland diet sometimes is recommended.[55] Unfortunately, there is little agreement on which foods should be included and which should be eliminated from the bland diet. Studies have shown that many foods formerly thought to be irritating were not. As a result, it is difficult to develop a rationale for the use of this diet.

Gastric atrophy in the chronic gastritis patient may involve loss of parietal cells and consequent decrease in intrinsic factor secretion. Since this increases the risk of vitamin B_{12} malabsorption, the patient's vitamin B_{12} status should be monitored and replacement provided if indicated.

Peptic Ulcer Disease

An *ulcer* is a circumscribed loss of tissue on the surface of the mucosa or skin. In the gastrointestinal tract, an ulcer is distinguished by the fact that it extends through the mucosa, submucosa, and sometimes, the muscle layer. It is distinct from an erosion in which the lesion is superficial and does not extend through the mucosa.

A *peptic ulcer* can occur in any area that is exposed to pepsin; the tissue must also be exposed to acid. Depending on location, peptic ulcers may be *gastric* (found in the stomach), *duodenal* (found in the duodenal bulb), or *esophageal* (occurring in the lower esophagus as a result of chronic reflux of gastric contents). If the patient's duodenum is surgically removed and the jejunum is joined to the stomach, a peptic ulcer may develop in the jejunum; this is called a *jejunal ulcer.* The creation of a passage between two normally separated organs is an *anastamosis.* Therefore, an ulcer in the area where stomach and jejunum are joined is an *anastamotic ulcer.* Most ulcers occur within 3 cm of the pylorus. Gastric ulcers are located most frequently on the lesser curvature in the antrum where it meets the body of the stomach. Usually, there is gastritis in the surrounding tissue.

Acute Ulcers

The cause of peptic ulcer is unknown. *Acute ulcers* or *stress ulcers* are associated with other conditions. For example, Curling's ulcer is secondary to severe burns, and Cushing's ulcer occurs in association with cerebral disease or brain surgery. Acute ulcers tend to manifest themselves by causing gastrointestinal bleeding or by perforation into the abdominal space, accompanied by pain, shock, and collapse. Management usually is with drugs or surgery.

Chronic Ulcers

Occurrence. Chronic peptic ulcer disease (PUD) is more common than acute ulcers, although the incidence of chronic duodenal ulcers has decreased in the last 20 years. Peptic ulcer disease occurs more frequently in men than women, but the incidence is increasing in women. Peptic ulcers can occur in children but are more usually found in the 35- to 55-year age group. Duodenal ulcers are four to five times more common than gastric ulcers. Duodenal and gastric ulcers vary somewhat in pathogenesis and in treatment. Both types of ulcer are discussed here for convenience even though, strictly speaking, a duodenal ulcer is not a disease of the stomach.

Predisposing Factors. Some genetic factors are believed to contribute to the incidence of chronic PUD. This belief is based on the observation that persons with blood group

O have a higher incidence of duodenal ulcers than do those with A, B, or AB blood groups, and those with blood group A have an increased incidence of gastric ulcer. Some persons secrete blood group mucopolysaccharides into gastrointestinal secretions. Nonsecretors are more likely to develop ulcers than are the secretors. It has been suggested that the blood group substances may protect against ulcerations.

It frequently is stated that some personality factors contribute to the incidence of PUD. It is commonly believed that tense, nervous, aggressive individuals are prone to the development of ulcers, but there is some contrary evidence that stress and personality factors are not associated with PUD.[56,57] Other possible predisposing factors are smoking and chronic drug ingestion of salicylates (aspirin), indomethacin, glucocorticoids, or caffeine. Diet has been thought to be involved, but there are no data to support this belief.

Pathogenesis. The pathogenesis of PUD is not entirely clear. It is generally agreed that there are parallel increases in acid and pepsin secretion, a decrease in resistance of the mucosa to digestion, or both. However, many questions remain to be answered.

High acid production does seem necessary for ulcer formation, since patients with achlorhydria almost never have gastric ulcers, but frequently the acid levels in the gastric juices of gastric ulcer patients are in the normal range. Two explanations have been offered for the absence of elevated hydrochloric acid in gastric ulcer patients: (1) An excess of acid is secreted but is reabsorbed by abnormal hydrogen ion diffusion that damages the mucosal barrier, or (2) a reflux of duodenal contents destroys the mucosal barrier and hydrogen ion is reabsorbed.[58]

Hypersecretion of acid commonly is associated with duodenal ulcer. The factors that cause hypersecretion are only partially understood. It is in the pathogenesis of duodenal ulcer that psychological factors are commonly believed to play a role.

A number of factors have been suggested as contributing to a decrease in mucosal resistance. These include:

1. Vascular factors in which *local ischemia* damages the mucosa.
2. An abnormality in the pylorus causing a delay in gastric emptying. The resultant distension of the antrum stimulates gastrin release, with consequent acid hypersecretion and mucosal damage (Fig. 5-7A). Excess acid delivered to the duodenum may overwhelm the neutralizing capacity of the pancreatic juice.
3. A disturbance in movement of materials through the pylorus, allowing the reflux of duodenal contents into the stomach. The bile acids present in the duodenal contents damage the gastric mucosa (Fig. 5-7B).
4. Ingestion of drugs such as salicylates, indomethacin, glucocorticoids, and caffeine, which causes mucosal damage similar to that caused by bile.

The *Zollinger-Ellison syndrome* is the cause of a particularly severe form of PUD. Zollinger-Ellison syndrome is due to a non-beta islet cell tumor of the pancreas, in the wall of the duodenum, or in locations outside of the gastrointestinal tract. The tumor is malignant in approximately 60 percent of the patients. Gastrin is secreted in large quantities by patients with Zollinger-Ellison syndrome. The gastrin, in turn, stimulates an enormous acid secretion and multiple ulcers result. The condition is treated by total gastrectomy.

When the mucosa is damaged, it is proposed that a sequence of events occurs which leads to ulcer formation. These events include entrance of acid through the broken mucosal barrier with destruction of cells of the mucosal lining and capillaries. Histamine is released, stimulating acid secretion.

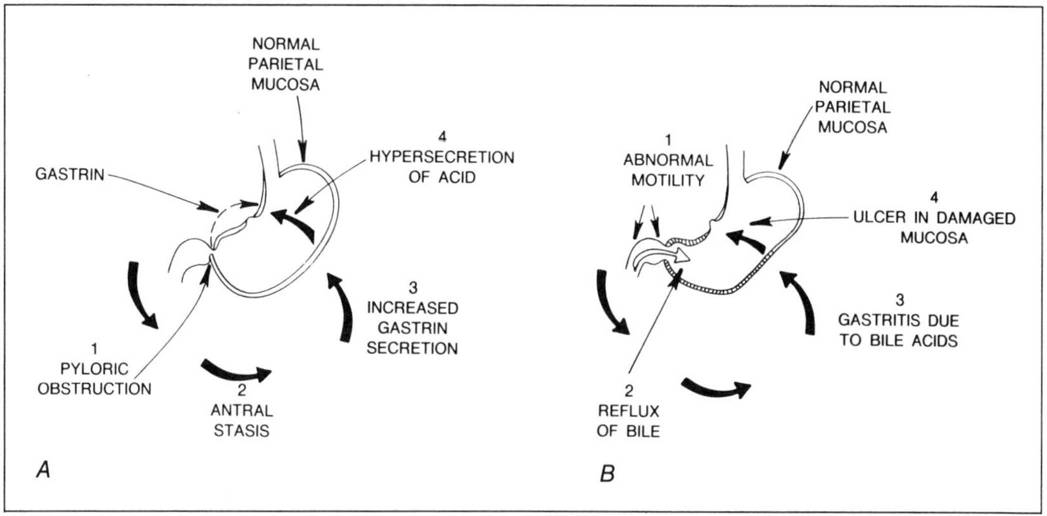

Figure 5-7. **A.** *The events that are postulated to account for gastric ulcer in patients with pyloric obstruction.* **B.** *The events that are postulated to account for gastric ulcer in patients who reflux bile into the stomach. The site of ulceration on the lesser curve is immediately adjacent to acid-secreting mucosa. (Reprinted with permission from Rhodes, J., and Callcraft, B., Aetiology of gastric ulcer with special reference to the roles of reflux and mucosal damage.* Clin. Gastroenterol. *2:227, 1973, p. 229.)*

Histamine also stimulates the intramural plexuses, and gastric motility increases. Damage to capillaries may cause an increase in permeability and protein loss into the lumen and sometimes causes hemorrhage.

Diagnosis. Chronic PUD can almost be diagnosed on the basis of the symptoms. When an ulcer is suspected from the history, the patient can be examined by roentgenography after swallowing a radiopaque mixture containing barium. Even more specifically, the ulcer may be seen directly by a procedure known as *fiberoptic endoscopy.* In addition, secretion rates, particularly of acid, may be studied.

Clinical Manifestations. The chronic gastric ulcer is characterized by upper gastrointestinal distress and pain which may radiate up the back. Patients with duodenal ulcer complain of epigastric pain when the stomach is empty. In both, pain is relieved by food or antacid medications. Dysphagia and heartburn are characteristic of esophageal ulcers. Jejunal ulcers cause left upper quadrant pain which is not relieved by food intake.

Patients with duodenal ulcers may gain weight from frequent food intake to counteract pain. The loss of weight is more common in patients with gastric ulcers. Duodenal ulcers may be complicated by hemorrhage, perforation, or stenosis (narrowing or stricture of the outlet) causing obstruction. They also tend to recur.

Conservative Treatment. The medical (conservative) management of PUD consists primarily of the use of medication and rest. These may relieve symptoms, and there is some evidence that certain drugs change the rate of healing of the ulcers. Modifications in diet have a supportive role.

Cimetidine is one of the newer and more effective drugs for the treatment of PUD. The drug is used in the treatment of duodenal ulcers but is not effective for gastric ulcers. Its mode of action is as follows: There are two receptors for the actions of histamine. The H_1 receptor controls smooth muscle contractions in the bronchi and gut. The H_2 receptor is believed to affect gastric secretions. Vagal stimulation causes the release of histamine from histamine-secreting cells in the gastric mucosa. The histamine acts on histamine H_2 receptors of the parietal cells, increasing hydrochloric acid production. Cimetidine is an antagonist to the H_2 receptor and thereby inhibits acid secretion. It accelerates the healing rate of duodenal ulcer and reduces pain.[59] It has few side effects and those that do occur are minor: mild transient diarrhea, slight gynecomastia, minor muscular pain, dizziness, and rash.[60,61] Cimetidine may decrease vitamin B_{12} absorption.[62] Therefore, the vitamin B_{12} nutritional status of the patient receiving long-term therapy should be monitored and a supplement provided if necessary.

Colloidal bismuth also accelerates healing by the action on the base of the ulcer, and it has no toxic side effects.[59] Its specific mode of action is unknown.

Antacids may be used in addition to or as an alternative to cimetidine. They neutralize gastric acid for relief of pain and to reduce mucosal damage. They buffer acid for only 30 minutes in an empty stomach but are effective for 3 to 4 hours if taken 1 hour after meals. It seems reasonable to assume that a neutral pH provides an environment that would promote the healing of the ulcer, and there is some evidence that antacids do, in fact, change the rate of healing.[63] There also is some evidence that it is a placebo effect.[64] Therefore, the question remains unresolved. Nutritionally relevant side effects of antacid treatment are listed in Table 5-7. The nutritional management of diarrhea and constipation, which are among the side effects, is discussed in the next chapter.

Carbenoxolone sodium also hastens healing but may cause sodium and fluid retention, hypokalemia, and hypertension.[65] Its use presently is limited.

Anticholinergic drugs sometimes are used in the management of duodenal ulcers, although there is evidence that they are ineffective.[66,67] They act on the nervous system to block the action of acetylcholine on the nerves and thereby decrease motility and the secretion of pepsin and acid. Side effects include a dry mouth, indicating a need for increased fluids to make the patient more comfortable.

Prostaglandins are currently being studied as a potential treatment of ulcers.

The use of *diet* in the conservative management of PUD has a long history. At one time, a common treatment consisted of the frequent feeding of milk and cream followed by a slow progression to a bland, nonirritating diet. It now is recognized that diet has no effect on the rate at which PUD heals.[68] Occasionally, however, extremely limited diets still are used for a few days in the acute stage of the disease.

In the past, patients had been advised to follow a bland diet for long periods in chronic disease, but the use of this diet is not supported by scientific evidence. Currently, it is believed that only a few diet modifications are helpful in making the patient more comfortable during the healing process, although, as previously stated, they have no effect on the rate of healing. There is some controversy on the best procedure to follow. Acidic foods and "gas formers" such as cabbage, onions, and turnips sometimes are excluded; however, many PUD patients tolerate these well. Consequently, patients usually are encouraged to eat any foods not associated with gastric distress.[69] Smaller, more frequent meals may be useful to neutralize acid, but there is some suspicion that frequent meals stimulate further acid secretion. The issue may be decided on the basis of the meal pattern with which the patient is most comfortable.

There seems to be general agreement that patients should be advised to eliminate caffeine and other methylxanthines (see Ap-

Table 5-7. Nutritionally Relevant Side Effects of Antacid Therapy

Side Effect	Types of Antacids and Their Involvement
Disturbed bowel function	Aluminum hydroxide and calcium carbonate cause constipation. Magnesium salts cause diarrhea.
Hypercalcemia and milk alkali syndrome	*Pathophysiology:* Large amounts of calcium in calcium antacids or as milk plus absorbable alkali induce hypercalcemia, reduced parathyroid hormone, phosphorus retention, elevated calcium phosphorus product, and precipitation of calcium. *Clinical manifestations: Acute* manifestations include nausea, vomiting, weakness, mental changes, headache, dizziness, and elevated calcium, blood urea nitrogen, and creatinine, after 1 wk. *Chronic* manifestations include asthenia, muscle aches, polydipsia, polyuria, band keratopathy, and nephrocalcinosis. Acute changes are reversible, but nephrocalcinosis is not. Renal calculi may develop with hypercalciuria.
Sodium retention	Most antacids contain 4 – 6 mEq of sodium per 100 ml. Riopan contains very little and should be used for patients in whom sodium intake is restricted.
Phosphorus depletion syndrome	Magnesium hydroxide and aluminum hydroxide impair phosphorus absorption, leading to hypophosphatemia, hypophosphaturia, increased calcium absorption, hypercalciuria, resorption of bone phosphorus and calcium, and debility with anorexia, weakness, bone pain, malaise, and involuntary movements.

pendix I) and alcohol, which stimulate acid secretion, and also pepper and aspirin, which are gastric irritants. Vinegar and mustard are eliminated if the patient finds them irritating. The nutritional care specialist should monitor the diet at intervals to assure that the patient does not restrict the diet excessively and so develop a nutritional deficiency.

Some patients find the elimination of coffee and alcohol a great hardship. Diets for these patients may be modified to allow for a glass of wine with meals and a limited amount of coffee following a meal. There is no specific evidence on this point, but it has been suggested that these practices lead to little acid secretion and little discomfort.[70] Large amounts of alcoholic beverages without accompanying food or repeated cups of coffee during the day should be avoided. It is important to point out to patients that a combination of alcohol and aspirin is particularly damaging. In addition, patients should be advised to avoid eating before bedtime to avoid stimulation of nocturnal acid secretion.

In gastric hemorrhage, nausea and *hematemesis* (the vomiting of blood) occur. When these subside, the patient should be returned to a normal diet as soon as possible. Feeding begins with foods such as milk, custards, gelatin desserts, and refined cereals and should be advanced to a more liberal diet as tolerated. This procedure has been found to result in a higher survival rate than the previous policy of not feeding the patient for several days.

Surgical Treatment. There are various indications for surgical treatment of ulcer disease.

Procedures. Total gastrectomy (removal of the whole stomach) may be indicated for gastric malignancy, Zollinger-Ellison syndrome, diffuse gastric polyposis, Menetrier's disease, and, sometimes, hemorrhage. *Partial gastrectomy* (removal of part of the stomach) is used in the treatment of peptic ulcers that are resistant to healing during medical management or are complicated by hemorrhage, perforation, or obstruction of the outlet with retention of gastric contents. Surgical removal of a simple ulcer is not effective in place of conservative management, since another ulcer rapidly appears.

The surgical procedures have a common objective, the marked long-term reduction in acid and pepsin content of the stomach. The various procedures from which the surgeon must choose may be associated with different mortality rates, possible complications, and nutritional consequences.

Several surgical procedures include *vagotomy* (severing of the vagus nerves). Vagotomy reduces gastric acid, pepsin, and gastrin production. It also reduces peristalsis in the antrum and thereby controls gastric motility and emptying. There are three main types of vagotomy. In *truncal vagotomy*, the two main trunks of the vagus nerves and any accessory fibers are severed at the level of the hiatus of the diaphragm. Parasympathetic stimulation in the stomach, biliary system, pancreas, and the intestinal tract to the transverse colon is thus halted (Fig. 5-8A). In *selective vagotomy*, only the branches to the stomach are severed (Fig. 5-8B), whereas in *parietal cell vagotomy* (also known as *highly selective, selective proximal*, or *proximal gastric vagotomy*), the branches to the acid-secreting parts of the stomach are interrupted. The branches to the antrum and pylorus are left intact (Fig. 5-8C). The complications of vagotomy are related to the type (Table 5-8); those with nutritional implications will be discussed further.

Figure 5-8. Various types of vagotomy. Shading depicts extent of gastrointestinal denervation following each procedure. Disturbances in physiology that may occur relate to some degree to the extent of denervation. (Reprinted with permission from Passaro, E., Jr., and Stabile, B.E., Late complications of vagotomy in relation to alterations in physiology. Postgrad. Med. *63(4):136, 1978.)*

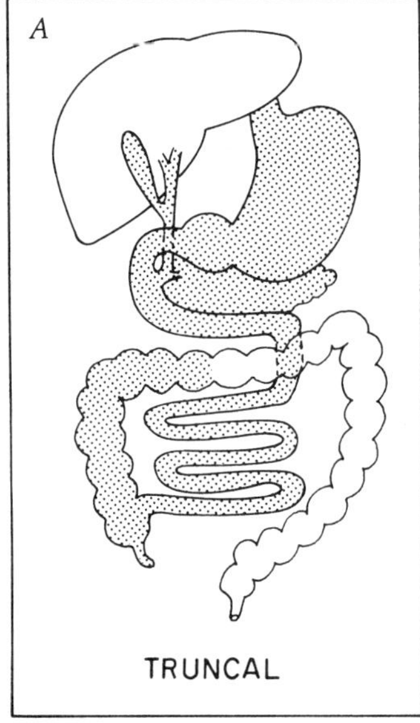

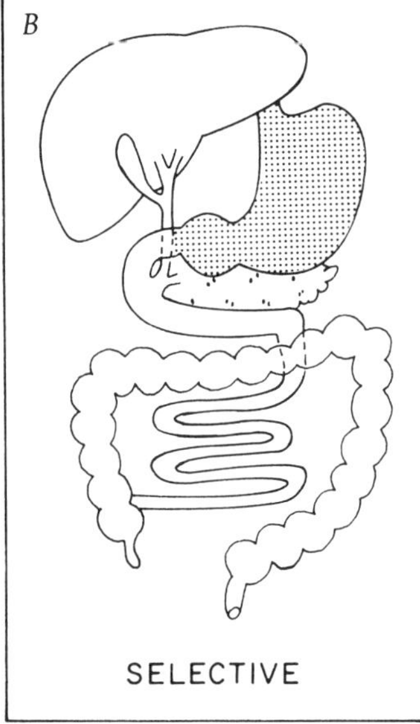

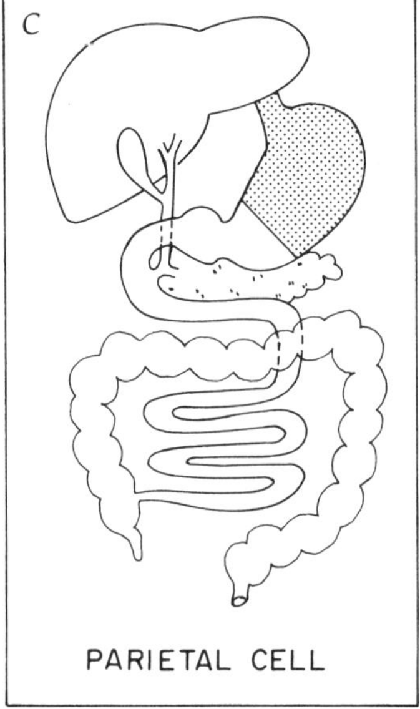

Table 5-8. Causes of Postvagotomy Syndromes

			Contributes to			
Procedure	Mechanism	Consequence	Gastric Retention	Dumping	Diarrhea	Duodenogastric Reflux
Denervation of proximal stomach (included in PCV, SV, TV)	Abolition of receptive relaxation → increased intragastric pressure	Accelerated initial emptying of liquids	No	++	++	No
	Early postoperatively: arrhythmia of gastric pacemaker → irregular antral motility	Delayed emptying of solids	+	No	No	No
Denervation of distal stomach (included in SV, TV)	Inhibition of antral motility	Delayed emptying of solids; delayed final emptying of liquids	+++	No	No	+
Intestinal denervation (included in TV)	Alteration of intestinal motility		No	No	+	+(?)
	Interruption of nervous intestinal regulation of gastric emptying	Accelerated emptying of liquids	No	+	+	No
Denervation of biliary tract (included in TV)	Increased capacity of gallbladder	Excessive bile acids in intestine	No	No	+	No
Drainage operation (pyloroplasty, gastrojejunostomy)	Decreased pyloric resistance	Accelerated emptying of liquids and solids	No	++	++	+++

Reprinted with permission from Hoelz, H.R., and Gewertz, B.L., Vagotomy. *Clin. Gastroenterol.* 8:306, 1979.
PCV = parietal cell vagotomy; SV = selective vagotomy; TV = truncal vagotomy; +, ++, +++ = relative severity of effect.

Truncal and selective vagotomies result in denervation of the gastric antrum and pyloric sphincter. This leads to gastric stasis, since the pump mechanism of the antrum and the valve function of the sphincter are lost. To compensate for this effect, vagotomy often is combined with a "drainage" procedure (Fig. 5-9, Table 5-9). Pyloroplasty (Fig. 5-9D), the most commonly used procedure, widens the pyloric opening. Gastrojejunostomy (Fig. 5-9C), which bypasses the pyloric sphincter, is not used frequently. Parietal cell vagotomy does not denervate the outlet, making concurrent drainage procedures unnecessary.

Resections or *surgical removal* are classified according to the site and extent of resected tissue. Gastric resections include:

1. Antrectomy (removal of the antrum), often with vagotomy (Fig. 5-9E).
2. Subtotal or partial gastrectomy. The amount removed varies. Vagotomy sometimes is done also (Fig. 5-9A and B).
3. Total gastrectomy

Some of the advantages and disadvantages of various drainage procedures and resections are compared in Table 5-9.

The type of *reconstruction* may be important in nutritional management. Two of these, used in partial gastrectomy or antrectomy, are shown in Fig. 5-9A and B. These methods are named after the surgeon who originated them. As indicated in the diagram, the *Billroth I* reconstruction consists of an anastamosis of the proximal end of the intestine to the distal end of the stomach. The original *Billroth II* reconstruction has been followed by several variations, one of which (Polya's operation) is shown. An important feature of this type is the *blind loop* or *afferent loop* created when the stomach is anastamosed to the side of the intestine some distance from its proximal end. The position of the afferent and efferent loops should be observed in the figure. Total gastric resections may simply restore the continuity of the tract, or a larger reservoir may be

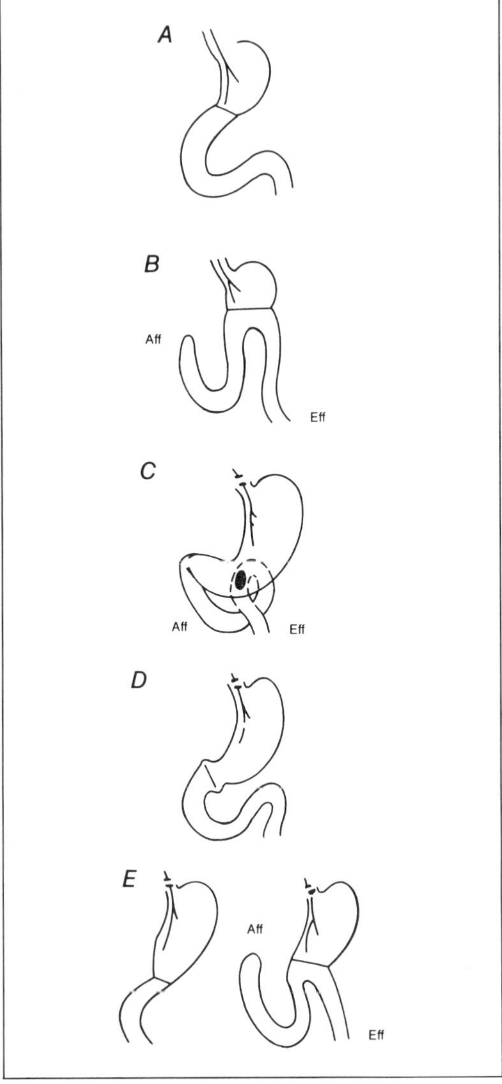

Figure 5-9. Operations for duodenal and gastric ulcers. **A.** *Partial gastrectomy with Billroth I reconstruction.* **B.** *Partial gastrectomy; Billroth II, Polya type reconstruction.* **C.** *Vagotomy and gastrojejunostomy.* **D.** *Vagotomy and pyloroplasty.* **E.** *Vagotomy and antrectomy.* **Aff** = *afferent loop;* **Eff** = *efferent loop. (Reprinted with permission from Naish, J.M., and Read, A.E.,* Basic Gastroenterology, *2nd ed. Bristol, Engl.: John Wright and Sons, 1974, p. 77.)*

Table 5-9. Comparison of Some Surgical Procedures for Gastric and Duodenal Ulcers

Operation	Advantages	Disadvantages
Partial gastrectomy, Billroth I reconstruction (see Fig. 5-9A)	Maintenance of normal food pathway guarantees minimum of nutritional disturbances afterward. Less "dumping." Ideal for gastric ulcer.	High rate (6% in men) or recurrent ulceration if done for duodenal ulcer.
Partial gastrectomy, Polya's operation (see Fig. 5-9B)	Combines removal of large part of acid-bearing area and antrum with neutralization of anastomotic area by alkaline duodenal juices. Low rate of recurrent ulcer (1–2%).	Poor mixing of food and enzymes. Weight loss and anemia are fairly frequent. "Dumping" symptoms in about 10%. Severe steatorrhea rarely.
Vagotomy and gastrojejunostomy (see Fig. 5-9C)	Simple. Low risk. Alkalinization of gastric contents by duodenal juice.	Difficult to make vagotomy complete. Fairly high rate of recurrent ulceration (5–8%).
Vagotomy and pyloroplasty (see Fig. 5-9D)	Cuts vagal acid secretion and drains stomach. Low risk. Maintains normal food pathway. Popular at present time.	No alkalinization of gastric contents. Fairly high rate of recurrent ulceration.
Vagotomy and antrectomy (limited resection) (see Fig. 5-9E)	Cuts vagally mediated and hormonally mediated (gastrin from antrum) secretion. Low risk.	Removes pH monitoring function of antrum, so gastrin secretion from outside may be permanently high.

Adapted with permission from Naish, J.M., and Read, A.E., *Basic Gastroenterology*, 2nd ed. Bristol, Engl.: John Wright and Sons, 1974, p. 77.

created using a section of jejunum to make a pouch to provide some space for storage of ingested food.

Postoperative nutrition. The *initial postoperative feeding* is important in preventing complications. Immediately following uncomplicated gastric surgery, the patient is given nothing by mouth (NPO), and a nasogastric tube is inserted. Suction is used to remove gastric contents until peristalsis resumes, and the patient is given fluid and electrolyte therapy to replace what is lost in the aspirate. Sometimes, a tube to be used for feeding is implanted into the jejunum during the surgery. If there are no complications, the typical patient may first be given 2 oz. low-carbohydrate clear liquids plus one-half slice toast or two crackers every 2 hours while awake. The clear liquids are chosen from broth, bouillon, decaffeinated coffee, unsweetened gelatin, or unsweetened fruit juice.[71] When gastrointestinal function has returned, a high-protein, low-carbohydrate, moderate-fat diet in small frequent feedings is used. Foods used should be low in fiber. Liquids are included in feedings separate from solid foods. Milk and carbonated beverages are eliminated. The patient may be fed every 1 to 2 hours. The purpose of these modifications is to prevent distension of the stomach and development of the dumping syndrome, a complication described later in this section. If no complications occur, other foods are added as tolerated. Some patients are able to have unrestricted intake within 2 to 3 weeks.

Sometimes the esophagus is damaged during truncal vagotomy. The patient may have pain and dysphagia for 1 or 2 weeks.[72] A soft diet, including the modifications previously described for patients recovering from gastric surgery, may be helpful.

Complications. Some patients develop complications following gastrectomy, several of which have nutritional implications. *Delayed gastric emptying* and *obstruction* are indicated by nausea and vomiting when oral feeding begins. When this occurs, feeding is stopped temporarily. When oral feeding is resumed, small liquid feedings may be tried, with the patient sitting up to take advantage of gravity. The condition usually disappears within a week; however, in some patients, delayed emptying may persist.

Other possible complications include the following:

1. *Dumping syndrome* is a group of symptoms that occur following eating in approximately 10 percent of gastric surgery patients. It has been divided into early and late phases, depending on how soon it occurs after eating.

Early dumping syndrome occurs during the meal or within 10 to 15 minutes after the meal is eaten. It occurs frequently after gastric resection and sometimes in patients in whom a drainage operation has been performed. The patient has a feeling of fullness in the epigastrium, flushing, sweating, weakness, tachycardia (excessive heart rate), diarrhea, and sometimes hypotension. The pathogenesis of early dumping syndrome is not understood entirely, but some facts are clear. The symptoms follow intake of high-carbohydrate foods. The loss of normal sphincter action, whether by resection, bypass, division, or denervation, allows rapid movement of hyperosmolar material (see Appendix H) from the stomach into the upper small intestine. Fluid is pulled into the intestine, causing intestinal distention and reduced plasma volume. The intestinal distension may cause the diarrhea. It also stimulates the argentaffin cells in the intestinal mucosa to secrete humoral agents such as serotonin, prostaglandins, bradykinin, and enteroglucagon. These may account for the gastrointestinal and vasomotor symptoms,[73-75] but there still is doubt on this point.[76-78]

The development of early dumping syndrome can often be avoided in gastric surgery patients by cautious postoperative feeding, as described earlier. If dumping syndrome does occur, the treatment is almost exclusively dietary. The rationale and main features of nutritional management are summarized in Table 5-10.

Table 5-10. Nutritional Management of Dumping Syndrome

Individualize the diet to the patient's tolerance. Consult the patient frequently concerning his or her response to individual food items and to portion sizes. The following items are general guidelines.
Reduce intake of carbohydrates to 100–200 g/day. Avoid simple sugars to prevent rapid movement of food into the jejunum with formation of a hyperosmolar solution. Use *unsweetened* fruits.
Increase fat content to 30–40% of calories to retard stomach emptying and to provide calories for weight gain.
Increase protein to 20% of calories for tissue formation and to supply energy. Include some protein in each meal.
Meals should be low in bulk, dry, and frequent: Six or more per day is common. Increase portion sizes as the patient's tolerance increases.
Provide low-carbohydrate fluids between meals, at least ½–1 hr after a meal, to retard gastric emptying. Avoid high-carbohydrate fluids.
All food and drink should be moderate in temperature. Cold drinks, especially, cause increased gastric motility.
Encourage the patient to eat slowly and then lie down for 20–30 min.
Encourage the patient to eat a variety of foods to provide an adequate diet and achievement of ideal body weight. It may be necessary to urge him or her to try foods that were being avoided preoperatively.
The possibility of lactose intolerance exists. Milk should be avoided until it is established that the patient tolerates milk (see Chapter 6).
To progress toward a more normal intake, add moderate amounts of carbohydrate with caution if the patient shows no symptoms of dumping in the first several days. Use sugar in the form of sweetened fruits and fruit juice and desserts such as sponge cake and cookies. If these are well tolerated, add more concentrated carbohydrates and foods at temperature extremes. Fresh fruits and vegetables may be added in 2–3 wk. They should be chewed thoroughly. The diet may be progressed rapidly in some patients and may be lifelong in others.

Late dumping syndrome or *alimentary hypoglycemia* develops 1½ to 3 hours following a meal. Patients feel faint and weak and perspire freely. There are varying degrees of effect on the central nervous system, and some patients lose consciousness. There are no gastrointestinal symptoms. The lack of the normal pyloric sphincter function allows the movement of carbohydrate into the upper small intestine. This carbohydrate is absorbed rapidly and the blood glucose level rises. As a result, a large amount of insulin is released and the blood glucose level falls. The symptoms are characteristic of low blood glucose.

Patients with late dumping syndrome should eat approximately every 2 hours, avoiding concentrated sweets. However, concentrated sweets should be available at all times and eaten if a hypoglycemic attack begins. Also, if protein foods are taken at this time, they may help to prevent another episode of hypoglycemia.

2. A change in bowel habits is common after gastric surgery, especially when vagotomy is included. Bowel function can vary from severe constipation to severe diarrhea. Severe incapacitating diarrhea, usually referred to as *postvagotomy diarrhea,* follows truncal vagotomy, especially if combined with antrectomy, more often than it does the more selective types.[79] It causes severe disability in approximately 2 percent of patients.

Treatment may include dietary changes as well as antispasmodic and antidiarrheal drugs and cholestyramine. If conservative treatment is unsuccessful, surgical correction may be necessary.

Mild diarrhea may be controlled by the use of small, frequent feedings and limitation of fluid with meals. An increase in dietary fiber may also be helpful.

3. *Weight loss* following subtotal gastric resection occurs in as many as 60 percent of patients, particularly those with a gastrojejunal anastamosis.[80–83] Total resection also results in weight loss. The causes are not understood entirely but probably are multiple.

In some patients, weight loss is clearly the result of inadequate food intake.[80] Patients with partial or total gastrectomy have a reduced storage capacity and a rapid development of the feeling of satiety. Those with dumping syndrome sometimes reduce their food intake to avoid the symptoms. It has also been speculated that the absence of a stomach decreases hunger sensations.[84]

Some patients develop a malabsorption syndrome as a late complication. In the stomach itself, the decreased production of acid and pepsin has an effect, but the significance of this change on overall fat and protein metabolism is not clear. Anatomic changes from surgery sometimes affect the availability of bile and pancreatic enzymes. The digestive and absorptive functions of the intestine are affected if emptying of the stomach and gallbladder and pancreatic secretion are incoordinated. Since many of these changes are similar to those seen in diseases of the intestine, pancreas, and gallbladder, their nutritional consequences and management are described in Chapter 6. If malabsorption is severe, it sometimes is surgically corrected by conversion to a different type of reconstruction.[85]

4. *Anemia* occurs late as a postoperative complication, sometimes several years later. The incidence varies greatly, depending on the definition of anemia used in the studies that are the source of the data. Several types of anemia are seen.[86]

Most cases of anemia following gastric surgery are *iron deficiency anemia.* This develops as a result of reduced food intake and possibly from impaired iron absorption. Patients may be unable to convert dietary iron to ferrous iron for absorption because of decreased gastric acid and decreased mixing with available acid. In addition, some surgical reconstructions cause the intestinal contents to bypass the duodenum where most iron absorption normally occurs.

Mild anemia may be asymptomatic, but some patients are apathetic, anorexic, and suffer from epigastric distress and weight loss. Treatment consists of supplementation with inorganic iron salts. The iron salts usually are given orally in patients with subtotal gastrectomy, although parenteral administration is necessary for some. Patients should be counseled on dietary sources of iron and meal planning, so that dietary iron deficiency does not contribute to the severity of the anemia.

Vitamin B_{12} deficiency anemia may occur also. Patients with total gastrectomy have lost the capacity to produce intrinsic factor, which is necessary for absorption of vitamin B_{12}. Some patients who have had a subtotal gastrectomy produce inadequate amounts of intrinsic factor. Only a few of these patients eventually develop macrocytic anemia.[87] Bacterial overgrowth in the proximal small intestine or afferent loop competes for vitamin B_{12} absorption and may contribute to the deficiency. Macrocytic anemia in these patients must be treated with supplemental vitamin B_{12}.

Folate deficiency may cause megaloblastic anemia following total or subtotal gastrectomy[88-90] and is believed to be the result of a deficient diet. Usually it is associated with the reduced food intake of patients with other complications such as dumping syndrome. Nutritional counseling may be helpful in prevention.

5. *Bezoars* are concretions of various materials sometimes found in the stomach or intestines. *Phytobezoars* are formed from plant fibers. They sometimes form in gastric surgery patients because of altered motility following vagotomy and possibly as a consequence of the reduced acid secretion. They are treated with digestive materials such as papain, cellulase, and pancreatic enzymes. A diet low in foods containing cellulose is used to prevent their reformation.[91]

6. Metabolic *bone disease*—osteomalacia or osteoporosis—occurs as a late complication of gastrectomy in 1 to 15 percent of patients.[92] Milder forms are much more common.[93,94] Bone disease has not been observed following vagotomy and pyloroplasty or vagotomy and gastroenterostomy.[79] *Osteomalacia* occurs in patients with a Billroth II reconstruction or gastrojejunostomy. It is believed to be the result of malabsorption of fat and fat-soluble vitamins, including vitamin D. Poor dietary intake may be another contributing factor. Patients are treated with vitamin D supplements. *Osteoporosis* occurs 10 to 20 years earlier in gastrectomy patients than in others.[95] There is no specific treatment, but it is reported that most of these patients are malnourished.[96] The following seem to be logical recommendations for nutritional management: Counsel the patient on adequate nutrient intake, and provide supplements if necessary to assure adequate intakes of calcium and vitamin D.

SPECIAL TECHNIQUES FOR NUTRITIONAL SUPPORT

In diseases of the alimentary tract, as well as those of other organ systems, it sometimes is not possible to provide adequate nourishment without the use of special products or special feeding techniques. These products and techniques can be classified in general as (1) supplements to oral feeding, (2) complete nutritional formulas taken orally or by tube in place of conventional meals, and (3) parenteral feeding. Since these procedures frequently present problems of nutritional care related to function of the digestive tract and since they also are used in management of diseases of the digestive system, the first two procedures will be described here. Parenteral feeding bypasses the digestive tract and will therefore be described in detail in Chapter 12.

Supplements are indicated for the patient whose food intake at meals is inadequate to meet nutritional needs. Some are liquid mixtures, emphasizing protein and carbohydrates, often served as beverage "snacks" between meals. Others are added to or substituted for foods in a conventional diet.

Liquid Supplemental Feeding

Some liquid supplements, such as milk shakes and malted milks, can be prepared from conventional ingredients. In addition, a wide array of commercial products are available. They are listed and described in Appendix J. Many of these supplements are intended to provide protein and kilocalories; others are an energy source but are low in protein or are protein-free for patients whose condition requires protein restriction. Some are lactose-free. These products are not intended to replace the diet and, therefore, not all provide all nutritional requirements. Products intended for addition to other foods or formulas to increase available energy or protein are listed in Appendix K.

An institution usually does not stock all the products listed. A given purpose may be served by any one of several products which differ only slightly. Factors that should be considered in choosing items to stock and in choosing a supplement for a specific patient include cost, availability, palatability, composition in relation to the nutrient requirements of the patient, and indications for the use of the product.

Complete Nutritional Formulas

When a patient is unable to take solid foods, it becomes necessary to provide the entire nutrient needs of the patient in liquid form. Conditions that may require the use of nutritional formulas are listed in Table 5-11. A variety of formulations are available for this purpose (see Appendix L). These formulas sometimes are used as oral supplements as well.

Although it would be possible to feed parenterally those patients who cannot take solid foods, the gastrointestinal tract should be used (*enteral feeding*) if possible. There are a number of reasons for this. The presence of food in the digestive tract helps to maintain the integrity of the mucosa of the gut. Enteral feedings are safer and considerably less expensive, and the procedure may be more acceptable to the patient, particularly if some conventional foods can be taken orally in addition.

Complete nutritional formulas are useful only in those patients who have sufficient gastrointestinal function to digest and absorb their ingredients. To some extent, a formula can be chosen that is suited to the digestive capacity of the patient.

Products Available

Formulas Containing Intact Nutrients. Some complete nutritional formulas contain intact ingredients such as whole protein, disaccharides, and triglycerides which require digestion. Many are low in osmolality; some are isotonic. They vary greatly in residue content. Therefore, these formulas are used for patients with an intact digestive and absorptive system, even though such patients may be unable to ingest conventional meals.

Formulas containing intact ingredients are categorized as *blenderized, milk-based,* or *lactose-free* (see Appendix L). Lactose-free formulas usually use soy as the protein source. Blenderized formulas may be prepared in the hospital by homogenizing a mixture of whole foods. Meat, eggs, fruits, vegetable, milk, oil, and other foods can be mixed in varying proportions to meet the nutritional needs of the individual patients. The nutritional care specialist may be called on to calculate formulas tailored to individual needs. Milk-based and lactose-free formulas can also be made from scratch to meet special needs. The hospital pharmacist may provide some of the ingredients for these formulas.

The purchase of commercial formulas saves time in preparation and may reduce the incidence of contamination. Commercial

Table 5-11. Indications for Use of Tube Feedings

- Inability to ingest food normally
  - Stupor, unconsciousness, coma
  - Cerebrovascular accidents
  - Inflammation in central nervous system
  - Cerebral neoplasms
  - Fracture of mandible
  - Oropharyngeal neoplasms
  - Head and neck surgery
  - Dysphagia
  - Radiation to head or neck
  - Chemotherapy
  - Multiple sclerosis
- Physiologic deterrents to food intake
  - Nausea or vomiting in pregnancy, drug reactions, radiation, or chemotherapy
  - Dumping syndrome
- Obstruction of gastrointestinal tract (if access is below obstruction)
  - Esophageal stricture or neoplasm
  - Spasm of pylorus
  - Neoplasm, foreign body, or other obstruction of stomach or intestine
- Psychiatric illness
  - Anorexia nervosa
  - Depression
- Diversion of flow (fistulas) (?)
- Impairment of digestion and/or absorption
  - Pancreatic insufficiency; carcinoma, chronic pancreatitis
  - Bile salt insufficiency
  - Bile acid–induced diarrhea: blind loop syndrome, Zollinger-Ellison syndrome
  - Short bowel syndrome
  - Gluten enteropathy (nontropical sprue)
  - Crohn's disease
  - Disaccharidase deficiency
  - Abetalipoproteinemia
  - Radiation damage
  - Whipple's disease
  - Obstruction of lymph flow
- Protein-calorie malnutrition
- Hypermetabolic states
  - Burns
  - Trauma
  - Surgery
  - Fever
- Intestinal surgery
  - Preparation for hemorrhoidectomy[a]
  - Preparation for intestinal surgery[a]
- Transition from total parenteral nutrition to conventional foods[a]
- Renal failure
- Hepatic failure
- Inborn errors of metabolism

Information gathered from *Dialogues in Nutrition* 1(2):1 (tape). Bloomfield, N.J.: Health Learning Systems, Inc., 1976; American Dietetic Association, *Handbook of Clinical Dietetics.* New Haven: Yale University Press, 1980; and Rombeau, J.L., and Miller, R.A., *Nasoenteric Tube Feeding: Practical Aspects.* Mountain View, Calif.: Health Development Corp., 1979.

[a] Defined formula diet.

products provide mixtures of known composition but have the disadvantage of affording reduced flexibility in composition which may not meet the needs of a patient who has unusual requirements. They may be modified only by altering the dilution or adding other materials.

Protein may provide 12 to 24 percent of the kilocalories in formulas containing intact nutrients. Casein often is the protein, but egg, beef, or soy is used in some. The carbohydrate may be corn syrup solids, fructose, sucrose, lactose, or from pureed fruits and vegetables. These carbohydrates markedly increase the osmolality. The patient's ability to tolerate lactose should be considered when lactose-containing formulas are used. Lactose intolerance is discussed in detail in Chapter 6.

The fat in the formula provides from 2 to 30 percent of the kilocalories. Fat adds to the caloric value and provides satiety without adding to the osmolality. It also improves the way a formula feels in the mouth when it is taken orally.

Vitamins and minerals are included in the commercial products to provide the Recommended Dietary Allowances (RDA). Additional supplements may be needed for those patients with significantly increased needs. It is important that the nutritional care specialist be alert to increased needs and recommend supplementation when necessary.

The most common caloric density is 1 kcal/ml, but a few commercial products, designed for severely debilitated patients, provide more calories per unit volume. These formulas are useful also for patients whose fluid intakes must be restricted or who are unable to tolerate a large volume of feeding. Those formulations that are used as infant formulas generally are more dilute.

Defined Formula Diets. A second type of complete nutritional formula is the *defined formula diet* (also known as the *chemically defined diet,* or *semisynthetic diet*). The older literature sometimes refers to them as *elemental diets,* an unfortunate term since the contents are not entirely in the form of separate elements. These formulas (see Appendix L) are useful in conditions in which the ability to digest and absorb nutrients has been reduced. They contain partially or completely digested nutrients and usually are almost completely absorbed, leaving little or no residue in the intestinal tract.

An important consideration in either oral or tube feeding is the osmolality of the mixture. Most formulas are hyperosmolar and cause water to be drawn into the gastrointestinal tract if the feeding is too rapid. Dumping syndrome and severe diarrhea then ensue.

The protein in defined formula diets provides 8 to 30 percent of the calories as egg albumin or amino acids. Carbohydrate appears in most formulations as glucose or dextrins and provides 60 to 90 percent of the calories. Fat may be present in small amounts to provide essential fatty acids, or in larger quantities, up to 28 percent, from vegetable oil. Vitamins and minerals are added to meet the Recommended Dietary Allowances, but RDA levels may not be adequate for the increased needs of some patients.

These formulas sometimes are taken orally, but their amino acid content makes most of them quite unpalatable. Flavor packets are provided which may improve acceptability somewhat but which increase the osmolality of the formula. For increased palatability, the product for oral use should be served chilled or on ice. It may be mixed with fruit juice to improve flavor, but fruit juice increases osmolality. A bent straw should be provided to the patient. If the straw is placed well back on the tongue, the flavor of the liquid is less noticeable. In general, however, oral feedings of these products is not successful.

Evaluation of Tube Feedings

The characteristics of an ideal tube feeding are given in Table 5-12. They should be

Table 5-12. Characteristics of an Ideal Tube Feeding

Low cost
Bacteriologic safety
Relatively low osmolality
Caloric density equivalent to 1 calorie per cubic centimeter
Suitable protein-calorie ratio
Adequate but not excessive nutrient intake, with nutrients present in nontoxic ratios and amounts
Balanced nutrient composition, including electrolyte composition, proper balance of amino acids, and well-utilized supplementary sources of nutrients
Nutritional adequacy for short-term use and, when indicated, for long-term feeding
Convenience and ease of administration
Suitable viscosity and homogenization

Reprinted with permission from Gormican, A., and Liddy, E., Nasogastric tube feedings: Practical considerations in prescription and evaluation. *Postgrad. Med.* 53(7):73, 1973.

considered in choosing items for use. It is interesting to find that taste may be important even when the patient is being fed by tube, since the feeding often is regurgitated. Patients frequently state that they can taste a tube feeding and request changes in flavor.

Techniques of Administration

Routes. The placement of tubes for feeding is shown in Fig. 5-10. *Intragastric* (or nasogastric or NG) tubes are used in problems of ingestion such as head and neck surgery. Longer mercury-tipped tubes may be *nasoduodenal,* reducing the incidence of vomiting or aspiration of regurgitated tube feeding into the lungs.

If the condition of the patient is such that access through the nose or mouth is not possible, an artificial opening or *stoma* may be created by the surgeon. The location of the stoma depends on the reason it was created. A *cervical esophagostomy* creates an opening into the esophagus at approximately the shoulder level. It has an advantage in that it does not require the patient to undress for feeding and the opening is easily concealed. Esophagostomies are dependable for long-term use and are easy to handle. A *gastrostomy* provides an opening directly into the stomach. It might be used for a patient whose esophagus has been removed. A *jejunostomy* creates access directly into the jejunum. A recent development is a *needle catheter jejunostomy,* in which a catheter is implanted into the jejunum for access rather than creating a stoma. The jejunostomy bypasses the duodenum and the duct system that provides bile and pancreatic enzymes. Therefore, a jejunostomy feeding must consist of predigested materials. With a jejunostomy, there is a high incidence of dumping syndrome and diarrhea, and adequate nutrient intake may be difficult to maintain.

Delivery Systems. The method of delivery of the feeding into the tube is very important. When an *Asepto syringe* is used, the nurse fills the syringe with the feeding and releases the material into the tube. The method provides a variable rate of delivery and is time-consuming for the busy nursing staff. As a consequence, there is a problem of missed feedings and an increased incidence of intolerance to the feeding.

In the *gravity drip* method, the feeding in its container is placed above the patient's head and connected to the tube. The flow rate is regulated with a stopcock but is variable, changing with the patient's position and the viscosity of the mixture. It is not usable for very viscous mixtures, but many commercial feedings are packaged so that they can be delivered by gravity drip.

An *infusion pump* can be used for some feedings. An infusion pump is primarily for parenteral feeding but can be adapted to enteral feeding. It controls the rate of flow electronically over a 24-hour period. Battery operation makes it possible for the patient to be ambulatory while being fed. Equipment costs are high, but labor cost is reduced and delivery of the formula is more dependable.

A *food pump* can deliver a blenderized diet. Like the infusion pump, it regulates the rate of flow over a 24-hour period. The equipment is expensive, but labor costs are reduced with the use of a food pump. The administration of the proper amount of formula also is more reliable.

Types of Tubes. The quality of feeding tubes has improved greatly in recent years. They are available in various diameters, and a tube must be chosen to suit the size of the patient and the nature of the feeding. The patient will be most comfortable with a tube of the smallest diameter that the feeding will pass through. As general guidelines, defined formula diets will go through No. 5, 6, or 8 French tubes, and lactose-free formulas, through a No. 5 or 6 Fr. if pumped or No. 7.3 Fr. by gravity drip. Milk-based formulas require a No. 7.3 to 9.6 Fr. by pump or No. 8 to 9.6 Fr. by gravity drip. Blenderized feeding requires a No. 8 to 9.6 Fr. by pump and a

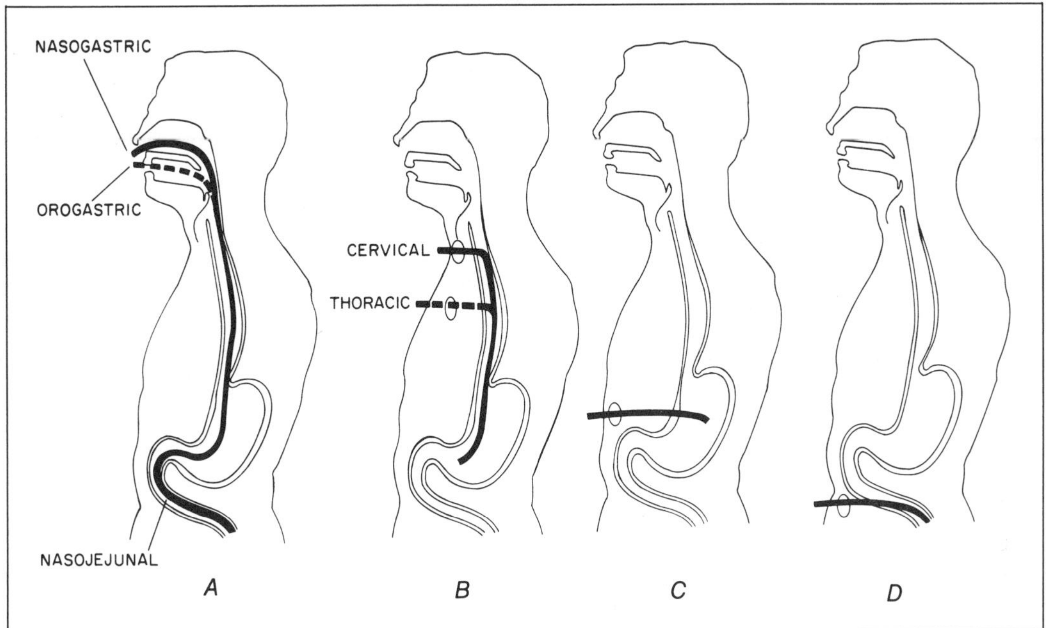

Figure 5-10. Types and sites of gastric feeding. **A.** *An intragastric tube, which is passed through the nose or mouth into the stomach and secured in place. (A tube passed through the mouth is more correctly called an* orogastric tube. *An orogastric tube ordinarily is inserted at mealtime and removed following the meal.)* **B.** *Esophagostomy. A temporary or permanent opening (stoma) is constructed at one of several sites to allow a tube to be introduced through the skin into the esophagus. The feeding tube usually is removed between meals.* **C.** *Gastrostomy: A temporary or permanent stoma is constructed allowing food to be introduced through the skin directly into the stomach.* **D.** *Jejunostomy. A stoma is constructed which gives direct access to the jejunum. This method of feeding may be used when the stomach must be bypassed. (Reprinted with permission from Suitor, C.W., and Hunter, M.F.,* Nutrition: Principles and Application in Health Promotion. *Philadelphia: J.B. Lippincott, 1980, p. 367.)*

No. 12 to 18 Fr. by gravity drip.[97] *French* is a scale used to denote the size of catheters and other tubes. Each unit is roughly equal to 0.33 mm in diameter.

A soft flexible tube is most comfortable for the patient. Polyvinyl and red rubber tubes tend to become hard and be uncomfortable. They may even cause intestinal perforation, esophagitis, or esophageal stricture.[98] Several new types of tubes made from Teflon or Silastic and polyurethane are available. They are more comfortable and do not harden with use. An enclosed mercury weight at the end of the tube assists in insertion and passage into the duodenum. Mercury weights also are visible on roentgenography, so that their proper placement can be confirmed.

Rate, Frequency, and Concentration of Feeding. If liquids high in osmolality are given rapidly, severe cramping and diarrhea are likely to occur. Therefore, tube feedings are begun cautiously, allowing an adjustment period. Intact nutrient feedings frequently are given first at one-half strength. Boluses may be begun at 50 to 100 ml and continuous drip at 40 to 60 ml/hr. The concentration and rate of feeding are increased to the desired objectives over 2 to 3 days. It is important not to increase concentration and rate at the same time.

Defined formula diets have a higher osmolality and must be approached with greater caution. They may be started at one-quarter strength and progressed to full strength in 4 to 5 days.

On a continuing basis, best results are obtained with the use of a constant feeding that provides a volume of 80 to 150 ml/hr. If equipment for continuous feeding is not available, bolus feeding may be given in lots of 200 to 350 ml, with each feeding given over a period of at least 10 minutes. Following the formula feeding, a volume of water half that of the tube feeding is given to prevent solute overload dehydration.

Contraindications to Tube Feeding

The primary contraindication to tube feeding is obstruction, unless access is available

Table 5-13. Nutrition-Related Problems in the Tube-Fed Patient

Problem	Possible Causes	Suggested Corrective Measures[a]
Nausea	Improper location of tube tip	Consult with physician or nurse on replacement of tube
	Excessive rate of feeding; excessive volume of feeding	Decrease volume or rate of feeding[a]
	Anxiety	Reassure patient
Vomiting	Excessive formula volume	Reduce volume of feeding[a]
Diarrhea	Very cold formula	Give formula near room temperature
	Too-rapid infusion	Give formula more slowly
	High osmolarity or high concentration of feeding	Adapt patient gradually; start with 1:2–4 dilution; add applesauce, pectin, banana flakes; add methylcellulose (for bulk); add paregoric, Lomotil, codeine, or Kaopectate to the feeding[a]
	Lactose intolerance	Use lactose-free formula[a]
Vomiting *and* diarrhea	Contamination	Check sanitation of formula and equipment; consult with bacteriologist
	Anxiety	Reassure patient; explain purpose and procedures
Constipation	High milk content	Use milk-free formula
	Lack of fiber	Use stool softeners or laxatives in formula
	Inadequate fluid intake	Increase fluid intake
Dehydration	Rapid infusion of carbohydrate leading to hyperglycemia and osmotic diarrhea	Administer tube feeding slowly; physician may prescribe insulin
	Excessive protein or electrolytes or both	Reduce protein, electrolytes, or increase fluid intake
	Inadequate fluid intake	Increase fluid intake
Edema	Excess sodium in formula	Use formula with less sodium
Gradual weight loss	Inadequate calories	Check if patient is receiving prescribed feeding; estimate caloric intake; possibly increase volume per day or concentration
Other signs of undernutrition	Nutrient content of formula inadequate for needs	Discuss appropriate supplements with physician
Gradual gain of excess weight	Excess calories	Dilute formula or decrease volume per day

[a] In consultation with physician or nursing staff if required by the policy of the institution.

below the area of the obstruction. Patients with obstruction of the esophagus, for example, may be fed through a gastrostomy. In cases of *paralytic ileus* (obstruction from inhibition of bowel motility), which is seen for a period following abdominal surgery and also occurs in burn patients, tube feeding should not be instituted until bowel sounds resume.

In addition, a highly osmolar defined formula diet is not used for patients with conditions that cause the patient to be unable to handle a high osmotic load, such as dumping syndrome, jejunal fistulas, and some hepatic and renal diseases. They should not be used for infants and only in very dilute form (12 percent weight by volume) for small children.

Patient Monitoring

Monitoring the tube-fed patient is the responsibility of the nutritional care specialist as well as that of the physician and nursing staff. The actual volume of intake, as well as the incidence of vomiting, diarrhea, or abdominal cramps, should be observed carefully. It is important to observe the patient for signs of dehydration, particularly if the formula is high in protein or electrolytes. The thirst mechanism may safeguard alert adult patients, but patients who are comatose, very weak, very ill, or have fever or drainage from a fistula, and all children should be observed with extreme care. Fluid intake and output and signs of edema and sudden weight gain should be noted. Values on the patient's chart to be monitored include blood urea nitrogen, glucose, albumin, and electrolyte concentrations in the serum, and urinary glucose and specific gravity. An estimate of nitrogen balance should be provided weekly by the nutritional care specialist. The nutritional status of patients who are tube-fed over an extended period should be assessed at regular intervals, using the methods described in Chapter 2.

Complications

A number of problems are associated with tube feeding. Those that may involve the nutritional care specialist and require corrective measures are listed in Table 5-13.

Parenteral Feeding

Parenteral feeding bypasses the digestive tract. Some nutritional support can be provided temporarily into a peripheral vein, most commonly in the nondominant arm. Such feedings are not nutritionally complete and are useful only for short periods. For long-term use, complete nutritional support can be provided into a central vein. The procedure, known as *total parenteral nutrition* (TPN), is described in Chapter 12.

Case Study: Lower Esophageal Sphincter Incompetence

W.M. was first seen at the age of 56 years. He complained of epigastric pain of several years' duration, dysphagia, and belching of uncertain duration. He described the dysphagia as a "feeling of fullness" and "food sticking in his chest" following ingestion of solid food. Sometimes he regurgitated this food but did not vomit. The symptoms were aggravated by lying down or bending over.

Physical examination and the complete blood cell count were normal. He denied any weight loss. X-ray films suggested lower esophageal sphincter incompetence and a sliding hiatal hernia.

The patient was given antacids and referred to the nutritional care specialist for diet counseling.

Subjective:
"I've got to have my morning cup of coffee."
24-hour recall:

Breakfast	4 oz. fruit juice
	2 eggs on toast
	Coffee, black

Snack (at work)	Coffee, black
	Sweet roll
Lunch (at work)	Steak sandwich
	French fries
	Tossed salad with French dressing
	Coffee, black
Snack (at work)	Ice cream, 1 scoop
Dinner	12 oz. beer
	Tuna noodle casserole
	Buttered frozen peas
	Fruit salad of canned pineapple, orange sections, sliced banana
	8 oz. milk
Snack	12 oz. soft drink
	20 pretzel sticks

Five years later, the patient returned complaining of dysphagia of 6 months' duration and persistent burning epigastric pain. He was able to eat only soft foods or liquids. His appetite was good, but he had lost 20 lb. Laboratory test values were as follows:

Hematocrit	31 percent
Hemoglobin	8.1 g/dl
Others	Within normal limits

Esophagoscopy showed a constricting lesion 39 cm from the incisors. A biopsy and esophageal washings showed no tumor cells. Attempts to dilate the stricture were unsuccessful. In the meantime, the patient lost additional weight.

The nutritional care specialist was asked to see the patient and suggest nutritional care necessary to prepare the patient for surgery.

Exercises

1. What clinical manifestations would alert the physician to the possibility of LES incompetence?
2. Evaluate the patient's diet from the 24-hour recall.
3. What is the significance of the values obtained for hematocrit and hemoglobin?
4. Describe the nutritional care you would suggest for this patient and explain the rationale.

Case Study: Dumping Syndrome

K.L., a 45-year-old man, was admitted to the hospital for surgery following 15 years of treatment for a gastric ulcer. The ulcer was no longer responding to medical management. A subtotal gastrectomy with a Billroth I anastomosis and a vagotomy was performed. Postoperatively, the patient was at first given nothing by mouth. When feeding was begun, he was given low-carbohydrate clear liquids and toast every 2 hours and progressed to a high-protein, low-carbohydrate diet in six small feedings. Fluids were given at separate feedings.

A week following discharge from the hospital, the patient called his physician complaining of nausea, diarrhea, and abdominal cramping an hour after meals. The physician referred the patient to the nutritional care specialist who obtained the following 24-hour recall information:

7:00 A.M.	1 c. pineapple juice
	2 slices buttered toast with jelly
	2 scrambled eggs
	Coffee with sugar
10:00 A.M.	Coffee with sugar
	Danish roll
12:30 P.M.	Hamburger on bun
	French fries
	Tossed salad with French dressing
	Lemon meringue pie
	Coffee with sugar
6:00 P.M.	6 oz. pork chop
	1 small sweet potato
	½ c. peas with butter
	Sliced tomato salad with Thousand Island dressing
	8 oz. milk
	Tea with sugar
9:30 P.M.	12 oz. soft drink
	½ c. strawberry ice cream

Exercises

1. Explain the rationale for the postoperative diet.
2. Name foods in the diet recall that the patient should eliminate from his diet.
3. Explain the mechanism by which the symptoms of dumping syndrome are produced.

References

1. Almy, T.P. The gastrointestinal tract in man under stress. In M.H. Sleisenger and J.S. Fordtran, Eds., *Gastrointestinal Disease: Pathophysiology, Diagnosis, Management,* 2nd ed. Philadelphia: W.B. Saunders, 1978.
2. Almy, T.P., Kinkle, L., Burke, B., and Kern, F. Alterations in colonic function in men under stress. *Gastroenterology* 12:437, 1949.
3. Almy, T.P., and Fielding, J.F., Eds. The GI Tract in Stress and Psychosocial Disorder. *Clin. Gastroenterol.* 6(3), 1977.
4. Jenkins, G.N. *The Physiology of the Mouth,* 4th ed. Oxford: Blackwell Scientific, 1978.
5. Mason, D.K., and Chisholm, D.M. *Salivary Glands in Health and Disease.* London: W.B. Saunders, 1975.
6. Kreitzman, S.N. Nutrition in the process of dental caries. *Dent. Clin. North Am.* 20:491, 1976.
7. Gould, R.F., Ed. *Dietary Chemicals vs. Dental Caries.* Washington, D.C.: American Chemical Society, 1970.
8. Menaker, L., and Navia, J.M. Effect of undernutrition during the perinatal period on caries development in the rat: II. Caries susceptibility in underfed rats supplemented with protein or calorie additions during the suckling period. *J. Dent. Res.* 52:680, 1973.
9. Menaker, L., and Navia, J.M. Effect of undernutrition during the perinatal period on caries development in the rat: III. Effects of undernutrition on biochemical parameters in the developing submandibular salivary gland. *J. Dent. Res.* 52:688, 1973.
10. Menaker, L., and Navia, J.M. Effect of undernutrition during the perinatal period on caries development in the rat: IV. Effects of differential tooth eruption and exposure to a cariogenic diet on subsequent dental caries incidence. *J. Dent. Res.* 52:692, 1973.
11. De Paola, D.P., and Kuftinec, M.M. Nutrition in growth and development of oral tissues. *Dent. Clin. North Am.* 20:441, 1976.
12. Sognnaes, R.F., Shaw, J.H., and Bogorock, R. Radiotracer studies on bone, cementum, dentin, and enamel of Rhesus monkeys. *Am. J. Physiol.* 180:408, 1955.
13. De Paola, D.P., and Alfano, M.C. Triphasic nutritional analysis and dietary counseling. *Dent. Clin. North Am.* 20:613, 1976.
14. Harris, R.S., Nizel, A.E., and Walsh, N.B. The effect of phosphate structure on dental caries development in rats. *J. Dent. Res.* 40:290, 1967.
15. Gustaffson, G., Stelling, E., Abramson, E., and Brunius, E. Experiments with various fats in a cariogenic diet. *Acta Odontol. Scand.* 13:75, 1955.
16. Williams, W.L., Broquist, H.P., and Snell, E.E. Oleic acid and related compounds on growth factors for lactic acid bacteria. *J. Biol. Chem.* 170:619, 1947.
17. Dawes, C. Effects of diet on salivary secretion and composition. *J. Dent. Res.* 49:1263, 1970.
18. Weiss, M.E., and Bibby, B.G. Effects of milk on enamel solubility. *Arch. Oral Biol.* 11:49, 1966.
19. Alfano, M.C. Controversies, perspectives and clinical implications of nutrition in periodontal disease. *Dent. Clin. North Am.* 20:519, 1976.
20. Jenkins, C., and Ferguson, D.B. Milk and dental caries. *Br. Dent. J.* 120:472, 1966.
21. Enwonwu, C.O. Role of biochemistry and nutrition in preventive dentistry. *J. Am. Soc. Prev. Dent.* 4:6, 1974.
22. Henrickson, P. Periodontal disease and calcium deficiency. *Acta Odontol. Scand.* 26 (Suppl. 50), 1968.
23. Krook, L., Lutwak, L., and Whalen, J.P. Human periodontal disease. Morphology and response to calcium therapy. *Cornell Vet.* 62:32, 1972.
24. Nizel, A.E. *Nutrition in Preventive Dentistry: Science and Practice,* 2nd ed. Philadelphia: W.B. Saunders, 1981.
25. Mann, A.W., Mann, J.M., and Spies, T.D. A clinical study of malnourished edentulous patients. *J. Am. Dent. Assoc.* 32:1357, 1945.
26. Greene, H.I., Dreizen, S., and Spies, T.D. A clinical survey of the incidence of impaired masticatory function in patients of a nutrition clinic. *J. Am. Dent. Assoc.* 39:561, 1949.
27. Shannon, I.L., Trodahl, J.D., and Starcke, E.N. Remineralization of enamel by a saliva substitute designed for use by irradiated patients. *Cancer* 41:1746, 1978.
28. Arey, L.B., Tremaine, M.H., and Monzengo, F.L. The numerical and topographical relations of taste buds to human circumvallate papillae throughout the lifespan. *Anat. Rec.* 64:9, 1935.
29. Schiffman, S. Food recognition in the elderly. *J. Gerontol.* 32:586, 1977.
30. Tomlinson, B.E., and Henderson, G. Some quantitative cerebral findings in normal and demented old people. *Neurobiology of Aging* 3:183, 1982.
31. Smith, C.G. Age incidence of atrophy of olfactory nerves in man. *J. Comp. Neurol.* 77:589, 1942.
32. Liss, L., and Gomez, F. The nature of senile

changes of the human olfactory bulb and tract. *Arch. Otolaryngol.* 67:167, 1958.
33. Scheibel, M.E., and Scheibel, A.B. Structural changes in the aging brain. In B.H. Brody, D. Harman, and J.M. Ardy, Eds., *Aging. Vol. I: Clinical, Morphological, and Neurochemical Aspects in the Aging Nervous System.* New York: Raven Press, 1975.
34. Castell, D.O., and Harris, L.D. Hormonal control of gastroesophageal sphincter strength. *N. Engl. J. Med.* 282:886, 1970.
35. Lipshutz, W., and Cohen, S. Physiological determinants of lower esophageal sphincter function. *Gastroenterology* 61:16, 1971.
36. Lipshutz, W., Tuch, A., and Cohen, S. A comparison of the site of action of gastrin I on lower esophageal sphincter and antral circular smooth muscle. *Gastroenterology* 61:454, 1971.
37. Cohen, S., and Lipshutz, W. Hormonal regulation of human lower esophageal sphincter competence: Interaction of gastrin and secretin. *J. Clin. Invest.* 50:449, 1971.
38. Lipshutz, W., and Cohen, S. Interaction of gastrin I and secretin on gastrointestinal circular muscle. *Am. J. Physiol.* 222:775, 1972.
39. Resin, H., Stern, D.H., Sturdevant, R.A.L., and Isenberg, J.I. Effect of the C-terminal octapeptide of cholecystokinin on lower esophageal sphincter pressure in man. *Gastroenterology* 64:946, 1973.
40. Fisher, R.S., Di Marino, A.J., and Cohen, S. Mechanism of cholecystokinin-induced inhibition of lower esophageal sphincter pressure (abstract). *Clin. Res.* 22(3):358A, 1974.
41. Jennewein, H.M., Waldeck, K., Siewert, R., et al. The interaction of glucagon and pentagastrin on the lower oesophageal sphincter in man and dog. *Gut* 14:861, 1973.
42. Goyal, R.K., and Rattan, S. Neurohormonal, hormonal and drug receptors for the lower esophageal sphincter. *Gastroenterology* 74: 598, 1978.
43. Sigmund, C.J., and McNally, E.F. The action of a carminative on the lower esophageal sphincter. *Gastroenterology* 56:13, 1969.
44. Babka, J.C., and Castell, D.O. On the genesis of heartburn. The effects of specific foods on the lower esophageal sphincter. *Am. J. Dig. Dis.* 18:391, 1973.
45. Hogan, W., Viegas de Andrade, S.R., and Winship, D. Ethanol induced acute esophageal motor dysfunction. *J. Appl. Physiol.* 32:755, 1972.
46. Hurwitz, A.L., Duranceau, A., and Haddad, J.K. *Disorders of Esophageal Motility.* Philadelphia: W.B. Saunders, 1979.
47. Harris, J.B., Nigon, K., and Alonso, D. Adenosine 3′5′ monophosphate: Intracellular mediator for methyl xanthine stimulation of gastric secretion. *Gastroenterology* 57:377, 1969.
48. Cohen, S., and Booth, G.H. Gastric acid secretion and lower esophageal sphincter pressure in response to coffee and caffeine. *N. Engl. J. Med.* 293:897, 1975.
49. Trounce, J.R., Deuchar, D.C., Kauntze, R., and Thomas, G.A. Studies in achalasia of the cardia. *Q. J. Med.* 26:433, 1957.
50. Ellis, F.H., Jr. Management of oesophageal achalasia. *Clin. Gastroenterol.* 5:89, 1976.
51. Cohen, S., Fisher, R., Lipshutz, W., et al. The pathogenesis of esophageal dysfunction in scleroderma and Raynaud's disease. *J. Clin. Invest.* 51:2663, 1972.
52. Van Thiel, D.H., Gavaler, J.S., Joshi, S.N., et al. Heartburn of pregnancy. *Gastroenterology* 72:666, 1977.
53. Gunning, A.J., and Marshall, R. Replacement of the esophagus. *Clin. Gastroenterol.* 8:292, 1979.
54. Doniach, D., and Roitt, I.M. An evaluation of gastric and thyroid autoimmunity in relation to hematologic disorders. *Semin. Hematol.* 1:313, 1964.
55. Fein, H.D. Nutrition in the stomach, including related areas in the esophagus and duodenum. In R.S. Goodhart and M.E. Shils, Eds., *Modern Nutrition in Health and Disease,* 6th ed. Philadelphia: Lea and Febiger, 1980.
56. Piper, D.W., Greig, M., Thomas, J., and Skinners, J. Personality pattern of patients with chronic gastric ulcer. Study of neuroticism and extroversion in a gastric ulcer and a control population. *Gastroenterology* 73:444, 1977.
57. Piper, D.W., Greig, M., Skinners, J., et al. Chronic gastric ulcer and stress. A comparison with a control population regarding stressful events over a lifetime. *Digestion* 18:303, 1978.
58. Luckmann, J., and Sorenson, K.C. *Medical-Surgical Nursing,* 2nd ed. Philadelphia: W.B. Saunders, 1980.
59. Piper, D.W. The treatment of chronic peptic ulcer. *Front. Gastrointest. Res.* 6:109, 1980.
60. Burland, W.L. Evidence for the safety of cimetidine in the treatment of peptic ulcer disease. In W. Creutzfeldt, Ed., *Cimetidine: Proceedings of the International Symposium on Histamine H_2 Receptor Antagonists.* Amsterdam: Excerpta Medica, 1978. P. 238.
61. Kruss, D.M., and Littman, A. Safety of cimetidine. *Gastroenterology* 74:484, 1978.

62. Barbezat, G.O., and Bank, S. Effect of prolonged cimetidine therapy on gastric acid secretion in man. *Gut* 19:51, 1978.
63. Peterson, W.L., Sturdevant, R.A.L., Frankl, H.D., et al. Healing of duodenal ulcer with an antacid regimen. *N. Engl. J. Med.* 297:341, 1977.
64. Sturdevant, R.A.L., Isenberg, J.I., Secrist, D., and Ansfield, J. Antacid and placebo produced similar pain relief in duodonal ulcer patients. *Gastroenterology* 72:1, 1977.
65. Lewis, J.R. Carbenoxolone sodium in the treatment of peptic ulcer. *J.A.M.A.* 229:460, 1974.
66. Piper, D.W. Antacid and anticholinergic drug therapy. *Clin. Gastroenterology* 2:361, 1973.
67. Ivery, K. Anticholinergics: Do they work in peptic ulcer? *Gastroenterology* 68:154, 1975.
68. Lennard-Hones, J.E., and Barbouris, N. Effect of different foods on the acidity of gastric contents in patients with duodenal ulcer: I. A comparison between two therapeutic diets and freely chosen meals. *Gut* 6:113, 1965.
69. Ingelfinger, F.J. Let the ulcer patient enjoy his food. In F.J. Ingelfinger, A.S. Relman, and M. Finland, Eds., *Controversy in Internal Medicine.* Philadelphia: W.B. Saunders, 1966.
70. Taylor, K.B. Gastroenterology. In H.A. Schneider, C.E. Anderson, and D.B. Coursin, Eds., *Nutritional Support of Medical Practice.* New York: Harper and Row, 1977.
71. Clinical Dietetics Section, Hospital Food Service. *Manual of Clinical Dietetics.* Los Angeles: University of California, 1977.
72. Hoelz, H.R., and Gewertz, B.L. Vagotomy. *Clin. Gastroenterol.* 8:305, 1979.
73. Jesseph, J.E. Serotonin and the dumping syndrome. A reappraisal. *Surgery* 63:536, 1968.
74. Thomford, N.R., Sirinek, K.R., Crockett, S.E., et al. Gastric inhibitory peptide: Response to oral glucose after vagotomy and pyloroplasty. *Arch. Surg.* 109:177, 1974.
75. Wong, P.T., Talamo, R.C., Babior, B.M., et al. Kallikrein-kinin system in postgastrectomy dumping syndrome. *Ann. Intern. Med.* 80:577, 1974.
76. MacDonald, J.M., Webster, M.M., Tennyson, C.H., and Drapanas, T. Serotonin and bradykinin in the dumping syndrome. *Am. J. Surg.* 117:204, 1969.
77. Stahlgren, L.H. The dumping syndrome: A study of its hemodynamics. *Hosp. Pract.* 5:59, 1970.
78. Schultz, K.T., Neelon, F.A., Nilsen, L.B., and Lebovitz, H.E. Mechanisms of postgastrectomy hypoglycemia. *Arch. Intern. Med.* 128: 240, 1971.
79. Small, W.P. The long-term results of peptic ulcer surgery. *Clin. Gastroenterol.* 2:427, 1972.
80. MacLean, L.D., Perry, J.F., Kelly, W.D., et al. Nutrition following subtotal gastrectomy of four types (Billroth I and II, segmental and tubular resections). *Surgery* 35:705, 1954.
81. Lundh, G. Intestinal digestion and absorption after gastrectomy. *Acta Chir. Scand.* (Suppl.) 231:1, 1958.
82. Hillman, H.S. Postgastrectomy malnutrition. *Gut* 9:576, 1968.
83. Pryor, J.P., O'Shea, M.J., Brooks, P.L., and Datar, G.K. The long-term metabolic consequences of partial gastrectomy. *Am. J. Med.* 51:5, 1971.
84. Bradley, E.L., III. Total gastrectomy. *Clin. Gastroenterol.* 8:354, 1979.
85. Alexander-Williams, J., and Hoare, A.M. Partial gastric resection. *Clin. Gastroenterol.* 8:321, 1979.
86. MacLean, L.D. Nutritional complications in the surgical patients. In C.P. Artz and J.D. Hardy, Eds., *Complications in Surgery and Their Management,* 2nd ed. Philadelphia: W.B. Saunders, 1969. P. 243.
87. Alexander-Williams, J. Partial gastrectomy. The late nutritional and metabolic effects. *Am. J. Proctol.* 17:288, 1966.
88. Bradley, E.L., III, and Isaacs, J.T. Postresectional anemia. *Arch. Surg.* 111:844, 1976.
89. Gough, K.R., Thirkette, J.L., and Reed, A.E. Folic acid deficiency in patients after gastric resection. *Q. J. Med.* 34:1, 1965.
90. Mahmud, K., Ripley, D., Swaim, W.R., and Doscherholmen, A. Hematologic complications of partial gastrectomy. *Ann. Surg.* 177:432, 1973.
91. Harris, A.I., and Janowitz, H.D. Medical management of problems following peptic ulcer surgery. *Postgrad. Med.* 63:127, 1978.
92. Fourman, P. Effects of gastrectomy on bone. In R.H. Gerdwood and A.N. Smith, Eds., *Malabsorption.* Medical Monographs 4. Edinburgh, University Press, 1969. Pp. 59–62.
93. Clark, C.G. Nutritional and Metabolic Consequences of Partial Gastrectomy. In A.G. Cox and J. Alexander-Williams, Eds., *Vagotomy on Trial.* London: William Heinemann Medical, 1973. P. 53.
94. Alexander-Williams, J. Some sequelae of gastric operations including the dumping syndrome and metabolic disorders. In R. Maingot, Ed., *Abdominal Operations.* New York: Appleton-Century-Crofts, 1974. P. 491.

95. Nilson, B.E., and Wastlin, L.E. The fracture incidence after gastrectomy. *Acta Chir. Scand.* 137:533, 1971.
96. French, J.M., and Crane, C.W. Undernutrition, malnutrition and malabsorption following gastrectomy. In F.A.R. Stammars and J. Alexander-Williams, Eds., *Complications and Metabolic Consequences.* London: Butterworth, 1963.
97. Rombeau, J.L., and Miller, R.A. *Nasoenteric Tube Feeding: Practical Aspects.* Mountain View, Calif.: Health Development Corp., 1979.
98. Shils, M.E. Enteral nutrition by tube. *Cancer Res.* 57:2432, 1977.

Bibliography

Alfano, M.C., and De Paola, D.P., Eds. Symposium on Nutrition. *Dent. Clin. North Am.* 20:441, 1976.

Artz, C.P., and Hardy, J.D., Eds. *Management of Surgical Complications,* 3rd ed. Philadelphia: W.B. Saunders, 1975.

Brooks, F.P. *Control of Gastrointestinal Function.* New York: Macmillan, 1970.

De Paola, D.P., and Alfano, M.C. Diet and oral health. *Nutrition Today* 12(3):6, 1977.

Field, M., Fordtran, J.S., and Schultz, S.G., Eds. *Secretory Diarrhea.* Bethesda, Md.: American Physiological Society, 1980.

Gould, R.F., Ed. *Dietary Chemicals vs. Dental Caries.* Washington, D.C.: American Chemical Society, 1970.

Guyton, A.C. *Textbook of Medical Physiology,* 6th ed. Philadelphia: W.B. Saunders, 1979.

Kirsner, J.B., and Winans, C.S. The stomach. In W.A. Sodeman and T.M. Sodeman, Eds., *Pathologic Physiology.* Philadelphia: W.B. Saunders, 1979.

Koretz, R.L., and Meyer, J.H. Elemental diets — facts and fantasies. *Gastroenterology* 78:393, 1980.

Lifshitz, F., Ed. *Clinical Disorders in Pediatric Gastroenterology and Nutrition.* New York: Marcel Dekker, 1980.

Lipshutz, W.H., Gaskins, R.D., Lukash, W.M., and Sode, J. Pathogenesis of lower-esophageal-sphincter incompetence. *N. Engl. J. Med.* 289:182, 1973.

Menguy, R. Surgery of peptic ulcer. In P.A. Ebert, Ed., *Major Problems in Clinical Surgery.* Philadelphia: W.B. Saunders, 1976.

Nizel, A.E. *Nutrition in Preventive Dentistry: Science and Practice,* 2nd ed. Philadelphia: W.B. Saunders, 1981.

Paige, D.M., and Bayless, T.M., Eds. *Lactose Digestion: Clinical and Nutritional Implications.* Baltimore: Johns Hopkins Press, 1981.

Skinner, D.B. The esophagus. In W.A. Sodeman and T.M. Sodeman, Eds., *Pathologic Physiology.* Philadelphia: W.B. Saunders, 1979.

Sleisenger, M.H., and Fordtran, J.S., Eds. *Gastrointestinal Disease: Pathophysiology, Diagnosis, Management,* 2nd ed. Philadelphia: W.B. Saunders, 1978.

Turnberg, L.A. The pathophysiology of diarrhea. *Clin. Gastroenterol.* 8:551, 1979.

Vander, A.J., Sherman, J.H., and Luciano, D.S. *Human Physiology: The Mechanisms of Body Function,* 3rd ed. New York: McGraw-Hill, 1980.

van der Reis, L., Ed. The stomach. *Front. Gastrointest. Res.* Vol. 6, 1980.

6. The Intestinal Tract and Accessory Organs

- I. Normal Anatomy and Physiology
  - A. Small intestine
    - 1. Normal structure
    - 2. Normal physiology
      - a. motility
      - b. secretion
      - c. digestion and absorption
      - d. protective mechanisms
  - B. Biliary tract
  - C. Pancreas
  - D. Large intestine
- II. Conditions Common to Many Gastrointestinal Disorders
  - A. Malabsorption syndromes
    - 1. Pathogenesis of malabsorption
      - a. lipids
      - b. carbohydrate
      - c. protein
      - d. vitamin B_{12}
      - e. drug-induced malabsorption
    - 2. General symptoms
    - 3. Diagnosis
    - 4. Treatment
  - B. Intestinal antigen absorption
    - 1. Absorptive mechanisms
    - 2. Related diseases
    - 3. Nutritional management
  - C. Diarrhea
    - 1. Pathophysiology and classification
    - 2. Diagnosis
    - 3. Metabolic consequences
    - 4. Therapy
  - D. Protein-losing enteropathies
  - E. Intestinal fistulas
- III. Diseases Affecting Primarily the Small Intestine
  - A. Gluten enteropathy
    - 1. Clinical manifestations
    - 2. Pathogenesis
    - 3. Treatment
  - B. Tropical sprue
  - C. Crohn's disease
    - 1. Clinical manifestations
    - 2. Causes and predisposing factors
    - 3. Treatment
  - D. Short bowel syndrome
    - 1. Etiology
    - 2. Pathophysiology
    - 3. Treatment
  - E. Carbohydrate intolerance
    - 1. Lactase deficiency
      - a. pathophysiology
      - b. forms and incidence
      - c. diagnosis
      - d. treatment
    - 2. Sucrase-isomaltase deficiency
    - 3. Glucose-galactose malabsorption
  - F. Intestinal lymphangiectasia
  - G. Abetalipoproteinemia
  - H. Endocrine-secreting tumors
    - 1. Foregut tumors
    - 2. Midgut and hindgut tumors
      - a. pathogenesis and manifestations
      - b. diagnosis
      - c. treatment
- IV. Diseases of the Gallbladder and Bile Ducts
  - A. Types of gallbladder diseases treated by diet
  - B. Nutritional management
- V. Diseases of the Pancreas
  - A. Diagnosis
  - B. Acute pancreatitis
  - C. Chronic pancreatitis
    - 1. Pathogenesis
    - 2. Clinical manifestations
    - 3. Nutritional management
  - D. Cystic fibrosis
    - 1. Pathophysiology and clinical manifestations
    - 2. Nutritional management
- VI. Diseases of the Large Intestine
  - A. Fiber and related substances
  - B. Intestinal gas
  - C. Constipation
  - D. Chronic ulcerative colitis
  - E. Diverticular disease
    - 1. Cause
    - 2. Clinical manifestations
    - 3. Management
  - F. Colon surgery
    - 1. Ileostomy
    - 2. Colostomy
  - G. Rectal surgery
- VII. Case Studies

The intestine, exocrine pancreas, and gallbladder are discussed in one chapter since they are involved simultaneously in the digestion and absorption of many nutrients. The nutritional consequences of liver disease are described in Chapter 11.

NORMAL ANATOMY AND PHYSIOLOGY

The Small Intestine

Normal Structure

The small intestine is approximately 15 ft long and consists of the *duodenum* (10 in.), the *jejunum* (9.5 ft), and the *ileum* (4 ft), in that order. Bile and secretions of the pancreas enter the duodenum via a duct system which penetrates the duodenal wall a few centimeters below the pyloric sphincter.

Three features of the structure of the small intestine increase the surface area that is in contact with the intestinal contents. These are *Kerckring's folds* or *plicae circularis,* the *villi,* and the *microvilli* on the luminal borders of the absorptive cells of the villi. Approximately twenty *crypts of Lieberkühn* lie at the base of each villus and penetrate down to the muscularis mucosae to a depth of approximately one-quarter of the height of the villus. The villi are covered with a single layer of cells, which also extend down into the crypts. Most of the cells in the crypts are undifferentiated and multiply rapidly, maturing as they move up the sides of the crypts and onto the walls of the villi. The ability of the cells to divide is lost as they leave the crypts. A small number of the cells differentiate into *goblet cells,* which secrete mucus, but most become *enterocytes* or *absorptive cells.* As they differentiate, the absorptive cells develop a brush border, enzymes, receptor sites, and carrier proteins, all of which function in digestion and absorption. The cells continue to migrate toward the tips of the villi and, after 3 to 7 days, they are extruded from the tips of the villi into the lumen of the intestine. The intestinal mucosa thus is renewed constantly.

The crypts of Lieberkühn also contain other cells that are nonmigrating. These include *Paneth cells,* the function of which is unknown, and *enterochromaffin, argentaffin,* or *basal granular cells.* There are several distinct populations of cells within the group of enterochromaffin cells. Some have an endocrine function, but the functions of others is unknown.

In the duodenum, elaborately branched *Brunner's glands* extend down from the mucosal surface. The secretion of these glands is high in mucus and bicarbonate. These substances lubricate chyme and neutralize gastric hydrochloric acid.

The luminal surface of the microvilli is coated with a mucopolysaccharide called the *glycocalyx.* Several digestive enzymes are located in this area. Above the glycocalyx is a stagnant layer of water, the so called unstirred layer, through which molecules in the lumen must move to be absorbed.[1,2] The *lamina propria* is the connective tissue layer that lies below the epithelium and its basement membrane. It carries blood and lymphatic capillaries close to the epithelial tissue. Absorbed materials thus move from the absorptive cells through the lamina propria and into the blood or lymph.

Normal Physiology

The functions of the intestinal tract include (1) motility to provide mixing and propulsion of intestinal contents, (2) secretion of enzymes, hormones, and other materials, (3) digestion and absorption of ingested materials, (4) protection of other organs' and its own integrity, and (5) excretion of waste products. Simultaneous normal bile production in the liver and normal gallbladder and pancreatic function are essential for normal intestinal function.

Motility. Mixing is accomplished mostly by *segmentation,* a kneading action resulting from contractions of the circular muscles. *Pendular movements,* longitudinal contractions that shorten the length of the gut, also contribute to mixing. The major function of the wormlike motion known as *peristalsis* is to propel the food through the tract although it, too, may have some mixing effects. Movements of the villi also contribute to mixing and propulsion. Intestinal motor activity is under hormonal and nervous control. Sympathetic nervous system stimulation inhibits propulsive activity and increases sphincter tone.

Secretion. The intestinal mucosa secretes enzymes, hormones, mucus, electrolytes and water. The enzymes include the disaccharidases, such as maltase, sucrase, and lactase, some *peptidases,* and *enterokinase* (Table 6-1).

In addition, the duodenal mucosa secretes gastrointestinal hormones. *Secretin* is released when the low pH of the gastric contents comes into contact with duodenal mucosa. It decreases intestinal motility and stimulates pancreatic secretion of bicarbonate into the duodenum, neutralizing the gastric acidity.

Cholecystokinin-pancreozymin (CCK-PZ) also is secreted by the duodenal mucosa. Its release is stimulated by the presence of fat in the duodenum. Cholecystokinin-pancreozymin increases production of pancreatic enzymes and stimulates contraction of the gallbladder to deliver bile to the intestinal lumen.

The secretion of fluid and electrolytes into the intestinal lumen is greater in magnitude than their movement into any other organ system. The combined volume of ingested and endogenous fluid that reaches the intestinal lumen has been estimated to be approximately 9 liters/day in the average adult. Approximately 2 liters of this is exogenous fluid taken in food and drink. Table 6-2 shows the typical amounts and sources of fluid and also the sites where the fluid normally is absorbed.

Digestion and Absorption. Although digestion and absorption are separate functions in concept, they are somewhat intertwined in fact and will therefore be discussed together.

Most digestion of protein, fat, and carbohydrate takes place in the duodenum and the first 3 ft of jejunum and involves the action of bile, pancreatic enzymes, and intestinal enzymes. The resulting fatty acids, monosaccharides, and amino acids are absorbed mostly in the first 60 to 100 cm of the jejunum. Materials and vitamins also are absorbed in the duodenum and jejunum, except for vitamin B_{12}, which is absorbed in the ileum. The ileum apparently is capable of absorption of other nutrients, but most are absorbed in more proximal portions of the gut and therefore are not present in the lumen of the ileum. The usual sites of absorption of the various nutrients are shown in Fig. 6-1.

Absorption is the translocation of materials from the lumen into the portal and lymphatic systems. The four possible modes by which it is believed to occur are *passive diffusion, active transport, facilitated transport,* and *pinocytosis.* Following one of these absorptive processes, the material is transported across the cell, released across the basal or lateral membrane of the cell, crosses the basement membrane, and moves into the capillaries or lacteals.

There is almost total absorption of digested protein, fat, and carbohydrate. Absorption is obligatory; that is, it does not depend on the body's need. Efficiency of absorption of water and of monovalent ions—sodium, potassium, chloride, iodine, and fluoride—also is very high, while absorption of divalent and trivalent ions, in-

Table 6-1. Summary of Digestive Processes

Source of and Stimulus for Secretion	Enzyme	Method of Activation and Optimal Conditions for Activity	Substrate	End Products or Action
Salivary glands of mouth: Secrete saliva in reflex response to presence of food in mouth	Salivary amylase	Chloride ion necessary; pH 6.6–6.8	Starch Glycogen	Maltose plus 1 : 6 glucosides (oligosaccharides) plus maltotriose
Stomach glands: Chief cells and parietal cells secrete gastric juice in response to reflex stimulation and chemical action of gastrin	Pepsin	Pepsinogen converted to active pepsin by HCl; pH 1.0–2.0	Protein	Proteoses Peptones
	Rennin	Calcium necessary for activity; pH 4.0	Casein of milk	Coagulates milk
Pancreas: Presence of acid chyme from stomach activates duodenum to produce (1) secretin, which hormonally stimulates flow of pancreatic juice; (2) cholecystokinin, which stimulates production of enzymes	Trypsin	Trypsinogen converted to active trypsin by enterokinase of intestine at pH 5.2–6.0; autocatalytic at pH 7.9	Protein Proteoses Peptones	Polypeptides Dipeptides
	Chymotrypsin	Secreted as chymotrypsinogen and converted to active form by trypsin; pH 8.0	Protein Proteoses Peptones	Same as trypsin; more coagulating power for milk
	Carboxypeptidase	Secreted as procarboxypeptidase, activated by trypsin	Polypeptides at the free carboxyl end of the chain	Lower peptides; free amino acids
	Pancreatic amylase	pH 7.1	Starch Glycogen	Maltose plus 1 : 6 glucosides (oligosaccharides) plus maltotriose
	Lipase	Activated by bile salts, phospholipids, colipase; pH 8.0	Primary ester linkages of triacylglycerol	Fatty acids, monoacylglycerols, diacylglycerols, glycerol

	Ribonuclease		Ribonucleic acid	Nucleotides
	Deoxyribonuclease		Deoxyribonucleic acids	Nucleotides
	Cholesteryl ester hydrolase	Activated by bile salts	Cholesteryl esters	Free cholesterol plus fatty acids
	Phospholipase A_2		Phospholipids	Fatty acids, lysophospholipids
Liver and gallbladder: Cholecystokinin, a hormone from the intestinal mucosa—and possibly also gastrin and secretin—stimulates gallbladder and secretion of bile by liver	(Bile salts and alkali)		Fats—also neutralize acid chyme	Fatty acid–bile salt conjugates and finely emulsified neutral fat—bile salt micelles
Small intestine: Secretions of Brunner's glands of duodenum and glands of Lieberkühn	Aminopeptidase		Polypeptides at the free amino end of the chain	Lower peptides; free amino acids
	Dipeptidases		Dipeptides	Amino acids
	Sucrase	pH 5.0–7.0	Sucrose	Fructose, glucose
	Maltase	pH 5.8–6.2	Maltose	Glucose
	Lactase	pH 5.4–6.0	Lactose	Glucose, galactose
	Phosphatase	pH 8.6	Organic phosphates	Free phosphate
	Isomaltase or 1:6 glucosidase		1:6 Glucosides	Glucose
	Polynucleotidase		Nucleic acid	Nucleotides
	Nucleosidases (nucleoside phosphorylases)		Purine or pyrimidine nucleosides	Purine or pyrimidine bases, pentose phosphate

Reprinted with permission from Martin, D.W., Mayes, P.A., and Rodwell, V.W., *Harper's Review of Biochemistry,* 18th ed. Los Altos, Calif.: Lange Medical, 1981, p. 528.

Table 6-2. Daily Volume of Fluid Circulation Through the Human Intestinal Lumen

Entering		Leaving (Absorbed)	
Source	Volume (liters)	Source	Volume (liters)
Diet	2	Jejunum	4.5
Saliva	1	Ileum	3.5
Gastric juice	2	Colon	1
Bile	1		
Pancreatic juice	2		
Small intestine	1		
Total	9	Total	9[a]

[a] Water content of stool is approximately 100 to 200 ml. Overall efficiency of water absorption is approximately 99 percent.

cluding calcium, iron, and zinc, is less complete. It is regulated according to need, thus protecting the body from toxic effects.

Triglycerides. In considering their digestion, the triglycerides must be considered in two categories, the digestion and absorption of which differ with the length of the fatty acid chains. One of these categories contains the *long-chain* triglycerides.

Most dietary fat is triglyceride with smaller amounts of other lipids. The fatty acids present in largest quantity in triglycerides are long-chain fatty acids containing twelve carbons or more. The most common fatty acids, palmitic (C16:0) and stearic (C18:0), are saturated, while the unsaturated fatty acids, oleic (C18:1) and linoleic (C18:2), have one or two unsaturated bonds, respectively.

Pancreatic lipase is required for digestion of these lipids. The action of pancreatic lipase on a triglyceride (*lipolysis*) results in the production of three fatty acids plus glycerol or a beta-monoglyceride plus two fatty acid molecules.

When fat enters the intestinal lumen, the action of bile comes into play. Bile, containing bile salts, is secreted by the liver and

Figure 6-1. Sites of absorption of major nutrients across the small intestinal mucosa. (Reprinted with permission from Greenberger, N.J., Gastrointestinal Disorders: A Pathophysiologic Approach, *2nd ed. Copyright © 1981 by Year Book Medical Publishers, Inc., Chicago. P. 128.)*

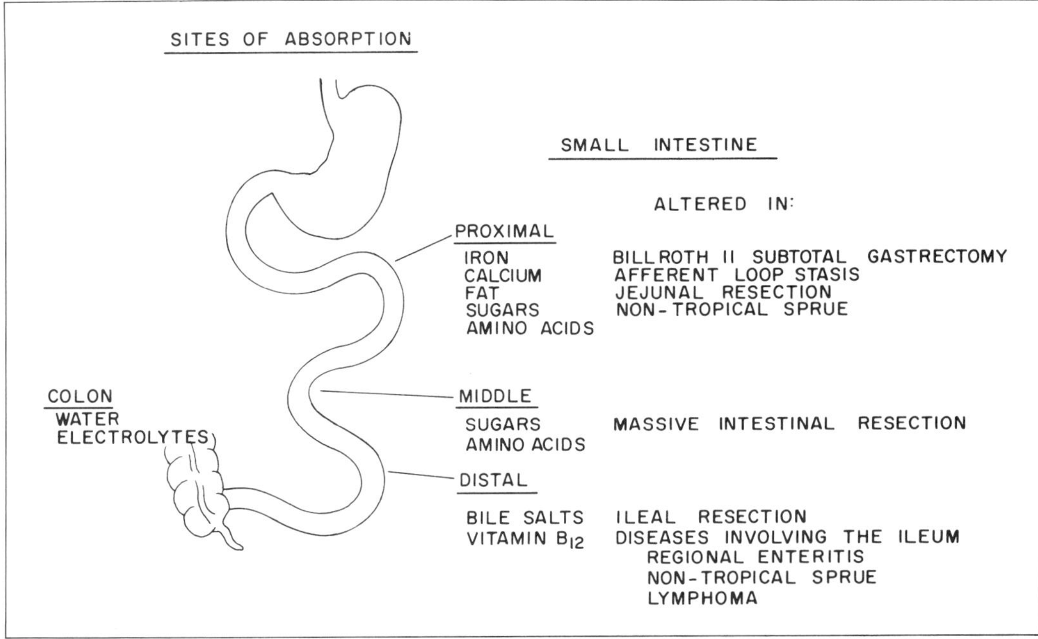

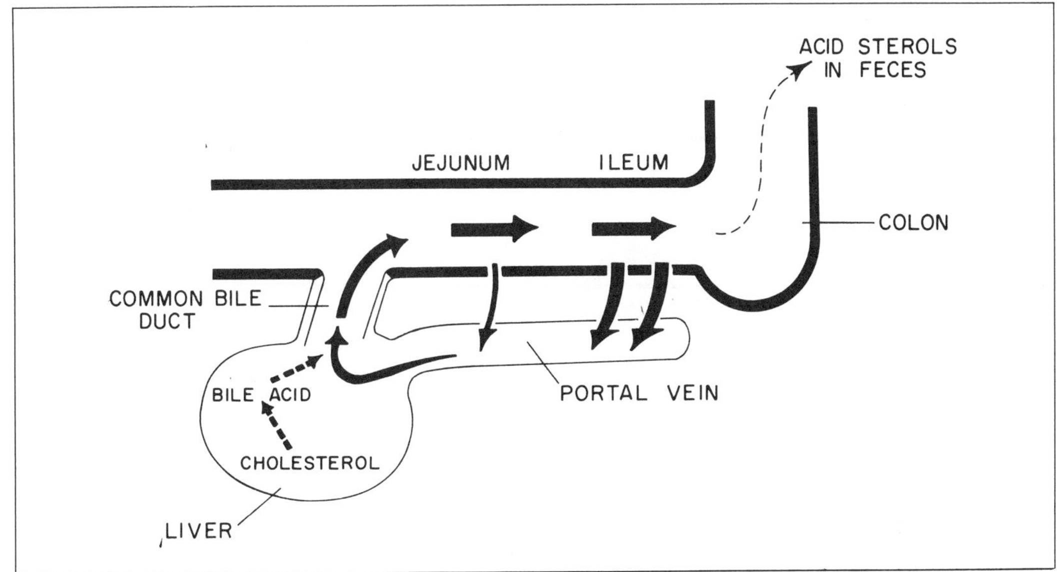

Figure 6-2. The enterohepatic circulation of bile salts. (Reprinted with permission from Riley, J.W., and Glickman, R.M., Fat malabsorption—advances in our understanding. Am. J. Med. *67:982, 1979.)*

stored in the gallbladder until needed. Cholecystokinin-pancreozymin stimulates contraction of the gallbladder and increases the delivery of bile to the intestinal lumen. When the bile salts reach the *critical micellar concentration* (0.15 M), they aggregate with the fatty acids and beta-monoglycerides to form *micelles,* small particles 3 to 10 nm in diameter with the hydrophilic polar group oriented on the surface. Micelles make it possible for the lipid to be solubilized in the contents of the intestinal lumen, forming a clear aqueous solution. They make enzymatic lipolysis possible in an aqueous environment and increase the rate of lipolysis by removing the end products of the reaction. Micelles also increase the rate at which the lipids can be diffused through the unstirred water layer, preliminary to absorption. Bile acts only in fat digestion and has no role in the digestion of protein or carbohydrate.

The micelle is believed to dissociate at the jejunal cell surface. The fatty acids and beta-monoglycerides cross the cell membrane by passive diffusion. The bile salts released from the micelles in the jejunum are carried to the ileum and reabsorbed, creating a cycle known as the *enterohepatic circulation* (Fig. 6-2). Approximately 2 to 4 g of bile salts exist in the body pool, but they are recycled six to ten times per day so that the ileum normally is presented with 20 to 30 g to reabsorb. The pool must recycle several times to absorb the lipid in a single meal.[3] The liver synthesizes and the intestine excretes 200 to 600 mg of bile salts daily.

The lipids are reesterified rapidly in the enterocyte (Fig. 6-3). The resulting triglycerides become associated with cholesterol, cholesteryl esters, phospholipid, and protein to form *chylomicrons.* The chylomicrons then are released from the cell and enter the lacteal by a process that is not completely understood, possibly by pinocytosis or through gaps at junctions of cells in the wall of the lacteal. The chylomicrons enter the blood via the thoracic duct. Their further metabolism and their relationship to cardiovascular disease is described in Chapter 8. Phospholipids and cholesterol also are absorbed via the lacteals.

In contrast to the rather complex sequence of events described for long-chain triglycerides, the procedure for digestion and

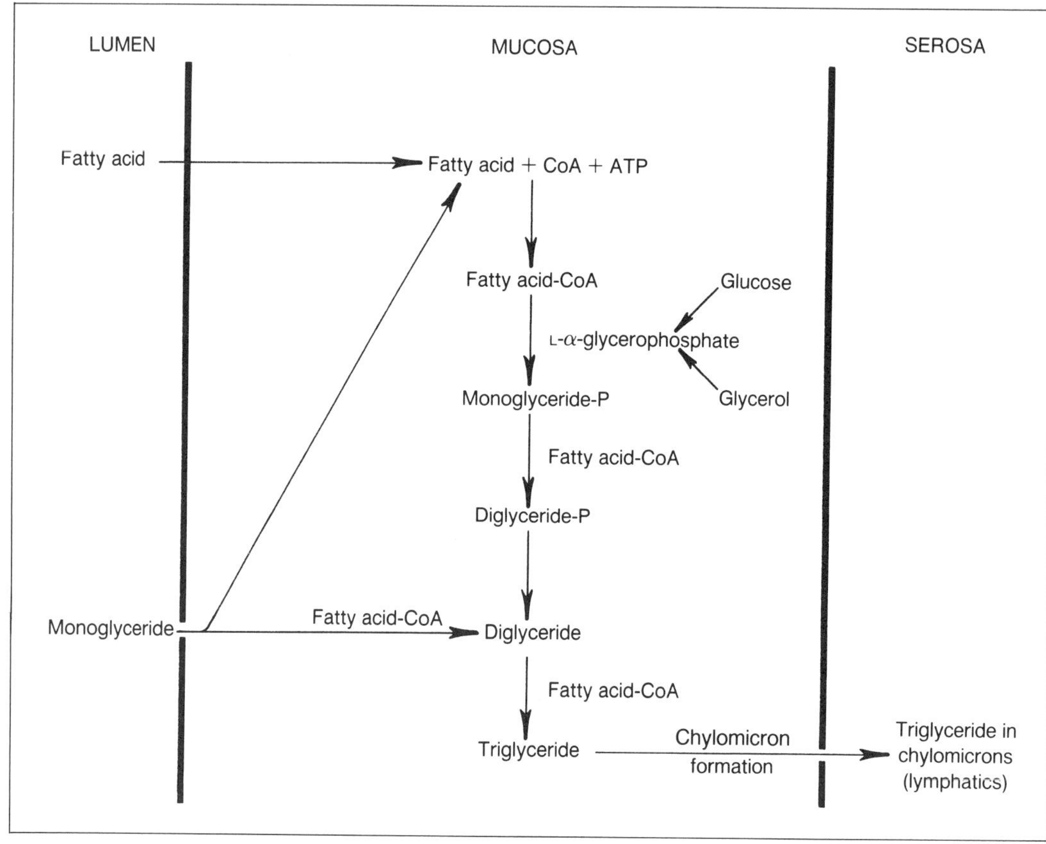

Figure 6-3. Major reactions in mucosal cells during fat absorption. P = phosphate. (Reprinted with permission from Isselbacher, K.J., Biochemical aspects of lipid malabsorption. Fed. Proc. *26:1421, 1967.)*

absorption of the *medium-chain* triglycerides, which contain shorter fatty acids (C6 : 0 to C10 : 0), is fairly simple. They are hydrolyzed easily by pancreatic lipase to free fatty acids. Very little beta-monoglyceride is produced. Furthermore, bile salts apparently are unnecessary, since micelle formation is not required for the absorption of medium-chain fatty acids. They are transported into the capillaries and thence into the portal vein, bypassing the lymphatics. Approximately 30 percent may be absorbed unchanged. Consequently, medium-chain triglycerides are useful in diseases involving deficiencies of pancreatic enzymes, decreased availability of bile, or diseased lymphatic function. Their use in nutritional care in these conditions will be discussed in more detail later in this chapter.

Protein. Protein digestion results primarily from the action of pancreatic enzymes. The site of action of pancreatic proteases, released as a result of vagal stimulation of CCK-PZ action, is not entirely clear. Some hydrolysis of proteins may occur in the intestinal lumen, but some proteases adsorb to the enterocyte membrane and may act at that site. They produce peptides that consist of three to six amino acid residues. *Oligopeptidases* and *tripeptidases,* which have been identified in the brush border, digest the largest molecules to dipeptides and amino acids. There are a number of *dipeptidases,* but their location is not clear. These function in dipeptide hydrolysis to amino acids.

Dipeptides, as well as amino acids, can cross the cell membrane and enter the enterocytes. The nutritional significance of this action is not known. The transport mechanisms involved in amino acid absorption are not understood entirely, but it is known that there is more than one mechanism, affecting various groups of amino acids. The rate of transport can apparently be affected to some degree by dietary manipulation.[4]

Carbohydrate. In the duodenal lumen, pancreatic amylase attacks the 1,4 linkages of starch, producing maltose, maltotriose, and alpha-dextrins. The alpha-dextrins contain the branching points with 1,6 linkages and usually consist of approximately eight glucose units. These products of pancreatic enzyme action plus dietary lactose and sucrose are further digested at the surface of the brush border in the intestinal phase. The enzymes, maltases, alpha-dextrinase, lactase, and sucrase are located in the area of the plasma membrane and glycocalyx. Most of the glucose, galactose, and fructose produced is absorbed into the enterocytes and thence into the capillaries, although a small amount may diffuse back into the lumen. Glucose and galactose are absorbed by a sodium-dependent active transport system. Fructose apparently is absorbed by facilitated diffusion.

Folic acid. Most folic acid in food occurs bound to additional L-glutamic acid residues. It is converted in the small intestine to the free monoglutamate form by the action of *conjugase,* the exact site of action of which is unknown. Absorption of folate occurs in the proximal small intestine, but the mechanism is not clear. Within the enterocyte, it is converted to reduced methylfolate and then is absorbed into the capillaries and carried to the portal vein.

Vitamin B_{12}. Dietary vitamin B_{12} is protein-bound and is released by the action of gastric acid and digestive enzymes. *Intrinsic factor* (IF) is produced by gastric parietal cells, then binds the free vitamin B_{12} to produce a vitamin B_{12}–IF complex. This form is required for the absorption of vitamin B_{12} to occur. Formation of the complex is believed to protect the vitamin from utilization by intestinal bacteria and possibly from digestion.

In the terminal ileum, the complex attaches to receptors in the plasma membrane–glycocalyx. This process is enhanced by calcium ion.[5] The vitamin is released from IF in or on the membrane and is transported into the cell and then into the portal circulation bound to a carrier known as *transcobalamin.* The fate of IF is unknown.

Other vitamins. The processes of absorption of other water-soluble vitamins are largely unknown. Most are believed to be absorbed by simple diffusion, although thiamine, which ionizes slowly, may be poorly absorbed. Absorption of fat-soluble vitamins parallels lipid absorption in general. Bile salts apparently are required for absorption by passive diffusion.

Water and mineral elements. Most of the 9 liters of water presented to the intestine daily are reabsorbed into the portal blood with only 200 ml or so appearing in the feces. Approximately 20 percent of the ingested water is absorbed per minute at locations indicated in Table 6-2.[6] Both passive and active absorption of water are likely, but the driving forces are uncertain. The absorption of water from the intestinal tract is obligatory, as is that of most monovalent ions. Excesses are excreted in the urine, so the kidney, not the intestine, provides the primary homeostatic mechanisms. It is not possible, for example, to cause diarrhea by water intakes in excess of need. Instead, excess water is excreted by increasing urine flow.

Electrolyte transport is an active process. A free exchange of Na^+, H^+, and Cl^- ions occurs across the duodenal mucosa. As a consequence, meals of varying composition are rendered iso-osmolar in Na^+ content with plasma, and isotonic and neutral in pH by mechanisms that are not understood completely. Approximately 50 percent of the water, Na^+, K^+ and Cl^- are absorbed in the jejunum.

In the ileum, Na^+ can be absorbed against a concentration gradient. A model linking exchange of Na^+-H^+ and $Cl^--HCO_3^-$ has been described by which the ileum absorbs approximately 75 percent of the load.[7] The colon absorbs the remaining Na^+ and Cl^- very effectively against a gradient into the portal blood, so that normal stools may contain only 1 to 2 mmole/day. Cl^- and HCO_3 are exchanged. The colonic mucosa is relatively impermeable to the diffusion of Na^+ back into the lumen. It maintains a large negative electric potential which provides a driving force for diffusion of K^+ into the lumen. Monovalent ions, such as sodium and chloride, are absorbed more rapidly than polyvalent ions, such as Ca^{++} and Fe^{++}.

Iron absorption usually is proportionate to the needs of the body. However, ferric iron, commonly found in food, appears to be reduced to the ferrous form before it is absorbed. Following absorption, ferrous iron is oxidized to the ferric form in the mucosal cells and binds to *apoferritin,* a binding protein found in the mucosa. It then crosses the cell membrane and is released into the portal blood. When the apoferritin is saturated with iron, absorption decreases. It has also been observed that certain iron-sugar complexes may move across mucosal cells without binding to apoferritin.

Calcium absorption involves the action of vitamin D metabolite and parathyroid hormone. Approximately 10 to 30 percent of dietary calcium is absorbed in the acid environment of the proximal duodenum. Details of the complexities of the processes involved in calcium absorption as well as absorption of other mineral elements are found in texts of normal nutrition.

Protective Mechanisms. A number of actions of the intestinal tract serve to protect the intestine itself and other cells of the body from damage. The bactericidal or bacteriostatic effects of saliva and gastric juice have already been described. The normal bacterial flora in the intestine may serve to counteract the growth of pathogenic bacteria, yeasts, and fungi. Vomiting and diarrhea may protect the body by eliminating toxic materials. It is postulated that the intestinal mucosa also serves as a barrier to the absorption of materials that would have a deleterious effect on other cells in the body via the immune system. Several mechanisms protect the integrity of the intestine itself. These include secretion of mucus, dilution, neutralization, and buffering of intestinal contents, and the constant renewal of mucosal cells.

The Biliary Tract

Functional Anatomy

The *hepatocytes* of the liver daily produce 600 to 800 ml of bile which flows into a duct system leading to the *hepatic duct.* The *gallbladder* is a hollow, pear-shaped sac with a capacity of 30 to 50 ml. It communicates with the hepatic duct via the *cystic duct.* These two ducts converge to form the common bile duct which enters the duodenum at the *ampulla of Vater. Oddi's sphincter* regulates the flow of bile into the intestine.

Normal Physiology

The bile, synthesized by the liver, contains bile salts, cholesterol, and phospholipids. The primary function of the gallbladder is to concentrate and store bile. The rate at which this concentration occurs is extremely rapid. Almost 90 percent of the original fluid volume can be reabsorbed in 3 to 6 hours. As a result, there is a sharp increase in the concentration of bile salts, cholesterol, and phospholipids. The cells of the gallbladder have an active sodium and chloride transport system, and water is reabsorbed as a

Table 6-3. The Composition of Hepatic and of Gallbladder Bile

Constituents	Hepatic Bile (as secreted) % of Total Bile	% of Total Solids	Bladder Bile (% of total bile)
Water	97.00		85.92
Solids	2.52		14.08
Bile acids	1.93	36.9	9.14
Mucin and pigments	0.53	21.3	2.98
Cholesterol	0.06	2.4	0.26
Fatty acids and fat	0.14	5.6	0.32
Inorganic salts	0.84	33.3	0.65
Specific gravity	1.01		1.04
pH	7.1–7.3		6.9–7.7

Reprinted with permission from Martin, D.W., Mayes, P.A., and Rodwell, V.W., *Harper's Review of Biochemistry*, 18th ed. Los Altos, Calif.: Lange Medical, 1981, p. 528.

consequence of the action of the sodium pump. Thus, the concentration of bile may be increased ten to fifteen times, making it possible to store a day's bile production. The composition of bile as secreted and of bile in the gallbladder is given in Table 6-3.

There are two primary acids (Fig. 6-4) that are synthesized in several steps from cholesterol. They are the trihydroxy bile acid, *cholic acid,* and the dihydroxy acid, *chenodeoxycholic acid.* Both conjugate with *glycine* and *taurine.* Deoxycholic acid, a "secondary" acid formed from cholic acid, also conjugates with taurine and glycine. *Lithocholic acid* is formed similarly from chenodeoxycholic acid, but in very small amounts. The secondary acids are products of bacterial action and take up approximately 20 percent of the total pool of bile salts. The bile contains large quantities of Na^+ and K^+, and the bile acids are assumed to exist as bile salts with these cations.

It is important to remember that, although bile salts circulate through the intestine over and over again during a day, they are very well conserved (see Fig. 6-2). Most are reabsorbed via the portal vein and returned to the liver to be resecreted. Only a small fraction of bile salts is lost each day; however, if the ileum, which is the main site of bile salt absorption, is removed, the pool is depleted rapidly.

The Pancreas

Normal Anatomy

The pancreas is both an exocrine and endocrine organ, but this chapter will deal only with the exocrine function of the gland. The basic secretory unit of the exocrine pancreas is the *acinus,* a group of cells that form a saclike unit. The apical surfaces of the cells of an acinus share a common lumen into which they secrete the pancreatic enzymes (Fig. 6-5). The lumen of the acinus empties into a duct which drains, successively, into the intralobular and interlobular ducts. The ducts actually extend into the center of the acinus. The cells in this portion of the duct are known as *centroacinar cells.* The interlobular ducts ultimately fuse to form the *duct of Wirsung,* the main pancreatic duct. Sometimes there is also an accessory *duct of Santorini.* The pancreatic ducts usually drain into the common bile duct but occasionally open into the duodenum directly.

Normal Physiology

The enzymes listed in Table 6-1 are synthesized by the acinar cells of the pancreas into membrane-bound structures called *zymogen granules* and eventually are discharged into the lumen of the acinus. The *duct cells* secrete a thin watery fluid high in bicarbonate. The pancreatic juice also contains Na^+, K^+, Ca^{++}, Mg^{++}, Cl^-, $SO_4^=$, $HPO_4^{\equiv}$, albumin, and globulin. Daily volume is usually approximately 2 liters.

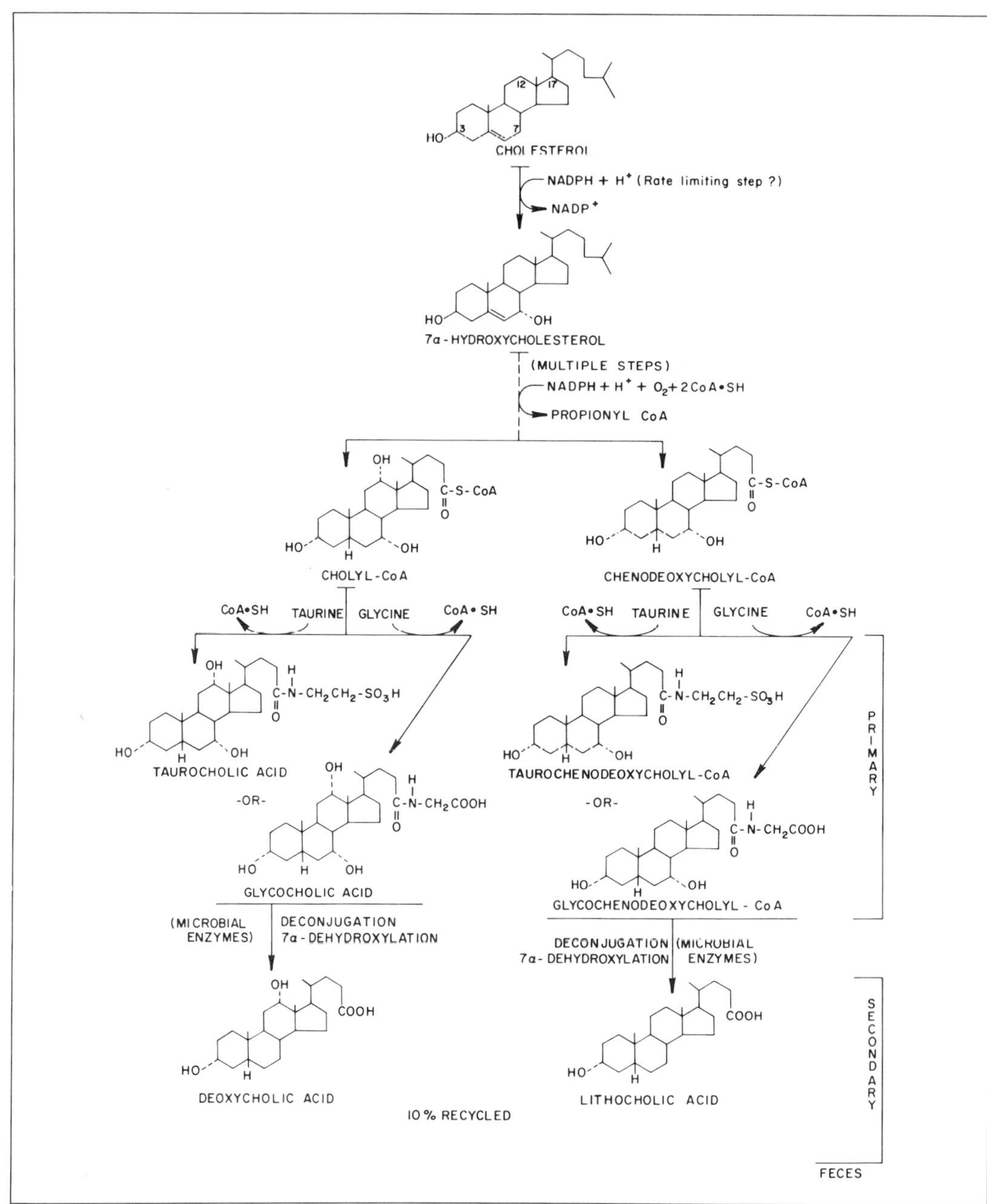

Figure 6-4. Bile acid metabolism.

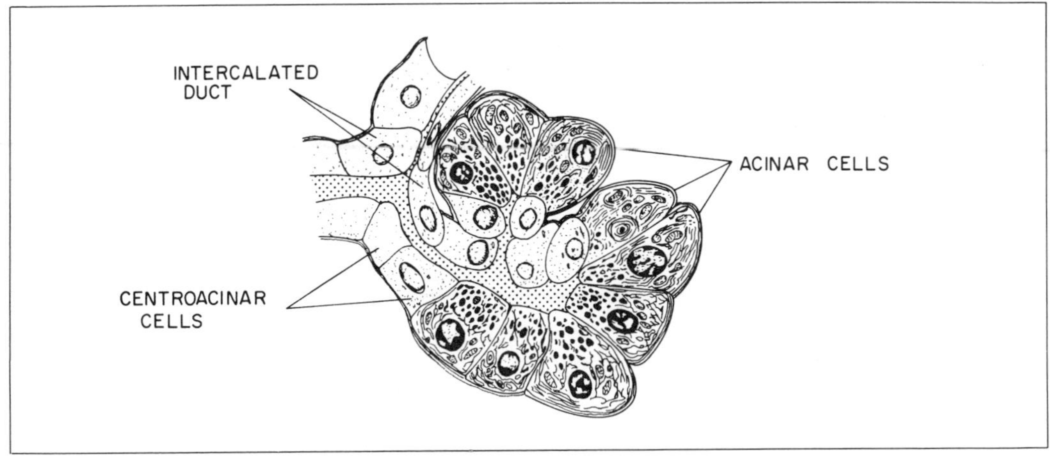

Figure 6-5. The relationship of a terminal branch of the duct system and centroacinar cells to the acinus. (Reprinted with permission from Bloom, W., and Fawcett, D.W., A Textbook of Histology, *10th ed. Philadelphia: W.B. Saunders, 1975, p. 738.)*

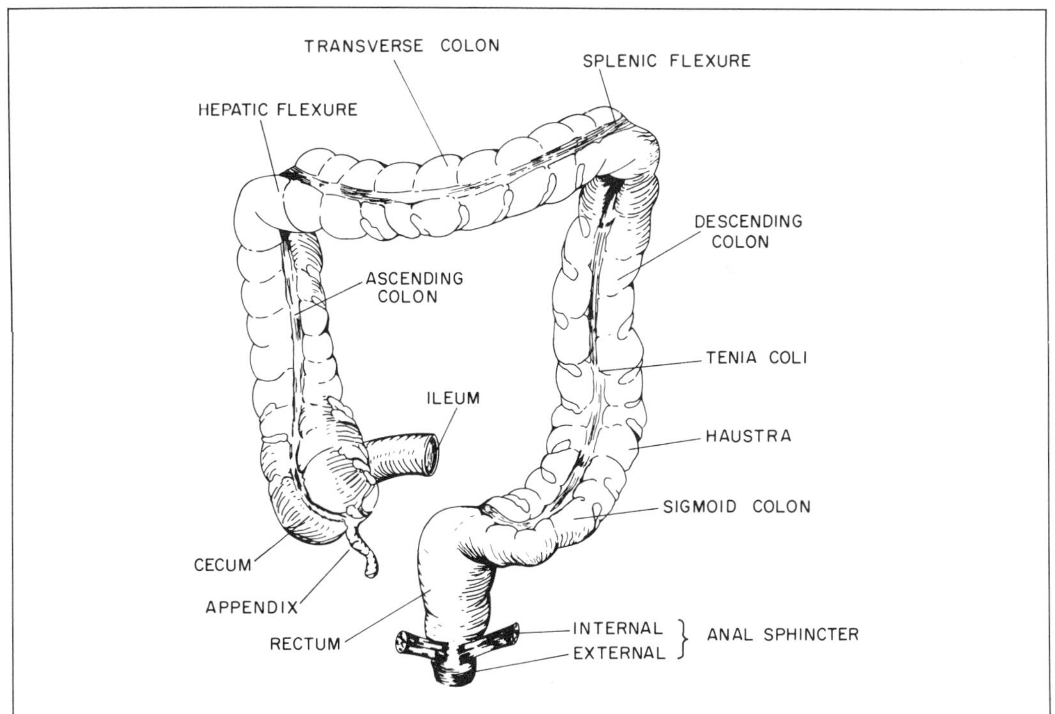

Figure 6-6. The human colon. (Reprinted with permission from Ganong, F.W., Review of Medical Physiology, *10th ed. Los Altos, Calif.: Lange Medical, 1981.)*

The Large Intestine

Normal Anatomy

The *large intestine* is approximately 5 ft long, with a diameter greater than that of the small intestine. It attaches to the ileum at the ileocecal valve and consists of the cecum, the ascending, transverse, descending, and sigmoid colon, and the rectum, and ends at the anus (Fig. 6-6). Three longitudinal muscles, the *teniae coli,* extend the length of the colon. The wall of the colon forms *haustra coli* or outpouchings between these muscles. The colonic glands, which extend into the mucosal layer, secrete large quantities of mucus.

Normal Physiology

No enzymatic digestion occurs in the colon, but the large number of bacteria that normally exist in the colon digest some resistant materials. The colon absorbs water, electrolytes, and some vitamins. Na^+ is absorbed by active transport, and potassium can be excreted. The colon also stores and eliminates wastes as feces. The fecal materials include water, indigestible fiber, dead mucosal cells, bacteria and products of their activity, bile salts, bilirubin, small amounts of unabsorbed nutrients, and nonfood items that may have been swallowed. The fat content of the feces is usually less than 5 percent.

CONDITIONS COMMON TO MANY GASTROINTESTINAL DISORDERS

The conditions discussed in this section are common to a number of disorders. Specific diseases in which they occur are described in succeeding sections.

Malabsorption Syndromes

The term *malabsorption* often is used to include abnormalities of either digestion or absorption or both. It almost always refers to conditions that cause decreased or inadequate function. As a result, maintenance of good nutrition often is difficult and patients tend to be undernourished.

The cause of malabsorption may be centered in any organ or tissue that contributes to the digestive or absorptive process—the liver, gallbladder, pancreas, intestinal mucosa, lymphatics, or combinations of these. Sometimes the problem involves a whole organ and, sometimes, only a part or a specific tissue within an organ. On occasion, the problem lies in the duct system. A particular problem may cause malabsorption of one nutrient or of many nutrients. The effects on nutritional status of the patient and the requirements for nutritional care are related to the organ or tissue involved, the extent of involvement, and the nutrients affected.

Many conditions that produce malabsorption are listed in Table 6-4. Although the list is long, the pathologic processes leading to malabsorption are much more limited in number.

Pathogenesis of Malabsorption

Lipids. Malabsorption of lipid occurs more often than with any other nutrient and the effects are more severe. It can result from abnormalities in any of the steps of and any of the organs and tissues involved in fat digestion and absorption.

In cases of *pancreatic insufficiency* (a deficiency or absence of pancreatic enzymes), most fat is not digested and, therefore, is not absorbed. The lipid then appears in the stools (*steatorrhea,* defined as fecal fat levels greater than 6 g/day). Normal fecal fat is 5 to 6 g/day. The large amounts of fat that appear in the colon in steatorrhea are hydroxylated by the bacteria of the colon. The hydroxylated fats act on the mucosa of the colon, increasing motility and decreasing water and electrolyte absorption in the colon, thus producing *diarrhea.*

Table 6-4. Causes of Malabsorption

Abetalipoproteinemia
Amyloidosis
Bacterial overgrowth
Blind loops
Intestinal diverticulosis
Intestinal motility disturbances
Strictures
Celiac disease
Dermatitis herpetiformis
Diffuse ileojejunitis
Drug-induced malabsorption
Dysgammaglobulinemias
Endocrine disorders
Addison's disease
Carcinoid
Diabetes mellitus
Hyperthyroidism
Hypoparathyroidism
Systemic mast cell disease
Zollinger-Ellison syndrome
Enteroenteric fistulas
Gastrectomy (Billroth II)
Intestinal lymphoma
Ischemic bowel disease
Atherosclerosis
Polycythemia vera
Vasculitis
Liver disease
Extrahepatic obstruction
Intrahepatic cholestasis
Hepatocellular disease
Lymphangiectasia
Pancreatic insufficiency
Chronic pancreatitis
Cystic fibrosis of the pancreas
Pancreatic carcinoma
Pancreatic resection
Parasitic disease
Radiation enteritis
Scleroderma
Short bowel
Tropical sprue
Whipple's disease

Decreased fat absorption in the *jejunum* may occur under several circumstances. There may be decreased absorptive surfaces such as occurs in damage to absorptive cells from disease, resection of the jejunum, or surgical bypass of the jejunum. Alternatively, disease may cause decreased function of absorptive cells. The failure to absorb fat results in steatorrhea and diarrhea.

Liver and gallbladder function may also be involved in lipid malabsorption, since a number of pathologic processes can cause malabsorption by altering the action of bile:

Intraluminal binding of bile acids. Occasionally, patients are given the resin cholestyramine as a medication. If given in large amounts, the resin binds bile acids and can produce bile acid insufficiency, interfering with micellar formation and lipid digestion. Steatorrhea and diarrhea can result.

Biliary tract obstruction. The obstruction of the bile duct—by a stone or tumor, for example—also produces a deficiency of bile salts. The formation of micelles is compromised, with resultant interference with digestion and absorption. Fecal fat levels may be 25 g/day, accompanied by diarrhea. If the obstruction is also in a position to block the pancreatic duct, there will be a simultaneous deficiency of pancreatic lipase. Lipid digestion then is compromised, and the steatorrhea will be much more severe.

Bacterial overgrowth. The upper part of the small intestine usually contains very few microorganisms, whereas the microbial population of the ileum and the colon is normally very high. The cleansing action of the movement of the intestinal contents normally controls the bacterial population. However, any abnormality that causes stasis or recirculation of intestinal contents may result in bacterial proliferation. Circumstances in which this may occur include anatomic defects such as strictures, fistulas, diverticula, and blind loops. For clarification, these are diagrammed in Fig. 6-7. Other causes of bacterial proliferation include disorders of motility and reduced antibacterial capacity.

When bacterial overgrowth occurs, there is an increase in the population of those strains of bacteria that reduce the concentration of conjugated bile salts in the intestinal lumen. The bacteria deconjugate bile salts, and the deconjugated molecules are

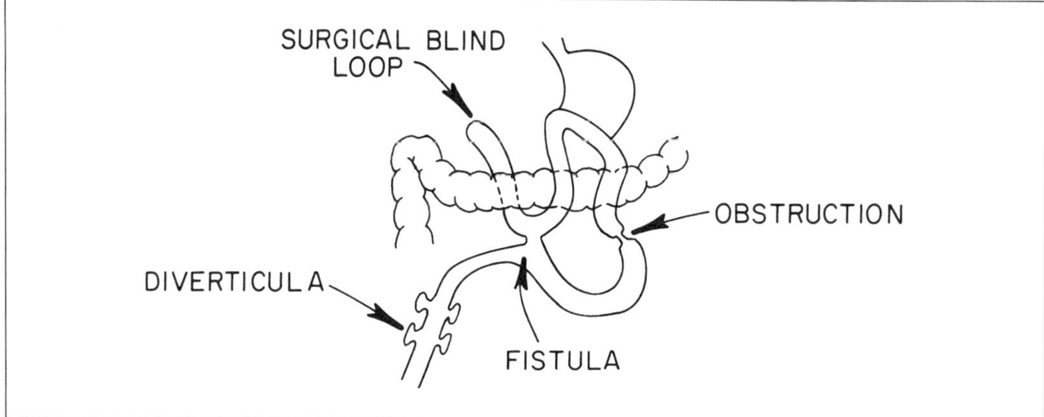

Figure 6-7. Anatomic lesions leading to bacterial overgrowth.

reabsorbed high in the intestinal tract before they function in fat absorption. Bacterial action also decreases the pH of intestinal contents and reduces the proportion of bile salts that are ionized. Un-ionized salts tend to precipitate out. The resulting decrease in intraluminal concentration of bile salts causes a decrease in micelle formation and thus contributes to fat malabsorption.

In addition, under conditions of bacterial overgrowth, bacterial action can alter the hydroxyl groups at the 3, 7, and 12 positions on the bile salt molecules (see Fig. 6-4), converting cholic to deoxycholic acid and chenodeoxycholic to lithocholic acid. It has been suggested that large amounts of deoxycholic and lithocholic acids produced during bacterial overgrowth alter the metabolism of absorptive cells and interfere with their absorptive capacity.

A third means by which bacterial overgrowth may affect fat absorption is through the effect of toxin produced by bacterial metabolism. The toxins may interfere with absorption by direct effects on the enterocytes.

The condition resulting from bacterial overgrowth is known also as *contaminated bowel syndrome.* When it involves stasis of intestinal contents, the terms *intestinal stasis syndrome* or *stagnant loop syndrome* are applied. The syndrome includes other functional impairments as well, although lipid malabsorption usually is most prominent.

Reduction of pH of duodenal contents. In the Zollinger-Ellison syndrome, gastric production of HCl is magnified and may overwhelm the capacity of the duodenum for neutralization. The resulting low pH in the duodenum may also result in precipitation of bile salts similar to that which occurs in bacterial overgrowth.

Ileal dysfunction. The enterohepatic circulation of bile salts depends on their reabsorption in the ileum. If ileal reabsorptive capacity is reduced, bile salts will be excreted in larger quantities. The liver is capable of approximately five times normal production of bile salts, but this capacity may be exceeded if losses are high. The net result, again, is an eventual reduction in bile salt concentration. When the critical micellar concentration is not achieved, leading to deficient micelle formation, steatorrhea and diarrhea result. High losses of bile salts can occur when the ileum is diseased and also when ileal tissue has been surgically removed or bypassed.

When deconjugated bile salts are not reabsorbed, they are carried to the colon where they have a cathartic effect. This is an additional factor contributing to the diarrhea in ileal dysfunction.

Fat malabsorption sometimes is the result of abnormalities in the *lymphatics*, where long-chain fatty acids normally are absorbed. Fat malabsorption may occur in patients with primary intestinal lymphangiectasia (tumor or fibrosis of the lymphatics), Whipple's disease (cause unknown; possibly infection), intestinal lymphoma (tumor), or Crohn's disease.

Carbohydrate. Malabsorption of carbohydrate is less common than fat malabsorption. It can occur when pancreatic exocrine secretion is deficient or absent following pancreatectomy (surgical removal of the pancreas) or obstruction of the duct. The digestion of starch is reduced as a result of the absence of pancreatic amylase. A diet low in starch may be used with increased monosaccharides and disaccharides. The diet is difficult to plan satisfactorily. In addition, the patient should be advised on dental care, since the diet will be high in sugar content.

It is more usual for disorders of carbohydrate absorption to be related to deficiencies of intestinal mucosal enzymes, resulting in intolerances to specific oligosaccharides. These are discussed in detail under Diseases Primarily Affecting the Small Intestine.

Protein. Some degree of protein malabsorption may occur as the result of deficiencies of pancreatic or intestinal enzymes. However, the degree of malabsorption and the severity of the consequences usually are less than those that occur in the case of fat or carbohydrate malabsorption.

Vitamin B_{12}. Malabsorption of vitamin B_{12} may occur for a variety of reasons, most of which can be anticipated based on a knowledge of the steps in normal absorption. Malabsorption of vitamin B_{12} can be expected to follow these conditions:[8]

1. Deficiency of IF, as seen in atrophic gastritis or total gastrectomy, with a reduction in IF-synthesizing cells
2. Bacterial overgrowth with increased binding or metabolism of the vitamin B_{12}–IF complex by the bacteria
3. Destruction or absence of ileal receptor sites for absorption, resulting from ileal disease or surgical resection
4. Intake of certain drugs or toxins, such as neomycin, colchicine, and aminosalicylic acid
5. Inappropriate pH or ion concentration in the ileal lumen

Calcium ions are necessary for absorption of the vitamin B_{12}–IF complex at the ileal receptor site. In chronic pancreatic disease with decreased bicarbonate secretion, calcium soaps are formed in the low pH environment, resulting in decreased availability of calcium. Low ileal pH due to Zollinger-Ellison syndrome has a similar effect.

Drug-Induced Malabsorption. A number of drugs are known to cause malabsorption (see Chapter 3), but those that cause major changes at usual doses are cholestyramine, neomycin, and antacids.

Malabsorption of many nutrients is common in chronic alcoholics.[9] Dietary folic acid and protein deficiency, pancreatic insufficiency, and decreased bile secretion contribute to malabsorption in alcoholics. In addition, alcohol has a direct effect on the intestinal mucosa (Table 6-5). Many of these abnormalities are reversed when the patient's nutritional status is improved, even if alcohol intake continues.[10]

General Symptoms of Malabsorption

Early symptoms of malabsorption include a change in bowel habits, fatigue, apathy, and a smooth surface on the lateral tongue. The patient usually does not seek treatment until

Table 6-5. Factors Contributing to Malabsorption and Diarrhea in Chronic Alcoholics

Factor	Effects
	Mucosal
Folic acid deficiency	Diffuse functional disturbance; morphological changes
Direct alcohol effects	Intestinal damage (cellular and subcellular); altered cellular metabolism (reduced sodium potassium ATPase, ATP); malabsorption (vitamin B_{12}, amino acids, thiamine); inhibition of sodium and water absorption; net secretion sodium and water; disaccharide deficiency → lactose intolerance
Protein malnutrition(?)	
	Luminal
Pancreatic insufficiency	Due to protein malnutrition and alcohol; alcohol-induced pancreatitis
Liver disease	Decreased bile salt secretion
Increased intestinal motility	

Reprinted with permission from Green, P.H.R., and Tall, A.R., Drugs, alcohol and malabsorption. *Am. J. Med.* 67:1070, 1979.

ATPase = adenosine triphosphatase; ATP = adenosine triphosphate.

the symptoms become more severe. In addition to steatorrhea and diarrhea, the patient frequently has clinical manifestations that are characteristic of specific nutritional deficiencies. These are listed in Table 6-6, with an explanation of the pathophysiology.

Diagnosis

Table 6-7 lists procedures used to diagnose malabsorption. Some tests are useful also in defining the cause of the condition.

The *fecal fat assay* measures the amount of fat that appears in the stool and is a screening test for overall malabsorption syndrome. It is most useful if done in relationship to a specified fat intake. Typically, the diet contains 100 g of fat per day. The excretion of more than 6 g of fat per day over a 3-day period is considered to indicate fat malabsorption. In some disease states, 40 g of fat per day may be excreted. The test does not distinguish between malabsorption of fat caused by pancreatic disease and that caused by intestinal disease. Simultaneous determination of *fecal nitrogen* suggests pancreatic insufficiency if the content is more than 6 g/day. An acid pH indicates bacterial fermentation of carbohydrates.

The *D-xylose absorption test* is used to distinguish intrinsic intestinal malabsorption from pancreatic insufficiency. In the test, 25 g of D-xylose, which is not metabolizable, is given orally. Urine is collected for 5 hours and tested for xylose. Normal excretion is 4.5 g/5 hr. Absorption of xylose does not require pancreatic enzymes or bile. In intestinal malabsorption, xylose concentration in blood and urine is diminished, whereas pancreatic insufficiency does not affect the ability of the enterocytes to absorb xylose.

The *Schilling test* is of use in differentiating intrinsic factor deficiency from dysfunction in the distal ileum. The patient is given radioactively labeled vitamin B_{12}. Two hours later, a large unlabeled flushing dose is given parenterally. Normally, 10 percent of the dose will be excreted in 48 hours. A diminished amount of radioactivity in the urine indicates malabsorption. If the vitamin is absorbed normally, ileal disease and pernicious anemia are ruled out. If the vitamin is absorbed only when intrinsic factor is given along with the vitamin, a diagnosis of pernicious anemia is suggested. Patients with severe bacterial overgrowth sometimes fail to absorb the vitamin either with or without intrinsic factor.

Other diagnostic tests include the lactose tolerance test (described on p. 193), tests for pancreatic function, roentgenography of the abdomen, and intestinal biopsy.

Table 6-6. Pathophysiologic Basis for Symptoms and Signs in Malabsorptive Disorders

Symptom or Sign	Pathophysiology
Generalized malnutrition and weight loss	Impaired absorption of fat, carbohydrate, and proteins → loss of calories
Diarrhea	Dihydroxyl bile acids and hydroxyl fatty acids cause decreased colonic absorption of sodium and water; excess load of fluid and electrolytes presented to colon may exceed its absorptive capacity
Bulky, frothy, voluminous stools	Excess fat content of feces
Weakness and easy fatigability	Anemia: electrolyte depletion (hypokalemia; hypomagnesemia)
Glossitis, cheilosis	Deficiencies of iron, vitamin B_{12}, folate, and other vitamins
Amenorrhea, decreased libido	Protein depletion → secondary hypopituitarism
Bleeding problems (oral, genitourinary, gastrointestinal, cutaneous)	Vitamin K malabsorption, hypoprothrombinemia
Tetany, paresthesias	Calcium malabsorption → hypocalcemia; magnesium malabsorption → hypomagnesemia
Peripheral neuropathy	Deficiency of vitamin B_{12}
Skeletal pain	Calcium malabsorption → osteomalacia; protein depletion → osteoporosis; vitamin D malabsorption → impaired absorption of calcium
Nocturia	Delayed absorption and excretion of water; hypokalemia
Edema	Impaired absorption of amino acids → protein depletion → hypoproteinemia
Anemia	Impaired absorption of iron, folate, and vitamin B_{12}
Eczema	Cause uncertain
Night blindness	Impaired absorption of vitamin A

Reprinted with permission from Greenberger, N.J., and Winship, D.H., *Gastrointestinal Disorders: A Pathophysiologic Approach.* Copyright © 1976 by Year Book Medical Publishers, Inc., Chicago. P. 116. (Modified from Greenberger, N.J., and Isselbacher, K.J., Disorders of absorption. In Isselbacher, K.J., et al., Eds., *Harrison's Principles of Internal Medicine,* 7th ed. New York: McGraw-Hill, 1974, pp. 1460–1461.)

Treatment

Any or all of the following may be used as required to treat malabsorption syndromes: surgical resection or repair, replacement of missing or deficient substances, such as pancreatic enzymes, antibiotics, and antidiarrheal drugs.

Nutritional care can be of great importance. It must be adjusted to the cause, symptoms, and severity of the underlying disease and its clinical manifestation and must be integrated with the other aspects of treatment. The objectives of nutritional care are relief of symptoms with an increase in the comfort of the patient and repletion and maintenance of good nutritional status. Relief of symptoms often involves the use of diets restricting nutrients that cause symptoms when not absorbed. The diet restricted in fat is useful for patients with fat malabsorption. All types of fat are restricted, but the degree of restriction is varied as needed. Useful levels of restriction which have been suggested are as follows:[11]

Mild fat restriction, in which fat comprises 35 to 40 percent of total kilocalories

Table 6-7. Tests Useful in the Diagnosis of Malabsorptive Disorders

Test	Normal Values	Typical Findings		Comment
		Malabsorption (nontropical sprue)	Maldigestion (pancreatic insufficiency)	
Stool examination				
Qualitative				Reliable screening test if properly performed; not sensitive enough to detect minimal steatorrhea
Neutral fat	1+	Normal	↑↑	
Fatty acid	1+	↑↑	↑	
Undigested muscle fibers	<5	<5	>5	
Quantitative determination of stool fat	≤6 g/24 hr; 95% coefficient of fat absorption	>6 g/24 hr	>6 g/24 hr	Most reliable test for documenting presence of steatorrhea
Carbohydrate absorption				
D-Xylose absorption test (25-g dose)	Urinary excretion ≥4.5 g/5 hr; blood level ≥30 mg/dl	↓	Normal	Good screening test for carbohydrate absorption; spurious low values may be obtained with incomplete urine collections, renal failure, ascites, bacterial overgrowth of small bowel, and certain drugs (indomethacin)
Oral glucose tolerance test (GTT)	USPHS criteria; O'Sullivan criteria	Frequently flat	Frequently diabetic	Approximately 10% of normal subjects have a flat GTT
Gastrointestinal roentgenograms of stomach and small bowel		Malabsorption pattern	May see malabsorption pattern or pancreatic calcification	Malabsorption pattern is nonspecific; may be present in several disorders
Peroral jejunal mucosal biopsy		Abnormal	Normal	
Pancreatic function tests				
Secretin test	Volume ≥1.8 ml/kg/hr; $[HCO_3] \geq 80$ mEq/L	Normal	Abnormal	A sensitive test for demonstration of exocrine pancreatic insufficiency
Duodenal perfusion with essential amino acids	Trypsin and lipase output	Frequently normal	↓	Abnormal volumes found when ≤10% of the exocrine pancreas is functioning
Schilling test for vitamin B_{12} absorption	>10% urinary excretion ^{60}Co in 48 hr	Frequently	Frequently	Useful in screening for gastric disorders (pernicious anemia), bacterial overgrowth, and ileal diseases (regional ileitis)

Blood tests				
Serum iron	80–150 μg/dl	Frequently ↓	Normal	Blood tests are fairly satisfactory screening tests for malabsorption; abnormalities should raise the question of malabsorption; however, such tests provide little help with regard to differential diagnosis
Serum calcium	9–11 mg/dl	Frequently ↓	Usually normal	
Serum cholesterol	150–250 mg/dl	Frequently ↓	Frequently ↓	
Serum albumin	3.5–5.5 g/dl	Frequently ↓	Occasionally ↓	
Prothrombin time	12–15 sec	Frequently prolonged	Occasionally prolonged	
Serum carotenes	100 IU/dl	↓	Frequently ↓	
Serum vitamin A	100 IU/dl	↓	Occasionally ↓	
Urine test: urine 5-hydroxy-indoleacetic acid (5-HIAA)	2–9 mg/24 hr	Frequently ↑	Normal	Greatly increased values characteristic of carcinoid syndrome; slightly increased levels (12–18 mg/24 hr) frequently found in sprue
Specialized tests				
Culture of jejunal contents	≤ 10^3 organisms per ml	Negative cultures	Negative cultures	Abnormal cultures (≥ 10^7 microorganisms per ml) characteristically found in bacterial overgrowth syndromes
Duodenal or jejunal fluid analysis				
Conjugated bile salts	≥ 2 mM/ml	Usually normal	Normal	May be decreased in sprue due to sequestration in gallbladder; characteristically decreased in ileal inflammatory disease and ileal resection
Unconjugated bile salts	Not present	Not present	Normal	Increased with bacterial overgrowth
Micellar lipid	≥ 50% dietary lipid ingested in micellar phase	Usually normal	Decreased	Decreased with a deficiency of steapsin or bile salts
^{14}C-glycolic acid breath test	<1% of dose excreted as $^{14}CO_2$ in 4 hr	Normal	Normal	Increased $^{14}CO_2$ excretion with bacterial overgrowth syndromes or bile acid malabsorption; determination of fecal bile acids aid in identifying the latter
Breath hydrogen test (after 50 g lactose)	Minimal breath hydrogen	Maybe ↑	Normal	Secondary to lactase deficiency

Reprinted with permission from Greenberger, N.J., *Gastrointestinal Diseases: A Pathophysiologic Approach,* 2nd ed. Copyright © 1981 by Year Book Medical Publishers, Inc., Chicago. (Modified from Greenberger, N.J., and Isselbacher, K.J., Disorders of absorption. In Isselbacher, K.J., et al., Eds., *Harrison's Principles of Internal Medicine,* 9th ed. New York: McGraw-Hill, 1980, pp. 1392–1409.)

USPHS = U.S. Public Health Service.

Moderate fat restriction, in which fat comprises 25 percent of total kilocalories
Severe fat restriction, in which fat comprises 10 to 15 percent of total kilocalories

The degree of restriction applied to a given patient is related to the severity of the malabsorption. Foods restricted on these diets are listed in the diet manuals of most hospitals.

Some patients with severe steatorrhea and diarrhea are more comfortable if the fiber content of the diet is reduced. Dietary fiber will be discussed later in this chapter.

The maintenance of good nutrition in the patient with malabsorption presents a great challenge to the nutritional care specialist. The following techniques are applied where appropriate:

1. In fat malabsorption, use the highest fat content possible consistent with control of steatorrhea and pain to maintain adequate kilocaloric intake for weight maintenance or gain. Divide the dietary fat equally among the three meals to avoid excessive fat at one meal.
2. Supplement the diet with vitamin and mineral medications. Representative dosages which may be prescribed by the patient's physician are shown in Table 6-8.
3. Add medium-chain triglycerides to the diet of patients with malabsorption of long-chain triglycerides if the fat-restricted diet provides insufficient energy.
4. Use chemically defined diets to supplement or replace the diet.

Medium-chain triglycerides are prepared by steam hydrolysis of coconut oil to separate them from the shorter-chain, more volatile fatty acids. They are available as MCT Oil (see Appendix K).[12] MCT Oil contains C8 and C10 fatty acids and provides 8.3 kcal/g. It is useful in increasing the available energy in patients with pancreatic lipase and bile deficiencies, deficiencies of chylomicron formation, or abnormalities of lymphatic transport. Some patients find the product somewhat unpalatable. They say it tastes "fishy" and, therefore, it must be disguised. It can be used only in limited quantities and should be distributed throughout the day, or it will cause diarrhea. MCT Oil does not help meet the need for linoleic acid or fat-soluble vitamins. It may be used in cooking in place of other oils in sauces, salad dressings, and baked goods. It can also be incorporated into milk shakes, casseroles, and juices. The manufacturer provides a recipe booklet which may be helpful to the patient using

Table 6-8. Representative Dosages for Agents Used in the Management of Patients with Malabsorption Syndrome

Calcium: Normal replacement is 1 to 2 g/day. Calcium carbonate may be given as Titralac (400 mg calcium per 5 ml) or Os-Cal (250 mg calcium per tablet).

Magnesium: Magnesium gluconate, 500 mg four times daily. Each tablet contains 29 mg of magnesium.

Iron: Ferrous sulfate, one 320-mg tablet four times daily. Each tablet contains 64 mg of iron.

Fat-soluble vitamins

Vitamin A: 25,000-unit tablets; for severe deficiency, 25,000–100,000 units/day. Maintenance dose is 3,000–5,000 units/day.

Vitamin D: Initial dose is 50,000 units two to three times per week. Dosage varies considerably, based on patient response as determined by serum and urinary calcium.

Vitamin K: Vitamin K_1 (water-miscible), 10 mg orally or intramuscularly per day, or vitamin K_3 (menadione), 10 mg orally per day.

Folic acid: 1–5 mg orally per day for 4–5 weeks is adequate to replenish stores and correct anemia. Maintenance dose is 1 mg orally per day.

Vitamin B_{12}: 100–1,000 μg/day intramuscularly for 2 weeks as a loading dose (if required). Maintenance dose is 100–1,000 μg/mo.

Vitamin B complex: Any multivitamin preparation that contains daily requirements (thiamine, 1.6 mg; riboflavin, 1.8 mg; niacin, 20 mg) should be administered twice daily.

Reprinted with permission from Stenson, W.F., Gastrointestinal diseases. In Freitag, J.J., and Miller, L.W., Eds., *Manual of Medical Therapeutics*, 23rd ed. Boston: Little, Brown, 1980, p. 268.

MCT Oil at home.[13] Other recipes have also been published.[14–19] The development of acceptable methods for its use represents an opportunity for the nutritional care specialist to show imagination and initiative. Since MCT Oil is very expensive, it is not practical to recommend (in the interests of efficiency in food preparation) that it be used for the whole family.

MCT Oil is also available in two casein-based formulas under the trade names of Portagen and Pregestimil. Information on these products and indications for their use are given in Appendix L.

Intestinal Antigen Absorption

Absorptive Mechanisms

In some diseases, the intestinal mucosa is thought to have lost its ability to act as a barrier to antigens. As a consequence, the patient absorbs toxic amounts of antigens in the diet or toxic products of bacterial metabolism. These may be important in the pathogenesis of disease.

Newborn infants are known to be capable of ingesting macromolecules,[18,19] and there is evidence that some adults normally retain a limited ability to do so.[20] The immunoglobulin A (IgA) antibody in the mucus coating the luminal surface normally complexes with the antigen and prevents its attachment to the membrane and subsequent ingestion. When a small amount of antigen crosses the enterocytes, macrophages and plasma cells in the lamina propria constitute a second line of defense and interact with the antigen, reducing the amount that reaches the general circulation.

In some diseases, excessive quantities of antigen cross the mucosal barrier. Some patients are deficient in secretory IgA, the predominant immunoglobulin in the intestine. In other diseases, the patients are deficient in the secondary defenses. The antigen then may reach the general circulation and cause a toxic or allergic reaction.[21] Patients with combined immunodeficiency disease or with secretory IgA deficiency have been shown to have an increased incidence of malabsorption-related diseases.[22,23] Newborn infants have no antibody in the small intestine or any plasma cells in the lamina propria. Until the immune system in this area matures, they are prone to increased antigen absorption.

Alteration in mucosal permeability also predisposes one to antigen absorption. Inflammation and ulceration are contributing factors. Conditions that enhance absorption of antigen to the mucosal surface, such as some drugs and some factors in human milk, have been shown in animals to increase antigen uptake.[24,25] The immature enterocytes of the newborn infant have an increased ability to take up antigens by pinocytosis.[26] Patients have an increased number of immature enterocytes following viral gastroenteritis, possibly accounting for their increased antigen uptake.[27]

Lysosomal enzymes sometimes are released inappropriately. Corticosteroids, for example, stabilize the lysosomal membrane.[28] This could result in decreased antigen breakdown within the cells and an increase in their transport into the general circulation.

In villous atrophy or ulceration, ingested antigens may diffuse across the mucosal barrier. Ionizing radiation, antibiotics, and antimetabolite drugs can alter mucosal function and antigen absorption.

Conditions that increase the concentration of macromolecules in the intestinal lumen may contribute to enhanced antigen absorption. Thus, it has been suggested, but not proved, that pancreatic insufficiency causes increased macromolecule absorption.

Related Diseases

A number of gastrointestinal diseases are suspected to be associated with abnormal antigen absorption. These include gastrointestinal responses to allergy, inflammatory bowel disease, celiac disease, and toxicogenic diarrhea from infection.[28] Those in which nutritional care is important are discussed in this chapter. It is important to remember that the association of these diseases to antigen absorption is somewhat speculative.

Nutritional Management

Prevention of excess antigen uptake in susceptible patients may be beneficial. Procedures suggested to accomplish this objective include encouraging breast feeding in early infancy and decreasing antigen load by using chemically defined formulas based on protein hydrolysates.[28]

Diarrhea

Diarrhea is defined as an increase, as compared to the usual pattern in an individual, in the frequency of bowel movements or excess water content of the stools or both. Usual habits vary, but more than four soft or watery bowel movements per day is considered abnormal in most individuals. Sometimes, the stools are small in volume but frequent. Diarrhea most directly involves the large intestine, but the pathogenesis frequently involves disease of the small intestine, pancreas, or gallbladder. *Acute diarrhea* of bacterial origin is relatively common and often is self-limiting. Specific therapy is not often required, except in infants. The adult patient usually can maintain his or her fluid and electrolyte balance with a clear liquid diet in diarrhea of short duration. A urine flow of 1,500 ml/day indicates adequate fluid intake. *Intractable diarrhea,* chronic or recurrent, has a greater nutritional impact.

Pathophysiology and Classification

Major mechanisms in the pathogenesis of diarrhea include the presence of excessive amounts of osmotically active substances in the intestinal lumen, secretion into the lumen, and derangement of intestinal motility.

Osmotic diarrhea results from the presence in the intestinal lumen of excessive numbers of osmotically active particles. Sources of these include saline laxatives, some antacids, the maldigestion of an unabsorbable osmotically active nutrient such as lactose, or failure to absorb an osmotically active nutrient. In the presence of these substances, there is a greater fluid *efflux* (movement of fluid into the lumen) than *influx* (absorption of fluid from the lumen). The total amount of fluid lost can be very great. The patient may have more than 1,000 ml of stool per day. Osmotic diarrhea stops when the intake of osmotically active substances stops. Therefore, osmotic diarrhea subsides during fasting.

Secretory diarrhea occurs when disease causes the secretion of large amounts of fluid into the intestinal lumen. This can occur in either the small or large intestine. Two mechanisms may be involved. *Passive secretion,* caused by increased tissue pressure or hydrostatic pressure, is believed to be the cause of increased secretion in obstruction and in intestinal inflammations. The other mechanism postulates *a stimulant* for secretion, which binds to a receptor on the membrane of cells in the crypts of Lieberkühn and stimulates adenyl cyclase. The action of adenyl cyclase increases the production of cyclic adenosine monophosphate (cAMP) in the cell. Cyclic AMP may inhibit sodium absorption by villous cells and induce secretion of the chloride and bicarbonate anions by crypt cells. Sodium, potassium, and water follow the movement of the anions.

An important related issue is the identity of stimulants to secretion. A number of substances are classifed as activators of adenyl cyclase. Many of these are enterotoxins, produced by bacteria that colonize in the intestine or have multiplied in food. *Escherichia coli,* causing traveler's diarrhea, and *Vibrio cholerae,* causing cholera, produce enterotoxins in the intestine. *Staphylococcus aureus* causes food poisoning by producing a toxin in the food in which it multiplies.

Prostaglandins have also been shown experimentally to stimulate adenyl cyclase. The diarrhea of some tumors of the intestine may be partly the result of the action of these substances.

Hormone-producing tumors may cause diarrhea. For example, the excess of gastrin produced in Zollinger-Ellison syndrome may stimulate adenyl cyclase. The acid inactivation of lipase leading to steatorrhea also contributes to the diarrhea.

Both bile salts and fatty acids stimulate adenyl cyclase. Bile salts are found in the colon when ileal reabsorption is decreased. The fat which then reaches the colon is hydrolyzed by bacteria to produce fatty acids. Thyrocalcitonin is the secretory stimulus in thyroid medullary carcinoma.

Secretory diarrhea causes a greater volume of fluid loss than does osmotic diarrhea and tends to persist during fasting. An exception is the secretory diarrhea resulting from unabsorbed fatty acids and bile salts.

Diarrhea also may result from alterations in intestinal motility. Circular muscle contractions normally retard the movement of intestinal contents. Loss of circular muscle tone may then contribute to diarrhea. Increased longitudinal muscle activity, which may occur in intestinal tumors and in emotional disorders, also causes diarrhea.

Sometimes diarrhea is a mixed type that simultaneously involves decreased fluid absorption and changes in secretion and motility. Some diseases of this type are infectious. Organisms involved include viruses, bacteria, protozoa, and helminths. Sometimes the basic disease is *idiopathic* (of unknown origin), whereas others are *iatrogenic* (resulting from treatment). For example, some patients given antibiotics develop diarrhea. When intestinal bacteria die as a result of antibiotic therapy, other bacteria can overgrow and produce an enterotoxin.

Table 6-9. Diagnostic Procedures for Diarrhea

Culture for microorganisms
Examinations for parasites
Examination for fecal leukocytes, which are present in colitis if bacterial, ulcerative, or antibiotic-associated
Determination of electrolyte content and osmolality of stool
If 2 × [sodium + potassium] is approximately equal to serum osmolality, diarrhea is secretory.
If difference is more than 100, diarrhea is osmotic.
A pH of less than 5 suggests disaccharidase deficiency.
Proctosigmoidoscopy
Radiologic tests: flat plate of abdomen; barium enema
Biopsy
Serum gastrin, vasoactive intestinal peptide, thyrocalcitonin
Urinary 5-hydroxyindoleacetic acid to detect carcinoid syndrome

Diagnosis

Many of the procedures described for diagnosis of malabsorption are applicable to the diagnosis of diarrhea in general. Others that may be indicated are listed in Table 6-9.

Metabolic Consequences

With diarrhea, fluid losses may reach 15 liters/day, with accompanying losses of sodium, potassium, and bicarbonate. The pattern of fluid and electrolyte loss is somewhat variable. For example, in osmotic diarrhea, water loss is greater than sodium loss. In persistent mild diarrhea, potassium deficiency can develop. If appropriate replacements are not provided, the patient may develop *dehydration, hyponatremia* (low serum sodium), *hypokalemia* (low serum potassium), and *acidosis.*

Therapy

The first step in treating diarrhea is to eliminate the underlying disease if possible. Fluid and electrolyte disturbances must be corrected (see Chapter 12). Nonspecific antidiarrheal agents may be used but are not appropriate in all conditions. Among the drugs which sometimes are prescribed by physicians are bismuth preparations, absorbents such as Kaopectate, narcotic agents such as paregoric or codeine, diphenoxylate hydrochloride with atropine sulfate (Lomotil), and antispasmodics such as belladonna preparations. Some of these may be accompanied by nutritionally relevant side effects:

Paregoric: Dry mouth, nausea, occasional abdominal distension
Codeine: Nausea, vomiting, anorexia, constipation
Lomotil: Nausea, vomiting, anorexia, constipation, bloating, dry mouth

If diarrhea is severe, food may be withheld for 24 hours or restricted to clear liquids followed by a soft diet in frequent small amounts as tolerated. Raw fruits and vegetables, whole grains, and concentrated sweets may be avoided and added as tolerated as the patient convalesces.

Chronic diarrhea leads to nutritional deficiencies if adequate replacement is not provided. High-protein, high-kilocalorie diets and supplements are useful. Patients may need vitamin supplements as well.

Protein-Losing Enteropathies

The leakage of protein into the intestine is considered to be a normal event in the metabolism of plasma proteins.[28,29] It has been estimated that 10 to 20 percent of the normal plasma protein loss occurs via this route. Protein losses may, however, reach excessive proportions in many diseases (Table 6-10),[29,30] and may be the consequence of increased mucosal permeability, inflammatory exudate, excessive turnover of cells, or leakage of lymph from obstruction of lacteals.[31]

Table 6-10. Classification and Therapy of Diseases Associated with Enteric Loss of Plasma Protein

Disease	Therapy
Mucosal ulceration	
Gastric carcinoma	Surgical resection
Gastric lymphoma	Surgical resection
Multiple gastric ulcers	Surgical resection
Colonic cancer	Surgical resection
Granulomatous enteritis	Surgical resection
Diffuse nongranulomatous ileojejunitis	Corticosteroids
Mucosal disease without ulceration	
Rugal hypertrophy (Menetrier's disease, etc.)	Resection, if local
Celiac sprue disease	Gluten elimination
Tropical sprue	Antimicrobials; folic acid
Whipple's disease	Antimicrobials
Allergic gastroenteropathy	Elimination diet; steroids
Bacterial or parasitic enteritis	Antimicrobials
Gastrocolic fistula	Resection
Villous adenoma of colon	Resection
Lymphatic abnormalities	
Capillaria philippinensis	Thiabendazole
Primary lymphangiectasia	Low-fat diet or medium-chain triglycerides
Lymphenteric fistula	Resection
Lymphoma	Chemotherapy
Constrictive pericarditis	Pericardiectomy
Tricuspid valvular disease	Treatment of heart failure

Reprinted with permission from Sleisenger, M.H., and Jeffries, G.H., Protein metabolism and protein-losing enteropathy. In M.H. Sleisenger and J.S. Fordtran, Eds., *Gastrointestinal Disease: Pathophysiology, Diagnosis, Management.* Philadelphia: W.B. Saunders, 1973, p. 36.

Loss of lipid, calcium, iron, and copper also may occur. The patient usually has edema and hypoproteinemia. Clinical signs of other deficiencies appear. Increases in protein intake and supplementation with vitamin and minerals often are necessary. Primary treatment, however, is directed to the underlying disease.[31]

Intestinal Fistulas

Fistulas are abnormal communications between two epithelial surfaces. They are classified according to their location or volume of output. They may be *internal,* between two hollow epithelium-lined organs, including two loops of intestine (*enteroenteral*) (see Fig. 6-7), or *external,* between a hollow organ such as the intestine and the skin (*enterocutaneous*). An intestinal fistula may result from a disease process or may be created surgically in the treatment of inflammatory or malignant bowel disease or for the treatment of obesity (see Chapter 15). Spontaneous fistulas may occur as a complication of peptic ulcers, tumors, inflammatory bowel disease, or trauma.

External gastrointestinal fistulas are classified further by volume of output. *High-output fistulas* produce 200 ml/day or more of effluent. Sometimes total volume is 5 liters. *Low-output fistulas* produce less than 200 ml/day of effluent. Fistulas of the stomach, duodenum, pancreatic duct, or proximal bowel are high-output. Low-output fistulas are in the distal small bowel and colon. They often are created surgically for excretory purposes and are discussed later in this chapter with other conditions affecting the colon.

When a patient has a fistula involving the small intestine, absorptive surface is lost by resection or by short-circuiting. If a fistula is formed between the small intestine and colon, the small intestine may become contaminated with colon bacteria. Fat malabsorption, steatorrhea, extreme weight loss, and protein-calorie malnutrition can result.

In gastric, duodenal, or jejunal fistulas, the fluid is isotonic and large amounts of sodium are lost. In addition to the resulting fluid and sodium depletion, alkalosis may develop if gastric fluid is lost. Loss of duodenal fluid containing bicarbonate can result in acidosis. Jejunal fistulas seldom cause acid-base problems since the fluid lost has a nearly neutral pH. Digestive enzymes in the jejunal effluent can cause digestion of the abdominal wall. Biliary fistulas result in water and sodium loss, but the losses are not severe. Pancreatic fistulas can involve fluid losses of 1 liter/day, acidosis from bicarbonate loss, and autolysis of the abdominal wall, a particularly troublesome complication.

Nutritional management involves replacement of fluid and electrolyte losses as a first priority of the physician.[32] Total parenteral nutrition (TPN) begins in 2 or 3 days and has been useful in reducing the mortality rate from high-output fistulas. In a week or more, it may be possible to begin tube feeding as an alternative or supplement to TPN.[32] A jejunostomy tube is advanced beyond the fistula or a feeding jejunostomy is constructed for this purpose. Patients with colonic fistulas can often be fed orally. It is important for all patients to be provided a high-kilocalorie diet with a fluid volume sufficient to maintain normal hydration.

Most external fistulas close spontaneously if the patient is well nourished, although some must be closed surgically.[33] Internal fistulas often lead to malabsorption of fat or bile and thence to alterations of water and electrolyte absorption. A low-fat diet usually is helpful if the patient can be fed orally, but TPN or tube feeding may be necessary.

DISEASES AFFECTING PRIMARILY THE SMALL INTESTINE

Gluten Enteropathy

Gluten enteropathy has also been known as *nontropical sprue, celiac disease, gluten-induced sprue,* and *idiopathic steatorrhea.* It typically appears in infancy when cereals are added to the diet, or in adults, primarily at 20 to 30 years of age. Sometimes, a child has a remission of the disease in adolescence, and then the disease recurs. It is a life-long condition. Gluten intolerance may occur as a transitory condition secondary to intestinal damage in other disorders.

Clinical Manifestations

The patient with gluten enteropathy has steatorrhea and diarrhea with frequent, foul-smelling, bulky stools. This is accompanied by failure to thrive in children, and, in both children and adults, weight loss and irritability are typical. The enterocytes are damaged, with a resultant decrease in disaccharidases and a secondary lactose intolerance. The damage to the cell also alters enterocyte permeability, resulting in active secretion of potassium and other electrolytes into the intestinal lumen.

There is a generalized decrease in villus length, so that the mucosa becomes partially or totally flattened. The lamina propria is infiltrated with lymphocytes and plasma cells. The surface epithelial cells become extensively vacuolated and lose their brush border.

Protein, fat, and carbohydrates are malabsorbed, as are fat-soluble vitamins. The consequent deficiencies of fat-soluble vitamins can lead to osteomalacia, rickets, tetany, bleeding tendencies, and night blindness. The patient may also have deficiencies of vitamin B_6 and of trace elements. Malabsorption of iron, folate, and vitamin B_{12} may cause microcytic or macrocytic anemia.

Pathogenesis

The small intestinal mucosa is damaged when the patient eats foods containing toxic *gluten,* a protein found in wheat, rye, barley, and possibly oats. Wheat gluten may be fractionated into two parts, *gliadin,* the damaging fraction, and *glutenin.* The basis for the toxicity of gluten in these cereal products is unknown but may be related to their content of amide and bound glutamine or proline. The toxic glutens, for example, have a higher percentage of amide nitrogen than is found in the well-tolerated corn and rice. Wheat gliadin contains a high proportion of glutamine and proline.

The exact mechanisms by which the disease is produced are not entirely clear, but there are several theories.[34] One suggests that there is an enzyme deficiency, allowing toxic products of gliadin degradation to accumulate and damage the enterocytes; however, the enzyme has not been identified. Another theory suggests that the enterocytes have surface receptors which bind to gluten, or gliadin, causing cell death. Thirdly, a large proportion of gluten-intolerant patients have a histocompatibility marker HLA-8 (see Chapter 4); the evidence indicates that immune factors are important. This last theory appears to have the most support at the present time.[35] There is infiltration of the jejunal mucosa with small lymphocytes and plasma cells[36] and changes in serum immunoglobulin concentrations,[37] particularly a reduction in secretory IgA and resulting antigen uptake.[23] Antibodies to gluten are found in the serum of these patients,[38] and many have autoantibodies to connective tissue.[39] There also is some evidence of an abnormal cell-mediated immune response.[40,41]

Treatment

The primary treatment of gluten enteropathy is the strict avoidance of gluten in the diet. Foods containing wheat, rye, barley, and oats must be carefully eliminated. An important function of the nutritional care specialist is to help the adult patient, or parents of a child patient, to identify sources of gluten or its derivatives in foods in which its presence is not obvious. Examples of foods that may contain gluten are meats prepared with cereal fillers, salad dressings, ice cream, candies, gravies and sauces containing fillers, malted milk, beer and ale which are prepared from barley, paste products, and foods containing bran or labeled *graham,* as in graham crackers. Hospital diet manuals usually contain a detailed list of foods to be avoided. Recovery from intestinal damage may take as long as 6 months. In primary disease, the gluten-free diet is a life-long requirement. If the patient eats gluten, the symptoms recur. For patients whose gluten intolerance is secondary to another condition, symptoms will not recur if the primary disease no longer exists.

The patient tolerates corn, rice, and millet. Cornmeal and flours from rice, arrowroot, potato, soy, and wheat starch can be used to prepare baked products. However, they cannot be substituted freely for wheat flour in recipes. As a consequence, special recipes must be provided to the patient.

For several months early in the dietary treatment, a restriction of fat and avoidance of lactose in the diet may be necessary. When the normal villus architecture returns, steatorrhea subsides and the tolerance to lactose returns, making these restrictions unnecessary. In the interim, however, the patient needs assistance in planning an adequate diet in the face of multiple restrictions. Sometimes MCT Oil is prescribed.

Until the villus architecture returns to normal, the patient is likely to require supportive treatment in the form of mineral and vitamin supplements prescribed by the attending physician. Complete reversion to normal is more likely in children than in adults. Residual effects in the adult may require continuing nutrient supplementation.

Tropical Sprue

Tropical sprue is a diarrheal disease which occurs primarily in the tropics. It also is seen in the temperate zone in patients who have visited the tropics. The cause of tropical sprue is unknown; it is believed to be due to microorganisms, but no single organism has been identified. The disease responds to antibiotics and folate, but it does *not* respond to a gluten-free diet. Nutritional care includes a high-calorie diet to restore and maintain normal body weight, at least 1 g of protein per kilogram of body weight, and replacement therapy, including folate and vitamin B_{12}.

Crohn's Disease

Crohn's disease is known also as *regional ileitis* or *regional enteritis.* The terminology varies somewhat with the location of the lesion. The condition sometimes affects the colon as well as the small intestine. Crohn's disease can occur at any age but is more common between the ages of 15 and 35 years. It usually is insidious in onset and becomes chronic and intermittent.

Clinical Manifestations

Patients with Crohn's disease complain of abdominal pain and have secretory diarrhea with weight loss and fever. There is a chronic inflammation of the affected bowel, often with granulomas. The terminal ileum is typically the primary site. The involved tissue may be discontinuous, with areas of healthy tissue interspersed among areas of diseased tissue. All layers of the intestinal wall are affected, and the mesentery and the lymph nodes in the area may also be involved. Possible complications include mechanical obstruction, ulcers, abscesses, and fistulas to the bladder or vagina. The incidence of colon or rectal cancer is increased.

Malnutrition frequently accompanies Crohn's disease, for several reasons. First, food intake usually is decreased. In addition, malabsorption may result from loss of bowel function due to inflammation, resection, or bypass surgery. Blood, protein, water, electrolyte, and bile salt losses are increased.

Causes and Predisposing Factors

The cause of regional enteritis is unknown. Genetic, infectious, and immunologic factors have been suggested. No specific pathogenic organism has been identified. Abnormal antigen absorption may be involved in its pathogenesis.[28]

Treatment

During an acute attack, bed rest is required. The diarrhea and abdominal pain are treated with medication. Often, immunosuppressants are prescribed by the physician. Nutritional therapy in Crohn's disease is supportive and very important. It must also be individualized. Sometimes, patients are given nothing by mouth for short periods to allow the bowel to rest. When fed, many patients are more comfortable with a diet that is reduced in fiber to reduce fecal output and avoid obstruction. Foods that are known to stimulate peristalsis, such as prunes and coffee, should be avoided. Low-fat meals to reduce steatorrhea, with increased protein and carbohydrate, may be helpful, and patients may better tolerate smaller, more frequent meals.

Vegetables and fruits sometimes are tolerated poorly, especially if raw, and their intake is reduced if the fiber of the diet is restricted. The guidelines for restricted fiber diets in many diet manuals list specific fruits and vegetables that may have to be limited in amount. Ascorbic acid and folate intake particularly may need to be supplemented if the diet is fiber-restricted. If the disease especially affects the ileum, parenteral vitamin B_{12} may be needed. Poor absorption of calcium, magnesium, and iron indicates a need for supplements of these elements. If there is a secondary lactase deficiency, lactose should be avoided. If the patient has bile salt deficiency as a consequence of ileal disease, medium-chain triglycerides may be useful.

Between acute attacks, the patient should be encouraged to eat as wide a variety of foods as possible. The intake should be monitored at intervals to assure adequate nutrition.

Surgical procedures usually are reserved for treatment of complications, since the disease tends to recur in 25 percent or more of the patients following resections. The general nutritional care of surgical patients is described in Chapter 12. The nutritional care of the chronic presurgical patient is continued after surgery in view of the recurrence rate. The care of patients who have had resections of large portions of the bowel is described in the next section.

Short Bowel Syndrome

Etiology

The short bowel syndrome is created when a large portion of the small intestine is resected. Extensive intestinal resection may be necessary in the following conditions:

1. Regional enteritis (the most common)
2. Thrombosis (formation of a blood clot in a blood vessel) or embolism (transfer of a mass in the vascular system), causing obstruction of the mesenteric artery
3. Volvulus of the small intestine (torsion of a loop), causing ischemia and gangrene
4. Neoplasm
5. Trauma
6. Intestinal bypass for obesity
7. Congenital atresia (absence of normal-sized lumen at birth)
8. Congenital Peutz-Jehgers syndrome (multiple polyps)
9. Radiation injury

Pathophysiology

The consequences of intestinal resection depend on the site and extent of bowel loss. Resection of small lengths of the jejunum does not result in any significant malabsorption, and resection of 40 to 50 percent of the small intestine usually is well tolerated if the proximal duodenum, the ileocecal valve, and the distal half of the ileum are not removed. The removal of the ileocecal valve and ileum results, however, in severe diarrhea, even if less than 30 percent of the intestine is removed. The loss of more than 50 percent of the small intestine usually produces significant malabsorption, while re-

Table 6-11. Intestinal Adaptation After Small Bowel Resection

Structural changes
Increased diameter of intestine
Increase in villus height
Increase in crypt depth
Hyperplasia-increased cell proliferation and migration rate
Increased rate of DNA synthesis; increased total DNA, RNA and protein concentration
Functional adaptations
Increase in water, electrolyte, and nutrient transport per centimeter of small intestine
Increase in mucosal enzymes per centimeter of small intestine
Changes in tissue metabolism accompanied by regeneration and growth

Reprinted with permission from Sheldon, G.F., Role of parenteral nutrition in patients with short bowel syndrome. *Am. J. Med.* 67:1026, 1979. (Adapted from Weser, E., *Viewpoints on Digestive Diseases,* No. 10. Chapel Hill, N.C.: American Gastroenterologic Association and Digestive Disease Foundation, 1978, p. 1.)

Table 6-12. Mechanisms of Intestinal Adaptation After Small Bowel Resection

Stimulation by intraluminal nutrients
Stimulation by bile and pancreatic secretions
Trophic effects of gut hormones
Altered intestinal blood flow
Altered innervation

Reprinted with permission from Weser, R., Nutritional aspects of malabsorption. Short gut adaptation. *Am. J. Med.* 67:1017, 1979.

moval of more than 70 percent makes survival questionable unless TPN is used.

The deficit causing malabsorption in the short bowel syndrome is probably a combination of deficiency of digestion, deficiency of absorbing area, and increase in transit speed, but the relative importance of these factors is unknown. Malabsorption of many nutrients follows resection. Most patients are able to absorb glucose efficiently if dumping syndrome is not induced. Protein absorption often is poor early in the postoperative period, but some improvement usually occurs in time. Lipid malabsorption is a common problem. If more than 100 cm of ileum are removed, hepatic synthesis of bile salts cannot be increased sufficiently to compensate for their increased loss, and steatorrhea ensues.[42] Fat-soluble vitamins, too, usually are lost in large quantities. Ileal resection, if very extensive, results in vitamin B_{12} deficiency unless parenteral replacement is provided. Other water-soluble vitamins generally are absorbed adequately.[43] Calcium and magnesium may be lost in large quantities in the form of soaps during steatorrhea, with consequent hypocalcemia and hypomagnesemia. Deficiencies of iron, potassium, and folate may occur, with the accompanying expected deficiency symptoms. If the malabsorption is severe, it can be crippling or life-threatening as a result of starvation.

The patients also have an increased incidence of gallstones. The presence of bile acids and unabsorbed fatty acids increases oxalate solubility and increases colon permeability to oxalate. The resultant increase in oxalate absorption contributes to an increased incidence of kidney stones.[44]

In time, some adaptive changes occur.[45] Structural changes (Table 6-11) in the intestine provide a more absorptive surface.[46,47] In addition functional adaptations (see Table 6-11) result in more efficient active transport.[47] The mechanisms of this adaptation are listed in Table 6-12. It is important to note that stimulation by intraluminal nutrients is one of the adaptive mechanisms, providing a rationale for feeding the patient enterally as soon as possible.

For several weeks postoperatively, a severe watery diarrhea occurs.[48] As a consequence, fluid, electrolyte, and acid-base balances can present problems. The causes of the diarrhea may include any of the following, depending on the site and extent of the resection.

1. The jejunal absorptive surface is reduced and the transport capacity of the remaining tissue is overwhelmed. Larger

amounts of fluid reach the colon. Many patients have partial removal of the colon, reducing its ability to absorb the added load.

2. Nutrients normally absorbed in the jejunum reach the colon. Carbohydrates are metabolized by colonic bacteria to short-chain fatty acids. The increased osmotic load contributes to an osmotic diarrhea. Long-chain fatty acids from the diet inhibit colonic absorption, especially if hydroxylated by bacteria.[49,50]

3. Bile acids normally absorbed in the ileum may alter colonic absorption and induce colonic secretions.[51]

4. The loss of the ileocecal valve may allow bacterial overgrowth in the remaining jejunum.

5. Gastric hypersecretion, which occurs in approximately 50 percent of the patients,[52] may aggravate the diarrhea by inactivating pancreatic enzymes. Changes in hormones affecting HCl secretion or hyperplasia of HCl-secreting cells may be reponsible for this effect.

Treatment

Nutritional Management. The patient with massive resection of the small bowel usually needs TPN for 3 weeks to 3 months, depending on the extent of the resection. Procedures for TPN are described in Chapter 12.

Oral feeding must be resumed gradually in order to avoid causing diarrhea. Frequently, the feedings are begun with the use of a dilute chemically defined diet containing amino acids and small-molecule carbohydrates administered by tube. A pump is used to deliver a constant low volume over the 24-hour period to make maximum use of the remaining absorptive surface. Gradually, these feedings are increased in volume and in concentration, but not simultaneously. The diet may then be progressed gradually to feedings containing polypeptides and small carbohydrates. Electrolyte and vitamin supplements are taken orally by some patients. The earliest trial of inclusion of lipid in the feeding often is more successful if medium-chain triglycerides are the lipid of choice. As the tube feedings are increased in caloric content, parenteral feedings should be diminished sufficiently so that the combined feedings provide adequate nutrition without loss of appetite.

The transition to conventional foods may begin with low-fiber foods in small frequent feedings. Lactose restriction is needed if insufficient lactase secretion has resulted from loss of secreting cells. If blood oxalate is increased, foods high in oxalate should be avoided. The size of the meals should be increased as tolerated. A low-fat diet with added medium-chain triglycerides often are helpful if the diarrhea continues to be a problem.[53] The fat content should be as high as can be tolerated without aggravating the diarrhea, usually 30 g or less.[53] As the intake of the foods is increased, the administration of tube feeding volume is decreased. Supplements taken between meals are helpful in achieving an adequate calorie intake when the patient is no longer being tube-fed.

After several months, the patient may be able to take all of his or her caloric requirements in the form of conventional foods by mouth, but the lactose restriction sometimes is still needed. Six to eight small meals are recommended.

An occasional patient has such extensive resection of the small intestine that maintenance of life with oral intake is not possible. Parenteral nutrition becomes a permanent necessity.

Drug Treatment and Nutrition. Drugs that may be prescribed by the physician for the patient include antiperistaltic drugs to prolong the time available for absorption. Cholestyramine binds bile salts and reduces their diarrhea-stimulating effect. Antibiotics may be prescribed if bacterial overgrowth is found. Cimetidine reduces gastric acid hypersecretion, and pancreatic enzymes are provided for replacement if gastric hypersecretion inactivates the endogenous enzymes. Sometimes antacids are prescribed.

The nutritional care specialist must be alert to drug-nutrient interactions in these patients. In addition, the patients have usually been given narcotics for several months for the purpose of reducing intestinal transit time, and it is important also to be aware of the possibility of drug addiction. Vomiting, poor intake, abdominal distension, and cramping may be the result of narcotic addiction rather than intolerance to the diet.

Carbohydrate Intolerance

An intolerance to a carbohydrate is most commonly the result of a deficiency of a disaccharidase necessary for digestion of a disaccharide to monosaccharides. Intolerances to monosaccharides do occur, but they are very rare.

Lactase Deficiency

The most common of the carbohydrate intolerances is caused by a deficiency of lactase. In the lactase-deficient patient, lactose taken in the diet cannot be digested to monosaccharides and absorbed. The lactose remains in the intestinal lumen where it has an osmotic effect. It has been estimated that 50 g lactose results in 150 ml of added fluid load. The increased fluid stimulates peristalsis, producing a watery diarrhea in which fluids and electrolytes are lost. It also contributes to a feeling of distension and discomfort. Bacterial action on the lactose in the colon metabolizes lactose to lactic acid and volatile fatty acids. These irritate the intestinal mucosa and also add to the osmotic effect and increased peristalsis. Carbon dioxide and hydrogen are produced, causing bloating and flatulence.

Forms of Lactose Intolerance. Lactose intolerance occurs in several forms which vary in their severity and incidence. *Congenital lactose intolerance* is present at birth and is severe. It occurs as *Holzel's syndrome* or as *Durand's syndrome.* In both, vomiting and diarrhea begin within a few days after birth. In Holzel's syndrome, lactase activity is approximately 10 percent of normal. Durand's syndrome is more severe. It differs from Holzel's syndrome in that, accompanying the symptoms previously described, a large quantity of lactose in the urine (*lactosuria*) and usually albuminuria, aminoaciduria, and acidosis are present. The prognosis is poor. Congential lactose intolerance in either form is rare.

Primary lactose intolerance is more common. Ethnic origin apparently is important in its occurrence, the condition being more prevalent in blacks, Orientals, Jews, and Indians than in whites of North European ancestry.[53] Those of Mediterranean ancestry and Arabs also show an increased incidence. The condition rarely is present at birth but may develop as early as weaning or at various times thereafter.[53] Sometimes, it does not develop until adulthood. The loss of lactase activity is an autosomal recessive trait and is a permanent condition.

Patients who have diseases of the intestinal tract that involve damage or removal of the intestinal mucosa may develop a *secondary intolerance,* the severity of which varies with the severity of the underlying cause. If enterocyte damage is repaired following treatment, secondary lactose intolerance subsides.

In either primary or secondary intolerance, the severity is variable. In patients with primary intolerance, for example, some patients have no symptoms unless lactose intake is very high. Many can tolerate at least 12 g of lactose, the amount in 1 c. of milk.

Diagnosis. Congential lactase deficiency is diagnosed by *intestinal biopsy* and *enzyme assay.* For suspected primary or secondary deficiencies, a *lactose tolerance* test often is used. In this test, 50 g of lactose is given to an adult orally. The dose for children is 2 g/kg. Blood samples are taken at intervals of 1, 15, 30, 60, and 120 minutes. An increase in plasma glucose of 30 mg/dl indicates normal lactase activity in which glucose is produced, whereas an increase of less than 20 mg/dl suggests lactase deficiency, especially if associated with symptoms. Increases of between 20 and 30 mg/dl are questionable.

An even more accurate test is the *breath hydrogen test.* Breath is collected for the measurement of hydrogen content before and after an oral load of 50 g of lactose. In lactase deficiency, some of the unabsorbed lactose is metabolized to hydrogen in the colon. The hydrogen diffuses into the blood and then into the air in the lungs. Breath hydrogen levels greater than 51 ml/4 hr is indicative of lactase deficiency.

Some physicians simply prescribe a diet free of lactose for a trial period as a diagnostic procedure. If symptoms subside, lactose intolerance is assumed.

Nutritional Care. The essential aspect of nutritional care is a reduction of lactose intake to the level of tolerance. In congenital deficiency, the infant at birth must be given a formula free of lactose. Some acceptable products are Isomil, ProSobee, Pregestimil, or Nutramigen (see Appendix L). The patients require a lactose-free diet indefinitely, and the nutritional care specialist must instruct patients or families carefully on the "hidden" sources of lactose. Most hospital diet manuals include lists of lactose-containing foods to be excluded from the lactose-free diet.

Patients with less severe forms of lactase deficiency may be able to tolerate small to moderate amounts of lactose in the diet. This diet sometimes is called a *lactose-restricted diet* and must be planned for the individual tolerance of each patient. Most patients can tolerate ½ to 1 c. of milk each day without unpleasant symptoms, especially if the milk is taken with meals.[54] Some patients tolerate chocolate milk better than unflavored whole milk, since its higher osmolality delays emptying time. Cheeses usually are well tolerated, since their lactose is converted to lactic acid during fermentation. Aged cheese has 6 percent lactose and cottage cheese 14 percent, as much as white milk with an equal amount of protein. A lactase enzyme (Lact-Aid, SugarLo Co., Atlantic City, N.J.), derived from the yeast *Saccharomyces lactis,* can be used to hydrolyze much of the lactose in milk. It must be added a few hours in advance to allow time for hydrolysis. The amount of milk that can be tolerated thus is increased. When the enzyme is used, the resulting milk is higher in osmolality and sweeter but quite acceptable. Buttermilk and yogurt also are better tolerated by some patients. Some of their lactose is fermented, but a large proportion usually remains. Yogurt, for example, contains 75 percent of the lactose found in whole milk, with an equal amount of protein. The reason for the increased tolerance is unknown.

Prolonged use of a milk-free diet has been reported to result in calcium deficiency[55] and possible osteoporosis.[56] Lactose intolerance does not interfere with the absorption of calcium, and dietary sources of calcium that do not contain lactose should be stressed. Calcium supplements, prescribed by the physician, may be required. The effect of lactose intolerance on other nutrients has been investigated. No effect on nitrogen retention, nitrogen balance, or on fat, phosphorus, or magnesium absorption was seen.[54,57,58]

Sucrase-Isomaltase Deficiency

Congenital sucrase-isomaltase deficiency is a rare condition which probably is a recessive trait. The condition can also be *acquired* as a result of mucosal damage or extensive intestinal resection. The deficiency of sucrase usually is more severe than the deficiency of isomaltase. The patient is unable to digest sucrose or dextrins. Starch with a high proportion of *amylopectin* is not well tolerated.

Amylopectin is highly branched and its digestion produces large amounts of isomaltose. Starches with a large proportion of amylose, such as those from corn or rice, produce only small amounts of isomaltose and are better tolerated.

As the result of the presence of sucrose and isomaltose in the intestinal lumen, diarrhea and other clinical manifestions are produced which are similar to those seen in lactose intolerance.[59] The symptoms are more severe in infants and smaller children than in older patients.[60] The condition may be diagnosed by a sucrose tolerance test, intestinal biopsy, and the onset of symptoms when sucrose, dextrins, or starch are fed.

In feeding patients with this condition, the infant formula must be free of sucrose. Lactose or fructose may be used in place of sucrose for the added carbohydrate in commonly used formulas based on diluted evaporated milk. Foods fed in addition to the formula also must be free of sucrose. Sucrose is added to many prepared infant foods; therefore, it may be necessary for the mother to prepare these at home.

Older patients and some infants may be less severely affected. The sucrose content of the diet should be adjusted to the level of tolerance. For those severely affected, a *sucrose-free diet,* eliminating all sources of sucrose, including almost all fruits, vegetables, cereals, and all foods to which sucrose has been added in processing or preparation, must be used. A *sucrose-restricted diet,* allowing limited quantities of fruits, vegetables, and cereals containing very small amounts of sucrose, may be used for less seriously affected patients. Details of the content of these diets are contained in some diet manuals. An enzyme, *glucomylase,* may be prescribed by the physician. Patients taking this enzyme are able to tolerate a higher sucrose content in the diet. Diets low in sucrose usually are low in ascorbic acid, folic acid, thiamine, riboflavin, and iron, and supplements of these nutrients are recommended.

Glucose-Galactose Malabsorption

Glucose-galactose malabsorption is a rare inherited, congenital condition in which the infant has a watery diarrhea and other symptoms seen in disaccharidase deficiency following the intake of sucrose, lactose, glucose, or galactose. The basic defect may be an alteration in the glucose-galactose shared transport system, but the normal process of absorption is not understood entirely; therefore, the specific nature of the defect is unknown.

Infant formulas containing fructose as the carbohydrate or carbohydrate-free formulas are tolerated. Some tolerance for glucose and galactose develops as the child becomes older, but some degree of defect is permanent.

Intestinal Lymphangiectasia

Intestinal lymphangiectasia was known formerly as *primary protein-losing gastroenteropathy* and is a prototype for the protein-losing enteropathies. The infantile form may result from a congenital malformation of the lymphatic system. In adults, its occurrence sometimes is secondary to damage from other conditions. The cause is unknown. The disease usually manifests itself in children or young adults.

The patient has severe peripheral edema, which may be asymmetrical, plus hypoproteinemia and lymphocytopenia. Gastrointestinal symptoms usually are mild but occasionally are severe. Most patients have intermittent diarrhea and steatorrhea. A few have severe steatorrhea, nausea, vomiting, and abdominal pain and distension.

Electron microscopy has shown accumulation of lipids in the endothelial cells of the intestinal lymphatics and also in the absorptive cells. The fat malabsorption may be explainable on this basis. Alterations in the endothelial cells and surrounding structure may account for the increased pressure in the lymphatics. This increase in pressure causes a dilation of the lymphatics, which may change the architecture of the villi. With increased pressure, lymph, containing both protein and lipid, is forced into the lumen of the bowel. Peripheral lymphatics are hypoplastic, and the thoracic duct may be tortuous, obstructed, or absent.

The normal lymph flow is approximately 1,500 ml/day and contains 70 g of fat and 50 g of albumin. The presence of long-chain triglycerides stimulates lymph flow. Loss of fat may be as much as 40 g/day. Protein loss into the bowel may account for the hypoproteinemia and related symptoms. The patients also often have vitamin B_{12} malabsorption. Some become hypocalcemic.

The reduction of long-chain fatty acids in the diet reduces the lymph flow and reduces the transudation of protein and lipid into the bowel lumen. Serum calcium levels also improve. The fat level in the diet must be very low, less than 5 g/day. Medium-chain triglycerides may be used to improve the energy content of the diet. For infants, Portagen or Pregestimil may be used as the basis for a formula (see Appendix L).

Abetalipoproteinemia

Abetalipoproteinemia (*Bassen-Kornzweig syndrome; acanthocytosis*) is a rare inherited disorder affecting primarily individuals of Mediterranean or Jewish origin. There is a deficiency of beta-lipoprotein. The incorporation of triglycerides and beta-lipoprotein to form chylomicrons is depressed, and lipid accumulates in the enterocytes. It has been suggested that when triglyceride accumulation reaches a certain level in the enterocyte, steatorrhea ensues.[61]

Other clinical manifestations of this progressive disease include *ataxia* (incoordination), intention tremors, absence of reflexes, muscular and skeletal deformities, and retinitis pigmentosa leading to blindness. Often, growth is retarded and the patient is thin. Plasma cholesterol is less than 80 mg/dl. Serum triglycerides are very low or absent. The relationship between the neuropathy and retinitis, on one hand, and the beta-lipoprotein deficiency, on the other, is unknown.

A fat-restricted diet with added medium-chain triglycerides allows some weight gain and reduction of steatorrhea but does not improve the neurologic symptoms. The diet should be supplemented with fat-soluble vitamins. Folate, iron, and linoleic acid supplements may be necessary also.

The prognosis is poor. Patients have progressive disability and many die in childhood, often from congestive heart failure.

Endocrine-Secreting Tumors of the Gastrointestinal Tract

In recent years, there has been increasing recognition of the endocrine functions of the gastrointestinal tract and of the pancreas, biliary tree, and bronchus, all of which are derived embryologically from the same source. When tumors occur in the endocrine cells of these organs, a wide variety of metabolic and nutritional problems ensue. Some cells secrete abnormally large quantities of their usual hormones, whereas others produce *ectopic hormones* (a hormone of a different cell type), making their quantities excessive. These tumors are classified according to their location as foregut, midgut, and hindgut tumors.

Foregut Tumors

One example of the category of diseases known as *foregut tumors* in the stomach, duodenum, pancreas, and biliary tract is the Zollinger-Ellison syndrome, described previously. Another type is a tumor in those cells, located in the pancreas and bronchus, that secrete vasoactive intestinal peptide (VIP). It is thought to cause a condition known as *pancreatic cholera, Verner-Morri-*

son syndrome, or *WDHA syndrome* (*w*atery *d*iarrhea, *h*ypokalemia, and *a*chlorhydria), although there is some controversy as to the hormone involved. The patient has a massive watery diarrhea and extensive potassium losses.

Midgut and Hindgut Tumors

Midgut and hindgut tumors occur in the appendix, small intestine, and occasionally, in the colon, stomach, or bronchi. Tumors of the appendix, however, rarely cause symptoms. Those in the other organs involve the argentaffin cells, which secrete a variety of potent substances including serotonin, histamine, kinins, adrenocorticotropic hormone, and prostaglandins. Thyroid medullary carcinoma secretes serotonin as well as thyrocalcitonin.

Excess serotonin is the most common hormonal abnormality presently recognized. It produces a complex of symptoms known as *carcinoid syndrome* or *APUDoma* (*a*mine *p*recursor *u*ptake and *d*ecarboxylation). Its effects on the intestinal tract include malabsorption, diarrhea, hypermotility, nausea, vomiting, abdominal cramps, and sometimes, intestinal obstruction or *intussusception* (telescoping of one part of the intestine into an adjoining part).

The simultaneous occurrence of these clinical manifestations and excessive serotonin suggests a causal relationship, but serotonin may not be responsible for all the symptoms. Some symptoms may be attributable to excess secretion of prostaglandins. Carcinoid tumors also produce kallikreins, which lead to an increase in circulating bradykinins and then to flushing. The overall manifestations are summarized in Table 6-13.

Diagnosis of carcinoid syndrome is made by determination of the presence of 5-hydroxyindoleacetic acid, a metabolite of serotonin, in the urine; the normal value is 16 mg/24 hr. For 2 days prior to the test, foods containing serotonin must be eliminated from the diet. These foods are walnuts, bananas, avocados, mushrooms, shellfish, tomatoes, pineapple, red plums, eggplant, and papaya.

Table 6-13. Principal Manifestations of the Carcinoid Syndrome

Vasomotor disturbances—cutaneous flushes and cyanosis
Hepatomegaly—large nodular liver
Intestinal hypermotility—borborygmi, cramps, diarrhea, vomiting, nausea
Bronchial constriction—cough, dyspnea, wheezing
Cardiac involvement—endomyocardial fibrosis with valvular deformity
Absence of hypertension—incidences no greater than general population
Prolonged clinical course—patients survive years longer than those with other tumors with metastases

Reprinted with permission from Kowlessar, O.D., The carcinoid syndrome. In M.H. Sleisenger and J.S. Fordtran, Eds., *Gastrointestinal Disease: Pathophysiology, Diagnosis, Management.* Philadelphia: W.B. Saunders, 1973.

Surgical removal of the tumor and various medications are the primary forms of treatment. Nutritional care is supportive. The clinical course is prolonged, averaging 8 years, and nutritional care can make an important contribution to the quality of life during that period.

For patients with diarrhea, nutritional support for malabsorption and diarrheal losses is necessary. Vitamin and mineral supplements may be required. In conditions with excess serotonin, niacin supplementation is needed. Some patients complain that milk, cheese, eggs, and citrus fruits cause flushing and diarrhea, and they are more comfortable if these foods are eliminated from the diet. Ascorbic acid, riboflavin, and calcium may be needed as replacements. The patient should be instructed on choosing a nutritionally adequate diet in view of these omissions.

This is an active area of research, and additional information will undoubtedly be forthcoming. The nutritional care specialist should be alert to new developments in this field.

DISEASES OF THE GALLBLADDER AND BILE DUCTS

Abnormalities of the gallbladder and bile ducts are very common. They tend to be seen more frequently in women than in men, particularly those who are middle-aged, obese, and multiparous (having had more than one baby). Diabetes, female hormones, and heredity have also been implicated.

Gallstones (*cholelithiasis*) usually are formed from cholesterol and bile salts, but some consist of bile pigments or a combination of these. Some stones are asymptomatic; others can cause inflammation of the gallbladder or obstruction of the duct (*choledocholithiasis*).

Cholecystitis (inflammation of the gallbladder) may result from the presence of gallstones or from chemical irritation of the wall of the gallbladder. It formerly was thought to be the result of infection, but no infectious organisms have been found. Symptoms include epigastric pain, vomiting, and flatulence.

Biliary dyskinesia is the result of malfunction of Oddi's sphincter, which controls the opening of the bile duct into the duodenum. If the sphincter is in spasm or simply fails to open, a back pressure into the gallbladder can develop, causing vague discomfort and sometimes pain.

In the treatment of gallbladder or bile duct disease, a low-fat diet sometimes is recommended to give symptomatic relief. Fat tolerance is highly variable, and the diet should be individualized. Some patients report that they are more comfortable if pork, eggs, fried foods, pastries, and other high-fat foods are excluded. Others find it difficult to tolerate spicy foods, onions, cabbage, cucumbers, and a few other vegetables. If the patient is obese, weight reduction is recommended.

In an acute attack, which usually occurs as a result of bile duct obstruction, a clear liquid diet may be used temporarily, with solid foods and fats added as tolerated.

The current primary treatment of gallstones and cholecystitis is surgical removal of the gallbladder or *cholecystectomy*. A more conservative treatment, dissolving gallstones by medication with chenodeoxycholic acid (CDCA) or lecithin, is promising when stones are small, but the process may take from 6 months up to 2 to 3 years. In addition, the long-term metabolic effects of CDCA administration are unknown. A high-fiber diet is recommended during this period for cholesterol binding and weight reduction.[62]

The postcholecystectomy patient may be more comfortable with a low-fat diet for several weeks or months. Eventually, the bile duct dilates and takes over the function of the gallbladder, and the patient can return to an unrestricted diet. A few patients continue to have unpleasant symptoms, referred to as *postcholecystectomy syndrome*. The etiologies include stone in the common duct, strictures, tumors, stenosis of the biliary tree, and diseases of adjacent organs. A low-fat diet may give these patients some symptomatic relief.

DISEASES OF THE PANCREAS

Various diseases of the pancreas have pancreatic insufficiency as a common clinical manifestation. As a result, they have common clinical features. Those features of nutritional significance include steatorrhea, increased fecal nitrogen loss, and vitamin B_{12} malabsorption, as described earlier.

Diagnosis

A number of tests are used to assess pancreatic function and diagnose pancreatic disease.[63] *Serum amylase* and *serum lipase* determinations are increased in inflammations of the pancreas as is *urine amylase*. Normal values are given in Appendixes D and E.

The *secretin-pancreozymin test* measures the pancreatic response to these two hormones. The hormones are given intravenously, and secretions into the duodenum are collected. Normal values are:

Secretin response	Volume output 2.0 mg/kg/80 min.
	Bicarbonate output 10 mEq/30 min.
	Bicarbonate concentration 80 mEq/L
CCK-PZ response	Amylase, 50 to 175 units/dl serum

In pancreatic insufficiency, both HCO_3^- and enzyme responses usually are reduced.

The *Lundh test meal* or *synthetic tripeptide test* causes an increase in the release of CCK-PZ and then of enzyme output. Other tests include the measure of fecal levels of fat, nitrogen, or pancreatic enzymes, roentgenography, *ultrasound,* and *biopsy.*

Acute Pancreatitis

There are many conditions that cause acute pancreatitis. Two of the most common are biliary tract disease and alcoholism coupled with a genetic predisposition to damage. The mechanism by which the condition is produced is not well understood, however. One scenario suggests that alcohol stimulates secretin release, increasing pancreatic flow while the duct is blocked at the outlet by edema.[64] Gallstones also may block the ampulla of Vater. Given a duct obstructed by one of these mechanisms, the most commonly accepted current theory of pathogenesis of the disease is that of autodigestion. Pancreatic enzymes normally are secreted into the intestinal lumen in proenzyme form and are activated there. In acute pancreatitis, they may begin a sequence of activation of many enzymes which then accumulate in the pancreas sufficiently to overcome trypsin inhibitor. Trypsin is activated within the pancreas and digests the pancreas itself.

The major symptom is abdominal pain. Nausea, vomiting, fever, and abdominal distension are common. When the outflow of amylase and lipase is obstructed by inflammation, cellular debris, and edema, the enzymes diffuse into the blood and blood levels can become very high. Circulating enzymes affect the hormonal regulation of calcium, and hypocalcemia results. Serum calcium levels of less than 7 mg/dl indicate a poor prognosis. Other effects include exudates in the peritoneal and pleural spaces, necrosis of mesenteric fat, and increased permeability of alveoli of the lungs with resultant pulmonary edema. Urinary amylase is increased. The disease is self-limiting in some patients but may progress to chronic pancreatitis in others.

The patient is given nothing by mouth, since all food and drink, even water, stimulates pancreatic secretion and adds to the pain. Fluids, electrolytes, and colloids may be given intravenously. Oral feeding may begin with a clear liquid or chemically defined diet. The diet is advanced slowly, providing six small meals of low-fat, high-carbohydrate, high-protein foods. Alcohol is strictly prohibited.

Chronic Pancreatitis

Chronic pancreatitis is seen most frequently in patients who have a history of alcoholism. Pancreatic damage may progress without signs or symptoms for a long period, but eventually the damage becomes severe enough that acute attacks occur with periods of increased alcohol intake. The loss of 90 percent of the pancreatic tissues causes pancreatic insufficiency, with weight loss and steatorrhea.

Pathogenesis

Three types of action of alcohol on the pancreas have been suggested:

1. Direct toxic effects of alcohol on pancreatic cells
2. Stimulation of pancreatic secretion with simultaneous induction of spasm in the duct system and Oddi's sphincter

3. Precipitation of protein material, possibly from degenerating cells, in the small duct (the large ducts become involved later)

As a result of these changes, acinar cells atrophy. The pancreas becomes inflamed, necrotic, hemorrhagic, and edematous. Acini may be replaced by fibrotic tissue. The islets of Langerhans, especially beta cells, eventually become involved, and some patients become diabetic.

Clinical Manifestations

Abdominal pain is the chief complaint in chronic pancreatitis. It may be episodic at first but becomes continuous if alcohol intake continues. Vomiting is frequent. Progressive pancreatic insufficiency leads to malabsorption of multiple nutrients, diarrhea, and the accompanying symptoms. These are summarized in Fig. 6-8.

Serum amylase and lipase are elevated early but may be normal or even low in advanced disease when pancreatic tissue is destroyed. Roentgenography sometimes shows calcification of the pancreas. Other complications include pleural and pericardial effusions, *ascites* (accumulation of fluid in the peritoneal cavity), psychosis, and necrosis of the bone.[65]

Nutritional Management

Replacement pancreatic enzymes, taken orally with meals, are the mainstay of the control of maldigestion and malabsorption. Antacids are given simultaneously to reduce inactivation of the enzymes by gastric acid. A diet low in fat and high in protein and carbohydrate is helpful. It may be supple-

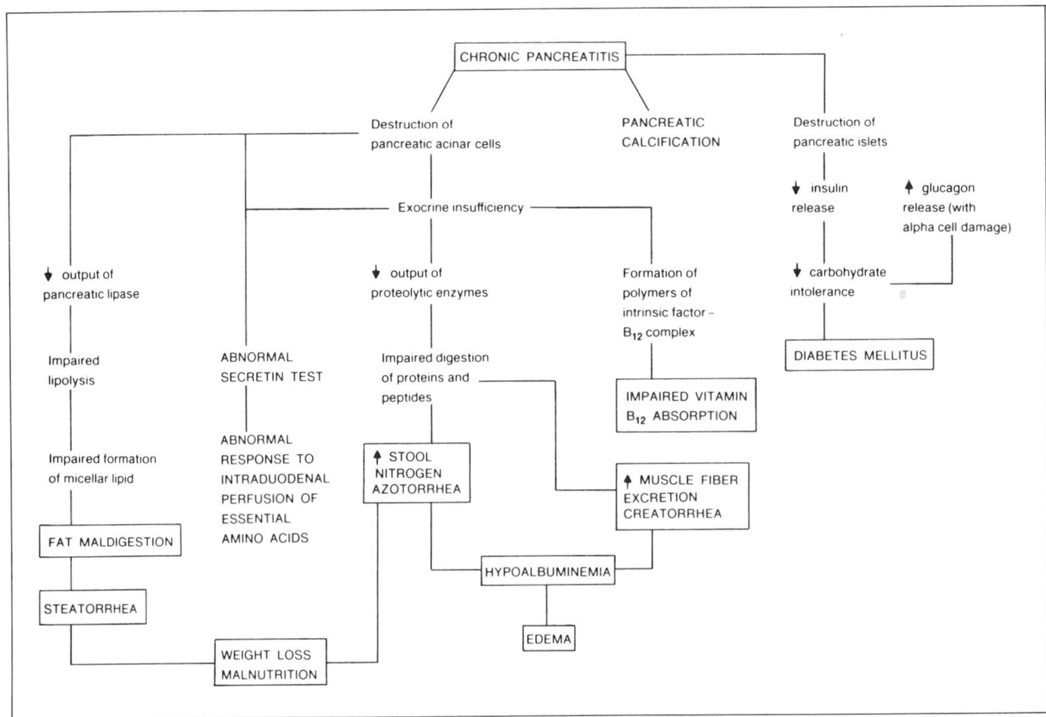

Figure 6-8. The pathophysiologic alterations in exocrine pancreatic insufficiency. (Reprinted with permission from Greenberger, N.J., Gastrointestinal Disorders: A Pathophysiologic Approach, *2nd ed. Copyright © 1981 by Year Book Medical Publishers, Inc., Chicago. P. 263.)*

mented with medium-chain triglycerides. Complete abstinence from alcohol is essential but difficult to achieve.

Cystic Fibrosis of the Pancreas

Cystic fibrosis (CF), also known as *mucoviscidosis,* is an inherited disorder of the mucus-producing glands in the pancreas, bronchi, intestines, and liver. The condition is an autosomal recessive trait that occurs about once in 1,600 live births. The pancreatic problems are prominent and are those most closely related to nutrition; therefore, discussion of the disease is included in this chapter.

Pathophysiology and Clinical Manifestations

The basic metabolic deficit in cystic fibrosis is unknown. An abnormally large amount of a very viscid mucus is secreted, and the sweat has three to five times the normal concentration of sodium and chloride. There are many manifestations of this disease, which are listed in Fig. 6-9. In the newborn, the meconium tends to be thick and sticky, causing intestinal obstruction known as *meconium ileus.* The incidence of volvulus, peritonitis, atresia, obstruction, and rectal prolapse also is increased.

Usually, but not always, pancreatic insufficiency is observed. When it is present, steatorrhea occurs along with maldigestion of protein and carbohydrate. Fat digestion is most severely affected. Duodenal assays for pancreatic enzymes shows them to be absent or reduced. The resulting malabsorption may be complicated by hepatic abnormalities.

The lungs usually are involved, with obstruction of the bronchi and increased incidence of *bronchiectasis* (chronic dilation with coughing and purulent exudate) and *atelectasis* (collapsed or airless portions of the lung), and pneumonia. The immune response appears to be normal. Other manifestations are listed in Table 6-14.

Table 6-14. Principal Clinical Manifestations of Cystic Fibrosis of the Pancreas

Viscid secretions/Small duct obstruction

Respiratory disorders
- Sinusitis, nasal polyposis
- Atelectasis
- Emphysema
- Bronchitis, bronchopneumonia, bronchiectasis, lung abscess, aspergillosis
- Respiratory failure
- Cor pulmonale

Intestinal disorders

Meconium ileus
- Volvulus
- Peritonitis
- Ileal atresia
- Obstruction

Pancreas
- Nutritional failure due to pancreatic insufficiency
- Steatorrhea and creatorrhea
- Diabetes mellitus
- Vitamin deficiencies
- Loss of bile salts

Hepatobiliary disorders

Mucous hypersecretion
Atrophic gallbladder
Focal biliary cirrhosis
Laennec's cirrhosis
Hepar lobatum
Portal hypertension
Esophageal varices
Hypersplenism

Reproductive system disorders

Males: sterility; absent vas deferens, epididymis, and seminal vesicles
Females: decreased fertility

Skeletal disorders

Retardation of bone age
Demineralization

Other disorders

Salt depletion
Heat stroke
Salivary gland hypertrophy
Retinal hemorrhage
Hypertrophy of apocrine glands

Reprinted with permission from Schwachman, H.L., and Grand, R.J., Cystic fibrosis. In M.H. Sleisenger and J.S. Fordtran, Eds., *Gastrointestinal Disease: Pathophysiology, Diagnosis, Management,* 2nd ed. Philadelphia: W.B. Saunders, 1978.

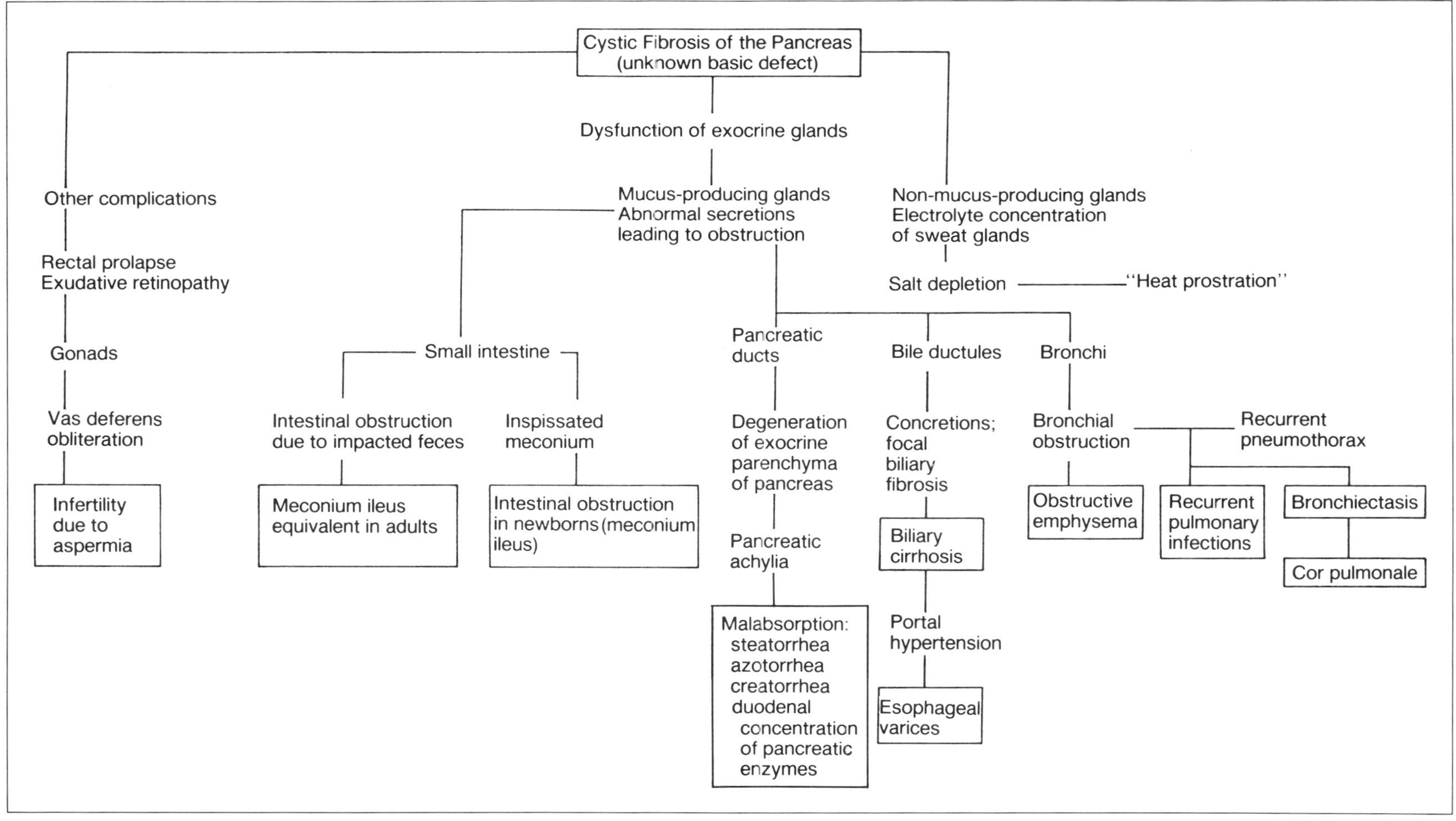

Figure 6-9. The pathophysiology and manifestations of cystic fibrosis of the pancreas. (Reprinted with permission from Greenberger, N.J., Gastrointestinal Disorders: A Pathophysiologic Approach, *2nd ed. Copyright © 1981 by Year Book Medical Publishers, Inc., Chicago. P. 276.)*

Nutritional Management

Currently, the average life expectancy of a cystic fibrosis patient is approximately 16 years, but some patients live to adulthood. Treatment is long-term and requires the cooperation of physicians, nurses, nutritionists, physical therapists, and social workers.

Nutritional management must be individualized, since the disease varies in severity. For pancreatic insufficiency, pancreatic enzyme extracts prescribed by the physician are taken with each meal. The dose is high and may be 0.1 to 0.3 g of pancreatin per kilogram of body weight per day. Products such as Viokase and Cotazyme are taken in relatively large quantities with meals. A low-fat, high-protein (3 to 4 g/kg), high-carbohydrate diet is used. Total kilocalorie content of the diet may have to be as high as 150 kcal/kg. MCT Oil, Polycose, and protein powders (see Appendix J) are added if necessary to provide sufficient energy.[66,67] Appetites sometimes are voracious but may diminish in response to pain and diarrhea.[68] For infants, Pregestimil may be needed in place of more commonly used formulas. Portagen is often used for children and adults as an alternative to milk. Total parenteral feeding sometimes is used for infants who are unable to achieve adequate caloric intake orally.[67] Multivitamin supplements in water-soluble form are necessary and are prescribed by the physician. Additional salt must be taken in hot weather, fever, or when the patient sweats excessively. Some patients do not have pancreatic insufficiency, and so diet modifications are unnecessary.

Postural drainage with clapping and vibrating, antibiotics, aerosols, expectorants, and exercise are included in the management of the respiratory disease.

DISEASES OF THE LARGE INTESTINE

There has been a great deal of confusion concerning the use of the terms *fiber, roughage, residue,* and *bulk.* It is important that these terms be understood when nutritional care in diseases of the large intestine is being considered.

Fiber and Related Substances

Available carbohydrates are those that are absorbed from the small bowel. *Unavailable carbohydrates* are those thought not to be absorbed. *Dietary fiber,* as the term is currently used, includes that portion of plant cells that are resistant to digestive enzymes in humans. The term is used to refer to a variety of plant materials that are resistant to digestion (Table 6-15). The definition has been expanded to include substances such as guar gum, which is used as an additive but does not occur naturally in food. Dietary fiber must be distinguished from *crude fiber,* the residue remaining after plant food has been treated with lipid solvent and dilute acid and alkali. Crude fiber includes only cellulose and lignin. The values that appear in food composition tables are for crude fiber. Unfortunately, values for dietary fiber, which would be more useful in diet planning, are not available because of a lack of adequate assay methods. It has been estimated that dietary fiber may equal two to six times the amount of crude fiber.

The terms *dietary fiber complex*[69] and *plantix*[70] have been suggested as useful terms that would be defined to include dietary fiber *plus* other materials, such as gums and mucilages associated with the structural compounds. A useful grouping might therefore consist of components that are considered to be fibers and those that are associated with fiber. The term *roughage* sometimes is used interchangeably with fiber. It stems from a belief that some foods have an abrasive quality. In the light of present knowledge, this term is not useful. *Residue* has been used to indicate the amount of material remaining from a food after digestion and absorption and has also been used as a synonym for fiber. The

Table 6-15. Classification of Dietary Fiber by Structure and Human Physiologic Function

Fiber Class	Chemical Structure of Main Chain	Human Function[a]
Noncellulosic polysaccharides		
Gums (secretions)	Galacturonic acid–mannose; galacturonic acid–rhamnose	1. May slow gastric emptying 2. Provide fermentable substrate for colonic bacteria, with production of gas and volatile fatty acids 3. Bind bile acids variably
Mucilages (secretions, plant seeds)	Galactose-mannose; galacturonic acid–rhamnose; arabinose-xylose	
Algal polysaccharides (from algae and seaweeds)	Mannose, xylose; glucuronic acid, glucose	
Pectin substances (intercellular cement)	Galacturonic acid	
Hemicelluloses (from the cell wall of many plants)	Xylose, mannose; galactose, glucose (branching chains)	1. Hold water, increase stool bulk 2. May reduce *elevated* colonic intraluminal pressure 3. Bind bile acids variably
Cellulose (principal cell wall constituent)	Polyglycan, unbranched glucose polymer	1. Depending on particle size, holds water 2. May reduce *elevated* colonic intraluminal pressure 3. May bind zinc
Lignin (woody part of plants)	Polymeric phenylpropane, noncarbohydrate	1. Serves as antioxidant 2. May bind metals

Reprinted with permission from Mendeloff, A.I., Dietary fiber and health. An introduction. In *Nutrition and Disease: Fiber.* Columbus, Ohio: Ross Laboratories, 1978.

[a] Incompletely understood.

relationship between food intake and fecal volume is unknown. Some foods, such as milk, are known to leave some residue in the intestinal lumen, even though they have little or no fiber. In addition, there is material containing water, mucus, bacteria, and desquamated intestinal cells present in the intestinal tract even if no food is eaten. *Bulk* refers to the capacity of some materials to hold water and increase the weight of the stool. It is used sometimes in discussing the action of some laxatives.

In nutritional science, given the present state of the art, *fiber* generally is considered to be the most useful term. It is important to realize, however, that the term refers to a mixture of substances the individual actions of which are unknown. The planning of high-fiber and low-fiber diets is a crude procedure at best.

Some digestion of dietary fiber does occur. Fermentation by microorganisms produces the volatile fatty acids acetic, propionic, and butyric, as well as hydrogen, carbon dioxide, methane, and ammonia gases.[71,72] Some proposed functions of dietary fiber are given in Table 6-15.

The effects of fiber on the function of the colon is complex and in need of further study. In addition, some evidence indicates that fiber affects carbohydrate and lipid metabolism. Therefore, it may be a consideration in the nutritional management of patients with diabetes mellitus and cardiovascular disease. Its relationships to these diseases are discussed in Chapters 8 and 9.

Intestinal Gas

Flatulence (excessive formation of gas in the digestive tract) and *eructation* or *belching* has been the basis for humor and social embarrassment. Flatulence also may be the cause of distension, bloating, and pain sufficiently severe to be mistaken for a heart attack. It may signal a serious disorder of the intestinal tract or may be benign.

Gas is present normally in the colon, but its volume and composition varies widely. The normal mean volume of gas passed from the rectum is 600 ml/day, but rates from 200 to 2,000 ml have been measured.[73] The amount in the intestinal tract at any one time usually is less than 200 ml.[74,75] The gas present consists almost entirely of various proportions of nitrogen, oxygen, carbon dioxide, hydrogen, and methane and is a combination of swallowed air and gas diffused from the blood and from intraluminal production.

The type of gas present suggests its source. Our atmosphere consists of approximately 80 percent nitrogen and 20 percent oxygen. These dissolve in the blood and then diffuse from the mucosal blood supply into the lumen. Swallowed air, too, is nitrogen and oxygen. One study indicated that 2 to 3 ml of air reaches the stomach with each swallow.[76] It is believed that most of this material normally is regurgitated, and diffusion from the blood accounts for most of the nitrogen seen in rectal flatus.[77]

Carbon dioxide is produced in large quantities from the reaction of normal gastric hydrogen ion and pancreatic bicarbonate. Most of it is reabsorbed. Hydrogen is produced by bacterial metabolism in the colon,[78] but some bacteria use hydrogen.[78,79] Bacteria also are believed to be the source of carbon dioxide found in the flatus since increases of both hydrogen and carbon dioxide usually are concurrent. Methane is produced by colonic bacterial metabolism but is not found in all individuals.

Studies have shown that some patients who complain of excess gas actually have a normal volume and composition of gas in the digestive tract.[80] Instead, they may have disorders of intestinal motility and increased sensitivity of the bowel to distension.[81] Disordered motility sometimes is treated with anticholinergics, but their effectiveness is unknown. Nutritional care includes methods to reduce intestinal gas to subnormal levels to avoid the patient's increased sensitivity. Patients can be advised to eat slowly and eat with the mouth closed. A straw should not be used for drinking. Chewing gum and smoking have been assumed to contribute to air swallowing. Although there is no supporting evidence, advice to the patient to eliminate these habits seems a logical step.

Foods reputed to increase intestinal gas may be eliminated. Foods containing carbohydrates that are not digestible by intestinal enzymes but are digestible by colon bacteria (such as some fruits and vegetables and whole grain cereals) and that provide substrates for gas production may be eliminated. Beans, which have a well-known reputation, contain the trisaccharide *raffinose* and the tetrasaccharide *stachyose,* both of which serve as a substrate for colon bacteria. Other vegetables reputed to be gas-forming include cabbage, cauliflower, broccoli, onions, turnips, corn, and cucumbers. No studies, however, have established that the reputation is deserved. If a diet history reveals that these food cause flatulence or that the patients believe they do, they may be eliminated from the diet. Foods that contain large amounts of gas, such as carbonated beverages, whips, and meringues, may be restricted. Sometimes a low-fat diet is useful in reducing the fatty acids that may serve as a source of hydrogen. It is important to monitor the patient's diet to assure adequate nutrient intake.

Some patients are believed to have excessive gas because of *aerophagia* (air swallowing). This often occurs in tense, nervous individuals whose main need is reassurance that there is no organic basis for the condition. Diet modification usually is unnecessary. Some patients may be cautioned against gas-containing foods and chewing gum and advised to eat slowly with closed mouth.

In those patients whose flatulence results from a malabsorption syndrome, the flatulence usually subsides with treatment of the basic disease.

Constipation

Constipation consists of the slow passage or retention of fecal matter until feces are too hard to pass easily or other uncomfortable symptoms occur. It can occur alone or as a symptom of other disease. Many drugs induce constipation, such as aluminum hydroxide antacids, anticholinergics, iron supplements, some antihypertensive agents, and some narcotics. Other circumstances that predispose to constipation include diabetes, hypothyroidism, colon cancer, prolonged immobilization, and conditions that cause pain on defecation, such as hemorrhoids and anal fissures.

The usual amount of time elapsed between eating and defecation varies greatly but most commonly is 24 to 72 hours. The normal number of bowel movements also may vary from several per day in some individuals to only once in several days in others. Given this wide variation, it is important to define constipation in terms of the usual habits of the individual and the presence of symptoms.

The types of constipation are categorized as obstructive, atonic, or spastic. *Obstructive constipation* occurs as a result of obstructions caused by adhesions, impaction, or tumors, including cancer. Impacted material may be feces or foreign materials and must sometimes be removed surgically. In preparation for surgery, the patient may need a low-residue chemically defined diet or TPN.

Atonic constipation is more likely to be the consequence of poor health habits. These include diets excessively low in fiber, inadequate water intake, irregular meals, habitually ignoring the defecation reflex, lack of exercise, and habitual use of cathartics. Sometimes atonic constipation accompanies hypothyroidism or the use of medications containing iron, aluminum, magnesium, or calcium compounds. It often occurs in the aged, the obese, and in pregnant women. Patients who are confined to bed for long periods may be chronically constipated. Constipation is a frequent problem in handicapped patients (see Chapter 16).

When no organic basis is found for atonic constipation, changes in diet are the primary mode of management. The patient is encouraged to increase his or her intake of fiber-containing foods, fruits, vegetables, and whole grain cereals. Prunes and prune juice are useful to stimulate peristalsis. The active principle in prunes is *dihydroxyphenyl isatin.* An increase in the intake of fluids also is helpful. At least 1 qt/day in fluid form is recommended. Sometimes 2 tsp. of bran with meals also is recommended. The increased undigested fiber absorbs water to increase the bulk of the intestinal contents and stimulate defecation. Therefore, the patient should be advised to eat breakfast to stimulate the gastrocolic reflex leading to defecation. In addition, the establishment of a regular pattern of food intake and exercise is helpful.

Spastic constipation occurs as one of the symptoms in the *irritable bowel syndrome,* also known as *mucous colitis, irritable colon,* or *spastic colon.* It is one of the most common gastrointestinal disorders presented for treatment. No organic abnormality is known to cause mucous colitis. Therefore, it is regarded as a functional disease and generally is believed to occur as the result of emotional stress. Other contributing factors that have been suggested include lack of sleep, insufficient fluid intake, excessive use of cathartics, coffee, tea, alcohol, or tobacco, and, sometimes, enteric infections and antibiotics. The condition possibly involves overstimulation of nerve endings, causing disturbances in motility, irregular contractions, and decreased sensitivity to the defecation reflex. The resulting symptoms include abdominal pain, heartburn, flatulence, and constipation which may alternate with episodes of diarrhea.

Treatment consists primarily of emotional support and establishment of regular habits as described for atonic constipation. The diet may be a basically normal adequate diet with increased amounts of fruits, vegetables, and whole grain cereals, with 2 tsp. of unprocessed bran with meals. During diarrheal episodes, avoidance of carbonated beverages and coffee may be recommended. It is not known if the effects of these diet changes are physiologic or psychological.

Constipated patients may be prescribed cathartics. Others will be seen to have acquired a habit of chronic laxative use by self-medication. In either case, the nutritional care specialist needs to be familiar with the major types, modes of action, and side effects of these drugs. Agents that promote defecation are *cathartics.* These may be classified by increasing intensity of their action as *laxatives, purgatives,* and *drastics.* They are also classified according to their modes of action.

Emollient laxatives are wetting agents that soften the fecal mass by allowing water and fat to penetrate the stool. *Dioctyl sodium sulfosuccinate* (*Colace*) and *dioctyl calcium sulfosuccinate* (*Surfak*) may cause nausea, vomiting, anorexia, and sometimes diarrhea. They have a bitter taste and are throat irritants and should, therefore, be taken with milk or fruit juice. Surfak is useful if the patient has a sodium-restricted diet.

Bulk-forming laxatives increase the moisture content of the stool and thus stimulate peristalsis. *Psyllium* (*Metamucil*) or *methylcellulose* should be taken with a large amount of water. They may cause steatorrhea, flatulence, and, if taken chronically, alterations in electrolyte absorption.

There are several *stimulant cathartics. Castor oil* is used in preparation for bowel examination almost exclusively. It is taken with juice on an empty stomach. *Bisacodyl* (*Dulcolax*) stimulates colon peristalsis. It may cause colic, diarrhea, and hypokalemia. A related compound, *phenolphthalein* (*Ex-Lax*), may decrease absorption of fat-soluble vitamins and other nutrients. If use is prolonged, it can cause dehydration and electrolyte imbalance. The incidence of allergy is high (5 to 7 percent). *Anthraquinone cathartics, extract of cascara,* and *extract of senna* (*Senokot*) stimulate the colon. They should be taken with meals or with at least 8 oz. of water. Chronic use may cause sodium and potassium depletion.

Saline cathartics are nonabsorbable salts with osmotic activity that causes water retention in the lumen of the colon. *Milk of magnesia,* for example, may cause nausea, colic, polyuria, and diarrhea.

Chronic Ulcerative Colitis

Chronic ulcerative colitis and Crohn's disease together are referred to as *inflammatory bowel disease.* The main features of Crohn's disease and its nutritional care were described under Diseases Primarily Affecting the Small Intestine (p. 189).

Chronic ulcerative colitis is an inflammatory disease of the colon and rectum. It primarily affects young adults. It is more common in women than men and in whites than in other races. The cause of the disease is unknown. Some patients improve when milk is removed from the diet, leading to the suggestion that the disease is immunologic in origin. Abnormal antigen absorption may be involved.[28] Many patients have been described as hostile, tense, and immature, suggesting an emotional etiology.

The onset of the disease usually is slow but can be sudden and severe. Chronic ulcerative colitis often is treated on an outpatient basis. It is characterized by remissions and exacerbations, but it can run a severe course in some patients. The patient has a bloody diarrhea and abdominal pain. During acute episodes, twenty to thirty bowel movements per day consisting of a mixture of mucus, blood, pus, and feces may be produced. The mucosa of the rectum is edematous and ulcerated with an exudate of mucus, pus, and blood. There may be fever, negative nitrogen balance, decreased serum albumin, nutritional edema, dehydration, and anemia. The patient often is extremely anorexic. Lesions elsewhere in the body include rash, hives, arthritis, and conjunctivitis, supporting the speculation that the disease is an immune response.[28]

The treatment includes drugs, diet, and sometimes surgery. Glucocorticoids are used to bring the patient into remission and sulfasalazine, to prolong remission. Side effects of sulfasalazine include nausea, vomiting, and diarrhea. These side effects must be considered in relation to the diet. The objectives of the diet are (1) to provide adequate nutrition, including nutrients for repair, (2) to reduce stool frequency, and (3) to make the patient more comfortable. A low-fiber diet sometimes is recommended to reduce pain and the number of stools. The major effort often needs to be expended in dealing with the anorexia and emotional problems of patients. Special effort should be made to cater to the patient's preferences and provide attractive service in cheerful surroundings to encourage the patient to eat. Small frequent meals often are used. If the patient's food intake is insufficient, tube feeding or TPN may be necessary.

Possible complications are hemorrhage, perforation, fistulas, obstruction, and *toxic megacolon,* in which the colon loses tone and dilates. Cancer develops more frequently in chronic ulcerative colitis patients than in the nonaffected population. Surgical resection of the affected parts is required in approximately 25 percent of the patients. Nutritional support is required to prepare the patient for surgery. Depending on the extent and location of the lesion, surgery may result in an end-to-end anastamosis or the colon may be resected, requiring the formation of an ileostomy or colostomy. Nutritional care of ostomy patients is discussed later in this chapter.

Diverticular Disease

The colon wall consists of the mucosal layer, a layer of circular muscle, and three longitudinal bands, the teniae coli (see Fig. 6-6). A *diverticulum* is a tiny pocket formed when a small portion of colon membrane is pushed out through weak spots in the muscle of the colon that exist in the circular layer where blood vessels penetrate the muscle. *Diverticulosis* is a common condition in the middle-aged and elderly in which diverticula are present in the intestinal tract. When first formed, the diverticula are reducible when intraluminal pressure falls and, therefore, their number varies. In time, they cannot be reduced or expel the feces they contain. The feces becomes *inspissated* (thickened) and may become stonelike formations known as *fecaliths. Diverticulitis* exists when the diverticula become inflamed. Only 10 to 15 percent of patients with diverticulosis develop diverticulitis.

Epidemiologic evidence indicates that these conditions occur in those eating a refined Western-type diet.[82] In less developed countries where food is not processed as extensively, the disease is almost unknown. In those countries, the colon tends to be quite enlarged and there is, instead of diverticulosis, a higher incidence of volvulus or intussusception.

One theory for the development of diverticula proposes that there is an increase in intraluminal pressure when the contents of the lumen is reduced or the lumen is narrowed, and segmentation increases. It has been suggested that these alterations occur more frequently in those eating a highly refined diet. It has also been suggested that sigmoid contractions in response to emotional stress contribute to intraluminal pressure.

Clinical Manifestations

Diverticulosis may be asymptomatic or the patient may have pain and constipation sometimes alternating with diarrhea. Diverticulitis involves inflammation with fever and pain. Sometimes there is ileus, anorexia, and nausea.

Management

Diet has recently become an important feature of long-term management of chronic diverticular disease. A high-fiber diet increases the bulk of the material reaching the colon. The diameter of the lumen of the colon is enlarged, decreasing the need for excessive segmentation and reducing the symptoms. Sometimes analgesics or tranquilizers are prescribed if the patient is in pain.

Between 10 and 15 g of bran and 200 g of fruits and vegetables are recommended to increase stool weight to at least 150 g/day. This diet is recommended for treatment of chronic diverticulosis but has not been shown to prevent diverticular disease or its symptoms.[83]

In diverticulitis, antibiotics and supportive therapy for water and electrolyte balance may be required. A liquid diet, used for a short time, is followed by a low-fiber diet as tolerated. When acute symptoms subside, the high-fiber diet as for diverticulosis may be used. Surgery occasionally is required, particularly for complications. Complications that sometimes occur include abscesses, peritonitis, fistulas, hemorrhage, or obstruction.[82]

Colon Surgery

A portion or all of the large intestine must sometimes be removed or rested. Diseases that make resection or rest necessary include chronic ulcerative colitis, Crohn's disease, and colon cancer. When part of the bowel is removed, it sometimes is possible to restore the continuity of the remaining bowel with an end-to-end anastamosis. In other cases, the location and size of the resection make that impossible. Then a *stoma* is made to provide a new exit for the intestinal contents; this stoma is permanent. However, when the purpose is to rest the bowel, the stoma may be temporary, and the continuity of the bowel may be restored at a later date. Temporary ostomies are closed in weeks, months, or sometimes, years.

Ileostomy

An *ileostomy* provides an opening from the distal ileum through the abdominal wall (Fig. 6-10). It bypasses the colon, rectum, and anus. The contents of the ileum is very liquid, since the colon's function of reabsorbing electrolytes and water is lost. The daily loss in excess of normal is approximately 500 ml of water and 30 to 50 mEq each of sodium and chloride.[84] At one time, all patients with an ileostomy had to wear an "appliance" or *ileostomy bag* into which the ileostomy drained constantly. Now, an internal reservoir may be created surgically. The result is called a *continent ileostomy*. It contains a nipple within the reservoir, formed from a length of ileum intussuscepted back into the reservoir. When the reservoir fills, the internal pressure closes the nipple. At intervals, the patient catheterizes the stoma and drains the reservoir.

Oral feeding postoperatively may begin with a clear liquid diet and progress to a low-fiber diet. Most ileostomy patients eventually can follow a normal diet. The diet they followed preoperatively is no longer needed, but some adjustments may be required to

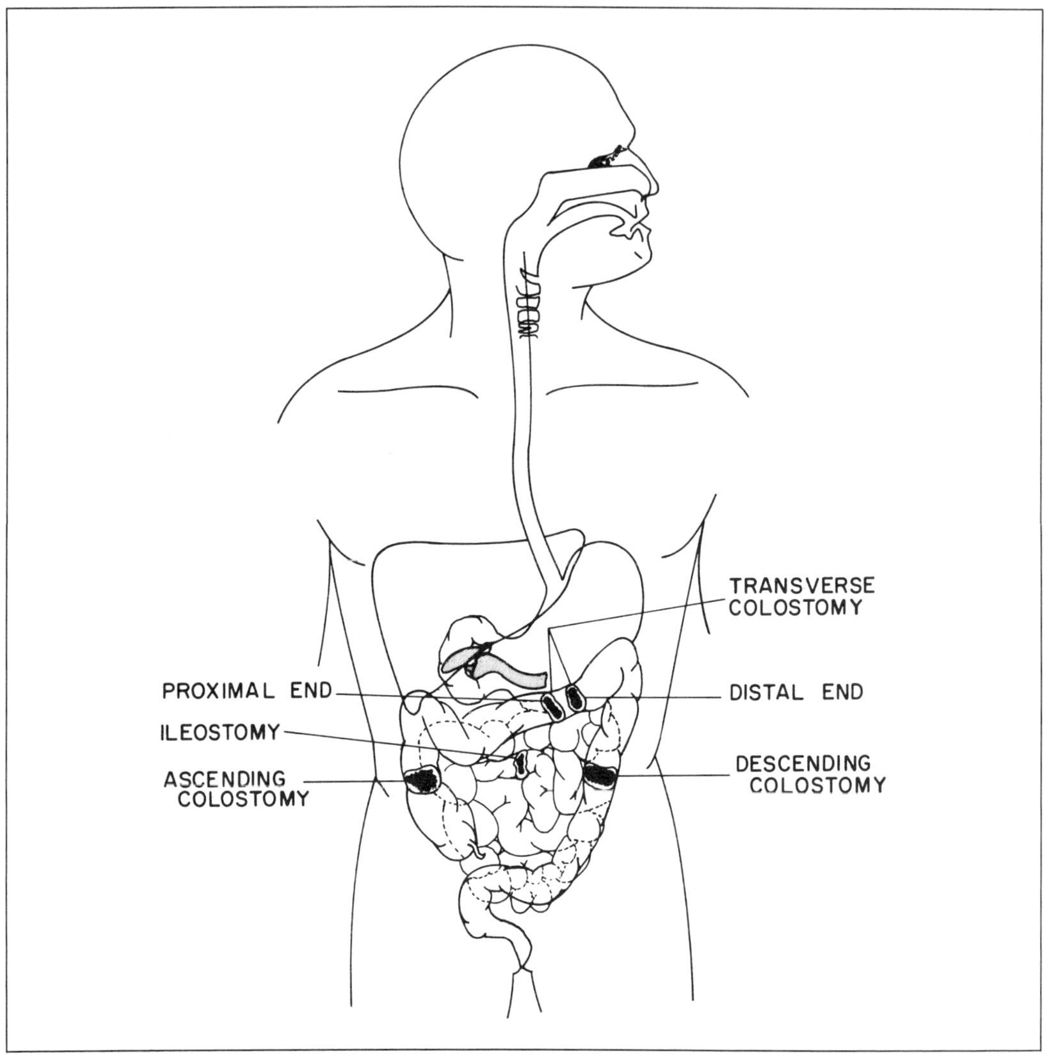

Figure 6-10. Ostomy sites. (Reprinted with permission from Tucker, S.M., Breeding, M.A., Canobbio, M.M., et al., Patient Care Standards, *2nd ed. St. Louis: C.V. Mosby, 1980, p. 242.)*

prevent obstruction, watery or an excessively large volume of discharge, and excessive odor and gas. The diet must be adjusted individually. Foods are added one at a time so that problem foods can be identified. A regular diet can usually be achieved in 2 to 3 weeks. Suggested procedures and problem foods are listed in Table 6-16.

The ileostomy patient should be advised to increase fluid and salt intake permanently. Salt and water are lost in varying amounts when the colon is removed, and dehydration can occur. If the volume of effluent exceeds 1,000 ml/day, the patient probably will need additional intake of fluid and sodium, which often is provided intravenously. If potassium losses are not large, small deficits can be replaced by encouraging the patient to increase intake of orange, grapefruit, or tomato juice, milk, or the various beverages advertised for use by athletes. It is important that the ileostomy patient understand that reducing his or her fluid intake causes dehydration, not a reduc-

Table 6-16. Some Procedures for Nutritional Management of an Ileostomy

Add foods one at a time to progress from a low-fiber diet to the unrestricted diet, so that problem foods can be identified.

To prevent obstruction:

- Increase fluid intake.
- Use prune juice and grape juice to increase liquidity of the effluent.
- Avoid foods high in fiber or with seeds or kernels.
- Chew foods thoroughly; be sure dentures are properly fitted.
- Approach with caution potential problem foods, including
  - Corn on the cob
  - Celery
  - Coleslaw
  - Lettuce
  - Chinese vegetables, such as bean sprouts and bamboo shoots
  - Peas
  - Mushrooms
  - Citrus fruit membranes
  - Nuts
  - Coconut
  - Peanuts
  - Tough meats
  - Fruits with seeds
  - Raw fruit
  - Tomatoes

To prevent watery discharge:

- Approach with caution potential problem foods, including
  - Prune juice
  - Beer
  - Baked beans
  - Green beans
  - Cabbage
  - Broccoli
  - Spinach
  - Highly spiced foods
  - Raw fruit

When a food causes a problem, it should be eliminated for a period and then tried again later. There is some adaptation in time.

To avoid flatulence with pain and odor:

- Eliminate gas-producing and odor-producing foods. These should be tried again at intervals.
  - Dried beans and peas
  - Beer
  - Mustard
  - Cabbage family
  - Spiced foods
  - Fish
  - Onions
  - Carbonated beverages
  - Melons
  - Eggs
  - Radishes
  - Cucumbers
  - Fatty foods, such as pastries and deep-fried foods
  - Pickles
  - Whips and meringues
  - Strong-flavored cheeses
- Avoid chewing gum.
- Do not use a straw.
- Chew food with mouth closed.
- Eat regular meals.
- Add cranberry juice, yogurt, and buttermilk.

tion in effluent volume. This is especially important when losses by other routes are increased, such as in fever and vomiting. If the patient is chronically dehydrated, urine volume decreases and the incidence of renal stones increases.

Vitamin supplements may be required. If the terminal ileum has been removed, parenteral vitamin B_{12} will be needed. If the patient also has lost large portions of the small intestine, supplements of fat-soluble vitamins may be necessary.

Common problems occurring a year or more postoperatively are excessive weight gain or weight loss. Long-term nutritional care should include monitoring body weight and giving advice on weight control or gain as necessary. The ileostomy does not preclude participation in active sports, including swimming and other water sports, running, tennis, and similar activities. Some physicians do advise against contact sports. The patient also is capable of relatively strenuous work. The patient's activity should be considered in advising him or her on caloric intake.

Colostomy

Colostomies are placed at various locations, depending on the location and amount of colon removed (see Fig. 6-10). If the stoma is in the cecum, it is called a *cecostomy.* Colostomies may be in the ascending, transverse, descending, or sigmoid colons. The solid or liquid state of the effluent depends on the location and has an important effect on management (Fig. 6-11).

A *right-sided colostomy,* in the ascending colon, is near the ileum and has a highly liquid effluent similar to that from an ileostomy. It also has a high content of irritating digestive enzymes. Unless a continent ileostomy is constructed, the patient must wear an appliance with a "faceplate" that attaches to the skin with an adhesive and a bag into which the effluent drains.

Left-sided colostomies, in the descending or sigmoid colon, are further from the ileum. Water is resorbed in the colon above the stoma, and the fecal matter thus is more solid. In addition, there is some storage capacity so that elimination can occur at regular intervals. The patient may wear a lightweight disposable pouch as a precaution, but a bag similar to that worn by some ileostomy patients is unnecessary.

Colostomies in the transverse colon are located at some point intermediate between those already described, and the consistency of the effluent depends on the specific location of the stoma.

The behavior of a colostomy in the ascending colon and, sometimes, in the transverse colon resembles that of an ileostomy, and the diet is managed in the same way (see Table 6-16). However, the stoma in a colostomy usually is larger and obstructions are less likely.

Postoperative feeding of patients with a colostomy in the descending or sigmoid colon usually begins with a clear liquid diet. The progression to a full diet is more rapid than it is for an ileostomy patient. Usually colostomy patients no longer require the modifications of the diet that were needed prior to surgery. However, the colostomy may present some problems that are amen-

Figure 6-11. Absorption and storage functions of the large intestine. (Reprinted with permission from Guyton, A.C., Textbook of Medical Physiology, *6th ed. Philadelphia: W.B. Saunders, 1981, P. 797.)*

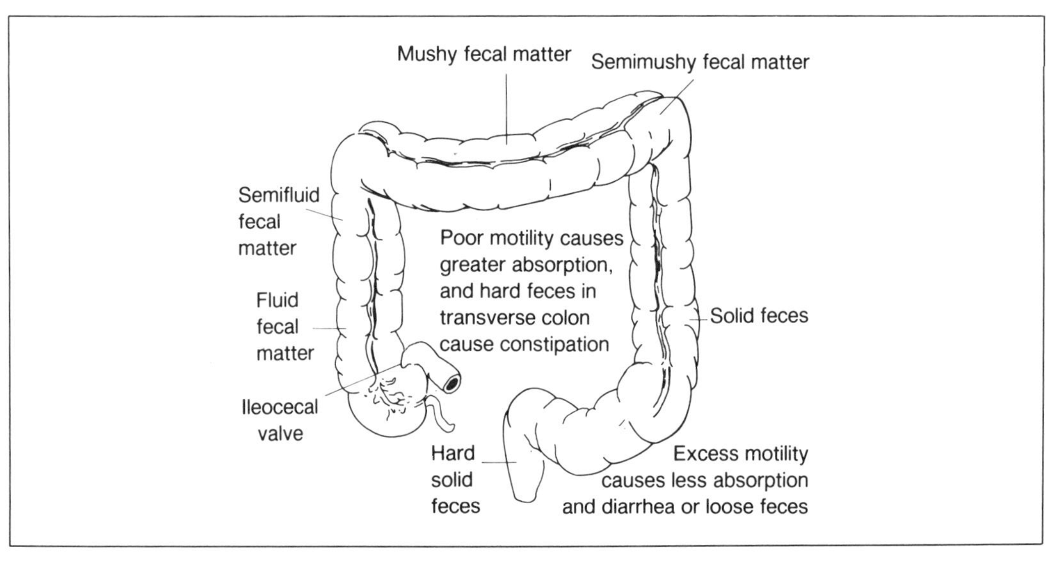

able to dietary manipulations, including constipation, diarrhea, flatus, and odor. Some procedures for management of these problems are given in Table 6-17.

Postoperatively, the ostomy patient must be carefully instructed in the care of the stoma. The process requires a team approach and should include the physician, nurse, and nutritional care specialist. Some institutions have specially trained nurses, known as *enterostomal therapists* (E.T.), who are important members of the team. The patient often needs a great deal of psychological support at first. Most can lead normal lives, including travel, marriage, and reproduction, once their stomas are "regulated." Contact sports may not be approved, but patients usually can participate in other sports. Special clothing is not required.

Table 6-17. Some Procedures for Management of a Colostomy

To prevent flatus and odor: see Table 6-16.

To prevent or treat constipation:

- Increase fluid intake, especially fruit juices. Use at least 1.5–2 liters/day of fluid.
- Increase intake of cooked fruits and vegetables.
- Add *soft* prunes, figs, and raisins.
- Add whole wheat and bran.

To prevent diarrhea or "loose bowels":

- Omit chocolate, licorice, fresh pineapple, figs, peaches, spinach, beer, and tomatoes.
- Add strained bananas, applesauce, boiled rice, tapioca, boiled milk, marshmallows, and cheese.
- Possibly, return to a low-fiber diet.

Rectal Surgery

Rectal or anal surgery may be required for *prolapse* (protrusion of the inverted rectum through the anus), incontinence, fecal impaction, chronic infection, anal fissure, fistulas, or *hemorrhoids* (rupture of blood vessels into the lumen in the anal area).

Hemorrhoids are fairly common. Causative factors include constipation and straining at defecation, prolonged use of laxatives or enemas, and pregnancy. Nutritional care for patients can provide some relief of symptoms during periods of acute pain. The diet should be low in fiber and the patient should be advised to drink a large quantity of fluids. Specific foods that the patient may identify as causing discomfort, such as highly spiced foods, may be eliminated. During remission, a high-fiber diet with intake of 1.5 or 2 liters of water per day is recommended to prevent constipation and straining at defecation. It is important that the patient understand that the high-fiber diet should be replaced by a low-fiber diet during an acute flare-up.

If the condition worsens, *hemorrhoidectomy* may be necessary. Following this procedure or other types of rectal surgery, the objectives of nutritional care are to reduce the number of bowel movements so that the surgical wound can heal without infection. At the same time, adequate nutrition should be maintained to support wound healing. A chemically defined diet that is low in fiber or fiber-free is useful in the early postoperative period following rectal surgery. The diet is progressed to a minimal fiber diet and then to a normal diet as tolerated. Some physicians recommend a high-fiber diet prior to discharge.

Case Study: Malabsorption

Mr. V.S., a 48-year-old man, presented with complaints of loss of appetite and up to four bowel movements per day with very bulky stools of 2 years' duration. In the last 3 weeks, he had experienced increasing abdominal and ankle edema. He had had a partial gastric resection for a peptic ulcer 4 years before.

Physical examination:

Normal vital signs
Muscle wasting
Upper abdominal scar
Pitting edema of the abdomen, genitalia, and legs
Soft mass to the right of the umbilicus in which peristaltic activity was visible.

Laboratory data:

Hematocrit: 28 percent
Macrocytic, hypochromic anemia
Stool smear: yellow globules of fat 15 to 70 μ in diameter
Serum albumin: 2.8 g/dl
Serum carotene: 85 μg/dl
5-g D-xylose dose: urinary excretion of 0.8 g/5 hr
Serum B_{12}: 65 pg/ml
Serum folate: 24 ng/ml
Schilling test without IF: 3.0 percent excretion per 24 hours
Schilling test following intake of 20 ml neutralized gastric juice: 3.2 percent excretion per 24 hours
72-hour stool collection: 40 g of fat/day on a 100-g fat diet
Duodenal fluid culture: *Escherichia coli*
Jejunal biopsy: fingerlike villi

The patient was treated with antibiotics, a monthly injection of vitamin B_{12}, and iron supplements.

The nutritional care specialist was asked to recommend a diet.

24-hour recall:

Breakfast	½ grapefruit, 1 tsp. sugar
	2 doughnuts
	coffee, cream
Lunch	Clam chowder, large bowl
	Grilled cheese sandwich
	8 oz. whole milk
Snack	Coffee, cream
	Danish roll
Dinner	2 pork chops, 4 oz. each, with fat
	¾ c. escalloped potatoes
	⅓ c. buttered green beans
	Orange and avocado salad
	Apple pie (⅙ pie)
	Tea with lemon and sugar
Snack	Lemonade
	Potato chips, approximately 2 oz.

Three weeks later, the laboratory results are as follows:

Hematocrit	45 percent
D-xylose excretion	1.1 g/5 hr
Fecal fat assay	20 g/day on a 100-g fat diet
Schilling test	16 percent excretion per 24 hours
Serum B_{12}	300 pg/ml
Serum folate	8 ng/ml
Serum albumin	4.5 g/dl

The edema has disappeared, and the patient reports that he feels better but has lost additional weight. His appetite is good.

Exercises

1. For each diagnostic test, state if the result is higher than, lower than, or within normal limits. For values not within normal limits, explain their significance.
2. Why was the patient given vitamin B_{12} and iron medications? Explain the process by which a deficiency of these nutrients could be created in this patient.
3. What diet modification should be recommended on the first visit? Assuming the patient followed this diet, what further modifications would you recommend on the next visit? Put your answer in a SOAP note.

Case Study: Gluten Intolerance

R.M. was admitted to the hospital, complaining of anorexia, weight loss, and abdominal cramps. She reported frequent, foul-smelling, light-colored stools. Physical examination showed a pale, weak, 24-year-old woman, 5 ft 8 in. tall and weighing 110 lb. The patient said she had recently had an intestinal infection.

A biopsy of the small intestine showed flattened villi. Fecal fat was 18 g/day. The D-xylose absorption test revealed 4 g excretion per 5 hours.

24-hour recall:

8 A.M.	4 oz. grapefruit juice
	1 slice white toast with butter
	½ c. bran flakes
	½ c. milk
10 A.M.	Coffee, black
	Sweet roll
12 noon	Chicken noodle soup
	Ham salad sandwich
	Coffee

6 P.M. 4 oz. roast lamb
½ c. buttered green beans
Molded fruit salad
2-in. square devil's food cake
Tea with lemon

Diagnosis: primary gluten intolerance, with fat malabsorption secondary to it. A gluten-free, low-fat diet was prescribed.

Exercises

1. Explain the rationale for the diet.
2. Evaluate the results of the laboratory tests and explain their significance.
3. Modify the patient's diet as given in the 24-hour recall to conform to the diet prescription.
4. If the patient had pancreatic insufficiency, what change would you expect in the results of the D-xylose absorption test?

References

1. Wilson, F.A., Sallee, V.L., and Dietschy, J.M. Unstirred water layers in the intestine: Rate determinant of fatty acid absorption from micellar solutions. *Science* 174:1031, 1971.
2. Wilson, F.A., and Dietschy, J.M. Characterization of bile and absorption across the unstirred water layer and brush border of the rat jejunum. *J. Clin. Invest.* 51:3015, 1972.
3. Bergstrom, B. On the importance of bile salts. *J. Lipid Res.* 16:411, 1975.
4. Adibi, S.A., and Allen, E.R. Impaired jejunal absorption rates of essential amino acids induced by either dietary caloric or protein deprivation in man. *Gastroenterology* 59:404, 1970.
5. Herbert, V., Cooper, B.A., and Castle, W.B. The site of vitamin B_{12}–intrinsic factor complex 'releasing factor' activity in the rat small intestine. *Proc. Soc. Exp. Biol. Med.* 110:315, 1962.
6. Code, C.F., Bass, P., McClary, G.B., Jr., et al. Absorption of water, sodium, and potassium in small intestine of dogs. *Am J. Physiol.* 199:281, 1960.
7. Turnberg, L.A., Bieberdorf, F.A., Morawski, S.G., and Fordtran, J.S. Interrelationships of chloride, bicarbonate, sodium and hydrogen transport in the human ileum. *J. Clin. Invest.* 49:557, 1970.
8. Corcino, J.J., Waxman, S., and Berbert, V. Absorption and malabsorption of vitamin B_{12}. *Am. J. Med.* 48:562, 1970.
9. Roggin, G.M., Iber, F.L., Kater, R.M.H., and Tabon, F. Malabsorption in the chronic alcoholic. *Johns Hopkins Med. J.* 125:321, 1969.
10. Green, P.H.R., and Tall, A.R. Drugs, alcohol and malabsorption. *Am. J. Med.* 67:1066, 1979.
11. Council on Foods and Nutrition. The regulation of dietary fat. *J.A.M.A.* 181:139, 1962.
12. Losowsky, M.S., Walker, B.E., and Kelleher, J. *Malabsorption in Clinical Practice.* Edinburgh: Churchill Livingstone, 1974.
13. *Recipes Using MCT Oil and Portagen.* Evansville, Ind.: Mead Johnson and Co., 1970.
14. Schizas, A.A., Cremen, A.A., Larson, E., and O'Brien, R. Medium-chain triglycerides—use in food preparation. *J. Am. Diet. Assoc.* 51:228, 1967.
15. Kalser, M.H. Medium chain triglycerides. *Adv. Intern. Med.* 17:301, 197.
16. Howard, B.D., and Morse, E.H. Muffins and pastry made with medium-chain triglyceride oil. *J. Am. Diet. Assoc.* 62:51, 1973.
17. Bowman, F. MCT cookies, cakes and quick breads; quality and acceptability. *J. Am. Diet. Assoc.* 62:180, 1973.
18. Greesky, F.L., and Cooke, R.E. The gastrointestinal absorption of unaltered protein in normal infants and in infants recovering from diarrhea. *Pediatrics* 16:763, 1955.
19. Rothberg, R.M. Immunoglobulin and specific antibody synthesis during the first weeks of life of premature infants. *J. Pediatr.* 75:391, 1969.
20. Korenblat, R.E., Rothberg, R.M., Minden, P., and Farr, R.S. Immune response of human adults after oral and parenteral exposure to bovine serum albumin. *J. Allergy* 41:226, 1968.
21. Ament, M.E. Immunodeficiency syndromes and gastrointestinal disease. *Pediatr. Clin. North Am.* 22:807, 1975.
22. Crabbe, P.A., and Heremans, J.F. Selective IgA deficiency with steatorrhea. A new syndrome. *Am. J. Med.* 42:319, 1967.
23. Savilahti, E., Pelkonen, P., and Visakorpi, J.K. A clinical study with special reference to intestinal findings. *Arch. Dis. Child.* 46:665, 1971.
24. Hardy, R.N. The influence of specific chemical factors in the solvent on the absorption of macromolecular substances from the small intestine of the newborn calf. *J. Physiol.* (Lond.) 204:607, 1969.
25. Leece, J.G., Morgan, D.O., and Matrone, G. Effect of feeding colostral and milk components on the cessation of intestinal absorption

of large molecules (closure) in neonatal pigs. *J. Nutr.* 84:43, 1964.

26. Gitlin, D., Kumate, J., Morales, C., et al. The turnover of amniotic fluid protein in the human conceptus. *Am. J. Obstet. Gynecol.* 113:632, 1972.
27. Kerzner, B., McClung, J., Kelly, M., et al. Intestinal secretion in acute viral enteritis. A function of crypt-type enterocytes? *Gastroenterology* 68:909, 1975.
28. Walker, W.A. Antigen absorption from the small intestine and gastrointestinal disease. *Pediatr. Clin. North Am.* 22:731, 1975.
29. Holman, H., Nickel, W.F., Jr., and Sleisenger, M.H. Hypoproteinemia antedating intestinal lesions and possibly due to excessive serum protein loss into intestine. *Am. J. Med.* 27:963, 1959.
30. Waldmann, T.A., Steinfeld, J.L., Dutcher, T.F., et al. Role of gastrointestinal system in 'idiopathic hypoproteinemia.' *Gastroenterology* 41:197, 1961.
31. Jeffries, G.H. Protein metabolism and protein-losing enteropathy. In M.H. Sleisenger and J.S. Fordtran, Eds., *Gastrointestinal Disease: Pathophysiology, Diagnosis, Management,* 2nd ed. Philadelphia: W.B. Saunders, 1978.
32. Reber, H.A. Abdominal abscesses and gastrointestinal fistulas. In M.H. Sleisenger and J.S. Fordtran, Eds., *Gastrointestinal Disease: Pathophysiology, Diagnosis, Management,* 2nd ed. Philadelphia: W.B. Saunders, 1978.
33. Kaminsky, V.M., and Deitel, M. Nutritional support in the management of external fistulas of the alimentary tract. *Br. J. Surg.* 62:100, 1975.
34. Falchuk, Z.M. Update on gluten-sensitive enteropathy. *Am. J. Med.* 67:1085, 1979.
35. Chandra, R.K., and Sahni, S. Immunological aspects of gluten intolerance. *Nutr. Rev.* 39:117, 1981.
36. Paulley, J.W. Observations on the aetiology of idiopathic steatorrhea. *Br. Med. J.* 2:1318, 1954.
37. Baklien, K., Brandtzaeg, P., and Fausa, O. Immunoglobulins in jejunal mucosa and serum from patients with adult coeliac disease. *Scand. J. Gastroenterol.* 12:149, 1977.
38. Taylor, K.B., Thomson, D.L., Truelove, S.C., and Wright, R. An immunological study of coeliac disease and idiopathic steatorrhoea. *Br. Med. J.* 2:1727, 1961.
39. Seah, P.P., Fry, L., Hoffbrand, A.V., and Holborow, E.J. Tissue antibodies in dermatitis herpetiformis and adult coeliac disease. *Lancet* 1:834, 1971.
40. Bullen, A.W., and Losowsky, M.S. Peripheral blood lymphocyte subpopulations in adult coeliac disease (CD). *Gut* 18:A408, 1977.
41. Allardyce, R.A., and Shearman, D.J.C. Leukocyte reactivity to α-gliadin in dermatitis herpetiformis and adult coeliac disease. *Int. Arch. Allergy Appl. Immunol.* 48:395, 1975.
42. Hofmann, A.F., and Poley, J.R. Role of bile acid malabsorption in pathogenesis of diarrhea and steatorrhea in patients with ileal resection: I. Response to cholestyramine or replacement of dietary long chain triglyceride by medium chain triglyceride. *Gastroenterology* 62:918, 1972.
43. Allcock, E. Absorption of vitamin B_{12} in man following extensive resection of the jejunum, ileum and colon. *Gastroenterology* 40:81, 1961.
44. Dobbins, J.W., and Binder, H.J. Derangements of oxalate metabolism in gastrointestinal disease and their mechanism. *Prog. Gastroenterol.* 3:505, 1977.
45. Williamson, R.C.N. Intestinal adaptation. *N. Engl. J. Med.* 298:1393, 1978.
46. Trier, J.S. The Short Bowel Syndrome. In M.H. Sleisenger and J. S. Fordtran, Eds., *Gastrointestinal Disease: Pathophysiology, Diagnosis, Management,* 2nd ed. Philadelphia: W.B. Saunders, 1978.
47. Obertop, H., Nundy, S., Malamud, D., and Malt, R.A. Onset of cell proliferation in the shortened gut. Rapid hyperplasia after jejunal resection. *Gastroenterology* 72:267, 1977.
48. Bochenk, W., Rodgers, J.B., and Alaint, J.A. Effects of changes in dietary lipids on intestinal fluid loss in the short bowel syndrome. *Ann. Intern. Med.* 72:205, 1970.
49. Soong, C.S., Thompson, J.B., Paley, J.R., and Hess, D.R. Hydroxy fatty acid in human diarrhea. *Gastroenterology* 63:748, 1972.
50. Ammon, H.V., and Phillips, S.F. Inhibition of colonic water and electrolyte absorption by fatty acids in man. *Gastroenterology* 65:744, 1973.
51. Mekhjian, H.S., Phillips, S.F., and Hofmann, A.F. Colonic secretion of water and electrolytes induced by bile acids: Perfusion studies in man. *J. Clin. Invest.* 50:1569, 1971.
52. Aber, G.M., Ashton, F., Carmalt, M.H.B., and Whitehead, T.P. Gastric hypersecretion following massive small bowel resection in man. *Am. J. Dig. Dis.* 12:785, 1967.
53. Weser, E. The management of patients after small bowel resection. *Gastroenterology* 71:146, 1976.
54. Committee on Nutrition, American Academy

of Pediatrics. The practical significance of lactose intolerance in children. *Pediatrics* 62:240, 1978.

55. Hadley, R.A. Calcium and hypoallergenic diets. *Ann. Allergy* 30:36, 1972.
56. Birge, S.J., Keutmann, H.T., Cautrecasas, P., and Whedon, G.D. Osteoporosis, intestinal lactase deficiency and low dietary calcium intake. *N. Engl. J. Med.* 276:445, 1967.
57. Bowie, M.D. Effect of lactose-induced diarrhea on absorption of nitrogen and fat. *Arch. Dis. Child.* 50:363, 1975.
58. Calloway, D.H., and Chenoweth, W.L. Utilization of nutrients in milk- and wheat-based diets by men with adequate and reduced abilities to absorb lactose: I. Energy and nitrogen. *Am. J. Clin. Nutr.* 26:939, 1973.
59. Bayless, T.M. Disaccharidase deficiency. *J. Am. Diet. Assoc.* 60:478, 1972.
60. Cornblath, M., and Schwartz, R. *Disorders of Carbohydrate Metabolism in Infancy,* 2nd ed. Vol. 3. *Major Problems in Clinical Pediatrics.* Philadelphia: W.B. Saunders, 1976.
61. vanBuchem, F.S.P., Pol, G., de Gier, J., et al. Congenital β-lipoprotein deficiency. *Am. J. Med.* 40:794, 1966.
62. Tangedahl, T. Dissolution of gallstones—when and how? *Surg. Clin. North Am.* 59:797, 1979.
63. Arvanitakis, C., Cooke, A.R., and Greenberger, N.J. Laboratory aids in the diagnosis of pancreatitis. *Med. Clin. North Am.* 62:107, 1978.
64. Cameron, J.L., Capuzzi, D.M., Zuidema, G.D., and Margolis, S. Acute pancreatitis with hyperlipemia. Evidence for a persistent defect in lipid metabolism. *Am. J. Med.* 56:482, 1974.
65. Greenberger, N.J., and Winship, D.H. *Gastrointestinal Disorders: A Pathophysiologic Approach,* 2nd ed. Chicago: Year Book Medical, 1981.
66. Holt, P. Medium chain triglycerides. *D.M.* June 1971. Pp. 1–30.
67. Schwachman, H. Gastrointestinal manifestations of cystic fibrosis. *Pediatr. Clin. North Am.* 22:787, 1975.
68. Chase, H.P., Long, M.A., and Lavin, M.H. Cystic fibrosis and malnutrition. *J. Pediatr.* 95:337, 1979.
69. Trowell, J. Definition of dietary fiber and hypothesis that it is a protective factor in certain diseases. *Am. J. Clin. Nutr.* 29:417, 1976.
70. Spiller, G.A., Fassett-Cornelius, G., and Briggs, S. A new term for plant fibers in nutrition. *Am. J. Clin. Nutr.* 29:934, 1976.
71. Cummings, J.H. Nutritional implications of dietary fiber. *Am. J. Clin. Nutr.* 31:5, 1978.
72. Mendeloff, A.I. Dietary fiber and human health. *N. Engl. J. Med.* 297:811, 1977.
73. Kirk, E. The quantity and composition of human colonic flatus. *Gastroenterology* 12:782, 1949.
74. Bedell, G.N., Marshall, R., Dubois, A.B., and Harris, J.H. Measurement of the volume of gas in the gastrointestinal tract. *J. Clin. Invest.* 35:336, 1956.
75. Levitt, M.D. Volume and composition of human intestinal gas determined by an intestinal washout technique. *N. Engl. J. Med.* 284:1394, 1971.
76. Maddock, W.G., Bell, J.L., and Tremaine, M.J. Gastrointestinal gas: observations on belching during anesthesia, operations and pyelography; and rapid passage of gas. *Ann. Surg.* 130:512, 1949.
77. Levitt, M.D., and Bond, J.H. Intestinal Gas. In M.H. Sleisenger and J.S. Fordtran, Eds., *Gastrointestinal Disease: Pathophysiology, Diagnosis, Management,* 2nd ed. Philadelphia: W.B. Saunders, 1978.
78. Levitt, M.D. Production and excretion of hydrogen gas in man. *N. Engl. J. Med.* 281:122, 1969.
79. Murphy, E.L., and Calloway, D.H. The effect of antibiotic drugs on the volume and composition of intestinal gas from beans. *Am. J. Dig. Dis.* 17:639, 1972.
80. Lasser, R.B., Bond, J.H., and Levitt, M.D. The role of intestinal gas in functional abdominal pain. *N. Engl. J. Med.* 293:524, 1975.
81. Ritchie, J. Pain from distension of the pelvic colon by inflating a balloon in the irritable colon syndrome. *Gut* 14:125, 1973.
82. Painter, N.S. *Diverticular Disease of the Colon.* London: William Heinemann Medical, 1975.
83. Eastwood, M.A. Medical and dietary management. *Clin. Gastroenterol.* 4(1):85, 1975.
84. Phillips, S.F. Absorption and secretion by the colon. *Gastroenterology* 56:966, 1969.

Bibliography

Dwyer, J.T., Goldin, B., Gorback, S., and Patterson, J. Dietary fiber and fiber supplements in therapy of gastrointestinal disorders. *J. Maine Med. Assoc.* 69:51, 1978.

Norman, A.W. Vitamin D metabolism and calcium absorption. *Am. J. Med.* 67:989, 1979.

Royal College of Physicians of London. *Medical*

Aspects of Dietary Fiber. Tunbridge Wells, U.K.: Pitman Medical, 1980.

di Sant'Agnese, P.A., and Davis, P.B. Research in cystic fibrosis (3 parts). *N. Engl. J. Med.* 295:481, 534, 597, 1976.

Sleisenger, M.H., and Fordtran, J.S., Eds. *Gastrointestinal Disease: Pathophysiology, Diagnosis, Management,* 2nd ed. Philadelphia: W.B. Saunders, 1978.

Sleisenger, M.H., and Glickman, R.M. Symposium on malabsorption. *Am. J. Med.* 67:979, 1979.

Weser, E. Nutritional aspects of malabsorption. Short gut adaptation. *Am. J. Med.* 67:1014, 1979.

Williamson, R.C.N. Intestinal adaptation. *N. Engl. J. Med.* 298:1393, 1978.

Sources of Current Information

Clinics in Gastroenterology
Digestive Diseases and Sciences
Pediatric Gastroenterology and Nutrition
Progress in Gastroenterology
Scandinavian Journal of Gastroenterology

IV. Diseases of the Renal and Cardiovascular Systems

7. The Urinary System

- I. The Normal Kidney
  - A. Renal anatomy
  - B. Renal physiology
    - 1. Urine formation
      - a. glomerular filtration
      - b. tubular reabsorption
      - c. tubular secretion
    - 2. Maintenance of homeostasis
      - a. regulation of osmolality and fluid volume
      - b. regulation of sodium balance
      - c. regulation of potassium balance
      - d. regulation of hydrogen ion concentration
      - e. regulation of calcium and phosphate balances
    - 3. Excretion of metabolic wastes
    - 4. Endocrine functions
- II. Renal Disease
  - A. Diagnostic tests
    - 1. Urinalysis
    - 2. Blood analyses
    - 3. Renal function tests
    - 4. Direct examination of kidney tissue
  - B. Renal failure
    - 1. Chronic renal failure
      - a. etiology
      - b. pathophysiology
      - c. natural history
      - d. manifestations
      - e. metabolic alterations and nutritional care in conservative management
        - (1) alterations in protein and nitrogen excretion
        - (2) energy needs
        - (3) abnormalities of sodium balance
        - (4) abnormalities of fluid balance
        - (5) abnormalities of potassium balance
        - (6) acidosis
        - (7) effects on other minerals
        - (8) vitamin needs
        - (9) calcium and phosphorus
        - (10) carbohydrate
        - (11) protein and amino acid metabolism
        - (12) lipids
        - (13) additional problems
      - f. the dialysis patient
        - (1) hemodialysis
        - (2) peritoneal dialysis
      - g. renal transplantation
        - (1) procedure
        - (2) nutritional management
    - 2. Acute renal failure
      - a. etiology
      - b. pathogenesis
      - c. pathology
      - d. pathophysiology
      - e. clinical course and prognosis
      - f. nutritional management
        - (1) sodium and fluid
        - (2) energy
        - (3) protein
        - (4) potassium
        - (5) other electrolytes
  - C. Glomerulopathy
    - 1. Etiology and pathogenesis
    - 2. Pathology
    - 3. Acute glomerulonephritis
      - a. clinical manifestations
      - b. treatment
      - c. clinical course
    - 4. Chronic glomerulonephritis
    - 5. Nephrotic syndrome
      - a. definition and etiology
      - b. clinical manifestations
        - (1) proteinuria
        - (2) hypoproteinemia
        - (3) edema
        - (4) hyperlipidemia
        - (5) lipiduria
        - (6) other
      - c. treatment
        - (1) diuretic drugs
        - (2) diet
  - D. Diabetic renal disease
  - E. Renal calculi
    - 1. Etiology
    - 2. Clinical manifestations
    - 3. Treatment
      - a. calcium oxalate calculi
      - b. calcium phosphate calculi
      - c. struvite calculi
      - d. uric acid calculi
      - e. cystine calculi
- III. Case Study

THE NORMAL KIDNEY

Renal Anatomy

The components of the urinary system are the *kidney, ureters, bladder,* and *urethra.* Each kidney is enclosed by a fibrous nonelastic *capsule* beneath which the renal *cortex* forms a layer 4 to 6 mm thick in an adult. The cortex is made up of *renal corpuscles, proximal and distal convoluted tubules,* and the *upper portions of the loops of Henle* and *collecting ducts.* The *medulla* lies beneath the cortex and is composed of several *pyramids* containing the remaining portions of the loops of Henle and the collecting ducts. Basement membrane surrounds the tubules and is supported by very delicate reticular fibers. There is very little connective tissue in the kidney.

The functional unit of the kidney is the *nephron* (Fig. 7-1). It has been estimated that each kidney contains 1 to 1.5 million nephrons, each of which includes a tuft of approximately fifty capillaries called the *glomerulus.* The glomerulus invaginates a *Bowman's capsule,* a blind-ended epithelial sac which, with the glomerulus, forms the *renal corpuscle.* Bowman's capsule is continuous with a tubular system, the parts of which

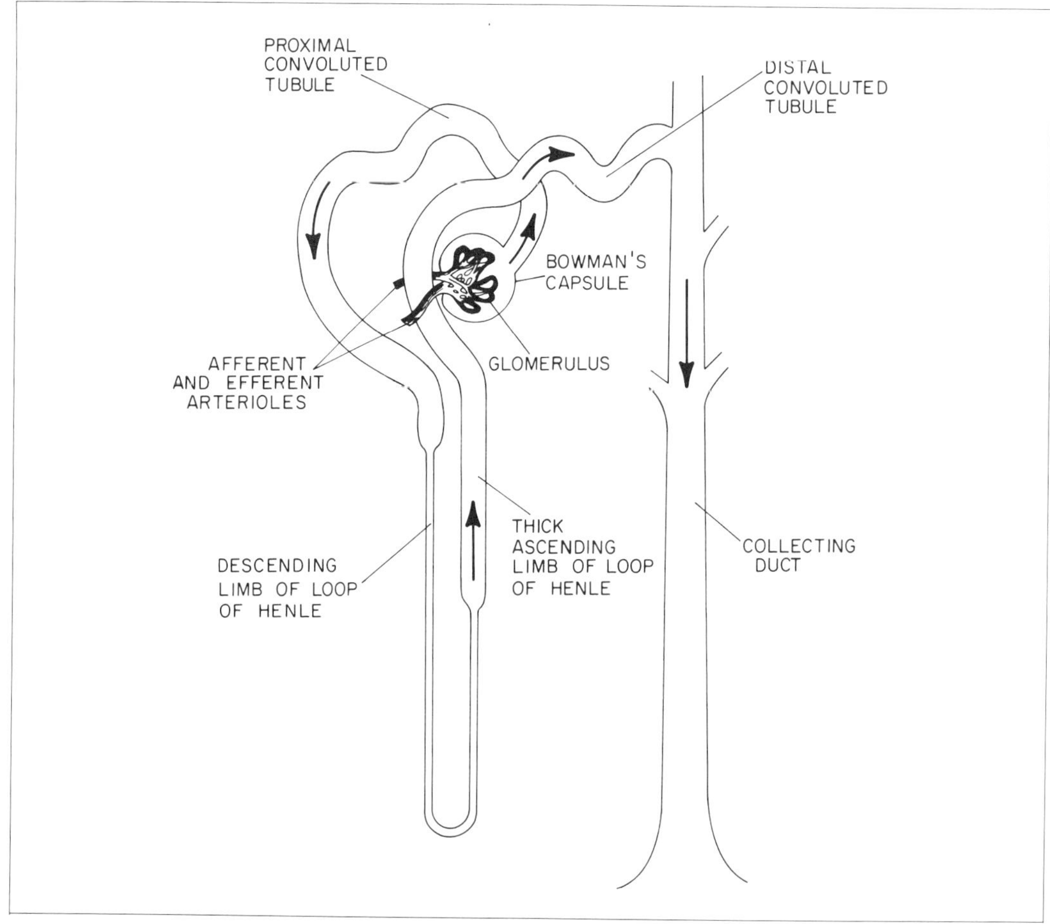

Figure 7-1. Relationships of component parts of the nephron. (Adapted from Vander, A.J., Sherman, J.H., and Luciano, D.S., Human Physiology: The Mechanisms of Body Function, *3rd ed. Copyright © 1980. Used with permission of McGraw-Hill Book Company, New York.)*

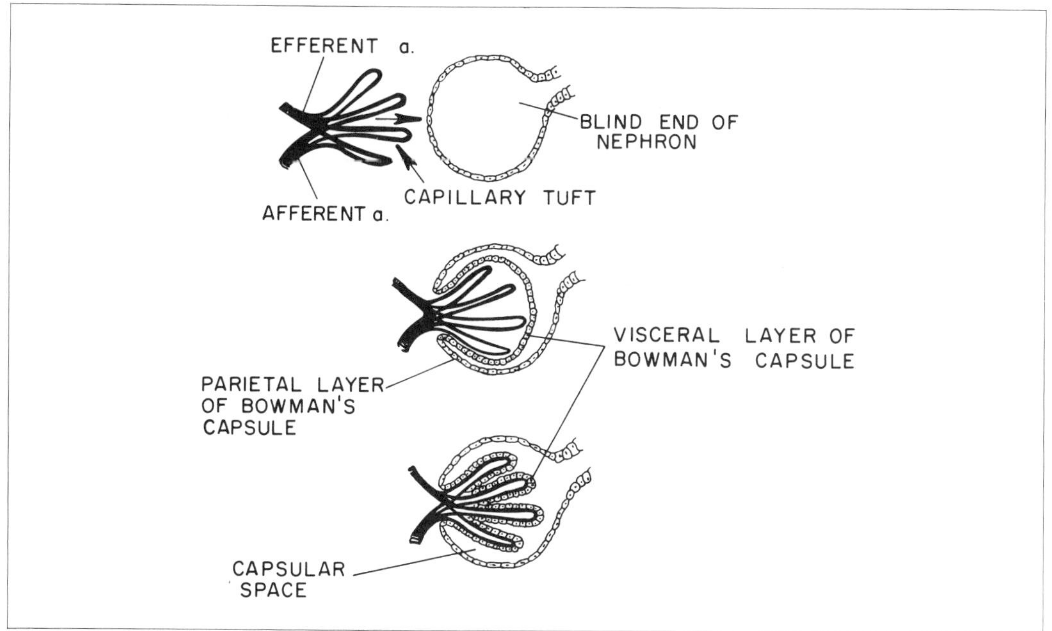

Figure 7-2. How the capillary loops between afferent and efferent vessels are invaginated into the blind end of the excretory tubule. The visceral layer of Bowman's capsule at first covers the group of capillary loops as a whole; later it covers each loop (lower picture), and finally it almost completely surrounds the outgoing and the incoming arms of each loop (not shown here). **a.** *= arteriole. (Reprinted with permission from Ham, A.W.,* Histology, *5th ed. Philadelphia: J.B. Lippincott, 1969, p. 773.)*

are, successively, the proximal convoluted tubule, the *loop of Henle,* the distal convoluted tubule, and the collecting duct. Urine flows through the collecting ducts to an opening in the *papilla* (the apex of the pyramid) and enters the *pelvis* of the kidney, which forms the funnel-shaped proximal end of the ureter through which the urine passes into the bladder.

A more detailed knowledge of the structure of the renal capsule is important to the understanding of some renal diseases. Bowman's capsule consists of an outer, *parietal layer,* which is continuous with the tubules. The parietal layer then is reflected back to form the *visceral layer,* which covers the capillaries. The area between the parietal and visceral layers is the *capsular space* (Fig. 7-2). The visceral layer is composed of *podocytes,* which have projections called *foot processes.* These are in contact with the basement membrane of the capillary endothelial cells. Mesangial cells, which are part of the reticuloendothelial system, are located between the capillaries. Together, they are enveloped by a basement membrane.

Another important feature of the nephron structure is the *juxtaglomerular apparatus.* It contains the *macula densa,* which is composed of specialized epithelial cells located in that part of the distal tubule nearest the afferent and efferent arterioles of Bowman's capsule, and specialized *granular* cells in the afferent arteriole. The juxtaglomerular apparatus functions in renin production for the control of blood pressure.

Renal Physiology

Those physiologic processes that are of major importance in a consideration of the renal diseases described in this chapter will be reviewed briefly. The references listed at the end of the chapter are sources of further details.

Urine Formation

Urine formation consists of three basic processes, *glomerular filtration, tubular secretion,* and *reabsorption.* It is by these processes that the kidney regulates the composition of the body fluids and removes metabolic wastes.

As blood flows through the glomerulus, water, smaller molecules, and a small amount of protein are filtered into the capsular space. Blood cells and large protein molecules, collectively called *colloids,* remain in the capillaries. An adult produces approximately 180 liters/day of glomerular filtrate from the 900 liters/day of blood that pass through the kidney. *Glomerular filtration rate* (GFR) is an important indicator of renal function. The normal rate is approximately 180 liters/(24 hours × 60 minutes), or 125 ml/min. The glomerular filtrate has the composition of blood plasma without blood cells and plasma proteins. Tubular secretion and reabsorption change the composition to maintain body homeostasis and form the final urine.

As the glomerular filtrate moves through the tubules, many components needed to maintain homeostasis are reabsorbed. These normally include approximately 99 percent of the water, all of the glucose, 99.5 percent of the sodium, 50 percent of the urea, and almost all of the calcium and amino acids. Potassium, phosphate, and lipid-soluble drugs also are reabsorbed. If all the water, glucose, electrolytes, and other materials filtered were excreted in the urine, the body would become depleted very quickly.

Homeostatic control of osmolality occurs in the distal convoluted tubules and collecting ducts. The movements of sodium and water may vary with the cell permeability, which is controlled by antidiuretic hormone (ADH). Changes in plasma osmolality are sensed by receptors in the posterior pituitary gland and hypothalamus, which alter the rate of secretion of ADH by the pituitary gland. An excess of body water causes a decrease in osmolality and inhibits ADH release. Then, permeability of the distal tubule cells is low and water is not reabsorbed, increasing both urine volume and plasma osmolality. When body water is decreased, osmolality increases and ADH secretion rises. In the presence of increased ADH, permeability is high and water is reabsorbed, reducing both urine volume and plasma osmolality. Sodium transport is not affected by ADH. These processes, therefore, can result in production of a hypoosmotic or isosmotic urine. Osmolarity of the urine may be as low as 50 mOsm/L.

By contrast, in order to produce a hyperosmolar urine, a *countercurrent system* in the loop of Henle is used. It creates an osmotic gradient from the cortex through the medulla to the papilla. The gradient is maintained by the parallel blood vessel structure known as the *vasa recta.* Water and solutes are reabsorbed from the tubules into the interstitium, then into the vasa recta, and carried into the general circulation. As the fluid flows through the collecting ducts, an osmotic gradient exists between it and the interstitial fluid. If the cells of the collecting ducts are permeable to water as a result of ADH action, water diffuses out of the ducts to equilibrate with the interstitial fluid. The net result is a hyperosmotic urine which may reach an osmolarity of 1,400 mOsm/L.

The body must excrete an approximate total of at least 600 mOsm of urea, sulfate, phosphate, and other waste products each day. This material, called the *solute load,* increases with increased intake of protein and electrolytes. In order to eliminate a solute load of 600 mOsm, a minimum of 600/1,400, or 0.444 liter/day of water will be used. This will be excreted as long as the kidneys function. More water is used to excrete an increased solute load. The amount of water needed to excrete the solute is the *obligatory water loss.* On the average, of the total 170 to 180 liters of glomerular filtrate,

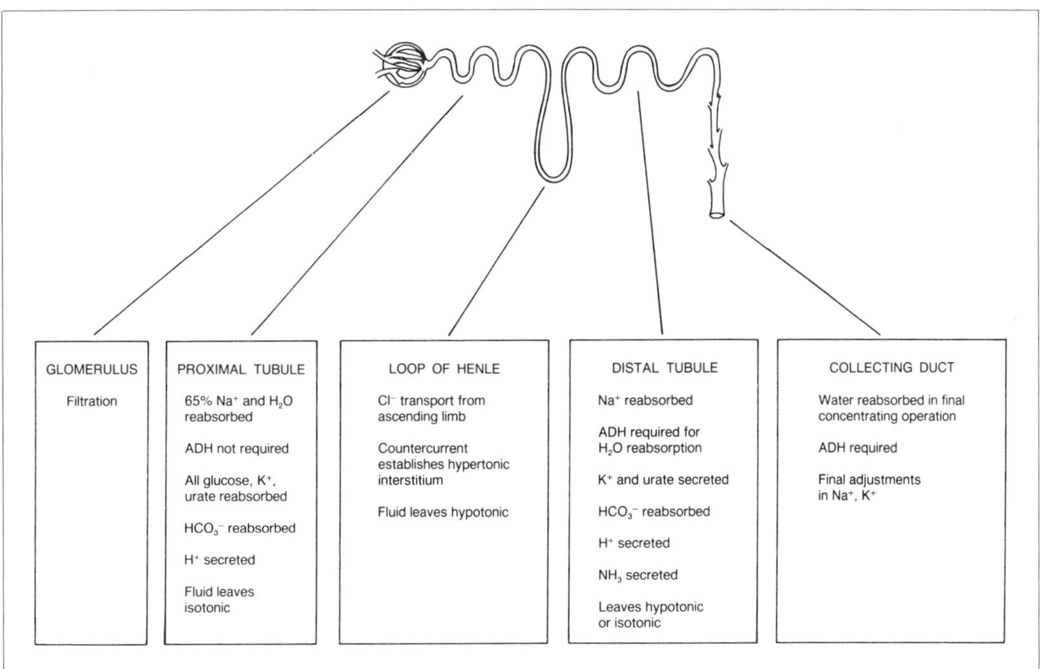

Figure 7-3. Major functions of each portion of the nephron. ADH = antidiuretic hormone. (Reprinted with permission from Papper, S., Clinical Nephrology, *2nd ed. Boston: Little, Brown, 1978, p. 52.)*

all but approximately 1.5 liters usually is absorbed.

At the same time as tubular reabsorption is occurring, some substances are secreted into the filtrate by cells of the tubular epithelium. Hydrogen ions, potassium, ammonia, and various organic acids and bases are secreted by the tubules. This process also is necessary to maintain homeostasis. It is important, for example, in acid-base balance.

Some substances secreted by the tubules are subsequently reabsorbed. Therefore, it is important to distinguish between *secretion* and *excretion.* Excretion occurs only for those materials that are contained in the final urine.

Maintenance of Homeostasis

In Fig. 7-3, the parts of the nephron are shown in an "extended" position, so that the functions of the various parts can be labeled. This figure gives an overview of the information included in this section.

Regulation of Osmolality and Fluid Volume. Water, sodium, and chloride are filtered freely from the glomerulus and then are largely reabsorbed in the tubules. Approximately 65 percent of the sodium and water in the glomerular filtrate is absorbed from the proximal convoluted tubules (see Fig. 7-3). Sodium is actively transported using a large portion of the great energy expenditure of the kidney. As sodium is reabsorbed from the tubules, the intercellular fluid becomes hyperosmotic. Water then is reabsorbed from the tubules as a consequence of the osmotic gradient produced. An increase in hydrostatic pressure resulting from the greater fluid volume forces movement of the fluid across the basement membrane and into the capillary.

The loops of Henle absorb approximately 25 percent of the sodium and 15 percent of the water of the glomerular filtrate, making the filtrate hypoosmotic to plasma. In the ascending loop, chloride is actively reabsorbed and sodium follows passively.

Regulation of Sodium Balance. The excretion of sodium is controlled separately from the regulation of osmolality. Normal plasma sodium concentration is 136 to 146 mEq/L; therefore, 140 mEq × 180 L/day or approximately 25,200 mEq of sodium are filtered each day. (See Appendix C for milliequivalent to milligram conversions.) Since daily sodium intake is only a small fraction of this amount, most of the filtered sodium must be reabsorbed, but an amount of sodium equal to intake must be excreted daily so that sodium does not accumulate.

The control of sodium is still being studied. Some factors that are important in control include variations in glomerular filtration rate and in tubular reabsorption. Most sodium is reabsorbed in the proximal tubules (see Fig. 7-3). An important additional factor in control of sodium reabsorption is *aldosterone,* produced by the *zona glomerulosa* of the adrenal cortex. Aldosterone stimulates the reabsorption of sodium in the distal convoluted tubules and collecting ducts, providing the "fine adjustments." It has been suggested that another hormone also controls sodium reabsorption, but the existence of this natriuretic hormone has not been proved.

Regulation of Potassium Balance. As with sodium, potassium balance is maintained by excretion of the amount ingested daily. Most of this excretion is urinary. Potassium is freely filtered at the glomerulus and is reabsorbed by the tubules. It is actively transported in the proximal convoluted tubules and loops of Henle. When the filtrate enters the distal convoluted tubules, it contains only 10 percent or less of the original filtered potassium. The distal convoluted tubules and collecting ducts may either reabsorb or secrete potassium. In the distal tubules, in the presence of adequate aldosterone and sodium, potassium is exchanged for sodium. There is a large reserve capacity for potassium excretion; therefore, potassium toxicity is difficult to produce if renal function is normal.

Regulation of Hydrogen Ion Concentration. The kidneys play an essential role in the maintenance of hydrogen ion homeostasis by means of their effects on secretion and excretion or on reabsorption of hydrogen, bicarbonate, ammonium, and phosphate ions. The kidney has a large reserve capacity for excreting acid.

In a normal person eating approximately 70 g of protein per day, the kidneys excrete approximately 40 to 60 mEq of hydrogen ion, most of which is produced by the oxidation of sulfur-containing amino acids and phosphorus to sulfuric and phosphoric acids. Approximately half of this hydrogen load appears in the urine in the form of ammonium ion created from glutamine. The remainder is buffered by phosphate. The kidney also replenishes the bicarbonate supply. These processes are summarized in Fig. 7-4.

Regulation of Calcium and Phosphate Balances. The regulation of calcium and phosphate balances involves interrelationships between the kidney, the gastrointestinal tract, the skeletal system, and parathyroid hormone (PTH).

Calcium is important in blood clotting, nervous system irritability, and muscle contractility. Phosphate is important in the formation of ATP. Thus, these substances have separate functions in general cellular metabolism. In bone, they unite to form crystals and provide rigidity if present in appropriate proportions. Thus, it is important that appropriate concentrations of each be maintained.

Parathyroid hormone is important in maintaining calcium and phosphorus homeostasis by increasing their absorption from the gut and reabsorption from the bone. In the kidney, approximately 50 percent of plasma calcium is protein-bound. The remainder is filtered and approximately

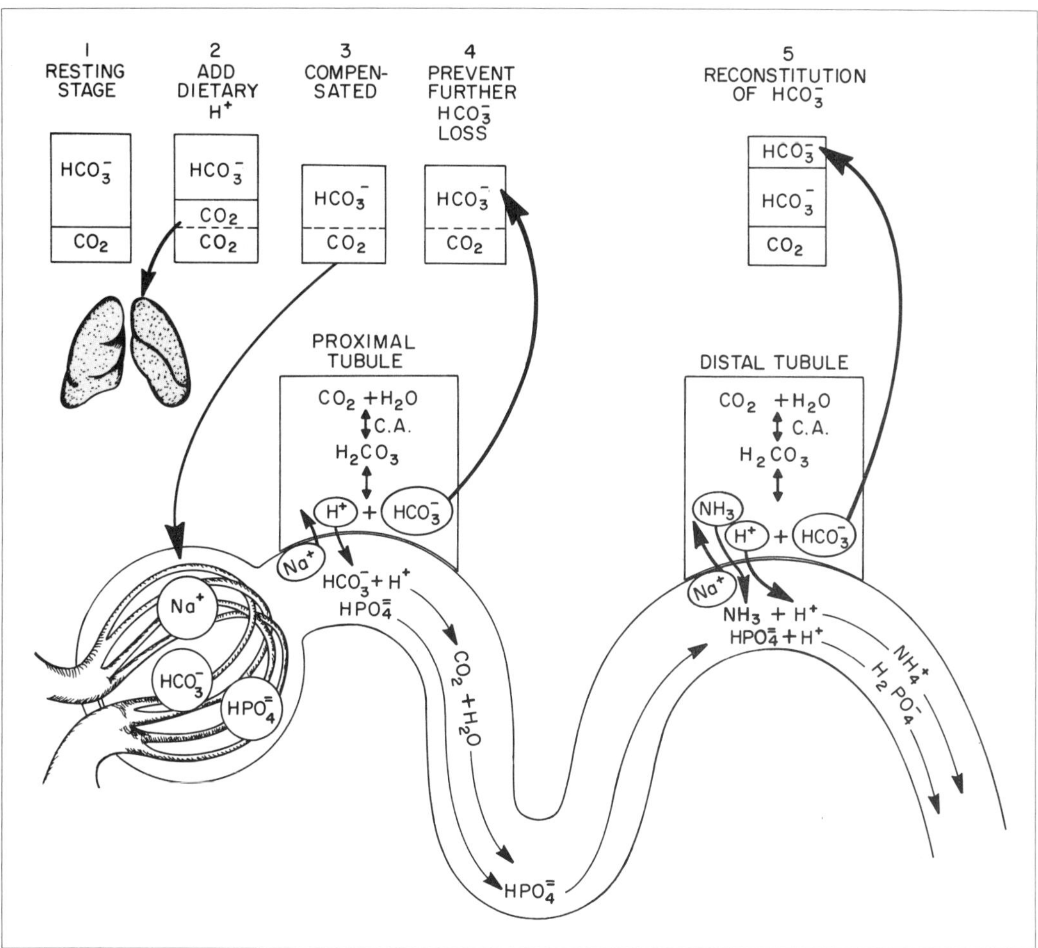

Figure 7-4. Renal handling of the daily dietary acid (hydrogen ion) load. (Modified with permission from Bricker, N.S., and Klahr, S., Treatment of disorders of acid-base metabolism. Mod. Treatment *5:637, July 1968.)* **C.A.** = *carbonic anhydrase.*

99 percent of this then is actively reabsorbed. When increased intake causes increased plasma calcium levels, more calcium is filtered and PTH secretion decreases. As a result, tubular reabsorption of calcium falls and the excess calcium is excreted. The PTH produced also reduces renal tubular reabsorption of phosphate, lowering its plasma concentration.

The final hydroxylation of vitamin D to the active hormone occurs in the kidneys (Fig. 7-5) and affects those processes of calcium metabolism in which vitamin D participates. These are calcium absorption from the gastrointestinal lumen and bone resorption. These actions of the kidney are of great importance in the maintenance of the skeletal system.

Excretion of Metabolic Wastes

In addition to excretion of excess water and electrolytes, the kidney also must excrete the waste products of metabolism. The elimination of the products of nitrogen metabolism are very important. Creatinine, urea, and uric acid are prominent among these, but there are many others, not all of which have been identified. The kidney is also important in the elimination of drugs and toxins.

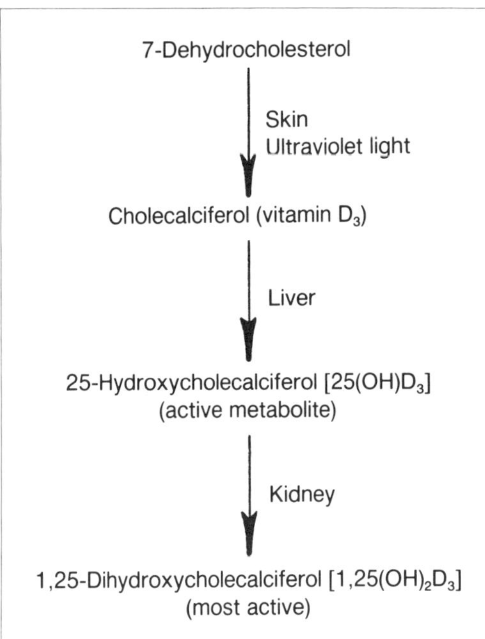

Figure 7-5. The role of the kidney in the metabolism of vitamin D. (Reprinted with permission from Papper, S., Clinical Nephrology, *2nd ed. Boston: Little, Brown, 1978, p. 87.)*

Endocrine Functions

The kidney has several endocrine functions which have a broad impact on body physiology. The activation of vitamin D and its relationship to the skeletal system have already been described. In addition, the kidney synthesizes *renin,* which functions in the renin-angiotensin system for control of blood pressure. It elaborates *prostaglandins* and *kallikreins,* which also affect blood pressure (see Chapter 8). An additional important renal function includes the maintenance of normal red cell production by stimulation via *erythropoietin.* The kidney also influences the action of other hormones, since it degrades and eliminates circulating hormones including insulin, glucagon, and PTH.

RENAL DISEASE

In the past 20 years, much progress has been made in the treatment of renal disease. Complex and expensive methods, such as dialysis and organ transplants, have extended the life of the patient whose kidneys fail; however, none of these methods is entirely satisfactory.

Most of the renal diseases in which nutritional care is important are those that are progressive and for which there is no available cure. Overall management of the disease is designed to prolong the patient's life and improve the quality of that life. The nutritional care specialist cooperates with other members of the health care team to achieve these objectives.

To a great extent, the purpose of nutritional management is to compensate for the loss of the function of the kidney in maintaining the constancy of the internal environment. Since food and fluid intakes normally make a large contribution to this variability, a major part of nutritional management is reducing the intake of substances that the kidney must excrete and providing replacements for those materials lost in abnormal quantities. While these modifications to the diet are being made, the patient must be provided with nutrients to maintain optimum nutritional status in the form of a diet that encourages acceptance by the patient. This represents a challenge to the skill of the nutritional care specialist, since the patient often suffers from anorexia, nausea, and vomiting. In summary, the overall objectives of nutritional care in most renal disease patients are: (1) to maintain optimum nutrition, (2) to minimize metabolic disorders and related symptoms, and (3) to relieve nausea and vomiting.

Diagnostic Tests

In order to understand the patient's needs and the rationale for the diet, the nutritional care specialist must be able to interpret the results of the relevant laboratory tests. This section describes a variety of tests used in the diagnosis of the disease and in the evaluation of its progress.

Urinalysis

The urine may be examined for the presence of materials not normally seen in the urine or for abnormal quantities of substances normally found in the urine. Substances that, when present in the urine, may indicate kidney or urinary tract disease include erythrocytes, leukocytes, microorganisms, and protein. Measurements of the pH and specific gravity of the urine are sometimes of diagnostic value as well, since they indicate the capacity of the kidney to maintain acid-base balance and a normal osmolality of body fluids.

Table 7-1. Tests of Renal Function

Function	Clinical Tests
Glomerular filtration rate	Blood urea nitrogen; creatinine clearance
Renal plasma flow	Phenolsulfonphthalein excretion; renal scan with isotopes
Transport in proximal tubules	Urinary excretion of amino acids, glucose, phosphate
Transport in Henle's loops and distal tubules	Maximum and minimum urine specific gravity and osmolality
Concentrating and diluting ability	Maximum and minimum urine specific gravity and osmolality

Blood Analyses

If the kidney is not functioning normally, substances usually excreted by the kidneys accumulate in the blood; however, it should be appreciated that the kidney has a large reserve capacity. Up to 50 percent of renal function may be lost without a change in concentration of many of the substances measured in clinical diagnosis. Nevertheless, blood analyses are simple and inexpensive and often are useful in evaluating the course of the disease.

Serum Creatinine. Phosphocreatine in muscles is formed from glycine, arginine, and methionine. Creatinine is a degradation product of phosphocreatine. It is produced in an amount proportionate to muscle mass and is excreted in the urine. Normal concentration in the serum is usually 0.6 to 1.5 mg/dl. If the kidney is unable to excrete nitrogenous waste products, the concentration of creatinine will increase in the blood.

Serum Urea Nitrogen (SUN) or Blood Urea Nitrogen (BUN). The deamination of amino acids results in the production of ammonia, a highly toxic substance. In the human liver, ammonia is converted to urea via the urea cycle and then is excreted in the urine. If the kidney is unable to excrete nitrogenous wastes, urea, too, will rise in concentration in the blood. The ranges of normal urea nitrogen concentrations are 5 to 20 mg/dl of blood and 6 to 20 mg/dl of serum.

Serum Uric Acid. Uric acid is a product of purine metabolism and normally appears in the serum in a concentration of 3 to 7 mg/dl in men or 2 to 6 mg/dl in women. Like urea and creatinine, it increases in concentration as renal function diminishes.

Renal Function Tests

Renal function tests evaluate specific aspects of the actions of the nephron, glomerular filtration, tubular function, or renal plasma flow. Several commonly used indicators of various aspects of renal function are listed in Table 7-1. The *creatinine clearance test* is used very frequently in clinical situations. It measures the amount of blood that can be cleared of creatinine per minute. Normal values are 110 to 150 ml/min. for men and 105 to 132 ml/min. for women when corrected to 1.73 m^2 of body surface area.

Direct Examination of Kidney Tissue

A number of means are available for direct examination of the kidney, including the following:

Plain radiography: A roentgenogram will show shadows indicating the size and location of the kidney. Calcified areas and renal calculi will be seen.

Sonography: Ultrasound can be used to show kidney size and the presence of cysts or masses in the kidney.

Intravenous pyelogram (*IVP*): A substance that is opaque to x-ray is injected into the vein and roentgenograms are taken at intervals as the dye is filtered by the kidney.

Isotopic renogram: A radioactive isotope–labeled material is injected into a vein, and its concentration and excretion is followed.

Renal arteriography: A radiopaque substance injected into the renal artery outlines the vascular system on the x-ray plate and detects abnormalities in renal blood flow.

Renal biopsy: A small core of renal tissue is obtained using a special needle. The tissue then is examined under a microscope.

Computerized axial tomography (*CAT*): This is a new noninvasive procedure used to visualize internal organs and structures, such as tumors.

Table 7-2. Causes of Chronic Renal Failure

Diseases in which kidney involvement is predominant
Glomerulonephritis
Interstitial nephritis
Renal calculi
Congenital nephritis
Polycystic disease
Renal hypoplasia
Renal tubular acidosis
Urinary tract obstructions that may *lead to renal failure*
Prostatic enlargement
Urethral stricture
Bladder neck obstruction
Neurogenic bladder
Malignancy
Conditions that often *cause renal failure*
Malignant hypertension
Periarteritis nodosa
Lupus erythematosus
Analgesic drug abuse
Potassium deficiency
Hypercalcemia
Cystinosis
Primary oxaluria
Lead or cadmium poisoning
Systemic diseases in which renal failure sometimes *occurs*
Benign essential hypertension
Atherosclerosis
Embolism
Gout
Diabetes
Heart failure

Renal Failure

Renal failure exists when the kidney is no longer able to maintain the constancy of the internal environment. Chronic renal failure will be discussed first, since nutritional management is of paramount importance in this condition. An abbreviated description of acute renal failure, particularly as it differs from chronic failure, will follow.

Chronic Renal Failure

Chronic renal failure (CRF) is the irreversible loss of the excretory capacity of the kidney which occurs over an extended period of time, from months to years. Endocrine and metabolic functions also are lost.

Etiology. A variety of renal and systemic diseases, some of which are listed in Table 7-2, can result in chronic renal failure. However, the cause of CRF in some patients is unknown.

Pathophysiology. The loss of nephron function has been shown by Bricker[1-3] to occur in an orderly fashion. Bricker's *intact nephron hypothesis* proposes that most of the nephrons of the diseased kidney in CRF fall into one of two categories.[1-3] They are either nonfunctioning nephrons, as a result of destruction of any portion of their structure, or nephrons that function normally. The changes in renal function occur as the result of a reduction in the number of functioning nephrons.

The kidneys continue to respond to the needs of the body insofar as they are able to do so. However, as the number of functioning nephrons diminishes, there are functional adaptations that occur in a regular sequence. The nature of the adaptive mechanisms varies with the solute that is controlled. The control systems functioning in these adaptations are still being investigated but are believed to be those that function in the normal kidney, not new systems produced as a result of the disease process.

Another important consideration is whether the adaptive mechanisms are always of positive value, or whether there sometimes are detrimental consequences. Bricker's *trade-off hypothesis*[4] suggests that some adaptations are detrimental but that they are the price to be paid to correct conditions that are more life-threatening. The body "trades off" one condition for a less serious one. Some examples will be cited in the discussion of individual solutes beginning on page 232.

Natural History of the Disease. The progression of CRF has been described as occurring in four stages which are not sharply separated but, rather, are phases in a continuing degenerative process with loss of more and more functioning nephrons. The four phases are (1) decreased renal reserve, (2) renal insufficiency, (3) renal failure, and (4) uremia or uremic syndrome.

Normally, the kidneys have a large reserve capacity. At least 55 percent of normal renal function must be lost before blood urea increases, although there may be some nephron hypertrophy during this first phase of *decreased renal reserve.* The GFR is greater than 55 ml/min., but less than the normal 125 ml/min. At this stage, the patient does not have any symptoms.

In *renal insufficiency,* up to 80 percent of nephron function may be lost, and the GFR is 30 to 55 ml/min. There is a mild *azotemia* (excessive amounts of nitrogen components in the blood). Serum urea and creatinine are thus above normal. The patient becomes more susceptible to the effects of stress, including large changes in intake of fluids, protein, and electrolytes. There is some loss of concentrating ability, producing *nocturia* (excessive urination at night). The patient may remain symptom-free if no overwhelming metabolic stress occurs. Symptoms occur if the patient is subjected to a stress such as infection.

In *renal failure,* loss of nephron function may reach 90 percent. The GFR is 12.5 to 30.0 ml/min. The patient shows moderate to severe azotemia and anemia, decreased concentrating ability, and impaired ability to maintain electrolyte and acid-base balance.

Loss of function in the final phase, uremia or uremic syndrome, is 90 to 100 percent. The GFR is less than 12.5 ml/min. The patient is *oliguric* (produces insufficient urine) or *anuric* (produces no urine), with uremic symptoms involving many organ systems.

Therefore, it is the patient with 20 percent or less of normal renal function who has lost the ability to adjust to the wide variations in fluid and nutrient intake that commonly occur in a healthy person.

Manifestations of Chronic Renal Failure. The onset of renal insufficiency and renal failure tends to be gradual and insidious. The patient may first present with *polyuria* (increased urine flow) and nocturia with a vague feeling of malaise. Nausea, vomiting, anorexia, and fatigue, possibly related to anemia and retention of organic acids, with some degree of breathlessness may follow. As the kidney function diminishes, many other organ systems become more clearly involved. These are summarized in Table 7-3, which illustrates the extent of the illness.

The development of methods of dialysis and of renal transplantation have revolutionized the treatment of CRF. However, these procedures often follow a long period of slow deterioration of kidney function. During the deterioration period, management is aimed at maintaining homeostasis with maximum possible function of the remaining nephrons. In these patients, it is particularly important that food and fluid

Table 7-3. Clinical Effects of Uremia

Central nervous system
Lethargy, poor concentration, weakness, coma, convulsions
Abnormal behavior, psychoses
Muscle weakness, atrophy
Neuropathy
Hematopoietic system
Bleeding tendencies, clotting defects, platelet abnormalities, anemia
Skin
Pruritus, urea frost, ecchymoses, purpura, easy bruising
Rashes
Cardiovascular system
Pericarditis, myocarditis, arrhythmias
Respiratory system
Uremic pneumonitis, pleurisy, hemoptysis
Gastrointestinal tract
Uremic fetor, dry mouth, hiccups, nausea, vomiting, stomatitis, gastritis, colitis, poor absorption, bleeding
Skeletal system
Poor bone growth or healing, osteomalacia, or rickets
Others
Decreased resistance to infection, impaired wound healing, carbohydrate intolerance, hypothermia

Reprinted with permission from Brackett, N.C., and Setter, J.G., Management of chronic renal insufficiency. *G.P.* 39:111, 1969.

intake be correlated with the functional capacity of the kidney. With appropriate treatment, many patients remain almost symptom free until the GFR decreases to approximately 10 ml/min. When the GFR falls below this level, it becomes very difficult to prevent the onset of severe complications of uremia and to maintain adequate nutrition. At this point, known as *end-stage renal disease,* dialysis or transplantation is necessary to prolong life.

Metabolic Alterations and Nutritional Care in Conservative Management. Chronic renal failure is a progressive, terminal disease which, if untreated, continues an inexorable course to the death of the patient. Conservative management was at one time the only treatment available. Some relief of symptoms and some prolongation of life was achieved with no change in the inevitable outcome.

With the advent of dialysis and renal transplantation, the role of *conservative management* with diet modification and medication has changed so that it now is used (1) for relief of symptoms and to improve the quality of life while delaying the necessity for dialysis; (2) to avoid irreversible physiologic changes and maintain the patient in the best possible condition prior to dialysis or transplant; and (3) to relieve symptoms and improve the quality of life for those patients for whom neither dialysis nor transplant is indicated. In order to understand the basis for the diet modifications, it is necessary to have a grasp of the metabolic alterations that occur.

Alterations in protein and nitrogen excretion. The diseased glomerulus may be unable to retain serum proteins, which are then lost in the urine (*proteinuria*). The protein lost is primarily albumin, and so the condition frequently is called *albuminuria.* Low serum protein levels occur (*hypoproteinemia* or *hypoalbuminemia*); and edema develops as serum protein falls. The triad of proteinuria, hypoproteinemia, and edema constitute the *nephrotic syndrome.* This syndrome occurs in relation to a number of renal diseases and is discussed in greater detail in the section on glomerulopathy (see pp. 255–261).

As the number of functioning nephrons declines, hypertrophy of the nephrons and osmotic diuresis, considered to be adaptive mechanisms, supervene. Adequate nitrogen excretion and normal serum levels of nitrogen metabolites thus are maintained. Eventually, as more nephrons are lost, those remaining can no longer carry the whole load. Blood levels of products of nitrogen metabolism (such as creatinine and urea) rise, producing nitrogen retention or azotemia. It now becomes important to reduce the demands on the remaining nephrons by reducing the amount of material that must be excreted.

The patient seems to feel well despite high levels of nitrogen metabolites until the GFR has decreased to about 15 to 20 ml/min.

At the same time, serum creatinine often has risen approximately 10 mg/dl, and serum urea, above 100 mg/dl. The patient then begins to show signs and symptoms of uremia. Although the severity of many symptoms of uremia seems to correlate well with blood urea levels, there is no evidence that either urea or creatinine is particularly toxic. Therefore, SUN and serum creatinine are used only as yardsticks to measure the severity of the disease and the effects of treatment.

The search for *the* uremic toxin has been long and futile. Many substances that accumulate in the blood of the uremic patient have been identified. These include phosphate, potassium, amino acids and other organic acids, amines, guanidines, indoles, phenols, nucleic acid metabolites, and the "middle molecules." Middle molecules have molecular weights of 400 to 5,000 and include some enzymes, such as transketolase, hormones, such as PTH, and some vitamins.[5,6] There is evidence that an increase in PTH levels in the serum is an important cause of a variety of hematologic, neurologic, and metabolic alterations in uremia.[7] None of these retained materials singly reproduces the clinical picture of uremia. It seems more likely that the complex of symptoms is produced by the accumulated disturbances resulting from renal failure and the interactions of these disturbances with one another.

In determining the protein content of the diet, a balance must be sought to reduce the accumulation of nitrogenous end products while maintaining a positive nitrogen balance. Provision of essential amino acids is required. Histidine is an essential amino acid for renal failure patients as well as for infants and must be supplied in the diet.[8]

Some degree of protein restriction is necessary in CRF. The minimal dietary protein requirement in uremia is not known, nor is there agreement on the time when protein restriction should begin. If the patient has a normal or increased urine volume, dietary protein usually is not restricted until the patient reaches the stage of renal failure with moderate to severe azotemia. Kopple[9] suggests that protein restriction should begin before the SUN reaches 90 mg/dl or even 60 mg/dl in order to avoid the symptoms that accompany higher levels. Recommended protein restrictions may be 60 to 90 g when the GFR is 20 to 25 ml/min. and may be lowered to 40 to 60 g/day (0.5 to 0.65 g/kg ideal body weight) as the GFR falls to 10 to 15 ml/min. At least 70 percent of this protein should be of high biologic value in order for the diet to be most effective in reducing SUN. If the patient has proteinuria, the protein in the diet should be increased sufficiently to provide replacement of the losses. This level of protein intake usually will prevent uremic symptoms until the GFR falls to approximately 4 to 5 ml/min. The diet should be planned for maximum anabolic effects of protein and maximum acceptability. Some general guidelines are given in Table 7-4.

Table 7-4. General Guidelines for the Management of the Protein-Restricted Diet

1. Distribute protein evenly throughout the day to minimize hepatic deamination.
2. Emphasize the use of proteins of high biologic value.
3. Provide energy needs from other sources to avoid the use of protein to provide energy.
   a. Use low-protein pasta products and wheat starch, if necessary, to meet energy needs. (See Appendix M for a description of available products.)
   b. Use low-protein, high-energy supplements if necessary. (See Appendix K for a description of available products.)
4. Use protein "stretchers"—combining protein foods with cereals, vegetables, mayonnaise, and so on. See *The Mayo Clinic Renal Diet Cookbook*[a] or similar volumes for recipes.
5. Use protein exchange lists in planning.
6. Encourage exercise within permissible limits to avoid muscle atrophy.

[a] Margie, J.D. *The Mayo Clinic Renal Diet Cookbook.* New York: Golden Press, 1974.

Prior to the availability of dialysis and transplantation, as oliguria supervened and azotemia increased in uremia, protein intake was restricted further, to 18 to 20 g/day, and the protein was almost entirely of high biologic value. The rationale for this very stringent protein restriction is based on the work of Giordano, Giovannetti, and Maggiore[10,11] which suggests that urea can supply amino groups which, along with carbon skeletons available in normal metabolic processes, can be used to form the nonessential amino acids. The diet, called the *Giordano-Giovannetti diet,* assumes that the patient is taking adequate calories, vitamins, and minerals. The net effect of the diet was to lower the urea levels to approximately 50 percent of the amount found in the patient who was fed 40 to 60 g of protein per day. There is now some doubt that recycling of significant amounts of urea actually occurs. It has been shown that the amino groups of urea provide little of the nitrogen for albumin synthesis.[12] Nevertheless, there was some relief of symptoms along with fewer complications and improved nutritional status.[13] Patient compliance with the diet was poor; patients were often in negative nitrogen balance and became wasted. The diet now is used less frequently. If possible, dialysis or transplant is undertaken before protein intake needs to be restricted to this extent.

Variations of this diet have been suggested to be of possible use with supplementary purified amino acids or a mixture of calcium salts of alpha-keto and alpha-hydroxyl analogues of the amino acids. Amino acid analogues provide the carbon skeletons of amino acids with a ketone or hydroxyl group in place of the amino group. Urea is used as the source of the amino group to form the amino acids, thus reducing SUN. The analogues of isoleucine, leucine, phenylalanine, methionine, and valine can be aminated to form the essential amino acid.[14,15] Lysine acetate, histidine, threonine, and tryptophan are given as the amino acids. Analogues of lysine and threonine cannot be transaminated. This procedure is still being evaluated. It appears to be more effective than the Giordano-Giovannetti diet but tends to be unpalatable and causes gastric irritation. Hypercalcemia and hypophosphatemia also occur.[16] Because a number of unanswered questions concerning this procedure remain, it is not generally available for clinical use at present but is for investigation only. The renal nutritionist should be alert to new developments in this area of research.

Energy needs. It is important to provide sufficient sources of kilocalories so that body protein is not metabolized to provide energy. The patient's loss of appetite plus the protein restriction tend to present problems in achieving this goal. If intake of sufficient kilocalories is to be achieved, the advice, skill, and encouragement of persons experienced in nutritional care are essential. A number of carbohydrate and lipid supplements intended to increase the caloric content of the diet are available. They are almost protein-free with low levels of electrolytes. Further information on these products is contained in Appendix K.

Abnormalities of sodium balance. As the number of functioning nephrons decreases and those remaining hypertrophy to compensate for the loss, sodium balance is maintained until impairment is significant. As renal function diminishes further, there is usually an impaired ability to conserve sodium. The obligatory loss of sodium may be 20 to 40 mEq/day, but some patients are less able to restrict renal losses of sodium. These so-called salt wasters lose salt as a result of either the osmotic diuresis resulting from the increased solute load (of urea) or specific damage to tubule cells. In addition, some patients lose sodium from vomiting and diarrhea.

Moderate sodium losses are replaced if the patient is given a diet containing 4 to 6 g of salt. When larger amounts of sodium are lost than can be replaced by normal sodium intake, the patient becomes sodium-depleted (*hyponatremia*). Extracellular fluid volume falls as the patient loses water to restore normal osmolality. The reduced plasma volume results in decreased cardiac output, further compromising renal function as blood flow to the kidney diminishes.

The sodium concentration must be maintained in these patients by adequate replacement. Additional sodium is provided in increased quantities of salty foods. If acidosis is being treated with sodium bicarbonate, some of the necessary sodium will be provided. Sodium chloride tablets, which might serve as a source of sodium, tend to cause gastric irritation, but some patients will put salt into capsules and take those.

With a further reduction in the number of functioning nephrons, the kidney's ability to excrete sodium is diminished, despite the adaptive mechanisms. Less sodium is filtered for excretion, and sodium retention (*hypernatremia*) results. This is accompanied by increased extracellular volume (fluid retention) to restore normal osmolality. The consequences of increased fluid volume may include peripheral edema, hypertension, congestive heart failure, pulmonary congestion, and pulmonary edema. It has been estimated that retention of 20 mEq/day of sodium will cause the retention of 1 liter of fluid per week, causing a weight gain of 1 kg.[17] It then becomes necessary to restrict sodium intake to a degree dependent on the hypertension and state of hydration.

The CRF patient is poised precariously between sodium depletion and sodium overload. The amount of sodium in the diet must be determined for each patient. It is important to allow the maximum amount of sodium that the patient can tolerate in order to maintain normal extracellular fluid volume and promote the maximum GFR of which the kidneys are capable.

Sodium-restricted diets are used in the nutritional care of patients with fluid retention or hypertension. These conditions are seen frequently, not only in patients with renal disease, but also in cases of liver and cardiovascular disease. Most institutional diet manuals contain copies of diets restricting sodium to varying degrees of severity. The most severe restriction is the 250-mg (11-mEq) sodium diet. It usually is used for a short period only. Patient compliance is difficult to maintain. Patients vary in their sensitivity to the taste of salt.[18] Those with reduced sensitivity generally find compliance with salt restriction more difficult. If at all possible, diets with higher sodium levels are used for these patients. The 500-mg (22-mEq) sodium diet is used to reduce edema, and the 1,000-mg (43-mEq) sodium diet to reduce very mild edema, for edema prevention, or for prevention of hypertension. Other sodium-restricted diets more commonly used contain 1,500, 2,000, 3,000, 4,000, or 5,000 mg of sodium. These are employed to prevent edema or hypertension and for patients receiving steroid therapy.

In choosing the appropriate sodium restriction level, the nutritional care specialist considers the immediate condition indicating the need for sodium restriction but also must take into consideration the need for protein in the diet. Since most protein foods are relatively high in sodium content, the need to increase dietary protein limits the extent to which sodium can be restricted. The patient's living conditions must also be considered in the nutritional care of outpatients. For example, the patient who must eat many meals in restaurants may need a more moderate sodium prescription with increases in drug dosage.

The nutritional care specialist must have a detailed knowledge of the sodium content of foods. Some foods contain significant amounts of sodium, even in the unprocessed state. These include meat, eggs, fish, poultry, milk, and milk products. A few vegetables, such as carrots, beets, greens, turnips, and celery, are also high in sodium content. Other foods may contain appreciable amounts of sodium because salt (sodium chloride) or some other sodium-containing compound has been added in processing or in preparation. The use of baked goods containing baking soda (sodium bicarbonate) or baking powder is limited on the more restrictive diets. Other sodium compounds used in food include monosodium glutamate, sodium nitrate, and sodium benzoate. There are many others, and therefore it is important to read labels carefully.

Drinking water contains appreciable amounts of sodium in some areas. Furthermore, the sodium content of the water in some homes is increased when water is softened. Many softeners act by exchanging the sodium cation for the calcium and magnesium ions that cause hardness.

Some dentifrices and mouthwashes contain significant amounts of sodium, as do some drugs, including nonprescription drugs. Sodium may be contained in laxatives, cough medicines, and antacids, and the labels must be read carefully by patients.

Diet manuals list foods to be eliminated or avoided by patients on sodium-restricted diets. Many contain exchange lists, which are used in a way similar to the diabetic exchange lists described in Chapter 9. These lists are particularly helpful in planning the more severely restricted diets.

Some special low-sodium products are available to provide additional variety and added nutrients. These include low-sodium milk, low-sodium baking powder, unsalted canned vegetables, unsalted meats and cheese, unsalted bakery products, and unsalted margarine and sweet butter. All tend to be more expensive than their salted equivalents.

Many commercial salt substitutes are available but should not be used without the consent of the physician, since most contain potassium chloride, which may be harmful to patients with renal disease. Others contain ammonium salts, hazardous in some liver diseases. Most salt substitutes are somewhat unpalatable and, if used, should be tried cautiously at first. The use of products consisting of 50 percent sodium chloride and 50 percent other salts must be discouraged unless planned into the diet. Patients should be encouraged to use other spices and flavorings instead. A number of recipe books and meal-planning guides are available for patients who need assistance in preparing palatable and varied menus. Some suggested methods and procedures for management of sodium-restricted diets are listed in Table 7-5.

A severe and prolonged sodium restriction may be harmful if the patient has excessive losses. The patient with renal disease who cannot conserve sodium and excrete a dilute urine is at risk. Patients on diets with severely restricted amounts of sodium should be observed for clinical manifestations of depletion. These signs and symptoms are:

Abdominal cramps and aching muscles
Weakness, lassitude
Anorexia and vomiting
Mental confusion

Abnormalities of fluid balance. When the number of functioning nephrons has decreased sufficiently to produce renal insufficiency in CRF, the remaining functioning nephrons are presented with a greater solute load, provoking a *solute diuresis.* More fluid must be provided if this load is to be excreted. The maximum efficiency of the kidney in excreting solutes is reached when urine volume is 2.0 to 2.5 liters, requiring an intake of approximately 3 liters of fluid. Polyuria and nocturia result. An increased thirst may provide the stimulus for the necessary water intake, but for some patients a specific intake must be prescribed to assure adequate fluids. The prescription often is written as *force fluids, encourage fluids,* or *push fluids.* Obviously, physical force should not be used. A day's fluid intake should be distributed throughout the 24 hours. Beverages should be offered frequently and should be those the patient particularly likes. Frozen and gelatin desserts, soups, and fruit juices also are helpful. Small frequent servings usually are more effective than large servings at less frequent intervals.

As fewer nephrons are available for filtration, the polyuric phase gives way to oliguria. Excess water that is ingested is

Table 7-5. Methods and Procedures for Nutritional Care of Patients Requiring A Sodium-Restricted Diet

1. Plan the diet for the individual patient's physiologic needs and life-style.
2. Specify amounts for only those foods that must be limited because of their sodium content.
3. A given level of sodium can be planned in many combinations, especially when the diet is more moderately restricted.
4. All foods should be cooked without the addition of salt in diets allowing less than 1,000 mg of sodium. In diets allowing 500 mg or less of sodium, foods containing high levels of naturally occurring sodium are carefully limited. Diets containing 1,000 mg of sodium may include ¼ tsp. of salt or specific amounts of salted foods. Diets allowing 2,000 mg or more of sodium may include some foods cooked with a limited amount of salt or other added sodium products, but no salt is added during meals.
5. Diet manuals and exchange lists give information on the sodium content of foods in each food group. These should be consulted in detail in diet planning. Outpatients must be instructed carefully about foods to be avoided and the use of exchange lists.
6. Plan the amounts of high-protein foods carefully.
   a. Meats, fish, and poultry that are smoked, cured, pickled, processed with sodium nitrite, or canned with salt must be used with special caution.
   b. In more restricted diets, used unsalted canned meat or fish.
   c. Use low-sodium milk in 250-mg sodium diets. Several products of variable palatability are available. They often are needed in diets of 500 mg or more of sodium. When low-sodium milk is used, serve it very cold, add flavorings that are low in sodium, or incorporate it in cooked dishes. Outpatients should be provided information on the source, cost, and preparation of this product and given recipes for its use.
   d. Kosher meats usually are high in sodium, 200 to 350 mg/oz., and generally must be avoided. Alternatives are meats that are broiled to allow the blood to drip away. Some meats can be boiled in water to reduce sodium content. The water is discarded.
   e. See diet manuals for the sodium content of cheese and cheese products and use them only as permitted by the degree of sodium restriction.
7. Avoid or limit foods containing the following:

   Baking soda or baking powder
   Sodium alginate (in some ice cream and chocolate milk)
   Sodium benzoate (a preservative)
   Sodium propionate (a mold inhibitor)
   Sodium sulfite (a fruit bleach and preservative)
   Sodium phosphate (in some cereals and cheeses)
   Monosodium glutamate (a flavor enhancer)

   Limited amounts of these products are acceptable on more moderately restricted diets.
8. Avoid obviously salty foods, such as potato chips, pretzels, pickles, and sauerkraut.
9. The more restrictive diets require low-sodium bread and sweet butter. The patient should be provided information on sources of these products.
10. Avoid most commercial seasonings, salad dressings, and condiments.
11. Consider the sodium content of drinking water in the area. Avoid locally bottled beverages if the sodium content of the water is high. Question the patient about water softeners in the home. It may be necessary to advise the patient to use distilled or bottled water for cooking and drinking.
12. Instruct the patient carefully on reading labels. Adjust instructions to the level of restriction required. Minor sodium sources may be ignored when the restriction is moderate.
13. Provide encouragement and emotional support. Remember that in some illnesses the patient has a reduced ability to taste salt.
14. Assist the patient in planning for variety in the menu. Provide recipes and information on special products, including low-sodium baking powder. Give instruction and encouragement on the use of spices, herbs, and other alternative flavoring agents.
15. Assist the patient in planning for home-prepared meals in place of presalted convenience foods.
16. Some synthetic detergents contain large amounts of sodium. Dishes should be rinsed carefully to remove the residue.
17. Sodium-restricted diets often are combined with modifications in potassium, protein, or fluid intake.
18. Provide the patient with a list of "free" foods.

retained, and the patient becomes overhydrated. Some renal patients eventually become anuric. If sodium intake is adequately controlled, the thirst mechanism at first serves as a good guide to fluid intake. Eventually, however, fluid taken out of habit and with medications, plus metabolic water, total an amount in excess of excretory capacity. When the GFR falls below 4 to 5 ml/min. and water begins to accumulate, it usually becomes necessary to restrict fluid intake. Fluid overload otherwise leads to hyponatremia and water intoxication, with muscle cramps, weakness, lassitude, anorexia, vomiting, and mental confusion. Fluid overload may also cause hypertension and pulmonary congestion.

To determine the amount of fluid to provide, dehydrated or overhydrated patients must first be brought to normal hydration. Fluid intake in the normally hydrated patient then is limited to an amount equal to the estimated total water loss. This frequently is based on urine volume for the previous day *plus* 500 to 1,000 ml to compensate for nonurinary losses. The estimates vary depending on environmental temperature and humidity, activity, body surface area, and other disease conditions. Body weight is monitored carefully. Sudden weight gain or loss indicates that fluid intake is inappropriate and should be corrected.

An allotment of fluid of less than 2,000 ml/day is considered to be a restriction. The anuric or severely oliguric patient obviously will require a severe restriction, sometimes to 500 to 600 ml/day. All beverages and liquid foods must be included within the prescribed allotment, including fruit juice, milk, soup, gruels, coffee, tea, soft drinks, and alcoholic beverages. The juice or syrup on fruits must be included as well as all items that are liquid at body temperature, such as gelatin mixtures, frozen desserts, and ice. The fluid content of solid foods is not included unless the fluid restriction is severe.

In the management of the hospitalized patient, conference and cooperation between the nursing service and nutritional care specialist usually is necessary, since fluid is needed for administration of medications. Some patients require fluid between meals because of a dry mouth or an unpleasant taste. Patients should be consulted regarding their preferences on the form in which their fluids are given. Some patients, for example, are willing to make other sacrifices in order to have that morning cup of coffee.

Abnormalities of potassium balance. In renal insufficiency, *hyperkalemia* (elevated serum potassium, greater than 5.5 mEq/L) usually does not occur as long as at least 1,000 ml of urine are produced, since the distal tubules have an enormous capacity to excrete potassium. Fecal excretion of potassium increases in renal insufficiency.[19] The secretion of potassium is increased by the greater aldosterone activity that is seen in some patients. The increased flow rate during polyuria also encourages potassium secretion. As a result, patients maintain serum potassium levels close to normal until late in the course of CRF.

When hyperkalemia does occur in these patients, food usually is not the main source of the excess potassium. Instead, potassium accumulates as a result of intercurrent conditions such as hemorrhage, acidosis, blood tranfusions, or catabolic stress such as occurs in surgery or trauma. The use of potassium-sparing medications or of salt substitutes containing potassium can be a precipitating factor. Since potassium is "exchanged" for sodium in the distal tubule, insufficient sodium may decrease potassium excretion with resultant hyperkalemia.

In late renal failure when oliguria supervenes, potassium balance becomes precarious. Control is essential, since high serum potassium levels cause cardiac arrest with disastrous results. Patients may be given ion exchange resins to reduce intestinal absorption of potassium and insulin to reduce release of cellular potassium. If hyperkalemia persists, dietary intake is limited to the extent indicated by serum potassium levels. Restrictions to 2,800 mg (70 mEq) or

2,000 mg (51 mEq) commonly are used. Sometimes, potassium is restricted to 1,000 to 1,500 mg (25 to 40 mEq) per day. A 40-g protein diet will include less than 70 mEq of potassium. The average daily diet in the United States contains 75 to 100 mEq of potassium. Hyperkalemia that persists when intake is restricted is an indication for dialysis.

There are many food sources of potassium. It is present in all living cells and therefore is found in all plant and animal foods except purified components such as sugar, starch, and oil. Potassium is very water soluble. Therefore, the potassium content of foods can be reduced by boiling them in large amounts of water and discarding the water. Baking, broiling, and frying do not affect the potassium content of foods. Processing also affects potassium content, depending on the water involved. Canned fruits are lower in potassium than fresh fruits if the syrup is not consumed, whereas dried fruits are higher in potassium content for equal weight, since all components are more concentrated. The potassium in cereals is found in the germ and bran. Therefore, highly refined cereal products contain less potassium.

In the potassium-restricted diet, intake of almost every food must be controlled, since there are few foods that are potassium-free. Occasionally, a potassium-free diet is required for an anuric patient with high serum potassium. For these patients, the commercial high-calorie, low-electrolyte supplements may be useful (see Appendix J). They carry with them, however, an appreciable amount of water.

For less seriously affected patients, potassium-restricted diets allow the consumption of more normal foods. Usually, though, a patient requiring potassium restriction also needs modification of protein and sodium intake. A group of exchange lists, found in almost all institution diet manuals, classifies foods simultaneously according to their contents of these three nutrients. The principles of the use of these exchange lists in planning are similar to those for the diabetic exchange lists (see Chapter 9).

It is important to remember, in planning the diet, that since dietary potassium is absorbed rapidly, the potassium must be distributed evenly throughout the day so that sharp increases in serum potassium do not occur. At the same time, it is important to maintain protein and energy intakes to levels that prevent tissue catabolism. Inadequate intakes result in tissue catabolism and release of intracellular potassium into the extracellular fluid. At least 40 percent of the kilocalorie content of the diet should come from carbohydrates. The movement of glucose into cells carries potassium with it. Patients should be encouraged to exercise as much as the physician allows. Exercise prevents muscle breakdown and increases movement of glucose into muscle cells. Both of these actions tend to reduce serum potassium.

Acidosis. In renal insufficiency, as the number of functioning nephrons diminishes, the ability to produce ammonium ion is impaired and the ability to excrete hydrogen ion thus is reduced. Diminished ability to reabsorb filtered bicarbonate also contributes to hydrogen ion retention. As a result, patients have a metabolic acidosis.

The excess acid is partially buffered by bone, contributing to skeletal abnormalities commonly seen in renal disease. In addition, acidosis causes nausea and fatigue. The patient breathes more deeply and more rapidly and may be breathless on exertion, but *Kussmaul respiration,* a deep gasping breathing seen in severe diabetic acidosis, is not common. These changes are compensatory mechanisms which lower the partial pressure of carbon dioxide and restore the bicarbonate–carbonic acid ratio to normal. However, the patient tends to remain in a state of mild acidosis.

Calcium carbonate, given as part of the treatment of the bone disease, partially corrects the acidosis. In addition, sodium bicarbonate or sodium citrate is given as a medication. Protein restriction reduces the production of acid, but there is no diet modification indicated that is specific for acidosis. Acidosis frequently is accompanied by nausea, adding to the problems of nutritional care.

Effects on other minerals. Anemia is a common finding in uremic patients. The major cause is believed to be bone marrow failure due to decreased erythropoietin production. Reduced iron absorption, gastrointestinal bleeding, and frequent blood sampling also contribute to anemia. Iron supplementation often is prescribed. Rather than oral supplements, iron sometimes is given parenterally to avoid loss from binding with the phosphate binders the patient may be taking. The use of iron-rich foods in the diet is helpful.

It has been suggested that dysgeusia in renal patients be treated with zinc supplements.[20] This may be of some importance in nutritional care, since it can be assumed to affect food intake.

Vitamin needs. The information on vitamin needs of patients with CRF is inadequate. A commonly recommended procedure is to provide the patients with daily supplements of 1.0 mg folic acid, 100 mg ascorbic acid, 5.0 mg pyridoxine hydrochloride, and the Recommended Dietary Allowances of the remaining water-soluble vitamins.

There is some evidence of changes in pyridoxine metabolism and an increased need for this vitamin.[21] It has been suggested that the etiology of the increased requirement includes the action of circulating inhibitors, increased clearance of pyridoxal phosphate, and drug-related impaired absorption.[22,23]

Serum vitamin A levels tend to be increased, and so vitamin A supplements are not indicated. Vitamin K sometimes is given. The need for vitamin D will be discussed in relation to bone disease.

Calcium and phosphorus. In renal disease, the alterations in vitamin D metabolism and in calcium and phosphorus homeostasis have far-reaching consequences. The skeletal system is seriously affected.

Calcium and phosphate concentrations in the extracellular fluid normally are close to those at which calcium phosphate salts would precipitate (calcium × phosphate product greater than 70 mg/dl). When the GFR decreases to 25 percent of normal or less, phosphate is retained and serum phosphate levels rise. Calcium phosphates are deposited both in bone and soft tissue, reducing the serum concentrations of phosphate and reducing serum calcium which was not elevated originally. The depressed serum calcium stimulates secretion of PTH, reducing tubular reabsorption of phosphate and restoring serum phosphate and calcium to normal. A new steady state thus is established until the GFR falls further.[24,25]

As the GFR falls, the process is repeated until the GFR decreases to approximately 20 ml/min. Then, phosphate levels increase and remain high and serum calcium is lower than normal. In an effort to keep serum calcium at normal levels, PTH secretion becomes chronically increased. Decreased renal clearance contributes to the maintenance of the high PTH levels.[24] Serum calcium is increased toward normal, but it remains somewhat depressed. Impaired calcium absorption from the intestine also contributes to the deficit in serum calcium. Intestinal absorption is affected when renal hydroxylation of the 25-hydroxycholecalciferol form of vitamin D to the 1,25 form, which stimulates calcium absorption, is depressed.

Acidosis, excess PTH, alterations in vitamin D metabolism, and reduced calcium absorption all contribute to the development of bone disease and other pathologic manifestations in patients with CRF. According to Bricker's trade-off hypothesis,[4] bone disease may be the price that is paid to maintain serum calcium levels near normal. Figure 7-6 gives a summary of mechanisms that contribute to the pathogenesis of the bone disease.

The bone disease, referred to as *osteodystrophy,* is a combination of four possible

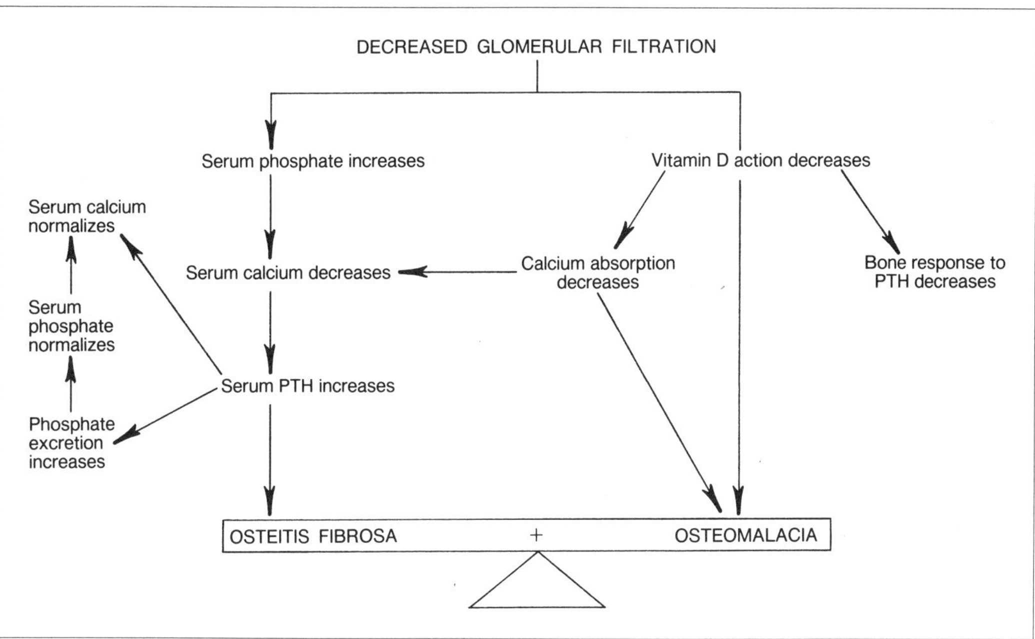

Figure 7-6. Pathogenesis of renal glomerular osteodystrophy. **PTH** *= parathyroid hormone. (Reprinted with permission from Genuth, S., Renal glomerular osteodystrophy.* Postgrad. Med. *52(3):212, 1972.)*

forms in varying proportion:[26]

1. *Osteitis fibrosa cystica:* classic hyperparathyroidism
2. *Osteomalacia:* excessive uncalcified bone matrix
3. *Osteopenia:* decreased bone mass
4. *Osteosclerosis:* increased bone density

The specific clinical features in a given patient depend on which of these four processes is dominant. The features include bone pain and an increase in fractures. Soft tissue calcification often occurs. High calcium levels in the skin cause severe itching. Other symptoms include muscle weakness and a variety of neurologic abnormalities.[24] Massry[27] has suggested that many of the manifestations of CRF are a consequence of hyperparathyroidism.

Diet modification is limited in effectiveness. An average adult's diet in the United States has been estimated to contain 1.0 to 1.8 g of phosphorus per day. In the renal patient with a diet of 40 g of protein per day, phosphorus intake is usually somewhat lower. A low-phosphate diet, with reduced intake of dairy products, provides 600 to 1,200 mg/day. This level alone is not sufficient to reduce serum phosphate to normal levels, and a phosphate restriction, superimposed on the other diet modifications, would further reduce the acceptability of the diet and patient compliance. In addition, planning for nutritional adequacy becomes exceedingly difficult. A low-phosphate diet also tends to be low in calcium. As a consequence of all these difficulties, aluminum gels, which act as phosphate binders to prevent phosphate absorption from the gastrointestinal tract, have commonly been used rather than diet to control hyperphosphatemia. The gels are taken *with meals* in the form of aluminum carbonate or aluminum hydroxide.

Some recent work showed that early use of phosphate binders prevents progression of bone lesions and may be useful in prevention of bone lesion formation.[28]

However, there are some problems that arise as side effects of the use of phosphate binders. Aluminum has recently been found to be elevated in tissues of patients receiving aluminum hydroxide or aluminum carbonate binders. It has been suggested that accumulation of aluminum in the brain may be related to a "dialysis dementia" sometimes seen in dialysis patients.[29] The source of the aluminum is uncertain but may be from water used in dialysis. A second problem consequent to the intake of phosphate binders is the occurrence of severe constipation and nausea. Large doses of antacids are not tolerated well because they are unpalatable. Products such as Amphojel (an aluminum hydroxide gel) have been incorporated into cookies to make them more acceptable.

Given the side effects and the unanswered question of the long-term safety of phosphate binders, there still may be a place for the low-phosphorus diet. A severe restriction is not possible, since phosphorus is present in almost all foods. If any restriction is ordered, it usually is in the range of 0.8 to 1.2 g of phosphorus per day. If the patient has a protein-restricted diet, the diet probably is already somewhat reduced in phosphorus content. It may then be sufficient to eliminate from the diet certain processed foods to which phosphorus compounds have been added (if the diet is already sodium-restricted, many of these items would already have been eliminated):

Cola beverages and other carbonated drinks made with phosphoric acid
Processed meats such as ham, Canadian bacon, hot dogs, and cold cuts
Processed cheeses
Instant puddings
Many commercial salad dressings
Refrigerated baked products
Fabricated potato chips

With the low-phosphorus diet, calcium supplements usually are given to prevent concurrent hypocalcemia, but it is important to reduce serum phosphorus levels first to avoid soft tissue calcification. A recommended dose of 1,000 mg of calcium is provided in 2,500 mg of calcium carbonate per day. Vitamin D also is supplemented. The most potent form is 1,25-dihydroxycholecalciferol (calcitriol [Rocaltrol]). The effects of long-term use of this material is unknown, since it is only newly available. There is evidence that other vitamin D analogues have separate effects from calcitriol and that CRF patients may need these as well.

Carbohydrate. A number of disorders of carbohydrate metabolism are associated with uremia, including fasting hyperglycemia and a glucose tolerance curve that strongly resembles the diabetic curve (see Chapter 9).[30] Circulating insulin levels often are high,[31] and there is evidence of peripheral insensitivity to insulin.[30,32,33]

The nature of the defect in the peripheral tissues is not understood completely. The binding of insulin to receptor sites appears to be normal, but there is some evidence that the metabolic steps following binding are abnormal.[33] The presence of circulating insulin antagonists has also been suggested but not proved.[31] The glucose intolerance is not sufficiently severe to present a clinical problem in most uremic patients. They do not develop ketoacidosis.

Protein and amino acid metabolism. A great deal of evidence points to alterations in protein and amino acid metabolism in uremia. Some of these alterations are characteristic of malnutrition, whereas others seem to be the consequence of uremia even in the absence of malnutrition.

An important element in the total picture of uremia which is of special interest to nutritionists is the *wasting syndrome.* In wasted uremic patients, body weight, adipose tissue, and muscle mass are decreased. Children are growth-retarded. Serum albumin, transferrin, and some immune system proteins are reduced. Poor dietary intake is believed to be a major cause of wasting, but blood losses and other concurrent illnesses may contribute. In addition to malnutrition, there are indications of other derangements that contribute to wasting and to other symptoms.

There is an increased synthesis and release of alanine and glutamine from the skeletal muscles, which contribute to the degradation of skeletal muscles and the wasting syndrome.[34] These changes also provide substrates for alterations in carbohydrate metabolism, including increased gluconeogenesis.

Aberrations in serum amino acid profile, with decreased essential amino acids and increased nonessential amino acids, have also been found. For example, the tyrosine-phenylalanine ratio is reduced, suggesting diminished activity of phenylalanine hydroxylase, which functions in the formation of tyrosine from phenylalanine. At the same time, other metabolites of phenylalanine are increased. The significance of these changes is unknown.

The essentiality of histidine in the uremic adult also indicates an alteration in metabolism. Histidine is important in the structure of hemoglobin, and the reduced plasma histidine in uremic patients may be related to hematologic changes. Supplementation with histidine has been shown to result in increased hematocrit and decreased reticulocytes (immature red blood cells).[35]

The cause of these metabolic alterations is not clear. It is conceivable that uremic toxins affect protein or amino acid metabolism in a variety of ways. High serum urea has been reported to inhibit urea cycle enzymes.[36] The concentration of some urea cycle intermediates may then increase and enter other metabolic pathways. Uremic toxins could also affect membrane transport and other aspects of amino acid metabolism. The various endocrine disorders and their interactions with nutrients may be significant. Alterations in the metabolism of carbohydrate, lipids, and some vitamins and minerals affect protein and amino acid metabolism. Our knowledge of these matters is sketchy at best. A better understanding may be useful in determining the ideal kind and amount of protein for the uremic patient and the ideal amino acid or analogue supplementation that should be used. The specialist in nutritional care should be alert to new developments in this field.

Lipids. Patients with CRF have hyperlipidemia and elevated triglycerides, usually of the type IV pattern and sometimes type II (see Chapter 8).[36] Uremic patients have a high incidence of atherosclerosis and coronary artery disease, which have been related to high triglyceride levels. Therefore, some attempts have been made to treat the hyperlipidemia by diet.[37,38] The effectiveness of these modifications in CRF is unknown.

Additional problems. The multiple dietary restrictions imposed on the uremic patient reduce the variety and palatability of the diet. Patients tend to complain that the diet is sweet and greasy. In addition, CRF patients often have ulcers of the mouth, nausea, and vomiting. The fluid restriction leads to thirst. Uremic patients suffer from anxiety, depression, and fear. Their feelings of frustration may result in noncompliance and antagonism. Under these circumstances, nutritional management of these patients is difficult and requires a great deal of skill.

The pediatric (child) patient presents some special problems. A decrease in growth rate frequently occurs when the GFR is 50 percent of normal or less, and uremia occurs earlier in the progress of the disease than in adults.[39] The child's protein intake per kilogram of body weight should, of course, be higher than in adults in order to support growth. Food to supply the higher energy requirement of the child will carry with it more sodium relative to body weight. Therefore, the use of other sources of sodium, such as salt added to foods, must be more severely restricted under otherwise equivalent conditions. The use of daily multivitamin preparations for pediatric patients is recommended.

The Dialysis Patient. Dialysis is a process of diffusion and filtration between solutions separated by a semipermeable membrane. In renal disease, blood is circulated on one side of the semipermeable membrane and a cleansing fluid, known as the *dialysate,* on the other. Dialysis has been shown to improve the condition of most patients in end-stage renal disease, but it cannot be used for all patients. It is employed in the treatment of both acute and chronic renal failure. In chronic disease, dialysis may be planned to continue indefinitely (*maintenance dialysis*) or for a short period prior to transplantation. It also is used sometimes after a renal transplant until the grafted kidney begins to function. Indications for beginning its use are hyperkalemia unresponsive to other treatment, severe metabolic acidosis, fluid overload, pericarditis, and uremia. In CRF, the patient usually begins dialysis treatments when the GFR is 5 to 10 ml/min. The patient who is dialyzed for an extended period is of most concern in nutritional care. There are two basic dialysis methods available, hemodialysis and peritoneal dialysis.

Hemodialysis. Hemodialysis involves the use of an artificial kidney machine or *dialyzer* to cleanse the blood of undesirable materials. The patient is connected to the dialyzer in such a way that the blood in an artery of an arm or leg circulates through the machine before being returned to the parallel vein. Various methods have been used to achieve this attachment. Originally, cannulas were placed surgically into an artery and a vein of an extremity and the exteriorized ends were connected by a bypass. The machine was connected when the bypass was removed. More recently, subcutaneous arteriovenous shunts have been created surgically. The shunts connect an artery and a vein so that arterial pressure enlarges the vein. This access site is less prone to accidents and provides less access to infection but does require puncture through the skin for each dialysis period. At present, arteriovenous shunts are the more commonly used method.

Although dialyzers vary in design, all are based on the same fundamental principle. Each machine has a semipermeable membrane made of a cellophane. The membrane material most widely used is marketed as Cuprophane but is familiar to lay people as sausage casing. This membrane is permeable to water and substances of low molecular weight, such as potassium, phosphates, sulfates, and the nitrogenous waste products, urea, creatinine, and uric acid. It also is permeable to the middle molecules. Substances of even higher molecular weights, up to approximately 40,000, cross the membrane slowly. The membrane is impermeable to blood cells and most plasma proteins.

Although the patient's physical condition usually is improved with hemodialysis, dialysis is not a perfect substitute for a normally functioning kidney. It has been suggested that results may be improved by removal of the middle molecules. For this purpose, the use of a more permeable membrane with a larger surface area and slower blood flow has been suggested. Excess water is removed by *ultrafiltration.* The hydrostatic pressure gradient across the membrane is increased with the use of pumps on the inflow of the blood and the outflow of the dialysate. Low-molecular-weight materials, such as urea and potassium, that are in high concentration in the blood and low in the dialysate are removed by *diffusion* across the membrane. At the same time, some low-molecular-weight substances may be maintained in the blood or even increased by having a high concentration in the dialysate, so that they diffuse in the opposite direction. Thus, the composition of the dialysate is very important. It has approximately the same composition as normal blood serum but with lower potassium and without urea or creatinine. Glucose is not always included in the dialysate, since it can serve as a medium for growth of bacteria.

Hemodialysis may be performed at various dialysis centers which often, but not always, are located in hospitals. Patients usually must be dialyzed two to three times per week for periods that may vary from 4 to

6 hours. Some patients may be dialyzed at home, but home dialysis requires a high degree of motivation, intelligence, and emotional stability in the patient. It also requires an appropriate home environment and the dedicated help of a family member or other person. Candidates for home dialysis and the persons assisting them must be carefully instructed.

As the availability of hemodialysis increases, there is a continuing tendency to undertake it earlier in the course of the disease to prevent some of the irreversible complications of uremia. This is not a procedure to be taken lightly. The effects on the patient and the patient's family have been vividly described by Campbell and Campbell[40] in a personal account.

Nutritional care is important in maintaining the best possible physical condition in the dialysis patient. The participation of a renal nutritionist is essential. It is important to remember that, since hemodialysis is intermittent, the substances normally excreted by the kidneys will accumulate between dialyses as they did prior to dialysis. Therefore, nutritional management must continue in a supportive role. It usually is possible, however, to liberalize the diet compared to that used in conservative management. The extent to which this may be done is variable. It is influenced by the frequency and effectiveness of the treatments, the amount of residual renal function, if any, and the psychological response of the patient.

Chronic hemodialysis is a catabolic process, and malnutrition is a continuing problem. The patient may lose amino acids, peptides, and some protein during each session, along with an amount of glucose that varies with the glucose content of the dialysate. The *protein* lost in hemodialysis, estimated to be 1 to 2 g/hr, must be replaced. An intake of 0.75 to 1.25 g/kg body weight has been recommended, at least 70 percent of which should be of high biologic value.[41] The diet may need to be more restricted if dialysis is limited to twice weekly; the degree of azotemia that develops between treatments will influence the choice.

Intake of sources of *energy* must be sufficient to spare protein and maintain body weight. Commonly recommended levels are 35 to 50 kcal/kg body weight. The hyperlipidemia and cardiovascular disease of renal failure does not respond to hemodialysis or transplantation.[42–44] Therefore, it often is considered desirable to adjust the diet to lessen these tendencies.[45,46] A diet containing 15 percent of total kilocalories from protein, 35 percent fat, and 50 percent carbohydrate, primarily from polysaccharides, has been recommended. It has been suggested that a 2:1 ratio of polyunsaturated-saturated fat be included (see Chapter 8), but this issue is controversial.

Usually *sodium* and *fluid* intakes must continue to be decreased moderately, since the accumulation of large amounts of these materials between treatments leads to hypertension, edema, and congestive heart failure. Sodium intake is restricted to the amount that limits weight gain from edema between dialyses to 0.5 kg/day. Sodium restriction varies from 2 to 4 g/day (85 to 170 mEq), and fluid may be limited to 500 to 1,500 ml in addition to that contained in solid food. Body weight and blood pressure are carefully monitored and used as indicators of the success of the restrictions.

Potassium usually is restricted to 2,000 to 3,000 mg/day (50 to 75 mEq), particularly if the patient is anuric. More severe restrictions are necessary in some patients.

Calcium and *phosphorus* levels should be controlled in the same manner as that used in conservative management. Hemodialysis does not correct the tendency to bone disease.

Water-soluble vitamins also are lost in dialysis, and patients become deficient if they are not given replacements. The permeability of the membrane to the various vitamins varies. Often, supplements of 1 mg of folate, 10 mg of pyridoxine, 100 mg of ascorbic acid, and Recommended Dietary

Allowances of other water-soluble vitamins are provided.

Iron supplementation also is given, either orally, bound to ascorbic acid, or intravenously. Clearly, it is important that the patient have an adequate diet to avoid increasing the severity of the malnutrition.

Additional problems in nutritional care that sometimes occur involve the emotional response of the patient. Some patients become very apprehensive; however, psychological, or even psychiatric, problems often regress as dialysis continues and uremic symptoms subside.

Food intake while dialysis is in progress is treated differently in different centers. Some dialysis centers serve meals during dialysis. Others do not do so because of the risk of hepatitis, but they allow patients to bring in their own food. Some units allow a "treat" the night before dialysis, reasoning that the dialysis will remove unwanted material. Others expect the patient's diet limitations to be strictly observed or only partially liberalized.

In some patients, complications of hemodialysis must be considered. *Anemia* generally does not soon improve when a patient is dialyzed. Transfusion of packed red blood cells at intervals may be necessary. Blood containing white cells and platelets is not used, since the patient may become sensitized and have an increased tendency to reject a transplant. The risk of hepatitis also is increased by transfusions. There is some evidence that, if a patient is not transfused, erythropoiesis improves slowly so that transfusion becomes unnecessary.[47] One of the objectives of nutritional care should be provision of optimum nutrition for erythropoiesis.

Hypertension is a frequent problem, particularly in patients who have high intakes of water and sodium. In many patients, these excesses can be treated by dialysis plus appropriate dietary sodium and fluid restriction. It often is a challenge in nutritional care to elicit patient cooperation in these restrictions. On the other hand, dialysis patients seem to be peculiarly sensitive to sodium and volume depletion; therefore, it is important that restrictions not be excessive. Some patients do not respond to these measures and require bilateral nephrectomy.

The various forms of *bone disease* are seen less frequently as we learn more about calcium, phosphate, and PTH metabolism. Parathyroid hormone levels sometimes remain above normal in dialyzed patients and may be reduced by increasing the magnesium levels in the dialysate. If this is ineffective, parathyroidectomy is necessary. The continued use of aluminum gels and restriction of intake of dairy products reduces phosphorus levels. These methods often are necessary, since phosphorus removal during dialysis is relatively inefficient. Calcium levels are manipulated by altering calcium concentrations in the dialysate or by regulating calcium intake. Dietary calcium should be 800 to 1,200 mg/day, but calcium supplements generally are necessary. A high-calcium diet is not feasible since it would also increase dietary phosphorus.

Other symptoms, such as peripheral neuropathy and central nervous system dysfunction, sometimes continue despite dialysis. Approximately 50 to 75 percent of the patients treated for 1 year or more can become normally productive.[17] Infections and vascular disease cause death in 4 to 15 percent of dialyzed patients, and dialysis is unsuccessful in another 10 to 15 percent of cases.

Special mention must be made of the problems of the pediatric patient. *Retarded growth* remains a concern. Inadequate protein and calorie intake are considered to be the major causes. The diet for pediatric patients on hemodialysis should provide 1.5 to 2.0 g of protein per kilogram of body weight, or 8 to 12 percent of the calories from protein with at least 70 percent of this of high biologic value. Recommended calorie intakes are 75 to 100 kcal/kg/day. Potassium intake is restricted to 1 to 3 g/day (25.6 to

77.0 mEq). Fluid is restricted to the amount that will limit weight gain between dialyses to 1.0 to 1.5 kg.

Peritoneal dialysis. Peritoneal dialysis, an alternative to hemodialysis, uses the membranes of the peritoneal cavity as the dialytic membrane. The *peritoneum* is the membrane that lines the abdominal cavity and surrounds the abdominal organs, forming a sac. The dialysate enters the sac via a catheter through the abdominal wall (Fig. 7-7) and is exchanged twenty to forty times at 20- to 60-minute intervals. A hyperosmolar solution causes fluid flow into the peritoneal cavity. Solute movement is thought to result from bulk flow or solvent drag or both.

This procedure is used for short periods in acute renal failure or in combination with conservative management of chronic renal failure when some reversible event, such as an infection, further reduces the GFR temporarily. It has also been used to maintain a patient who is waiting to enter a chronic hemodialysis program or for a transplant.

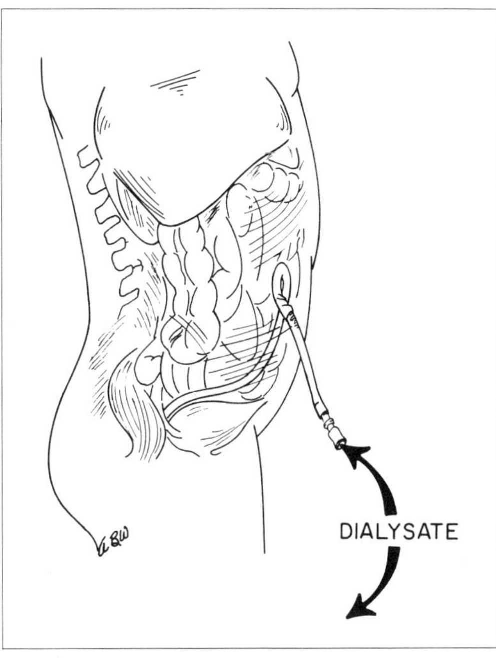

Figure 7-7. In peritoneal dialysis, the membranes of the peritoneal cavity are used as the dialytic membrane. The dialysate is exchanged through a catheter that enters the peritoneum through the abdominal wall. (Reprinted with permission from Johnson, W.J., Treatment of Irreversible Renal Failure by Dialysis and Transplantation. In F.G. Knox, Ed., Textbook of Renal Pathophysiology. *New York: Harper and Row, 1978, p. 315.)*

For some years, peritoneal dialysis for long-term use was in disrepute, largely because of a high incidence of infection and the hazard of intestinal perforation. The availability of improved equipment providing an automated delivery system, permanent catheters, disposable equipment, and sterile solutions have reduced infections and made peritoneal dialysis easier and more practical for home use. Long-term peritoneal dialysis is now being used more often. It is considered preferable to hemodialysis in elderly patients, diabetics, patients with systemic diseases, and children, and for home dialysis when the patient does not have adequate help.[48] It also is useful for patients who have exhausted their access sites for hemodialysis. Sometimes it is used for fluid and electrolyte disturbances unrelated to renal disease, such as diuretic-resistant congestive heart failure. The dialysate solution commonly used in uremia contains 1.5 g/dl of dextrose solution (350 mOsm/L), a concentration that is slightly hypertonic to plasma. If the patient is overhydrated, a dextrose solution with 4.25 g/dl (490 mOsm/L) can be used. Hyperosmolar solutions cause a net flow of water into the intraperitoneal space of as high as 300 to 500 ml per exchange. Lactate (35 mEq/L) is included as an alkalizing agent.[49] A recommended sodium content is 132 mEq/L. Potassium content varies greatly with need.

Generally, peritoneal dialysis is *intermittent* (IPD), commonly four times per week for 10 hours each, usually at night. A newer method, which has been used only on a limited number of patients to date, is *continuous ambulatory peritoneal dialysis* (CAPD). In this procedure, sterile dialysate in a plastic pouch is infused and drained by gravity at

4-hour intervals five times daily, 7 days/week. Because CAPD is only a few years old, its long-term effects are unknown.

The nutritional management of the peritoneal dialysis patient is handicapped by limited information. The rationale and current practices have been described by Blumenkrantz et al.[50] Protein losses may be extensive. They vary with dialysate volume and dwell time — that is, the time the dialysate remains in the peritoneal cavity. Protein losses in the patient without peritonitis have been estimated to be 5 to 20 g/day,[51] and these increase in patients with episodes of peritonitis.[52] Patients receiving intermittent peritoneal dialysis may have low body weight, with decreased body fat, muscle, and serum protein.[53] These parameters do not differ significantly from those seen in hemodialysis patients.[54] Most CAPD patients gain weight.

Recommendations for protein intake vary but normally are in the range of 1.0 to 1.5 g of protein (largely of high biologic value) per kg body weight per day. Kilocalorie intake should be at least 35 kcal/kg of ideal body weight per day. These estimates must be adjusted for body size and activity and for concurrent illnesses. As appetite improves in CAPD patients, obesity can occur. It is important to control the weight gain sufficiently early. Glucose absorbed from the dialysate may contribute to the gain. In addition, CAPD patients may have improved amino acid metabolism[55] and protein utilization and achieve positive nitrogen balance more readily.[56]

Triglyceride levels tend to remain high, for which several explanations have been offered:[53]

1. In the dialysate, an alpha-1-acid-glycoprotein, a cofactor for lipoprotein lipase, is lost.
2. Unlike patients receiving hemodialysis, peritoneal dialysis patients do not routinely receive heparin, which is a clearing factor.
3. Protein losses to the dialysate and increased glucose absorption may contribute to hyperlipidemia.
4. Patients may continue their former high-fat, high-carbohydrate diet.
5. It may be an unexplained side effect of the treatment.

In order to control triglyceride levels, it has been suggested that the carbohydrate in the diet be reduced and the polyunsaturated fat level be increased (see Chapter 8 for the rationale).[53] The effectiveness of this procedure is unknown.

Water-soluble vitamins may be lost in the dialysate. Recommendations for supplements are similar to those for hemodialysis patients.[53,55] *Vitamin D* supplements may also be indicated.

In IPD, *sodium* and *fluid* may be restricted in the same amounts as for hemodialysis. If the patient persists in a higher sodium intake, more frequent dialyses may be necessary. In addition, if the glucose content of the dialysate is increased, more water can be removed as a result of its higher osmotic effect. In contrast, CAPD patients may not need fluid, sodium, or potassium restriction, and some patients may require added salt to prevent hypotension.[56]

Serum phosphorus levels have been found to be elevated in both IPD and CAPD patients. Phosphorus uptake is limited by reducing the intake of dairy products and by using phosphate binders. Dietary phosphorus restriction makes possible a reduction in the dosage of phosphate binders, which cause constipation.[57] However, most high-protein foods contain phosphorus, and so phosphorus cannot be severely restricted without creating the hazard of protein depletion.

Acid-base balance is almost completely corrected by CAPD. The continuously available lactate in the dialysate can be converted to bicarbonate. Bicarbonate levels are higher in CAPD patients than in patients on hemodialysis or IPD.

Renal Transplantation. Transplantation of a healthy kidney from a donor to a patient in renal failure is very desirable for most patients, since the transplanted kidney more adequately performs the excretory and endocrine functions of the kidney than does dialysis. In addition, a transplanted kidney frees the patient from the time-consuming demands of intermittent dialysis. However, not all uremia patients are candidates for transplants. Risk factors include advanced age, malignancy, and infection. The availability of donor organs also is limiting. The transplanted kidney is implanted into the pelvis, not in the normal location of a kidney.

Donors may be either living relatives or cadavers. When a transplant is planned, *histocompatibility testing* (tissue typing) determines the amount of similarity or dissimilarity between the donor's and recipient's antigens. The donor-recipient matches are graded A (best) to E. Grade A indicates *HLA identity.* It is not common but exists in identical twins and sometimes occurs in other siblings. Not all antigens are identified in tissue typing, so it is possible for even a grade A–matched kidney to be rejected.

Failure of a transplant usually is the result of acute tubular necrosis or immune rejection, indicated by increased plasma creatinine, decreased urine volume, proteinuria, and hypertension. Patients are treated with immunosuppressant drugs to avoid rejection. The dose is reduced in time but must be continued for life.

Nutritional care of the transplant patient is divided into three periods: preparation for transplant, care in the early posttransplant period, and long-term posttransplant care.

In preparation for a transplant, it is important to avoid malnutrition during the periods of conservative management and hemodialysis. General nutritional care for surgery patients in the immediate postoperative period is described in Chapter 12. This must be integrated with specific needs of the transplant patient, since the patient is undergoing major surgery and will be treated with high doses of immunosuppressive agents.

Transplant patients usually are given *prednisone,* a corticosteroid, to suppress the inflammatory response and *azathioprine* to reduce the cellular immune response. Some side effects of these drugs, relevant to nutritional care, are listed in Table 7-6 with appropriate nutritional care procedures which must be integrated with the other diet modifications needed by the patient.

In the early postoperative period, transplant patients usually receive clear liquids for the first meal and progress to solid foods as tolerated thereafer. The specific diet order will depend on how well the transplanted kidney is functioning. The procedures for nutritional care vary from one transplant center to another and may be liberal or conservative. The following guidelines are examples of those in use, giving the liberal approach first, followed by a more conservative policy. The nutritional care specialist will follow the policies of the institution.

If renal function is adequate, as indicated by urine volume and specific gravity, blood levels of nitrogen metabolites, and a renal scan, a *sodium* content of 2 to 5 g may be prescribed. If renal function is poor, due to rejection or acute tubular necrosis, the sodium level is decreased to the extent indicated by increased serum sodium, diminished urine output, and weight gain. *Fluid* intake also is restricted. At more conservative institutions, the protocol provides a more severely restricted sodium intake, perhaps 500 mg, for the first few days. When the graft begins to function, a diuretic phase ensues, and the diet is liberalized as tolerated. Fluid also is restricted to 600 ml plus urine volume until the onset of the diuresis.

Serum *potassium* concentrations are used as guidelines for determining dietary potassium. Potassium is restricted only if serum potassium rises and if urine output decreases below 100 ml/day. In a more conservative approach, potassium intake is limited to 40 to 50 mEq/day until the onset of diuresis

Table 7-6. Some Associated Side Effects and Possible Nutritional Implications of Immunosuppression[a]

Side Effects of Specific Immunosuppressants[b]	Common Dietetic Considerations
Azathioprine (Imuran)	
Severe bone marrow depression	All foods served by reverse precaution or precaution technique when leukocyte count is extremely low
Infection (fungal, protozoal, viral, and uncommon bacteria)	Small frequent feedings—high-protein, high-energy foods
Toxic hepatitis or biliary stasis	Modified fat diet
Nausea, anorexia	Small frequent feedings
Diarrhea, vomiting	Fluid and electrolyte replacement
Steatorrhea	Low-fat diet
Negative nitrogen balance	High-protein, high-energy foods
Prednisone	
Sodium retention	Moderate to low sodium intake
Potassium loss	High-potassium foods
Peptic ulcer	Avoid caffeine, alcohol, pepper
Pancreatitis	Moderate to low fat intake
Abdominal distension	Small frequent feedings
Ulcerative esophagitis	Modified food consistency
Altered carbohydrate metabolism, manifestation of latent diabetes mellitus, higher insulin needs in patients with previous diabetes	Decreased concentrated sweets or American Diabetes Association diets
Negative nitrogen balance (secondary to protein catabolism)	High-protein, high-energy foods
Altered fat metabolism	Low-cholesterol or other appropriate diet for the specific type of hyperlipidemia

Adapted from Henry, R.R. The kidneys and urinary tract. In R.B. Howard and N.H. Herbold, Eds., *Nutrition in Clinical Care.* Copyright © 1978. Used with permission of McGraw-Hill Book Company, New York.

[a] The nutritional considerations stated here are general. As always, diets should be modified on an individual basis. Of course, kidney function also will influence the diet prescribed.

[b] *Physicians' Desk Reference,* 30th ed. Oradell, N.J.: Medical Economics, 1976, pp. 674, 1231–1235.

and then liberalized. Some patients need potassium supplements if diuresis is severe.

Because of the *protein* catabolism and negative nitrogen balance seen in transplant patients, protein usually is not severely restricted during the posttransplant period, even during rejection or tubular necrosis. Protein restriction may be required, however, if SUN rises and the patient shows symptoms of uremia. A more conservative approach begins with a 40-g protein diet with 1,500 kcal on the second postoperative day. The diet is increased as tolerated to 40 to 50 kcal/kg of ideal body weight per day and approximately 80 g of protein per day. Under ideal circumstances, this progression takes a week or so but is varied with the SUN concentration.

Whether the procedures in a given institution are liberal or more conservative, it is desirable to individualize the diet for each patient. If a transplant patient requires dialysis after surgery, the diet is somewhat more liberal and follows that for the chronic hemodialysis patient.

Over the long term, weight control is stressed because the patients have an increased appetite and a tendency to weight gain and body composition changes. The need for diet modification diminishes as drug dosage is decreased. Many transplant patients eventually need no diet modifications.

Table 7-7 provides an example of the guidelines for nutritional care of renal patients in one institution. It is important to remember that these are general guidelines only. The diet should be individualized for each patient.

Acute Renal Failure

Acute renal failure (ARF) refers to loss of the excretory functions of the kidney within a short time, a few minutes to days, with no opportunity for the adaptations seen in CRF. Usually, there is no previous history of impairment of renal function. It may, however, be superimposed on chronic renal disease by stress factors such as infection or dehydration. In contrast to CRF, it is reversible in some patients.

Etiology. The causes of ARF have been categorized as prerenal, intrarenal, and postrenal. *Prerenal failure* occurs as a result of decreased blood pressure which may follow hemorrhage, cardiac failure, dehydration, obstruction of renal arteries, use of vasodilating drugs, or abnormal sequestration of large amounts of body fluids. All of these factors decrease blood flow to the kidneys, resulting in a fall in the GRF.

Intrarenal failure can occur when the kidney tissue is damaged directly. Damage may be caused by nephrotoxic drugs or other chemicals and by antigen-antibody reactions. Hemolysis of blood, as from a mismatched transfusion, releases hemoglobin, which may precipitate in and injure the renal tubules. Crushing injuries and burns also cause release of hemoglobin and of myoglobin from damaged muscles, adding to the damage from ischemia. The mechanism of hemoglobin and myoglobin damage is not understood entirely. Additional intrarenal causes include acute glomerulonephritis, vasculitis, hypercalcemia, and hepatorenal syndrome, a disease of the liver that also damages the parenchymal tissue of the kidney.

Postrenal failure (*obstructive nephropathy*) results from obstruction to the excretion of urine. Obstructions may occur as a result of calculi, strictures, or malformations. As the hydrostatic pressure rises, it affects the tubule cells directly. It can also compress renal blood vessels, causing ischemia. When ARF is the result of ischemic or toxic injury, it is called *acute tubular necrosis* (ATN) or *acute tubular insufficiency.* The condition may affect the interstitium and the glomerulus as well as the tubules. Acute tubular necrosis is accountable for 80 percent of the cases of ARF.

Pathogenesis. The mechanisms by which ATN is produced are not understood entirely, but several explanations exist. Hypotension causes vasoconstriction in the kidney, particularly in the cortex. This could lead to the fall in the GFR that is seen in ATN. Damage to the tubules may occur as a result of ischemic hypoxia, which might, in turn, cause tubular edema, obstruction of tubules by cellular debris, and increased tubule cell permeability. It has also been suggested that tubular hypoxia results in decreased sodium reabsorption. When the sodium remaining in the tubule reaches the macula densa, it stimulates the release of renin and, via the renin-angiotensin system, precipitates a severe vasoconstriction and a decline in the GFR with further tubular damage.

Pathology. Two types of structural alterations have been observed. When nephrotoxic damage causes ATN, the proximal tubule cells are damaged but the basement membranes remain intact. In ATN caused by renal ischemia, there is patchy necrosis of the tubular epithelium and basement membrane throughout both proximal and distal tubules. Disruptions of the tubule cell result in openings between the tubular lumen and adjacent capillaries, loss of tubular secretory and reabsorptive functions, interstitial edema, and infiltration of inflammatory cells. Recovery is more rapid in nephrotoxic disease in which the basement membrane is intact.

Pathophysiology. Although in ARF there is a significant decline in tubular capacity for sodium and water reabsorption, oliguria usually is marked. The primary cause is believed to be a decrease in the GFR, which may be as low as 1 ml/min. The cause of the reduced GFR is not understood completely. It may follow vasoconstriction that results in decreased renal blood flow. The renin-angiotensin system possibly plays a role in

Table 7-7. Nutritional Recommendations for Various Stages and Treatments of Renal Failure

Nutrients and Electrolytes	Predialysis	Hemodialysis			Peritoneal Dialysis	Transplantation
		Average Adult Patient	Pediatric Patients	Diabetic Patients		
Maintenance calories	35–40 kcals/kg/day or BEE × 1.5	35–40 kcals/kg/day or BEE × 1.5	75–100 kcals/kg/day	35–40 kcal/kg/day or BEE × 1.5	35–40 kcal/kg/day or BEE × 1.5	35–40 kcal/kg/day or to maintain IBW
Protein	If GFR = 25 ml/min., no protein restriction If GFR = 20–25 ml/min., 1.3 g/kg/day If GFR = 15–20 ml/min., 1.0 g/kg/day If GFR = 10–15 ml/min., 0.7 g/kg/day If GFR = 4–10 ml/min., 0.5–0.6 g/kg/day	1 g/kg/day	1.5–2.0 g/kg/day	1 g/kg/day	1.5 g/kg/day	No restrictions; RDA = 0.8 g/kg/day
Carbohydrate	Unrestricted	Unrestricted	Unrestricted	50% of total kcal	Unrestricted	Unrestricted
Fat	Individualized	Individualized	Individualized	40% of total kcal	Individualized	Individualized

Sodium	Individualized (2 g)	Individualized (2–4 g)	Individualized (1–2 g)	Individualized (2–4 g)	Individualized	Individualized (2–5 g)
Potassium	Individualized (1.5–3.0 g)	Individualized (2–3 g)	Individualized (1–3 g)	Individualized (2–3 g)	Individualized	Usually unrestricted
Calcium	RDA (800–1,200 mg)	RDA (800–1,200 mg)	RDA (800 mg)	RDA (800–1,200 mg)	RDA (800–1,200 mg)	RDA (800–1,200 mg)
Phosphorus	Individualized	Individualized	Individualized	Individualized	Individualized	Individualized
Fluids	Equal to urine output	Individualized (500–1,000 cc)	Controlled by sodium intake	Individualized (500–1,000 cc)	Individualized (800–1,000 cc)	Individualized; usually unrestricted
Supplements	Individualized	General multivitamin (thiamin, riboflavin, niacin, pantothenic acid, pyridoxine, biotin); vitamins B_6, C, and folic acid	General multivitamin and vitamins B_6, C, and folic acid	General multivitamin and vitamins B_6, C, and folic acid	General multivitamin and vitamins B_6, C, and folic acid	Individualized

From Doris Dare, Department of Nutrition and Dietetics, University of California, San Francisco; Hospitals and Clinics, San Francisco, Calif. Compiled from information in Harvey, K.B., Blumenkrantz, M.J., Levine, S.E., and Blackburn, G.L. Nutritional assessment and treatment of chronic renal failure. *Am. J. Clin. Nutr.* 33:1586, 1980; Halliday, M.S., McHenry-Richardson, K., and Portale, A. Nutritional management of chronic renal disease. *Med. Clin. North Am.* 63:945, 1979; and the renal dietitians of the Renal Disease Network #3. Reproduced with permission.

BEE = basal energy expenditure; GFR = glomerular filtration rate; IBW = ideal body weight; RDA = Recommended Dietary Allowances.

producing the vasoconstriction, but this has not been proved. As a consequence of the low GFR, the patient retains sodium, water, nitrogen metabolites, and other waste products. A few patients produce a normal volume of urine (*high-output renal failure*). This occurs when the GFR is low but water reabsorption is even lower, so that urine volume appears to be satisfactory; however, retention of waste products occurs, since the total volume filtered is so small. The prognosis is better in high-output failure than in oliguria.

The onset of ARF follows exposure to the precipitating factor in 48 hours or less. Clinical manifestations include oliguria and sodium, water, potassium, and nitrogen retention. Potassium retention is a particular problem in ARF, an important difference from chronic failure. It is particularly severe in a patient whose renal failure was precipitated by extensive tissue damage with release of intracellular potassium. As the renal failure becomes more severe, clinical manifestations appear in other organ systems, including the central nervous system, gastrointestinal tract, and cardiovascular system. These manifestations are similar to those seen in CRF.

Clinical Course and Prognosis. The overall mortality rate is 40 to 50 percent but varies greatly depending on the cause. Obstruction to urine outflow or the renal blood supply may be corrected by surgery. The patient then may recover completely, since renal tubule cells are capable of regeneration. Other patients may make a partial recovery but then progress to severe chronic renal disease over a long period.

The clinical course is extremely variable. In ATN, it may be divided into three phases:

1. Oliguric phase: The urine volume is 400 to 500 ml/day or less for periods up to several weeks, with hematuria, proteinuria and isosthenuria.
2. Diuretic phase: As the patient begins to recover, he or she progresses to the diuretic phase. Urine flow increases, but the reabsorptive capacity of the tubules may still be depressed. As a result, urea clearance may still be decreased. Serum urea nitrogen and serum creatinine then remain high during part of this period.
3. Recovery phase: The patient may have some degree of decreased renal function for months. Others never fully recover.

Nutritional Management. In addition to identification and treatment of the underlying cause, protection from infection, and bed rest, the condition, if it persists more than a week, is treated by dialysis. Recent experience indicates that dialysis improves the survival rate.

Although it seems reasonable to assume that good nutrition will improve the survival rate of ARF patients, there are no unequivocal data to support this assumption. Patients with ARF often are incapable of oral intake and must be fed by tube or intravenously. A special tube feeding formula, Amin-Aid, is available for patients with renal disease (see Appendix L). Information on parenteral feeding of renal patients is included in Chapter 12. If the condition is mild or if dialysis is not available and the patient is capable of oral intake, a more *conservative management* with modification of the diet and fluids can be used. Essential features of the diet used in conservative management during the oliguric phase are as follows:

Sodium and fluid. If the patient is dehydrated, normal fluid balance must first be restored (see Chapter 12). As indicated in CRF, fluid intake is limited to the volume of urine output plus 500 ml/day for insensible losses, plus other measurable losses such as from drainage or vomiting. Metabolic processes produce approximately 400 ml of water per day, which must be considered as part of the intake. Some fluid must also be reserved for use by the nursing service in giving medication.

Sodium often is restricted to 20 to 40 mEq/day. Only enough sodium to replace losses is given. If fluid and sodium intake are appropriate, the patient whose caloric intake is severely depressed will lose 0.25 to 0.5 kg of body weight per day, and plasma sodium levels will be normal. The patient should be weighed daily. Weight gain indicates fluid retention and is counteracted with further fluid and sodium restriction to avoid congestive heart failure.

Energy. Ideally, kilocalories are provided in sufficient amounts to prevent protein catabolism. However, most ARF patients are severly catabolic. A 3,000-calorie diet for an adult is a useful objective, but is attained only occasionally and with difficulty. The amount of food that can be eaten is often limited by anorexia, nausea, and vomiting in the patient, and by the water content of the food in relation to the fluid restriction. As a result, the weight loss previously described is a common occurrence. Kilocalorie intake is improved with the use of protein-free, low-electrolyte, high-carbohydrate liquid supplements (see appendix K), hard candy, or "butterballs," a flavored butter and sugar mixture.

Protein. In the adult who does not have a catabolic condition such as traumatic injury, major surgery, or burns, protein intake is limited to 0.25 g/kg of body weight per day to minimize the azotemia. The protein should be of high biologic value. The patient who is severely catabolic, as indicated by an SUN value of 100 mg/day or more plus elevated serum potassium and acidosis, is given more protein. Severely catabolic patients are those for whom dialysis is indicated.

Potassium. Hyperkalemia develops rapidly as a result of decreased excretion, increased release of intracellular potassium during tissue breakdown, presence of blood at abnormal sites, and infection. A diet limited to 25 to 40 mEq of potassium to prevent hyperkalemia until urine volume increases during recovery is needed if the patient is fed orally. Uncontrollable hyperkalemia is an indication for dialysis.

Other electrolytes. An additional diet modification sometimes recommended for patients with ARF is restriction of dietary phosphate. Since a low-phosphate diet is poorly accepted, phosphate-binding antacids usually are used instead. Medications are commonly used also, instead of diet modification, for treatment of the accompanying hyperuricemia and hypocalcemia.

If the patient is being dialyzed, a more liberal diet is possible. During the diuretic phase, too, the diet is liberalized. Protein should be restricted until serum urea and creatinine fall. Frequently, high potassium intakes are required to replace potassium lost in diuresis. Fluid and sodium may be allowed as desired, since the patient's thirst is a useful guide to fluid and sodium intake during the diuresis phase.

Glomerulopathy

The term *glomerulopathy* includes a group of conditions in which the disease process begins in the glomerulus. Glomerulopathies have been categorized on the basis of their etiology when this is known, on the basis of morphological changes seen in biopsy specimens, and according to their symptoms and clinical manifestations. Such methods of categorization have resulted in a number of variable, and sometimes confusing, classifications. Our concern is with those glomerulopathies classified as *glomerulonephritis,* in which nutritional care is of particular importance.

Etiology and Pathogenesis

Glomerulonephritis frequently occurs following an infection and may also occur as part of the total clinical picture of a number of systemic diseases, including lupus erythematosus, Goodpasture's syndrome, hereditary nephritis (Alport's syndrome), and diabetes mellitus.

It now is believed that most, if not all, of the glomerulonephritides are the result of an immune response.[58-60] There are two general types of immune reactions that have been described.[61] In *immune complex glomerulonephritis,* an antibody is formed in the bloodstream in response to a bacterial or viral infection, to a foreign protein, or to the patient's own tissue in an autoimmune disease. An antigen-antibody-complement complex is formed and becomes trapped in the glomerulus when the circulatory system carries it to the kidney. Poststreptococcal glomerulonephritis is the most commonly occurring example of this form of the disease. In a smaller number of patients, antibodies to the glomerular basement membrane (GBM) develop and form a complex with the GBM and with complement. This is called *anti-GBM disease.* The reason for the development of antibodies to basement membrane is unknown. A classic example of anti-GBM disease is Goodpasture's syndrome. In this syndrome, the antibodies also react with basement membranes of alveoli of the lung, which may be antigenically similar.

In either type of disease, complement is transformed into a chemotactic factor that attracts neutrophils. The neutrophils attach to the GBM and damage it by releasing proteolytic enzymes and other mediators of inflammation.

Some forms of glomerulonephritis may not involve the immune system but instead may result from coagulation with deposition of fibrin in the capillaries, or from a dysfunction of the mesangium,[62] metabolic defects, or hereditary factors. Immune complex disease is thought to account for approximately 70 percent of the cases, anti-GBM disease for approximately 5 percent, and all other causes for the remaining 25 percent.

Pathology

The pathologic changes in the glomerulus in acute glomerulonephritis are characteristically (1) *proliferation* of epithelial, endothelial, or mesangial cells, (2) *exudation* of neutrophils in the glomerulus, and (3) *necrosis* of glomerular capillaries. The degree to which each of these appears is variable, as is the location. The lesions may be *diffuse,* involving all glomeruli, or *focal,* involving only some. They also may be *local* or *segmented* —that is, involving only parts of the affected glomeruli.

Proliferative changes also are seen in chronic glomerulonephritis. In addition, *membranous* changes, in which the basement membrane becomes thickened, frequently occur. Other chronic lesions include sclerosis, hyalinization, and scarring. Chronic insults may cause tubular damage and scarring in the interstitium (the space between the nephrons).

Acute Glomerulonephritis

Acute glomerulonephritis is most commonly the result of an infection with a type 4 or type 12 strain of *Streptococcus.* There are other causes, including other organisms and hypersensitivity. Sometimes the cause is unknown.

Clinical Manifestations. Clinical manifestations of acute glomerulonephritis include *hematuria, oliguria, proteinuria, hypertension,* and *edema.* The red blood cells and protein in the urine may coagulate and form plugs or *casts.* These may be washed out in the final urine by the force of the pressure of the filtrate behind them. The presence of casts sometimes is called *cylindruria* because the casts are cylindrical in shape. If a cast does not wash out, the nephron or nephrons "upstream" from it cease to function. The GFR is reduced and sometimes tubular function also is depressed.

Treatment. No specific treatment is certain to alter the course of the disease. Currently available treatment is intended to maintain the patient until recovery occurs from natural processes. The usual procedures include bed rest during the acute stage, with gradual ambulation during the recovery phase. Drug treatment may include antibiotics given to remove sources of antigen if the etiology of the disease so indicates. Hypertension is treated by the physician with those antihypertensive agents that do not reduce renal blood flow. Diuretics and digitalis may be useful in the treatment of edema and congestive heart failure. Glucocorticoids and cytotoxic drugs are used in some forms of the disease. The nutritional care specialist must be alert to possible drug-nutrient interactions when patients are receiving these drugs.

There is some controversy concerning the need for diet modification, but the following procedures sometimes are used.[63]

Fluid and sodium. Fluid retention, indicated by edema formation, oliguria, and weight gain of more than 3 kg, may be treated by restriction of sodium and fluid on the same basis as is used in chronic and acute renal failure. Oral fluids are limited to 500 ml/day plus the volume of urine output for the previous day. Sodium is limited to 500 mg or less.

Protein. Dietary protein restriction does not alter the course of acute glomerulonephritis; however, a moderate restriction, 40 to 70 g/day, for the azotemic patient sometimes is recommended until there is assurance that the patient is not developing renal failure.[61]

Potassium. Potassium restriction occasionally is indicated as a precaution against hyperkalemia when the patient is oliguric.

Clinical Course. Acute glomerulonephritis varies greatly in the severity of the attack and its further consequences. Most children and 50 to 75 percent of adults have a complete recovery. The course of the disease in the remaining patients appears to follow one of three forms: (1) progression to *chronic glomerulonephritis,* (2) rapid progression to *subacute glomerulonephritis* with nephron destruction and subsequent renal failure in 1 to 2 months, or (3) development of *acute renal failure.*

Chronic Glomerulonephritis

Chronic glomerulonephritis may follow as a consequence of acute poststreptococcal glomerulonephritis, but there are other etiologic factors. It is believed that, because it is so diverse in nature, chronic glomerulonephritis is not a single disease but is, instead, a group of conditions with some characteristics in common. Proteinuria and hematuria commonly occur. If proteinuria is not accompanied by symptoms of protein loss, probably no diet modification is needed. Many patients have *nephrotic syndrome* during the course of the disease. Nutritional care in this condition is reviewed in the next section.

There may be a long latent period, but nephron destruction progresses. Chronic renal failure may ensue in 10 years or more, and it is treated as previously indicated (see pp. 232–250).

Nephrotic Syndrome

Definition and Etiology. The nephrotic syndrome is not a single disease but is, instead, a combination of symptoms that occurs in relation to a number of renal and systemic diseases. Some of these diseases are listed in Table 7-8.

Clinical Manifestations. Nephrotic syndrome is commonly defined by the following clinical manifestations and symptoms. Other symptoms also occur, but vary in incidence and nature depending on the etiology.

Proteinuria. Proteinuria is present, with values of 3.5 g of protein or more per day up to as high as 30 g/day. Normal urinary protein is 150 mg/day or less, commonly 40 to 80 mg. The proteinuria apparently results from an increased permeability of the basement membrane, which allows the loss of protein into the glomerular filtrate. The

Table 7-8. Selected Causes of the Nephrotic Syndrome

Intrinsic renal disease
- Lipid nephrosis
- Membranous nephropathy
- Proliferative glomerulonephritis, acute or chronic
- Membranoproliferative glomerulonephritis
- Focal sclerosing glomerulonephritis
- Hereditary nephritis (Alport's syndrome)
- Congenital nephrotic syndrome
- Homograft rejection
- Nephrotoxins
  - Compounds of mercury
  - Bismuth
  - Gold
- Allergens
  - Bee stings
  - Pollen
  - Poison oak, poison ivy
- Drugs
  - Penicillamine
  - Anticonvulsants
  - Probenecid

Systemic diseases affecting the glomerulus
- Metabolic diseases
  - Amyloidosis
  - Diabetes mellitus
  - Myxedema
- Collagen vascular disease
  - Systemic lupus erythematosus
  - Periarteritis nodosa
  - Goodpasture's syndrome
  - Dermatomyositis
  - Schönlein-Henoch purpura
  - Erythema multiforme
- Infectious diseases
  - Syphilis
  - Malaria
  - Hepatitis B
  - Bacterial endocarditis
  - Cytomegalic inclusion disease
- Malignancies
  - Hodgkin's disease
  - Multiple myeloma
  - Carcinoma
  - Lymphocytic leukemia

Systemic diseases altering renal hemodynamic relationships (with severely increased renal venous pressure)
- Renal vein thrombosis
- Inferior vena cava stenosis or thrombosis
- Tricuspid insufficiency
- Cor pulmonale
- Constructive pericarditis
- Pulmonary artery thrombosis
- Severe congestive heart failure

From Schrier R.W., and Guggenheim, S., Nephrotic syndrome. In G.W. Thorn, R.D. Adams, E. Braunwald, et al., Eds. *Harrison's Principle of Internal Medicine,* 8th ed. Copyright © 1977. Used with permission of McGraw-Hill Book Company, New York.

mechanism of increased permeability is not understood completely. The size of the protein molecule in comparison to the size of pores through which they are filtered in the glomeruli seems to be of some significance.[62] In renal disease, the pores may enlarge, allowing protein molecules to be filtered; however, additional factors apparently are important.

There is some evidence that abnormal T-lymphocytes produce a factor that alters permeability of the glomerulus to protein.[64,65] Alternatively, it has been suggested that negative electric charges exist on the foot processes of the glomerular epithelium,[66,67] the loss of which permits the proteinuria of nephrotic syndrome.[67] Changes in hemodynamics also may cause proteinuria, even in the absence of alterations in glomerular permeability.[68]

Albumin is lost in the largest quantity, with relatively smaller losses of other proteins, such as gamma globulin, transferrin, ceruloplasmin, and thyroxine-binding protein. The protein loss is apparently the primary disease process, and the other abnormalities develop as a consequence.

Hypoproteinemia. Hypoproteinemia can be severe, with the serum protein concentration as low as 1 g/dl. To some extent, this is attributable to the urinary losses. However, the liver has been shown to be capable of synthesizing 50 g of albumin per day. It could provide replacement if urinary loss were the only abnormality. The presence of hypoalbuminemia in patients losing less than 50 g/day suggests that there are other modes of loss. One of these is increased catabolism of protein, which occurs in the tubule cells of the kidney.[69–72] In addition,

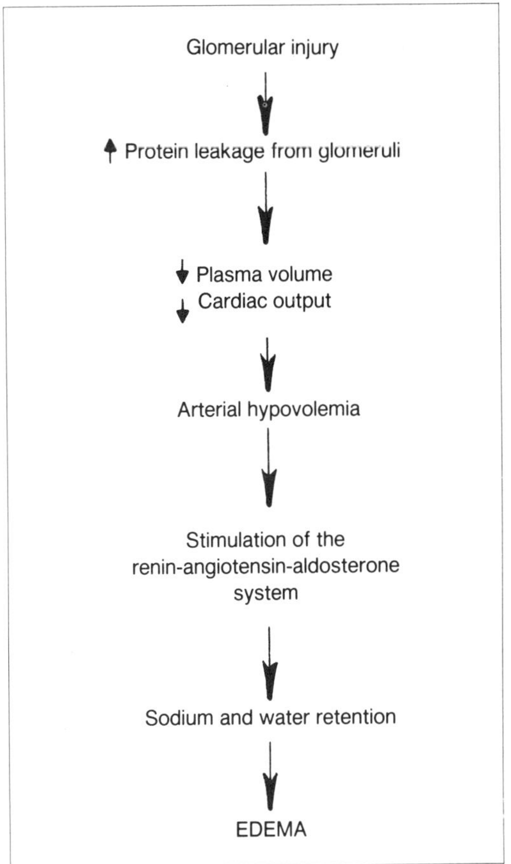

Figure 7-8. Physiologic processes leading to edema formation in nephrotic syndrome.

there is some evidence of loss by migration of protein out of the blood vessels.[73]

Edema. Edema often is the first manifestation noted by the patient and varies from slight to incapacitating. As serum albumin concentration falls, the colloid osmotic pressure falls, with transudation of fluid from the circulatory system to the interstitial space. The reduction in circulatory volume (*hypovolemia*) decreases renal blood flow and blood pressure, stimulating the renin-angiotensin-aldosterone system and resulting in increased retention of sodium and water by the distal tubules (*secondary hyperaldosteronism*). The retained sodium and water also leak into the interstitial space, aggravating the edema, until the increased hydrostatic pressure limits further edema formation. The mechanism is summarized in Fig. 7-8.

The edema appears first in areas of low tissue turgor and is affected by gravity. Although the edema is generalized (*anasarca*), some patients have edema in the face, particularly around the eyes (*periorbital edema*), in the morning. Later in the day, the fluid shifts, and the feet and ankles are particularly affected (*pedal edema*). Fluid also accumulates in the pleural cavity, resulting in dyspnea in some patients.

Hyperlipidemia. Hyperlipidemia (see Chapter 8) also occurs commonly in the nephrotic syndrome, but it is not present invariably. Serum cholesterol levels sometimes are as high as 1,000 g/dl. Phospholipids and triglycerides are elevated. Total serum lipids sometimes reach 5,000 mg/dl. It has been suggested that hypoproteinemia enhances hepatic synthesis of lipids, contributing to the lipids in the blood.[74] Increased synthesis of lipoproteins by the liver and decreased lipid clearance have been demonstrated in animals.[75,76] Patients with long-standing nephrotic syndrome have an increased incidence of coronary artery disease to which these alterations in lipid levels may contribute.[77]

Lipiduria. Lipiduria, too, is found in nephrotic patients. The urine contains free fat, oval fat bodies, and fatty casts.

Other manifestations. Other complaints of nephrotic patients include *weakness, anorexia,* and *headaches. Oliguria* is common while edema fluid is accumulating. The protein loss can cause *fatty degeneration of the liver* and *tissue wasting,* especially of muscle and cartilage, but edema may mask the tissue wasting. The loss of protein reduces levels of a number of biologically active proteins and of protein-bound trace elements. The clinical significance of these changes is not known.

Treatment. The main elements of therapy for nephrotic syndrome are diet and the use of diuretic drugs. Some patients receive steroids and other drugs. Specifically, the management of the syndrome includes the following:

Diuretic drugs. Diuretic drugs increase the volume of urine produced by inhibiting tubular reabsorption of filtered sodium. They then induce a contraction of urine volume, which leads to a decrease in renal plasma flow and the GFR and an increase in function of the renin-angiotensin-aldosterone system. This counteracts the drug effect, and a new steady state with less fluid is established. The patient is more comfortable, but diuretics are not known to alter the course of the disease.

These drugs are useful in the management of several forms of renal disease, including nephrotic syndrome, renal failure, and renal calculi. In addition, they are of value in the management of other chronic conditions, such as hypertension, chronic congestive heart failure, and cirrhosis of the liver with ascites. Since diuretics are used more frequently in the management of hypertension, details of their action and a list of available drugs is given in Table 8-3 (pp. 286–287).

Moderate sodium restriction often is prescribed for the patient receiving diuretic drugs, but the diet need not be as restricted as it was before diuretics were available. Therefore, the diet now is more acceptable and patient compliance is improved. Moderate salt restriction makes it possible to reduce the drug dosage, thus moderating any side effects of the drug. The use of a severely sodium-restricted diet in combination with a potent diuretic may increase the risk of hyponatremia and ARF.

A side effect of diuretic action is an increase in potassium excretion by one of two mechanisms. Diuretics increase the release of aldosterone which stimulates potassium excretion, or they increase the amount of sodium reaching the distal tubules and collecting ducts, where it may be exchanged for potassium. Potassium depletion occurs in some patients if dietary intake is inadequate for replacement. Mild symptoms of depletion can often be avoided by increasing the intake of foods high in potassium. Potassium supplements often are given by medication if depletion becomes more marked. The question of supplements versus diet for this purpose is discussed in more detail under Diet.

Immunosuppressants. Immunosuppressants may be prescribed for patients with various glomerulopathies. Table 7-6 lists the side effects of some of these drugs and appropriate nutritional care.

Diet. Increased *protein* intake usually is necessary for the nephrotic patient. The diet should have sufficient protein to provide for current needs, including continuing losses, and to replace any deficit created by earlier losses. This protein should be of high biologic value to reduce the accumulation of nitrogenous metabolites. The amount of protein needed for these purposes and to produce a positive nitrogen balance usually is approximately 1.5 g/kg of body weight per day for an adult. With a higher protein intake, proteinuria also can be expected to increase; the protein in the diet needs to be increased to a level which takes this into account. If, however, the patient becomes severely azotemic, it will be necessary to decrease the protein intake.

It is important that sufficient nonprotein sources of *energy* be supplied so that protein is not catabolized to meet the patient's energy needs, particularly if the patient is azotemic. Provision for 50 to 60 kcal/kg of ideal body weight per day is desirable.

If the patient is anorexic, assurance of adequate energy intake becomes a particularly challenging problem. Those patients who are receiving steroid drugs, however, usually have good appetites.

The high levels of serum *lipids* and the increased incidence of cardiovascular disease have led to the suggestion that the diet be modified to decrease the hyperlipidemia (see Chapter 8).[78] Although this seems logical, there is as yet no evidence that nephrotic

Table 7-9. Procedures for Planning the High-Potassium Diet

Increase the intake of fruit and vegetables that are high in potassium. These are listed in most diet manuals.
Substitute whole grain for refined cereals.
Increase high-protein foods, particularly milk and fish.
Reduce the servings of refined foods.
Prepare foods to conserve the potassium content. Use small amounts of water or cook with dry heat.
With the physician's concurrence, use a potassium-containing salt substitute.

patients benefit by such treatment. The effect of another modification on the acceptability of the diet and, thus, on protein and energy intake must be considered.

The comparative values of *sodium restriction* and of the use of diuretic drugs in nephrotic syndrome is a matter of controversy. In general, if the edema is mild or moderate, a moderate sodium restriction to 800 to 1,600 mg, combined with diuretic medication is considered useful. If edema is severe, dietary sodium might theoretically be reduced to as low as 250 mg/day but only at the expense of reduced protein intake, since protein foods contain appreciable quantities of sodium. If the patient complies with the sodium restriction, generally no fluid restriction is necessary. High protein and low sodium levels are difficult to plan in the same diet and are incompatible at the extremes. In addition, the diets tend to be unappetizing. Some patients increase their food intake if they are provided with a substitute for a salt. When a choice must be made between increasing protein and further restricting sodium, it usually is considered more important to provide sufficient protein in the diet and use diuretics to correct the edema.

Potassium loss and resultant hypokalemia (serum potassium less than 3.5 mEq/L) can result from the use of furosemide and thiazides in renal patients and in patients taking such drugs for other conditions. Hypokalemia can occur, for example, in the many patients taking thiazides for control of hypertension. It is a frequent practice to prescribe potassium supplements as medication for these patients. These supplements have an extremely unpleasant taste and are gastric irritants which can be the cause of gastric ulcers. However, noncompliance with the drug prescription can be hazardous.

Increased potassium can be supplied by appropriate modification of the diet, as a safe and more palatable alternative. The procedures listed in Table 7-9 are appropriate general guidelines.

Diabetic Renal Disease

It has been estimated that 50 percent of child diabetics will develop serious renal disease and that renal disease contributes to mortality in 25 percent of maturity-onset diabetes cases.[79] A typical sequence of events includes proteinuria approximately 17 years following the onset of juvenile diabetes, azotemia and hypertension in 2 more years, and death in uremia or fluid overload 3 years later.[80] Typical lesions of the kidneys include hyalinization of the glomeruli and thickening of the mesangium and the basement membrane of the glomeruli, Bowman's capsule, and the tubules. Nodules often develop on the glomeruli.[81,82] The typical disease with nodules is called *Kimmelstiel-Wilson syndrome.*

It is assumed that the metabolic alterations in diabetes cause the renal disease in some way, but the specific mechanisms are unknown. It also is assumed that control of the diabetes will prevent, or at least delay, the progress of the disease. However, actual evidence on this point is very scanty.

The diabetic diet must be combined with the diet modifications indicated during the period of declining renal function. The reduction of protein intake is accompanied by increases in carbohydrate and fat, a recommendation that many diabetic patients find startling and sometimes disturbing.

As renal function diminishes, the half-life of insulin increases, so that the diabetes becomes less severe. It is believed that this occurs because the kidney excretes insulin more slowly and because decreased insulinase production by the diseased kidney results in prolonged insulin action and amelioration of the diabetes.

When a patient receives a renal transplant, the insulin requirement increases significantly as corticosteroids are given for immunosuppression. Approximately 1 year postoperatively, the patient returns to nearly the same severity of diabetes that existed prior to the onset of manifest renal disease. The patient's appetite and activity often increase considerably following transplant.

It is necessary to monitor the nutritional status of the patient frequently during these various stages of his or her disease. The diabetic diet must be adjusted carefully to meet the patient's changing needs and must be modified according to the renal disease.

Renal Calculi

Renal calculi are known also as *nephrolithiasis, urolithiasis,* or as *kidney stones.* They vary from the size of a grain of sand to a large staghorn calculus that fills the entire pelvis of the kidney. Renal calculi form when salts precipitate out of the urine. They almost always are composed of calcium (85 to 90 percent), uric acid (10 percent), or cystine (0.7 percent). Calcium crystallizes with oxalate and phosphate, or occurs as mixtures of oxalate and phosphate or in *struvite* ($MgNH_4PO_4$), which usually is mixed with carbonate-apatite.

Etiology

There are three specific conditions that are postulated to cause calculus formation.

1. The urine is supersaturated with two or more of the ions previously listed. These ions then precipitate out of solution to form a calculus. A reduced urine flow, increased excretion of the ions, and changes in pH may increase the tendency to calculus formation.
2. Crystallization occurs around some organic material in the urine.
3. There is a decrease in some materials in the urine which otherwise would inhibit calculus formation.

A metabolic disease that predisposes to calculus formation is found in approximately half of the patients. These metabolic diseases include cystinuria, gout, hyperoxaluria, and those that increase calcium excretion, such as hyperparathyroidism, some bone diseases, excessive intake of vitamin D, renal tubular acidosis, and idiopathic hypercalciuria. Idiopathic calciuria may be absorptive or renal in form.[83] It is proposed that, in absorptive hypercalciuria, intestinal calcium absorption is increased, leading to decreased PTH secretion and thence to decreased tubule reabsorption of calcium. As a consequence, calcium levels in the urine increase. In the renal form, the pathogenesis is proposed to consist of decreased calcium resorption in the tubules, resulting in increased PTH secretion, increased 1,25-dihydroxycholecalciferol production, and increased calcium absorption in the intestine; hypercalciuria ensues.

Hyperoxaluria occurs in short bowel syndrome. Bile salts and fatty acids increase the permeability of the colonic mucosa to oxalate. Fatty acids also form soaps with calcium which otherwise would reduce oxalate absorption by formation of calcium oxalate. As a consequence, oxalate absorption occurs with resultant hyperoxaluria. Hyperoxaluria never occurs if the colon has been removed.

Prolonged immobilization also promotes calcium excretion. Urolithiasis may occur as a complication of gastrointestinal disorders. In many other patients, the cause of the disease is unknown. There may be genetic involvement, since calculus formation is found to occur in more than one member of some families. Urinary obstruction and infection also are predisposing factors. Bacterial infections predispose to struvite calculi in particular.

Clinical Manifestations

Kidney stones grow on the papillary surface. While attached to the papilla, they may cause hematuria or be asymptomatic. When they break loose, they may cause mild abdominal or flank pain or an agonizingly painful "renal colic." Renal calculi tend to recur; 67 percent of patients have a recurrence within 10 years.

Treatment

Most calculi are passed spontaneously. Others must eventually be removed by surgery. It is common practice to try to reduce calculus formation by increasing water intake to 3 to 4 L/day, even though the effectiveness of this treatment is unknown. An intake of 250 ml/hr while awake and when the patient voids at night will achieve this. Most of the fluid should be water.[84] Further measures may be undertaken depending on the composition of the stone.

Calcium Oxalate Calculi. Thiazide diuretics increase calcium reabsorption and decrease calcium concentration in the filtrate. When extracellular fluid is depleted under the influence of the diuretic, the proximal tubules are stimulated to reabsorb water, sodium, chloride, and calcium. Thiazides also stimulate calcium reabsorption in the distal tubules.[79] Therefore, mild salt restriction may be helpful.

For most patients, calcium intake should not be restricted severely unless intake is significantly higher than normal, since calcium restriction increases oxalate absorption from the intestine and, thus, its excretion. A moderate restriction to 600 mg of calcium per day may be useful for patients with *absorptive* hypercalciuria who are allergic to thiazides, are young, or who have not formed many stones. The patient with renal hypercalciuria is not treated with reduced calcium, because these patients would be forced into negative calcium balance and bone demineralization. A simultaneous calcium and oxalate restriction may be helpful.

Table 7-10. Treatment of Enteric Hyperoxaluria

Stage 1. All patients
- Maximum fluid intake
- Low-oxalate diet

Stage 2. Treatment for specific abnormalities
- Steatorrhea
  - Low-fat diet (40–50 g)
  - Calcium supplement (1 g/day)
- Bile-acid diarrhea
  - Cholestyramine (4 g four times daily)
  - Taurine (e.g., to 4 g three times daily)[a]
- Metabolic acidosis and hypocitruria
  - Alkali replacement (60–120 mEq of base per day)
- Magnesium deficiency
  - Magnesium replacement (must often be given intramuscularly)
- Uric acid calculi or epitaxy with uric acid or urates
  - Allopurinol (300 mg every day)

Stage 3. Combinations of stage 2 based on multiple abnormalities present

Reprinted with permission from Smith, L.H., Enteric hyperoxaluria and other hyperoxaluric states. In F.L. Coe, B.M. Brenner, and J.H. Stein, Eds., *Contemporary Issues in Nephrology,* vol. 5. *Nephrolithiasis.* New York: Churchill Livingstone, 1980, p. 151.

[a] The effectiveness of taurine in suppressing the urinary excretion of oxalate has not been established.

Some patients have *oxalosis,* an inborn error of metabolism in which oxalate calculi are formed. Oxalate calculi also form in patients with Crohn's disease and those who have had a jejunoileal bypass for obesity. The formation of the stones apparently is related to changes in glycine metabolism as well as to increased absorption of oxalic acid.

Treatment of patients with oxalate calculi that occur as a complication of gastrointestinal disease (enteric hyperoxaluria) is summarized in Table 7-10. Treatment begins with stage 1 and progresses to succeeding stages if necessary.

Ascorbic acid is a precursor to oxalate production. Doses of ascorbic acid of 4 g/day or more increase oxalate excretion and the tendency to form oxalate calculi. Hence, it seems logical to avoid such massive doses.

A deficiency of pyridoxine, a cofactor in the transamination of glyoxylate to glycine, results in increased oxalate excretion. In a deficiency, glyoxylate may be metabolized to oxalate rather than glycine. Significant hyperoxaluria resulting from pyridoxine deficiency is rare, but supplements of 200 to 400 mg of pyridoxine per day have been used in treatment of idiopathic calcium oxalate calculi. The effectiveness of this procedure has not been studied.

Maintenance of acidity in the urine (pH 6 or less) increases the solubility of calcium salts. The results of attempts to accomplish this by using an acid-ash diet were disappointing. Methionine or ammonium salts as medications are considered to be more effective.

Calcium Phosphate Calculi. Patients with calcium phosphate stones should be given a diet moderately low in calcium. A diet moderately low in phosphate has also been recommended but may be somewhat hazardous. Inadequate phosphorus intake can cause an increase in citrate excretion and formation of citrate stones.[85]

Struvite (Triple Phosphate) Calculi. The staghorn calculi that may form from struvite must be removed surgically. Nutritional aspects of care to minimize further stone formation may include restriction of dietary phosphate. Acidification of the urine is desirable, but the acid-ash diet is not very useful for that purpose since the diet contains a high level of phosphorus.

Uric Acid Calculi. Causes of excess uric acid in the urine include renal failure, diabetic acidosis, some neoplastic disease, glycogen storage disease, Lesch-Nyhan syndrome, starvation, some blood diseases, and the use of some drugs.[85] Patients with these conditions have an increased tendency to form calculi.

In addition to the use of allopurinol and bicarbonate medication, uric acid calculi may be treated by maintaining an alkaline urine. This actually may dissolve the stone. Usually bicarbonate or citrate are administered for this purpose. The alkaline-ash diet, formerly used, is not effective. Production of uric acid may be limited by the use of a low-purine diet; however, patient compliance with such a diet was found to be poor, and so its use has been discontinued in favor of drug treatment.

Cystine Calculi. The patient with cystine calculi usually has congenital cystinuria. The urine flow should be maintained at a high level with increased water intake. Maintaining a urinary pH of 7.8 with bicarbonate or citrate medication increases cystine solubility and decreases stone formation.

Cystine is produced from the metabolism of methionine. Therefore, low-protein or low-methionine diets have been proposed as treatment, but results have been inconsistent, and the diets may be hazardous, since methionine is an essential amino acid. The avoidance of *excess* protein may be useful.

Case Study: Renal Failure

Mary McCartney, age 12, developed strep throat. A week later her ankles and eyelids were puffy and her urine was reddish brown. She was hospitalized with gross hematuria, 4+ proteinuria, and oliguria of 400 ml/day. Her blood pressure was 155/108, and the hemoglobin was 10.2 g/dl. She was given bed rest and a low-salt diet. In 10 days, Mary's blood pressure was 125/87, she had lost 6 kg of body weight, and albuminuria was 1+.

Fifteen years later, Mary noted that she had swollen ankles and felt tired at the end of the day. She had nocturia and had gained 10 lb. in 6 weeks. Her blood pressure was 150/95. A renal biopsy showed hyalinized and sclerosing glomeruli. Laboratory test results were as follows:

SUN	45 mg/dl
Serum creatinine	2 mg/dl
Creatinine clearance	15 ml/min.
Serum phosphorus	5.9 mg/dl
Serum calcium	8.3 mg/dl
Hemoglobin	9.9 g/dl
Hematocrit	33 percent
Serum sodium	144 mEq/L
Serum potassium	4 mEq/L
Serum albumin	3.5 g/dl
Urine specific gravity	1.01
Urine volume	1,500 ml/day
Proteinuria	2+

She was given a diet with 40 g of high-biologic-value protein, 2,500 kcal, and 43 mEq of sodium. Drugs prescribed were 60 mg of furosemide (Lasix) per day, aluminum hydroxide (Amphojel) to be taken with each meal, and dioctyl sodium sulfosuccinate (Colace) as necessary.

After several more years, Mary began to experience headaches, nausea, and vomiting, weight loss, hypertension, polyuria, and muscle cramps. The furosemide dosage was increased, and methyldopa (Aldomet), 250 mg three times daily, was added as an antihypertensive agent. A solution of sodium citrate and citric acid was prescribed to correct acidosis. However, the patient became anemic and was weak, irritable, drowsy, and forgetful. Laboratory results were:

SUN	112 mg/dl
Serum creatinine	10 mg/dl
Creatinine clearance	6 ml/min.
Serum potassium	5 mEq/L
Serum phosphorus	7 mEq/L
Blood pH	7.35
Proteinuria	3+

Mary was scheduled for dialysis three times per week. A diet with 60 g of protein, 2,000 kcal, a sodium intake of 150 mEq/day, 1,500 ml of fluid, and 75 mEq of potassium was prescribed. Folate, pyridoxine, ascorbic acid, water-soluble vitamins, and iron were given as supplements.

Exercises

1. Explain the rationale for the diet modifications used during the original infection.
2. Compare the laboratory results with normal values.
3. Which laboratory values indicate
   a. Problems with solute reabsorption? Problems with excretion?
   b. Problems with protein homeostasis?
   c. Decreasing ability of the renal tubules to regulate fluid balance?
4. Explain the purpose for each medication.
5. Explain the rationale for each diet modification during renal failure.
6. Explain the pathogenesis of the following clinical manifestations in this patient: nocturia; polyuria; anemia; proteinuria; sodium retention; increased serum potassium; decreased creatinine clearance; increased SUN; acidosis.

References

1. Bricker, N.S., Klahr, S., Lubowitz, H., and Rieselbach, R.E. Renal function in chronic renal disease. *Medicine* (Baltimore) 44:263, 1965.
2. Bricker, N.S. On the meaning of the intact nephron hypothesis. *Am. J. Med.* 46:1, 1969.
3. Bricker, N.S., Bourgoignie, J.J., and Weber, H. The renal response to progressive nephron loss. In B.M. Brenner and F.C. Rector, Jr., Eds., *The Kidney.* Philadelphia: W.B. Saunders, 1976.
4. Bricker, N.S. On the pathogenesis of the uremic state: An exposition of the 'trade off' hypothesis. *N. Engl. J. Med.* 286:1093, 1972.
5. Welt, L.G., Black, H.R., and Krueger, K.K., Eds. Symposium on renal toxins. *Arch. Intern. Med.* 126:773, 1970.
6. Feldman, H.A., and Singer, I. Endocrinology and metabolism in uremia and dialysis: A clinical review. *Medicine* (Baltimore) 54:345, 1974.
7. Avram, M.M. Parathyroid hormone in kidney failure. *Contrib. Nephrol.* 20:1, 1980.
8. Bergstrom, J., Furst, P., Josephson, B., and Noru, L.O. Improvement of nitrogen balance in a uremic patient by the addition of histidine to essential amino acid solutions given intravenously. *Life Sci.* (II) 9:787, 1980.
9. Kopple, J.D. Nutrition and the kidney. In R.B. Alfin-Slater and D. Kritchevsky, Eds., *Human Nutrition: A Comprehensive Treatise,* vol. 4. New York: Plenum, 1979. P. 409.
10. Giordano, C. Use of exogenous and endogenous urea for protein synthesis in normal and uremic subjects. *J. Lab. Clin. Med.* 62:231, 1963.

11. Giovannetti, S., and Maggiore, Q. A low nitrogen diet with proteins of high biological value for severe chronic uremia. *Lancet* 1:1000, 1964.
12. Varcoe, R., Halliday, D., Carson, E.R., et al. Efficiency of utilization of urea nitrogen for albumin syntheses by chronically uraemic and normal men. *Clin. Sci. Mol. Med.* 48:379, 1975.
13. Berlyne, G.M., Bazzard, F.J., Booth, E.M., et al. The dietary treatment of acute renal failure. *Q. J. Med.* 36:59, 1967.
14. Walser, M., Coulter, A.W., Dighe, S., and Crantz, F.R. The effect of ketoanalogues of essential amino acids in severe chronic uremia. *J. Clin. Invest.* 52:678, 1973.
15. Walser, M. Ketoacids in the treatment of uremia. *Clin. Nephrol.* 3:180, 1975.
16. Walser, M. Principles of keto acid therapy in uremia. *Am. J. Clin. Nutr.* 31:1756, 1978.
17. Meneely, G.R., and Battarbee, R.D. Sodium and potassium. *Nutr. Rev.* 34:225, 1976.
18. Contreras, R.J. Salt taste and disease. *Am. J. Clin. Nutr.* 31:1088, 1978.
19. Kopple, J.D., and Coburn, J.W. Metabolic studies of low protein diets in uremia: I. Nitrogen and potassium. *Medicine* (Baltimore) 52:583, 1973.
20. Atkin-Thor, E., Goddard, B.W., O'Nion, J., et al. Hypogcusia and zinc depletion in chronic dialysis patients. *Am. J. Clin. Nutr.* 31:1948, 1978.
21. Kopple, J.D., Mercurio, K.C., and Card, B.K. Florence: The Sixth International Congress of Nephrology, 1975, Abstract no. 906.
22. Spannuths, C.L., Warnock, L.G., Wagner, C., and Stone, W.J. Increased metabolic clearance of pyridoxal-5-phosphate in uremia. *Clin. Res.* 24:412A, 1976.
23. Raskin, N.H., and Fishman, R.A. Pyridoxine-deficiency neuropathy due to hydralazine. *N. Engl. J. Med.* 273:1182, 1965.
24. Slatopolsky, E., Caglar, S., Pennell, J.P., et al. On the pathogenesis of hyperparathyroidism in experimental chronic renal insufficiency in the dog. *J. Clin. Invest.* 50:492, 1971.
25. Slatopolsky, E., Caglar, S., Gradowska, L., et al. On the prevention of secondary hyperthyroidism in experimental chronic renal disease using "proportional reduction" of dietary phosphorus intake. *Kidney Int.* 2:147, 1972.
26. Hanley, D.A., and Sherwood, L.M. Secondary hyperthroidism in chronic renal failure. *Med. Clin. North Am.* 62:1319, 1978.
27. Massry, S.G. Is parathyroid hormone a uremic toxin? *Nephron* 19:125, 1977.
28. Maschio, G., Tessitore, N., D'Angelo, A., et al. Early dietary phosphorus restriction and supplementation in the prevention of renal osteodystrophy. *Am. J. Clin. Nutr.* 33:1546, 1980.
29. Alfrey, A.C., and Smythe, W.R. Trace element abnormalities in chronic uremia. In B.B. Mackey, Ed., *Tenth Annual Contractors Conference of the Artificial Kidney and Chronic Uremia Program of the National Institute of Arthritis, Metabolism, and Digestive Diseases* [AKCUP-NIAMDD]. DHEW Publication no. 77-1442. Bethesda, Md.: National Institutes of Health, 1977. P. 37.
30. De Fronzo, R.A., Andres, R., Edgar, P., and Walker, W.G. Carbohydrate metabolism in uremia: A review. *Medicine* (Baltimore) 52:469, 1973.
31. Dzurik, T., Niederland, T.R., and Cernacek, P. Carbohydrate metabolism by rat liver slices incubated in serum obtained from uraemic patients. *Clin. Sci.* 37:409, 1969.
32. Lowrie, E.G., Soeldner, J.S., Hampers, C.L., and Merrill, J.P. Glucose metabolism and insulin secretion in uremic, prediabetic and normal subjects. *J. Lab. Clin. Med.* 76:603, 1970.
33. De Fronzo, R.A., and Alvestrand, A. Glucose intolerance in uremia: Site and mechanism. *Am. J. Clin. Nutr.* 33:1438, 1980.
34. Maillet, C., and Garber, A.J. Skeletal muscle amino acid metabolism in chronic uremia. *Am. J. Clin. Nutr.* 33:1343, 1980.
35. Giordano, C., De Santo, N.G., Rimaldi, S., et al. Histidine for treatment of uremic anemia. *Br. Med. J.* 4:714, 1973.
36. Bagdade, J.D., Porte, D., Jr., and Bierman, E.L. Hypertriglyceridemia: A metabolic consequence of chronic renal failure. *N. Engl. J. Med.* 279:181, 1968.
37. Lindner, A., Charra, B., Sherrard, D., and Scribner, B.H. Accelerated atherosclerosis in prolonged maintenance hemodialysis. *N. Engl. J. Med.* 290:697, 1974.
38. Bonomini, V., Feletti, C., Scolari, M.P., et al. Atherosclerosis in uremia: A longitudinal study. *Am. J. Clin. Nutr.* 33:1493, 1980.
39. Holliday, M.A., McHenry-Richardson, K., and Portale, A. Nutritional management of chronic renal disease. *Med. Clin. North Am.* 63:645, 1979.
40. Campbell, J.D., and Campbell, A.R. The social and economic costs of end-stage renal disease. *N. Engl. J. Med.* 299:386, 1978.
41. Kopple, J.D., Shinaberger, J.H., Coburn, J.W., et al. Evaluating modified protein diets for uremia. *J. Am. Diet. Assoc.* 54:481, 1969.
42. Daubresse, J.C., Larson, G., Loomteax, G., et al. Lipids and lipoprotein in chronic urae-

mia. A study of the influence of regular hemodialysis. *Eur. J. Clin. Invest.* 6:159, 1976.

43. McCask, E.J. Hypertriglyceridemia in patients with chronic renal insufficiency. *Am. J. Clin. Nutr.* 28:1036, 1975.
44. Hussey, H.H. Hyperlipidemia in children following long term hemodialysis or renal transplantation. *J.A.M.A.* 236:1387, 1976.
45. Gokal, R., Mann, D.M., Oliver, D.O., and Ledingham, J.G.G. Dietary treatment of hyperlipidemia in chronic hemodialysis patients. *Am. J. Clin. Nutr.* 31:1915, 1978.
46. Sanfelippo, M.L., Swenson, R.S., and Reaven, G.M. Response of plasma triglycerides to dietary changes in patients on hemodialysis. *Kidney Int.* 14:180, 1978.
47. Epstein, F.H., and Merrill, J.P. Chronic Renal Failure. In G.W. Thorn, R.D. Adams, F. Braunwald, et al., Eds., *Harrison's Principles of Internal Medicine,* 8th ed. New York: McGraw-Hill, 1977.
48. Aeropoulos, D.G. Chronic peritoneal dialysis. *Clin. Nephrol.* 9:165, 1978.
49. Vaamonde, C.A. Peritoneal dialysis. Current status. *Postgrad. Med.* 62:148, 1977.
50. Blumenkrantz, M.J., Roberts, C.E., Card, B., et al. Nutritional management of the adult patient undergoing peritoneal dialysis. *J. Am. Diet. Assoc.* 73:251, 1978.
51. Moncrief, J.W., and Popovich, R.P. Continuous ambulatory peritoneal dialysis. *Contrib. Nephrol.* 17:139, 1979.
52. Giordano, C., and De Santo, N.G. Dietary management of patients on peritoneal dialysis. *Contrib. Nephrol.* 17:17, 1979.
53. Blumenkrantz, M.J., Kopple, J.D., and V.A. Cooperative Dialysis Study Participants. Incidence of nutritional abnormalities in uremic patients entering dialysis therapy. *Kidney Int.* 10:514, 1976.
54. Coburn, J.W., Blumenkrantz, M.J., and Kopple, J.D. *Controlled Evaluation of Maintenance Peritoneal Dialysis.* Technical report no. 2, AKCUP-NIAMDD. Bethesda, Md.: National Institutes of Health, 1977. P. 120.
55. Bergstrom, J. Introductory remarks: Potential metabolic problems associated with continuous ambulatory peritoneal dialysis. In M. Legrain, Ed., *Continuous Ambulatory Peritoneal Dialysis.* Amsterdam: Excerpta Medica, 1980.
56. Lindholm, B., Aklberg, M., Alvestrand, A., et al. Nutritional aspects of continuous ambulatory peritoneal dialysis. In M. Legrain, Ed., *Continuous Ambulatory Peritoneal Dialysis.* Amsterdam: Excerpta Medica, 1980.
57. Nold, J.M., Kellman, B., Jabaz, O., and Areopoulos, D.G. The dietary treatment of patients on continuous ambulatory peritoneal dialysis: Practical aspects. In M. Legrain, Ed., *Continuous Ambulatory Peritoneal Dialysis.* Amsterdam: Excerpta Medica, 1980.
58. Unanue, E.R., and Dixon, F.J. Experimental glomerulonephritis: Immunological events and pathogenetic mechanisms. *Adv. Immunol.* 6:1, 1967.
59. McClusky, R.T. Immunologic mechanisms in renal disease. In R.H. Heptinstall, Ed., *Pathology of the Kidney,* 2nd ed. Boston: Little, Brown, 1974.
60. Wilson, C.B., and Dixon, F.J. Diagnosis of immunopathologic renal disease. *Kidney Int.* 5:389, 1974.
61. Dixon, F.J. Glomerulonephritis and immunopathology. *Hosp. Pract.* 2:35, 1967.
62. Schrier, R.C. Glomerular diseases. In G.W. Thorn, R.D. Adams, F. Braunwald, et al., Eds., *Harrison's Principles of Internal Medicine,* 8th ed. New York: McGraw-Hill, 1977.
63. Wrong, O.M. Glomerulonephritis. In P.B. Beeson, W. McDermott, and J.B. Wyngaarden, Eds., *Cecil's Textbook of Medicine,* 15th ed. Philadelphia: W.B. Saunders, 1979.
64. Shalkoub, R.J. Pathogenesis of lipoid nephrosis: A disorder of T-cell function. *Lancet* 2:556, 1974.
65. Giangiacomo, J., Cleary, T.G., Cole, B.R., et al. Serum immunoglobulins in the nephrotic syndrome. *N. Engl. J. Med.* 293:8, 1975.
66. Brenner, B.M., Hostetter, T.H., and Humes, H.D. Molecular basis of proteinuria of molecular origin. *N. Engl. J. Med.* 298:826, 1978.
67. Blau, E.B., and Haas, D.E. Glomerular sialic acid and proteinuria in human renal disease. *Lab. Invest.* 28:447, 1973.
68. Bohrer, M.P., Dien, W.M., Robertson, C.R., and Brenner, B.M. Mechanism of angiotensin II–induced proteinuria in the rat. *Am. J. Physiol.* 2:F13, 1977.
69. Gitlin, D., Janeway, C.A., and Farr, L.E. Studies on the metabolism of plasma proteins in the nephrotic syndrome: I. Albumin, globulin and iron-binding globulin. *J. Clin. Invest.* 35:44, 1956.
70. Kaitz, A.L. Albumin metabolism in nephrotic adults. *J. Lab. Clin. Med.* 53:186, 1959.
71. Jensen, H., Rossing, N., Andersen, S.B., and Jarnum, S. Albumin metabolism in the nephrotic syndrome in adults. *Clin. Sci.* 33:445, 1967.
72. Strober, W., and Waldman, T.A. The role of the kidney in the metabolism of plasma proteins. *Nephron* 13:35, 1974.
73. Walker, W.A., Ulstrom, R.A., and Lowman, J.T. Albumin synthesis rates in patients with hypoproteinemia. *J. Pediatr.* 78:812, 1971.

74. Rosenman, R.H., Friedman, M., and Byers, S.O. The causal role of plasma albumin deficiency in experimental nephrotic hyperlipemia and hypercholesteremia. *J. Clin. Invest.* 35:522, 1956.
75. Radding, C.M., and Steinberg, D. Studies on the synthesis and secretion of serum lipoproteins by rat liver slices. *J. Clin. Invest.* 39:1560, 1960.
76. McKenzie, I.F.C., and Nestel, P.J. Studies on the turnover of triglyceride and esterified cholesterol in subjects with the nephrotic syndrome. *J. Clin. Invest.* 47:1685, 1968.
77. Berlyne, G.M., and Mallick, N.P. Ischaemic heart-disease as a complication of nephrotic syndrome. *Lancet* 2:399, 1969.
78. Eiser, A.R., and Swartz, C. Nephrotic syndrome—Current concepts. In E.L. Coodley, W.W. Oaks, D.A. Major, and K. Bharadwaja, Eds., *Internal Medicine Update 1979–80.* New York: Grune and Stratton, 1979–1980.
79. Goetz, F.C., and Kjellstrand, C.M. The treatment of diabetic kidney disease. *Diabetologia* 17:267, 1979.
80. Kussman, M., Goldstein, H., and Gleason, R. The clinical course of diabetic nephropathy. *J.A.M.A.* 236:1861, 1976.
81. Lendrum, A.C., Sidders, W., and Fraser, D. Renal hyaline: A study of amyloidosis and diabetic fibrinous vasculosis with new staining methods. *J. Clin. Pathol.* 25:373, 1972.
82. Kimmelstiel, P., and Wilson, C. Intercapillary lesions in the glomeruli of the kidney. *Am. J. Pathol.* 12:83, 1936.
83. Coe, F.L., Canterbury, J.M., Firpo, J.J., and Reiss, E. Evidence for secondary hyperparathyroidism in idiopathic hypercalciuria. *J. Clin. Invest.* 52:134, 1973.
84. Smith, L.H., Van den Berg, C.J., and Wilson, D.M. Nutrition and urolithiasis. *N. Engl. J. Med.* 298:87, 1978.
85. Maude, D.L. *Kidney Physiology and Kidney Disease.* Philadelphia: J.B. Lippincott, 1977.

Bibliography

Blumenkrantz, M.J., Roberts, C.E., Card, B., et al. Nutritional management of the adult patient undergoing peritoneal dialysis. *J. Am. Diet. Assoc.* 73:251, 1978.

Bricker, N.S., Klahr, S., Lubowitz, H., and Slatopolsky, E. The pathophysiology of renal insufficiency: On the functional transformations in the residual nephrons with advancing disease. *Pediatr. Clin. North Am.* 18:595, 1971.

Burton, B.T. Current concepts of nutrition and diet in diseases of the kidney: I. General principles of dietary management; II. Dietary regimen in specific kidney disorders. *J. Am. Diet. Assoc.* 65:623, 1974.

Early, L.E. Edema formation and the use of diuretics. *Calif. Med.* 114:56, 1971.

Frazier, H.S., and Yager, H. The clinical use of diuretics (in two parts). *N. Engl. J. Med.* 288:246, 455, 1973.

Guttmann, R.D. Renal transplantation (in two parts). *N. Engl. J. Med.* 301:975, 1038, 1979.

Guyton, A.C. *Textbook of Medical Physiology,* 6th ed. Philadelphia: W.B. Saunders, 1981.

Kopple, J.D. Nutritional therapy in kidney failure. *Nutr. Rev.* 39:193, 1981.

Kopple, J.D., Massry, S.G., Bonomini, V., and Heidland, A. Symposium on nutrition in renal disease. *Am. J. Clin. Nutr.* 33:1343, 1980.

Kopple, J.D., Massry, S.G., and Heidland, A. Symposium on nutrition in renal disease (in two parts). *Am. J. Clin. Nutr.* 31:1531, 1742, 1978.

Kopple, J.D., and Swendseid, M.E. Vitamin nutrition in patients undergoing maintenance hemodialysis. *Kidney Int.* [*Suppl.*] 2:79, 1975.

Legrain, M., Ed. *Continuous Ambulatory Peritoneal Dialysis.* Amsterdam: Excerpta Medica, 1980.

Manis, T., and Friedman, E.A. Dialytic therapy for irreversible uremia (in two parts). *N. Engl. J. Med.* 301: 1260, 1321, 1979.

Merrill, J.P., and Hampers, C.L. Uremia (in two parts). *N. Engl. J. Med.* 282:953, 1014, 1970.

National Academy of Sciences. *Sodium Restricted Diets and the Use of Diuretics: Rationale, Complications and Practical Aspects of Their Use.* Washington, D.C.: National Research Council, 1979.

Nolph, K.D., Gahl, G.M., Kessel, M. *Advances in Peritoneal Dialysis. Proceedings of the Second International Symposium on Peritoneal Dialysis.* Berlin, June 16–19, 1981. Amsterdam: Excerpta Medica, 1981.

Papper, S. *Clinical Nephrology,* 2nd ed. Boston: Little, Brown, 1978.

Valtin, H. *Renal Dysfunction: Mechanisms Involved in Fluid and Solute Imbalance.* Boston: Little, Brown, 1979.

Vander, A.J. *Renal Physiology,* 2nd ed. New York: McGraw-Hill, 1980.

Sources of Current Information

Clinical Nephrology
Contributions to Nephrology
Kidney International
Nephron

8. The Cardiovascular System

- I. The Normal Circulatory System
  - A. Normal anatomy
    - 1. Heart
    - 2. Vascular system
      - a. systemic circulation
      - b. pulmonary circulation
      - c. circulation to specific areas
        - (1) coronary
        - (2) cerebral
        - (3) portal and splanchnic
        - (4) fetal
    - 3. Blood vessels
  - B. Normal cardiovascular function
    - 1. Cardiac output
    - 2. Peripheral vascular resistance
    - 3. Blood pressure
- II. Hypertension
  - A. Classification and pathogenesis
  - B. Risk factors
    - 1. Uncontrollable
    - 2. Controllable
      - a. sodium and potassium intakes
      - b. obesity
      - c. psychological factors
  - C. Pathophysiology of essential hypertension
  - D. Management
    - 1. Sodium-restricted diets
    - 2. Weight reduction
    - 3. Drugs
    - 4. Potassium
- III. Hyperlipidemia
  - A. Classification of lipoproteins
  - B. Cholesterol
  - C. Lipoprotein and cholesterol metabolism
    - 1. Exogenous transport system
    - 2. Endogenous transport system
    - 3. High-density lipoprotein
  - D. Effects of diet on serum lipids and lipoproteins
    - 1. Sterols and fats
      - a. dietary cholesterol and triglyceride
      - b. saturated and unsaturated fatty acids
    - 2. Excess calories
    - 3. Carbohydrate
    - 4. Alcohol
    - 5. Lecithin
    - 6. Protein
  - E. The hyperlipoproteinemias
    - 1. Classification and clinical features
    - 2. Lipoproteins, cholesterol, and atherosclerosis
    - 3. Management
      - a. nutritional management
      - b. drug treatment
- IV. Atherosclerosis
  - A. The lesion
    - 1. Early lesions
    - 2. Fatty streaks
    - 3. Fibrous plaques
    - 4. Complicated lesions
  - B. Pathogenesis
  - C. Etiology
  - D. Prevention
- V. Ischemic Heart Disease
  - A. Risk factors
  - B. Angina pectoris
    - 1. Clinical manifestations
    - 2. Diagnosis
    - 3. Management
  - C. Myocardial infarction
    - 1. Clinical manifestations
    - 2. Diagnosis
    - 3. Clinical course
    - 4. Management
- VI. Congestive Heart Failure
  - A. Pathogenesis
  - B. Salt and water retention
  - C. Clinical manifestations
  - D. Management
    - 1. Nutritional care
    - 2. Drugs
- VII. Cerebrovascular Disease
- VIII. Peripheral Vascular Atherosclerotic Occlusive Disease
- IX. Cardiac Cachexia
- X. Rheumatic Heart Disease
- XI. Congenital Heart Disease
- XII. Heart Disease and Alcoholism
- XIII. Pickwickian Syndrome
- XIV. Case Study

It is estimated that more than 28 million people in the United States have some form of cardiovascular disease, and diseases of the cardiovascular system are the leading cause of death. Although many questions remain concerning the cause, treatment, and prevention of the common cardiovascular diseases, it appears that nutrition is of major importance in both prevention and treatment.

THE NORMAL CIRCULATORY SYSTEM

The cardiovascular system consists of the heart and blood vessels. The heart pumps blood through the blood vessels and thereby transports oxygen, water, and nutrients to the body cells. It removes carbon dioxide and other waste products of cell metabolism for excretion and distributes endogenous metabolites within the body. In addition, the circulatory system is important in regulating body temperature.

Normal Anatomy

Heart

The heart, a hollow double pump, has a three-layered wall. The innermost layer, the *endocardium,* consists of squamous epithelium, which lines the interior hollows of the heart and forms the valves. The *myocardium* is the thick layer of underlying muscle, and the *pericardium* lines the outside of the heart. The pericardium also forms the lining of the pericardial sac containing the heart.

The two pumps in the heart each consist of an *atrium* and a *ventricle* so that the heart actually has four chambers. The right and left sides of the heart are separated by a *septum,* largely formed of myocardium. The part between the ventricles is called the *interventricular septum,* and that between the atria is the *interatrial septum.*

The route of the blood through the heart is shown in Fig. 8-1. Blood enters the heart from the systemic circulation at the right atrium, and passes through the *tricuspid* (or

Figure 8-1. The heart and great vessels and the route of blood flow through them. Dark shaded area indicates venous blood flow (low in oxygen). Light shaded area indicates arterial blood flow (high in oxygen). (Reprinted with permission from Memmler, R.L., and Rada, R.B., The Human Body in Health and Disease, *4th ed. Philadelphia: J.B. Lippincott, 1977, p. 172.)*

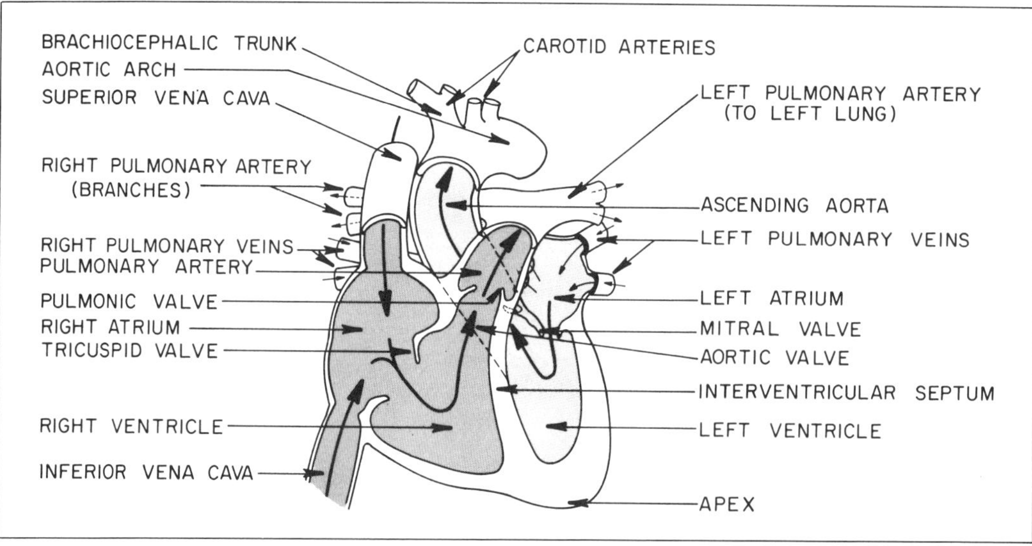

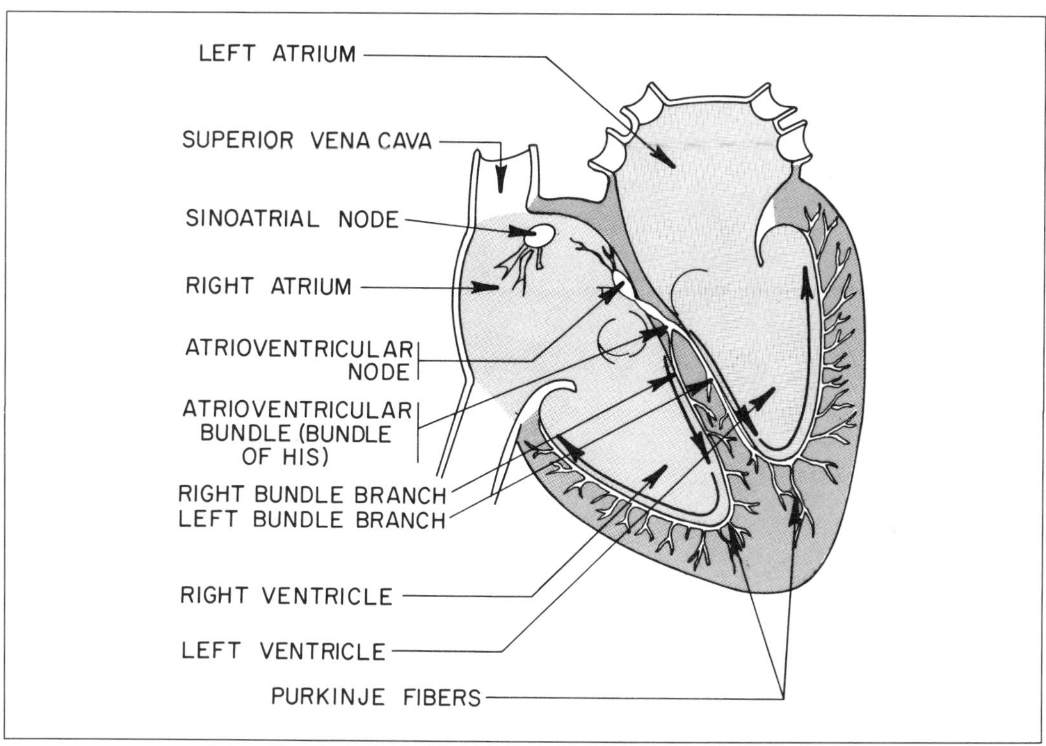

Figure 8-2. Conduction system of the heart: the Purkinje system. (Reprinted with permission from Memmler, R.L., and Rada, R.B., The Human Body in Health and Disease, *4th ed. Philadelphia: J.B. Lippincott, 1977, p. 175.)*

atrioventricular) valves to the right ventricle. The right ventricle pumps blood through the *pulmonic valves* to the *pulmonary arteries* and then to the lungs. Blood returns from the lungs via the four *pulmonary veins* to the left atrium. It then flows through the *mitral valves* into the left ventricle which, in turn, pumps the blood through the *aortic valves* into the *aorta* and thence back into the systemic circulation.

Specialized tissues in the wall of the heart form a conduction system (the *Purkinje system*) to stimulate the contraction of the cardiac muscle (Fig. 8-2). The *sinoatrial* (SA) *node,* in the upper wall of the right atrium, acts as a pacemaker. An electric impulse normally begins there and travels through the atrial muscles, causing them to contract, and also through bundles of *Purkinje fibers* in the *internodal pathway* to the *atrioventricular* (AV) *node* at the junction of the interatrial and interventricular septa. When the AV node is stimulated, it transmits the contraction wave via Purkinje fibers, which form the *atrioventricular bundle* (*bundle of His*). The *AV bundle* divides into *right* and *left bundle branches.* These subdivide further until Purkinje fibers terminate in a network in the subendocardial tissues of the ventricles. This conduction system makes it possible for the contraction of all parts of both ventricles to occur simultaneously. The changes in electric potential during the cardiac cycle are carried to the surface of the body by the body fluids and are recorded as an *electrocardiogram* (*ECG* or *EKG*).

Vascular System

Systemic Circulation. Blood is pumped by the left ventricle through the aorta (Fig. 8-3) to

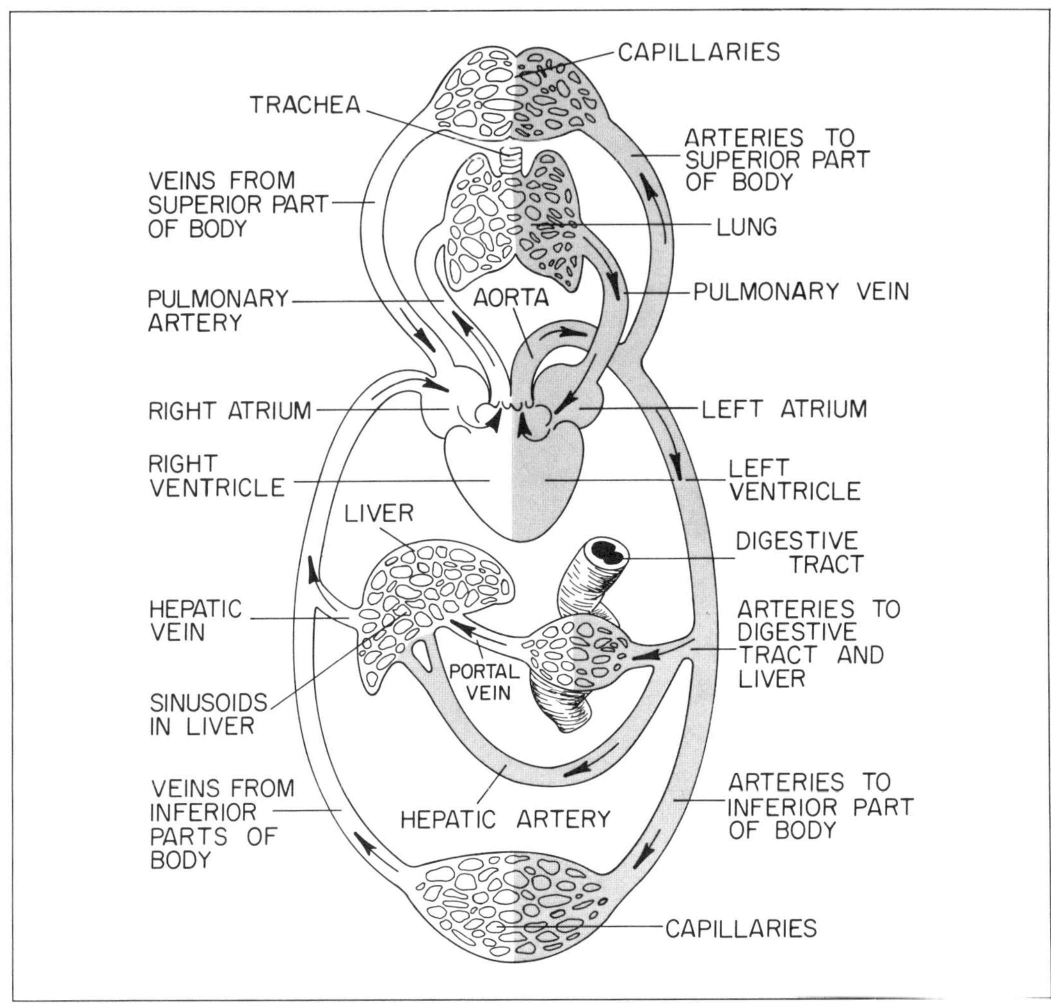

Figure 8-3. The pulmonary and systemic circulations in the adult human. Shaded areas indicate oxygenated blood; nonoxygenated blood is uncolored. Arrows indicate the direction of blood flow. (Reprinted with permission from Crouch, J.E., Functional Human Anatomy, *3rd ed. Philadelphia: Lea and Febiger, 1978, p. 404.)*

the large and medium arteries and thence to the arterioles. The arterioles branch into a network of capillaries in the brain, muscles, viscera, skin, and other tissues, including the heart itself. Blood in the capillaries then flows through the venules into successively larger veins and eventually into the vena cava, which drains into the right atrium. In total, this route is called the *systemic* or *major circulation.*

Pulmonary Circulation. The *pulmonary* or *lesser circulation* contains blood pumped from the right ventricle through the pulmonary arteries, arterioles, and capillaries of the lungs. Blood returns via venules and small and medium-sized veins to the large pulmonary veins to the left atrium of the heart.

Circulation to Specific Areas. The circulation to some organs or areas of the body is of particular importance in understanding cardiovascular diseases. These include coronary, cerebral, portal, and splanchnic circulations. Fetal circulation, too, is of special concern.

Coronary circulation. The heart itself must be supplied with blood. This blood is provided by three arteries that branch from the aorta. These arteries, collectively known as the *coronary circulation,* divide into arterioles and capillaries to vascularize the heart muscle, carrying approximately 5 percent of the cardiac output.

Cerebral circulation. The blood supply to the brain (*cerebral circulation*) contains approximately 15 percent of the cardiac output. Blood is supplied to the brain via the *internal carotid* and *vertebral arteries* which, along with connecting vessels, form an anastomosis known as the *circle of Willis* at the base of the brain. Three trunks, the *anterior, middle,* and *posterior cerebral arteries,* arise from the circle of Willis to supply each cerebral hemisphere.

Blood flow to the brain is relatively constant. It is thought to be regulated by local concentrations of oxygen and carbon dioxide. Excess carbon dioxide plays an important role in regulating cerebral blood flow, causing vasodilation as its concentration rises.

Portal and splanchnic circulations. The blood flow to the intestines and spleen and then through the portal vein to the liver is the *portal circulation.* If the arterial blood flow to the liver, stomach, and pancreas is included also, the total is the *splanchnic circulation.*

The splanchnic circulation can be reduced significantly during exercise when more blood is needed by the heart and skeletal muscles. In contrast, a large increase in blood supply is needed when food is digested. This becomes an important consideration in decisions on feeding patients with failing hearts. The portal circulation and its significance in liver disease is described in Chapter 11.

Fetal circulation. The fetal circulation is separated from that of the mother by the placenta and is, therefore, not truly part of the maternal circulation. Since some cardiovascular disease originates before birth, the circulation in the fetus and the changes that occur at birth are described briefly.

In the fetus, blood is oxygenated at the placenta rather than in the lungs. The blood returning from the placenta flows to the fetal liver. Most of it flows through the liver by a relatively direct route, the *ductus venosus* (Fig. 8-4), whereas a minor portion seeps through the swamplike liver tissue. All the blood eventually arrives at the right atrium of the heart. Since the fetal lungs are not yet functioning, not all the blood is pumped into the pulmonary circulation. Instead, a large portion is pumped through an opening, the *foramen ovale,* directly into the left atrium and from there into the left ventricle, the aorta, and its branches to the head. The head thus is supplied with well-oxygenated blood. When that blood returns to the right atrium, it mixes with the remaining portion of the blood from the placenta and ductus venosus. This blood is pumped from the right ventricle through an artery, the *ductus arteriosus,* which connects directly with the descending aorta to supply the lower body. The pulmonary circulation, because of the existence of the foramen ovale and ductus arteriosus, is bypassed almost completely.

At birth, this fetal system changes very rapidly to the pulmonary type of respiration as the placental circulation is interrupted. The intrathoracic pressure falls on the first inspiration, and pulmonary circulation is initiated. Blood pressure decreases in the pulmonary artery since it now supplies a large capillary network in the expanded lung. As a result, blood flow decreases in the ductus arteriosus, in which the muscle wall collapses. The ductus arteriosus closes completely in a few days. Pulmonary blood increases the pressure in the left atrium, pressing together the septa between the right and left atria and closing the foramen ovale. The circulatory system thus has assumed the adult form in which the major

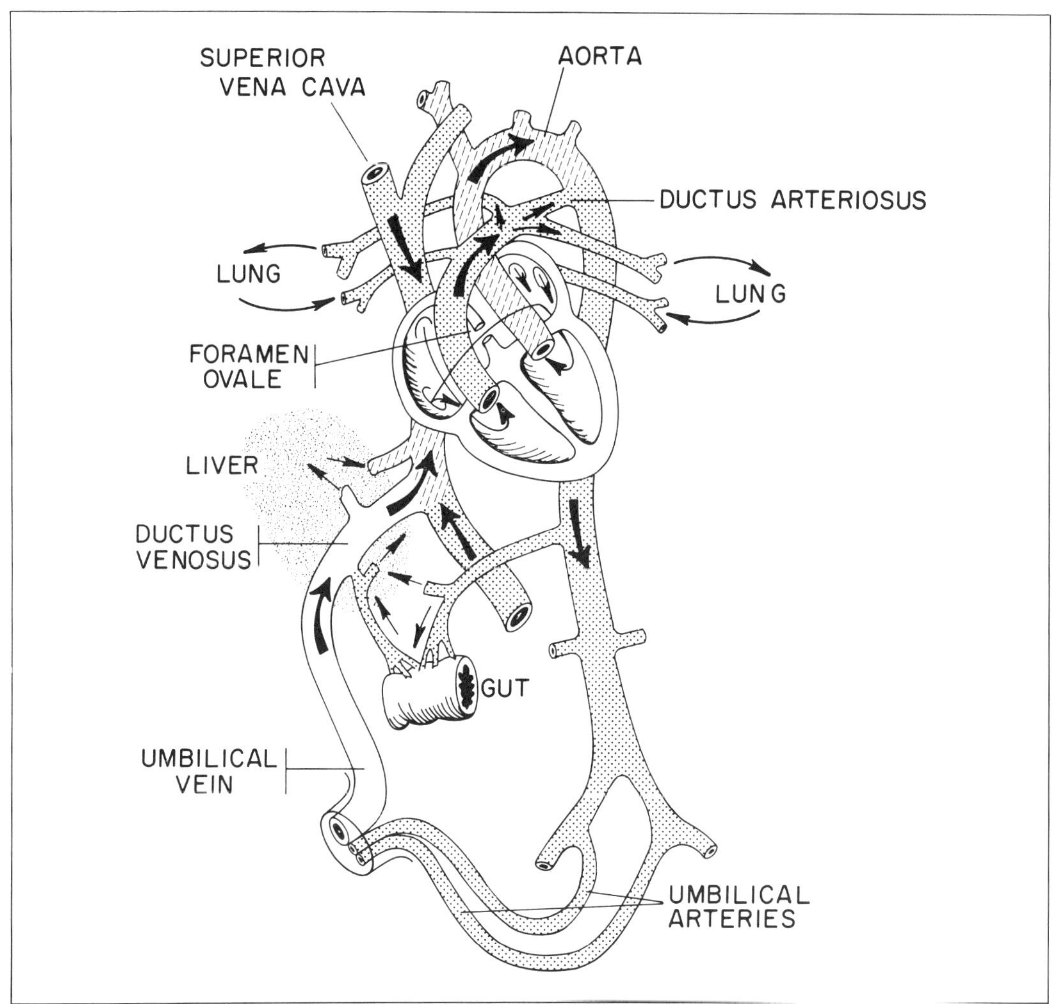

Figure 8-4. The fetal circulation. Most blood flows through the fetal liver via the ductus venosus. (Reprinted with permission from Guyton, A.C., Function of the Human Body, *4th ed. Philadelphia: W.B. Saunders, 1974, p. 457. Modified from Arey, L.B.,* Developmental Anatomy, *7th ed. Philadelphia: W.B. Saunders, 1974, p. 392.)*

and minor circulations are physiologically separated. Within a few weeks, the separation becomes anatomically complete with fibrous degeneration of the ductus arteriosus to form a ligament and fusion of the interatrial septa to form the definitive single interauricular septum. Congenital heart disease can result when the structure of the heart is abnormal and these changes do not occur.

Blood Vessels

Structure. A knowledge of the structure of the blood vessels, particularly the arteries, is important to an understanding of some forms of cardiovascular disease. In general, blood vessels are composed of three layers, the *tunica intima, tunica media,* and *tunica adventitia.* The tunica intima is the innermost layer, lining the lumen of the blood vessel. It is composed of an innermost thin layer of endothelial cells lining the lumen, beneath which there is the *subendothelium,* composed of a layer of loose connective tissue and its matrix and containing a few smooth muscle cells. Underneath the subendothelium lies a perforated *internal elastic lamina.* When the blood vessel contracts, this membrane has a scalloped appearance. As an individual ages, smooth muscle cells and matrix accumulate, increasing the thickness of the intima.[1]

The tunica media consists of smooth muscle cells arranged in a circular pattern, with interposed elastic tissue. The smooth muscle cells are surrounded by collagen and other matrix materials. The aorta contains a large amount of elastic tissue. The adventitia is composed of elastic connective tissue that fuses with the connective tissue surrounding adjacent organs. An *external limiting membrane* often is found within the adventitia, which also contains fibroblasts, collagen, glycosaminoglycans, and glycoproteins.

The cells of the blood vessels must themselves be nourished. Small arteries and the inner layers of large arteries can be nourished from the lumen. The adventitia of large arteries and veins contains small blood vessels known as the *vasa vasorum,* which supply the tissue of those vessels that are too thick to be nourished from the main stream of blood in the lumen. Since the blood in veins is poorer in nutrients, the vasa vasorum of veins is more richly branched. The outer portion of the tunica media is supplied by arterioles that originate at arterial branching points, and the tunica intima and the internal portion of the tunica media are nourished by diffusion.

Types of Blood Vessels. With this general structural plan in mind, we now can consider how various types of blood vessels differ. Arteries are classified according to their size and structure. The *large arteries* (*elastic arteries*) are the aorta and its large branches. The intima of these vessels is lined with endothelial cells and has a thick subendothelial layer. The media consists of concentric perforated elastic membranes interspersed with smooth muscle cells and fibroblasts. The adventitia does not have an external limiting membrane. These characteristics make it possible for these blood vessels to dilate and contract with the beat of the heart.

In contrast, *small* and *medium-sized arteries* (*muscular arteries*) have a thick muscle layer and are not so elastic. The arterioles are even smaller, usually less then 0.5 mm in diameter. They have endothelium but no subendothelial layer, a thin media of muscle cells, and a narrow adventitia.

The walls of the capillaries are a single endothelial cell in thickness. It is in this area that exchanges between blood and interstitial fluid occur, the true purpose of the cardiovascular system. Most cells are a distance of only 0.1 mm or less from a capillary blood supply.

Veins also are classified by size. The smallest are *venules.* Small and medium-sized veins have much thinner walls than do the arteries. Large veins have a thicker intima and adventitia and a thin media. The arterioles, capillaries, and venules are known collectively as the *microcirculation.*

Normal Cardiovascular Function

The cardiovascular system might be considered as a mechanical system containing a pump (the heart), a compression chamber (the elastic arteries), and a variable resistance to outflow (primarily arterioles). In order to keep the fluid flowing through the system, it is necessary to maintain a head of pressure.

Blood pressure (BP) is created because the inflow of blood from the heart (*cardiac output* [CO]) is pumped into a closed system containing a *resistance* (R) to outflow. The three variables—cardiac output, blood pressure, and resistance—are interdependent, so that a change in one is reflected in changes in another. The relationship can be expressed mathematically as follows:

$$CO = \frac{BP}{R} \quad or \quad BP = CO \times R$$

In an average man at rest, cardiac output is typically 5 L/min. Systolic blood pressure might be 120 mm Hg. Resistance is obtained by calculation: 120 mm Hg/5 L/min. = 24 mm Hg/L/min. Using these formulas, in a situation where cardiac output is constant but the resistance increases, as it does in some vascular diseases, it should be clear that the blood pressure will rise. On the other hand, if resistance decreases, as it does in exercise when blood vessels dilate, cardiac output must rise in order to maintain the blood pressure.

Since blood pressure is a function of cardiac output and peripheral resistance, influences on these factors will be reflected in the blood pressure. The control of blood flow to the tissues can thus be considered from the point of view of the control of blood pressure.

Cardiac Output

The heart muscles contract in a specified sequence to pump blood. Contraction begins in the thin-walled atria, followed by contraction of the thicker-walled ventricles. This contraction phase, *systole,* is followed by a short rest period known as *diastole.* During systole, so much blood is forced into the aorta and its elastic artery branches that they expand. Their contraction, during diastole, serves to maintain a moderate pressure in the system.

The heart has its own intrinsic rhythm and will beat automatically if its nerve supply is cut. Impulses from the nervous system are required to cause a faster or slower beat.

The amount of blood pumped to the tissues by the heart—the cardiac output—is expressed as liters of blood pumped per minute. It is the product of the *stroke volume* (amount ejected from the heart at each beat) and the *heart rate* (beats per minute). For example, if the stroke volume is 70 ml and the heart rate is 72 beats per minute, cardiac output would be 70 × 72 or 5,040 ml. The cardiac output can thus be varied by changing either the heart rate or the stroke volume. The heart rate can be increased two to three times by sympathetic stimulation, whereas parasympathetic stimulation decreases the rate. Both sympathetic and parasympathetic nerve fibers terminate on the SA node. The parasympathetic (vagal) fibers release *acetylcholine* on the SA nodal cells. Acetylcholine alters the permeability of the membrane and prolongs the time between beats by slowing the rate of membrane repolarization, thus slowing the heart rate (a *negative chronotropic effect*). Sympathetic fibers release norepinephrine and increase the heart rate (a *positive chronotropic effect*). Other factors, including various ions, hormones, and temperature, also influence the heart rate.

Filling of the ventricles is completed by middiastole and emptying is relatively complete by midsystole. Thus, shortening the intervals between beats, which must occur when heart rate increases, does not decrease stroke volume appreciably. Instead, with increased heart rate, up to 100 to 150 beats per minute, the cardiac output increases.

It is possible to vary cardiac output by changing the stroke volume. Within physiologic limits, an increase in the length of the muscle fibers, and thus an increase in the amount of blood in the ventricle, leads to an increase in the strength of the contraction of the normal heart. Thus, the heart normally will pump all the blood that is returned to it by the venous system, a principle known as the *Frank-Starling law.* At the same time, it is important to remember that there are limitations. A muscle fiber stretched beyond a given point will have weaker, not stronger, contractions. Increased sympathetic stimulation also results in stronger contractions *at a given length.* This reaction is known as an *inotropic response.* On the other hand, increased arterial pressure tends to cause a decrease in stroke volume.

Peripheral Vascular Resistance

The resistance to blood flow is the effect of the friction of the blood in the vessel. The narrower the tube, the more resistance there will be. If pressure is not changed, resistance decreases if a blood vessel dilates and increases if the blood vessel constricts. Conversely, if the vessel constricts, assuming constant cardiac output, pressure will rise, and if the vessels dilate, pressure will fall. This concept is very important in understanding the effects of atherosclerosis, which are discussed on pages 303–304.

Blood flow through the capillaries is regulated by the contraction and relaxation of the smooth muscle in the arterioles and of the sphincters at the entrance to some capillaries. These muscles always have some tone; that is, they always are partly constricted. By contracting and relaxing certain areas, the arterioles can shunt blood to areas of the body where the need is greatest. For example, more blood is supplied to the skeletal muscle during exercise and to the abdominal organs during digestion.

The control of blood supply in an organ or tissue may be acute or long-term. In either case, the response is primarily to the tissue's need for nutrition, especially for oxygen. In the skin, it also serves to dissipate heat. Local blood flow can be altered very quickly in response to oxygen deficit or to excess carbon dioxide, hydrogen ion, or other metabolites. There is controversy concerning the mechanism by which this occurs. The *oxygen demand theory* postulates that oxygen and other nutrients are needed to maintain muscle contraction. When these nutrients are lacking, the vascular muscles relax and the vessel dilates. The *vasodilator theory* is much in favor with physiologists at the present time. It postulates the formation of some vasodilator substances when oxygen and other nutrients are deficient. Various materials have been suggested to be the vasodilator substance, including carbon dioxide, lactate, histamine, hydrogen ion, potassium ion, adenosine, and adenosine phosphates. Adenosine currently is receiving much attention as a candidate.

If alterations in tissue requirements persist, a long-term alteration of local blood flow can develop. For example, if a tissue becomes chronically overactive, the blood supply gradually will increase. The mechanism involved probably is a change in the vascularity of the tissue. If the need for more blood becomes chronic, the size, and sometimes the number, of the blood vessels increases. This is important in the development of the *collateral circulation,* which is significant in some cardiovascular diseases.

Blood Pressure

A fairly narrow range of arterial blood pressures exists in a large proportion of the population. A systolic pressure of 120 mm Hg and a diastolic pressure of 80 mm Hg, usually expressed as 120/80 (read "120 over 80"), is very common and often is considered the standard of normalcy. However, blood pressures within a population are a continuous variable, and there is no definitive dividing line between normal and abnormal.

The pressure quoted in most clinical situations is the pressure measured in the arteries. There is a precipitous drop in pressure as blood flows through the arterioles so that mean pressure in the capillaries is approximately 25 mm Hg. As blood flows through the veins, pressure continues to fall until, when the blood returns to the right atrium, pressure is very nearly 0 mm Hg.

Short-Term Regulation. Nervous system control of the circulation occurs via the autonomic nervous system. It is very short-term, occurring in a few minutes or less. Sympathetic vasoconstrictor fibers innervate all parts of the arterial system and have an especially powerful effect on the kidneys, spleen, gut, and skin. In addition to its effect on the vasculature, sympathetic stimulation increases the heart rate and increases the heart's pumping strength. The overall effect, then, is to increase the blood pressure.

In the medulla of the brain, the *vasomotor center* transmits regulatory impulses. It is tonically active so that some muscle tone is maintained constantly. It can, in turn, be influenced by higher centers in the brain. When the vasomotor center is active, norepinephrine is secreted from the ends of vasoconstrictor nerves of the sympathetic nervous system and causes the smooth muscle of blood vessels to contract. The sympathetic impulses also stimulate the adrenal medulla to secrete epinephrine and norepinephrine. The usual result is vasoconstriction.

There are several mechanisms for reflex regulation of the pressure and volume of the circulation. When arterial pressure increases, it stretches the walls of the elastic arteries. In these arteries, particularly in the aortic arch and the area above the branching of the carotid arteries known as the *carotid sinus,* there are stretch receptors (*baroreceptors* or *pressoreceptors*) in the walls. These *carotid bodies* and *aortic bodies* are stimulated when the artery stretches and signals the vasomotor centers. The reflex action slows the heart and dilates the vessels, thus reducing the blood pressure to normal. Stretch receptors, located in the vena cava and right atrium, monitor atrial pressure. Increased atrial volume stretches the SA node and increases the heart rate. These receptors transmit signals to the medulla oblongata, eliciting stimulation of the heart rate and contractility (*Bainbridge reflex*). Nervous system regulation loses its ability to respond to a consistent blood pressure elevation in a few hours or days.

Another mechanism for short-term control of blood pressure, the *capillary fluid shift,* occurs when blood volume is inadequate or excessive. As pressures alter in the capillaries, fluid leaks out into the extracellular space or is retained by the capillaries, tending to return blood pressure to normal. This mechanism is, however, slower than neural control.

The kidneys also control blood pressure by controlling blood volume. They react very quickly to small changes in arterial pressure by increasing or decreasing urine formation. If blood pressure falls, for example, glomerular filtration declines and tubular reabsorption rises. Fluid and sodium accumulate until the blood volume increases sufficiently to restore normal pressure. On the other hand, if arterial pressure is too high, urinary output increases and blood volume decreases, thus returning the pressure to normal.

Long-Term Regulation. The kidneys also are important to the mechanisms that assure the long-term stability of the arterial pressure. The long-term regulation of blood pressure now is considered to involve the renin-angiotensin system, prostaglandins, and the kallikrein-kinin system.

The *renin-angiotensin system* is stimulated by decreased blood pressure in the renal artery accompanied by diminished blood flow. As blood flow through the kidneys falls, the cells of the juxtaglomerular apparatus (see Chapter 7) secrete *renin* (Fig. 8-5). Renin is an enzyme that splits the end from a substance in the plasma that is synthesized in the liver, known as *angiotensinogen* or *renin substrate.* The resulting compound is known as *angiotensin I.* In the plasma, a converting enzyme cleaves off a dipeptide to form *angiotensin II.* This reaction occurs largely in the lungs. The rate-limiting step in this series of reactions is renin production by the kidney; therefore, the kidney becomes the major controlling organ.

Angiotensin II causes (1) constriction of arterioles, (2) moderate constriction of veins, thereby increasing the venous return to the heart, (3) constriction of renal arterioles, and (4) increased secretion of aldosterone. These

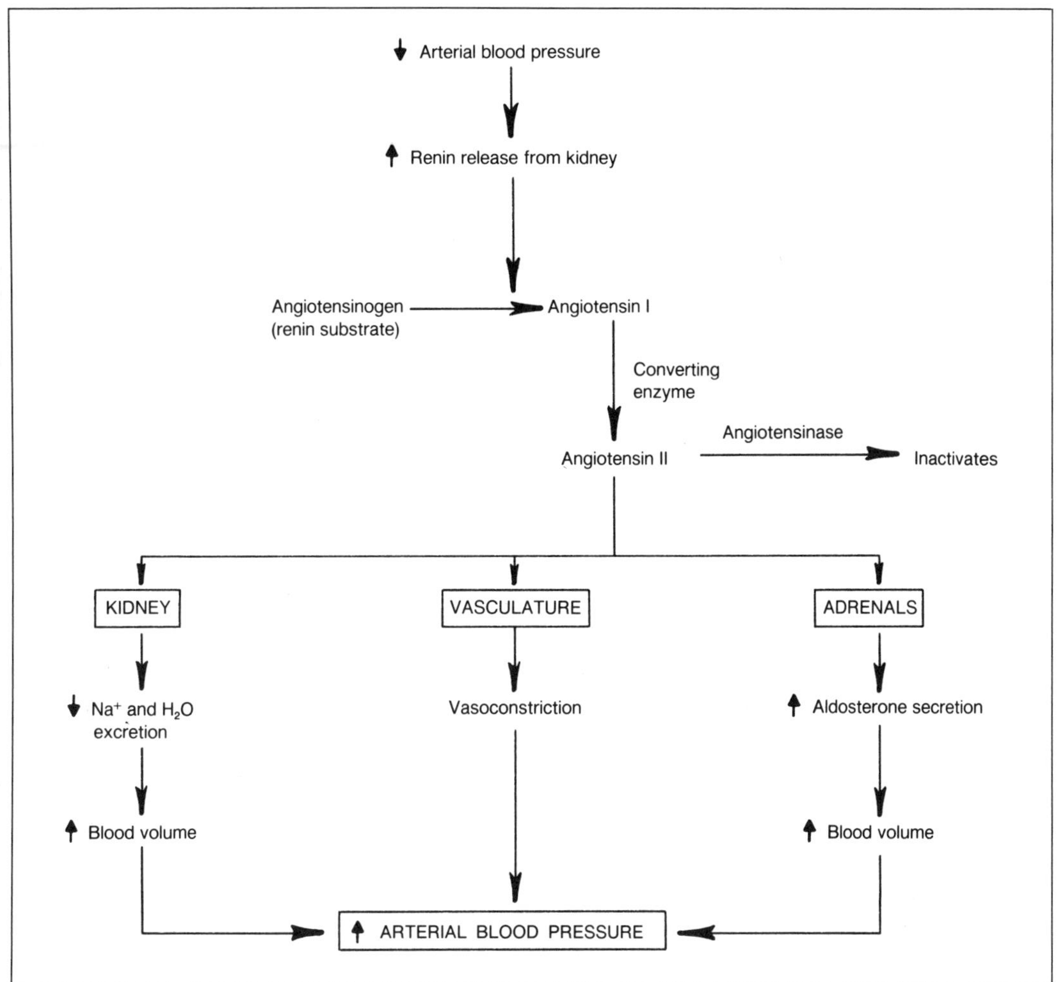

Figure 8-5. The renin-angiotensin system and its role in long-term regulation of arterial blood pressure.

actions cause the kidneys to retain water and salt, increasing the blood volume and also contributing to the rise in blood pressure. Angiotensin is inactivated by angiotensinase. The factors controlling renin release are not understood entirely, but renal perfusion, decreased sodium delivery to the macula densa, renal nerves, the adrenal medulla, and the autonomic nervous system all appear to play a role in controlling renin release.

A great deal less is known about the vasodilators that counteract this system. The *kinins* are potent vasodilators formed from kininogen, a component of plasma globulin (Fig. 8-6).[2] Kininogen is converted to kinins by the action of *kallikrein.* There are two kallikreins. *Prekallikrein* is formed in the liver and is converted to *plasma kallikrein* by the action of *Hageman factor* (a component of the blood coagulation system). *Glandular kallikrein* is found in the kidney, pancreas, intestine, other tissues, and urine. The kallikreins and kinins that appear in the urine are believed to be formed in the distal tubules.[3] Plasma kallikrein liberates *bradykinin* from kininogen, whereas glandular kallikrein liberates *lysyl bradykinin,* which is

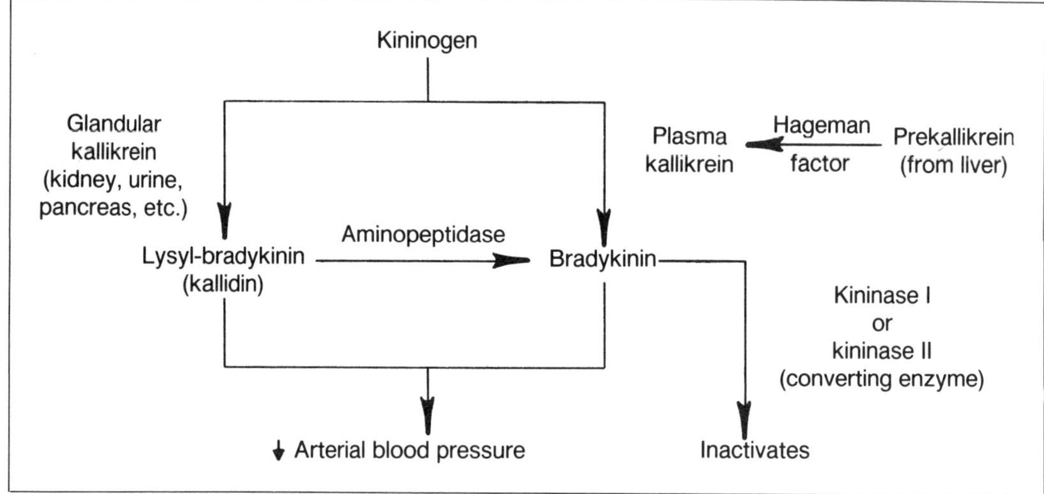

Figure 8-6. The kallikrein-kinin system and its role in long-term regulation of arterial blood pressure.

partially converted to bradykinin by *aminopeptidase.* Kinins act as vasodilators and thus lower the arterial pressure.[3]

Kinins are inactivated by the action of kininase I and II. Kininase II is reported to be the same as the converting enzyme that functions in the conversion of angiotensin I to angiotensin II, thus forming the connection between the two systems.[4]

Some *prostaglandins* increase water and sodium excretion by the kidney and may reduce blood pressure by reducing the blood volume.[5] However, most prostaglandins cause renal vasodilation and tend to lower the blood pressure by this means, although some are vasoconstrictors.

There are complex interactions between the renin-angiotensin-aldosterone system, the kallikrein-kinin system, and prostaglandins. The kallikrein-kinin system and prostaglandins contribute to the control of blood pressure by vasodilation, attenuating the effect of the renin-angiotensin-aldosterone system and influencing renal blood flow and salt and water excretion. For example, the synthesis or release of kallikrein may be regulated by aldosterone levels,[3] while kallikrein may promote activation of renin.[6] Prostaglandins may modulate the vasoconstrictive effects of angiotensin II.[7] Kinin stimulates the release of prostaglandin with a resultant increase in renal blood flow.[8] These and other interactions are a subject of current active research that will be of interest to those responsible for nutritional care of patients with cardiovascular disease.

Vasopressin or *antidiuretic hormone* also affects blood pressure. It is secreted by the hypothalamus and released by the posterior pituitary gland. It can be a potent vasoconstrictor in emergency situations such as hemorrhage, but the importance of its function in normal physiology is unknown.[9]

HYPERTENSION

Hypertension is defined as an arterial blood pressure that exceeds some arbitrarily established limit. The increase may be in systolic or diastolic pressure or both. Since the arterial blood pressure in a population is a continuously distributed variable and there is no generally agreed-on point that defines hypertension, the upper limit of normal arterial pressure sometimes is defined arbitrarily as 160/95 mm Hg.[9] Others have defined it as 130/90 for men younger than 45 years,

140/95 for men older than 45, and 160/95 for women.[10] A summary of epidemiologic studies demonstrated that hypertension is very common and increases with age.[11] It occurs more often in men younger than 50 years and in women older than 50 years, so that in total the condition occurs more often in women than in men. It is reported to be present in 20 percent of the population.[12]

Classification and Pathogenesis

Hypertension is associated with a number of conditions and can be classified in several ways. In one method, it is categorized according to whether systolic or diastolic pressure is increased. It can also be classified according to severity as *nonmalignant* or *malignant,* or by cause as *primary* (also called *essential*—that is, of unknown origin) or *secondary* to other conditions. Table 8-1 provides a classification of hypertension according to etiology, incorporating these categories. In 90 percent of cases, the condition is classified as essential hypertension and thus its cause is unknown. The kidney is believed, however, to have a central role in the etiology.

Secondary hypertension is treated by removal, if possible, of the basic cause. Nutritional care may be appropriate in removing the underlying cause and is described in other chapters (see Chapters 7 and 9). Secondary hypertension itself usually is not amenable to alterations in diet. Therefore, the remainder of this section will focus on essential hypertension.

As previously described, blood pressure may be increased by increasing the cardiac output or by increasing the peripheral resistance. Only in rare cases of secondary hypertension, such as pheochromocytoma, is cardiac output altered. In most hypertensives, cardiac output remains within normal range and is relatively stable. Therefore, the development of hypertension is usually the result of increasing peripheral resistance. Resistance is a function of the length of the tube, the viscosity of liquid flowing through it, and the radius of the tube. For practical purposes, in the circulatory system, the length of the tube (the arterial system) does not vary nor are there appreciable changes in the viscosity of the fluid (the blood). Therefore, a reduction in the size of the lumen of the blood vessels must be responsible for the increased blood pressure.

For many years, attention has focused on the function of the renin-angiotensin system and its effects on the constriction of the blood vessels as the cause of hypertension. Recently, it has been suggested that a deficit in the action of prostaglandins or the kallikrein-kinin system may contribute to the onset of the condition.[3] Research in this area is continuing.

Table 8-1. Etiologies of Hypertension

Systolic hypertension

Increased left ventricular stroke volume (e.g., patent ductus arteriosus, thyrotoxicosis, arteriovenous fistula, aortic regurgitation)

Decreased aortic distensibility (e.g., coarctation of the aorta, arteriosclerosis of the aorta)

Arterial hypertension (elevated systolic and diastolic pressures)

Essential hypertension

Renal hypertension
- Compression of kidney, as from trauma
- Renal artery disease (e.g., atherosclerosis, embolism, traumatic injury)
- Kidney disease (e.g., glomerulonephritis, pyelonephritis, polycystic kidneys, intercapillary glomerulosclerosis, interstitial nephritis, tumor, amyloidosis, radiation nephritis, some connective tissue and autoimmune disorders)

Endocrine hypertension
- Pheochromocytoma; excess catecholamine
- Excess mineralocorticoid (e.g., primary hyperaldosteronism, adrenal hyperplasia)
- Excess glucocorticoid (e.g., Cushing's syndrome)
- Oral contraceptives

Neurogenic hypertension
- Intracranial diseases (e.g., increased intracranial pressure, encephalitis, lead encephalopathy)
- Vasomotor center disturbances (e.g., bulbar poliomyelitis, decreased vascular supply)
- Spinal cord and peripheral nerve disorders (e.g., transection of spinal cord, polyneuritis, porphyria)
- Anxiety states (?)

Toxemia of pregnancy: preeclampsia or eclampsia

Risk Factors

It generally is believed that there are a number of *risk factors* that contribute to the incidence and to the severity of the consequences of essential hypertension.[13] They may be classified as uncontrollable and controllable.

Uncontrollable Risk Factors

In industrialized Western nations, blood pressure increases with age in men, for unknown reasons. In women, the rise occurs after menopause and may, therefore, be related to female hormones. The sensitivity of vasoreceptors decreases with age, but it is not known if this is a cause or effect of hypertension. As indicated, sex may be a risk factor, depending on age.

An individual's genetic background also may be a risk factor. It is believed that up to 20 percent of the population is genetically susceptible to hypertension. The mechanisms involved are not clear and are difficult to separate from environmental influences. Race is another risk factor; young black men have a high incidence of hypertension.

Controllable Risk Factors

Sodium and Potassium Intake. The possible relationship of sodium intake to hypertension is the subject of considerable debate. Recently, potassium intake has been added to the controversy. Because of the importance of sodium in regulating body fluids, including blood volume (see Chapter 7), it is assumed that alterations in body sodium can alter blood pressure. This relationship, however, does not prove that excess sodium intake causes hypertension.

A great deal of controversy exists concerning recommendations for changes in the diet of the general population for prevention of hypertension. Both animal and epidemiologic studies have implicated high sodium intake as a cause of hypertension.[14–16] However, within population groups studied epidemiologically, there appears to be no correlation between salt intake and blood pressure elevation. It has been suggested that a genetic predisposition in some individuals causes them to develop hypertension under the stimulus of a high-salt diet, while others are unaffected.[16]

Based on the incidence of hypertension, it seems reasonable to assume that 20 percent of the young population is at risk. As a consequence, it was suggested that the relatively high salt content of commercial baby foods be reduced as a public health measure.[17] This has been done by most manufacturers. Reduction of the salt intake in the population in general has also been suggested,[18,19] but there are those who believe that advocating a reduction in salt intake for everyone is not justified if the change would be helpful to only those people who are genetically susceptible.

Obesity. Hypertension is found in association with obesity in many patients, but there is no firm evidence that obesity causes hypertension. Rather, obesity may interact with other factors. It also increases the work load of the heart, which is already laboring against increased pressure.

Psychological Factors. Mental and emotional stress can cause a temporary rise in blood pressure, but there is no evidence that such stresses, or even psychoses, cause a sustained elevation. Some attempts have been made to lower blood pressure by mental relaxation or meditation. These methods often are associated with other changes in life-style, including diet, and have not been adequately evaluated yet.

Pathophysiology of Essential Hypertension

Early mild *benign hypertension* is asymptomatic. When it becomes more severe, it sometimes is associated with headaches.

However, headaches are a symptom of many diseases and cannot be used for a definitive diagnosis. Other symptoms of benign hypertension include *vertigo* (dizziness), *tinnitus* (noise in ears), *syncope* (fainting), and dimmed vision.

Hypertension is of concern primarily because it is associated with damage to the heart and arterial walls and, as a result, can damage the eyes, kidneys, brain, and other organs. It is a potentially life-threatening condition, but the condition usually progresses slowly. The extent of the damage is influenced by other risk factors, discussed in the section on risk factors for atherosclerosis (p. 307), that impair the ability of the circulatory system to withstand damage.[9]

In some patients, the blood pressure rises suddenly, representing a change from a slowly progressive benign hypertension to *malignant hypertension* (diastolic pressure greater than 130 mm Hg). Untreated malignant hypertension progresses rapidly and is associated with a mortality of 80 percent in the first year and 100 percent within 2 years.

In the progression of the disease, the cardiac cells increase in size, leading to gradual hypertrophy of the left ventricle to compensate for the excessive work load created by the increased pressure. Eventually, heart function deteriorates and the heart fails. Heart failure is discussed in more detail in the section Congestive Heart Failure (pp. 311–313).

The muscle cells in the tunica media of the arteries also thicken, reducing the lumen size. Peripheral resistance is a function of the fourth power of the radius of the vessel; therefore, a small reduction in lumen size can increase peripheral resistance significantly and increase blood pressure further.

The endothelium of the arterial wall is damaged by the retention of lipoproteins (*atherosclerosis*). The resultant thickening and fatty infiltration of the blood vessel walls have important effects on various organs of the body, depending on the site of the lesions. Lesions tend to appear in areas of turbulence such as at arterial junctions. For example, they occur at the junction of the aorta and carotid arteries, affecting blood supply to the brain, and at the junctions of the femoral arteries, affecting blood supplies to the leg. Thickening of renal arteries can cause renal failure. *Thrombus* (clot) or *embolus* (clot carried in the circulation) formation can impair circulation to various organs, including the eyes. Clearly, a wide variety of specific disorders can result from hypertension. Those with nutritional care implications will be discussed in detail later in this chapter.

Management

Management of hypertension has changed over the years from attempts to control hypertension only when it becomes severe to the present policy of controlling fairly mild increases in blood pressure. The present procedure is believed to be associated with a reduced incidence of complications and decreased mortality. Early treatment was largely dietary. With the development of more effective drugs, treatment now has evolved into a combination of drugs and diet. In addition, behavior modification (see Chapter 15) and physical exercise sometimes are components of treatment.

Sodium-Restricted Diets

The present average daily consumption of salt in the United States is estimated to be 10 to 12 g and exceeds the requirement by as much as ten times. Only 200 mg of sodium (9 mEq) are required to maintain sodium balance. It has been suggested that 50 to 150 mEq of sodium (1,100 to 3,300 mg) would be an adequate daily intake for the normal adult in all except the most unusual circumstances. In order to control hypertension using sodium-restricted diets alone, an individual's sodium intake would have to be limited to 250 mg/day. This is a very severe

Table 8-2. Sodium and Salt Content of Typical Sodium-Restricted Diets

Sodium (mg)	Sodium (approximate mEq)	Salt (approximate g)
250	12	0.6
500	22	1.3
1,000	43	2.5
1,500	65	3.8
2,000	87	5.0
2,400	100	6.0
3,000	130	7.6
4,000	174	10.2
4,500	200	11.5
5,000	215	12.6

restriction with which few patients are able to comply.

The use of oral diuretic drugs has removed the necessity for such severe dietary sodium restriction. Mild sodium restriction, although it does not appear to affect the blood pressure directly, does seem to increase the effectiveness of most antihypertensive drugs. As a consequence, a sodium restriction of 1,500 to 2,000 mg/day (65 to 87 mEq) accompanied by drug treatment has been recommended for mild hypertension. Contents of some typical diets are given in Table 8-2.

Sodium-restricted diets are used not only for the treatment of mild hypertension but for various other forms of cardiovascular disease, liver disease, and, as we saw in Chapter 7, renal disorders. The range of sodium restrictions will be described here.

1. *Mild* sodium restriction for the patient with moderate heart damage or mild hypertension controlled by drugs allows 2,400 to 4,500 mg or more of sodium per day, depending on the patient's specific food choices. It omits very salty foods and salting food at the table but allows a limited amount of salt in cooking.

2. *Moderate* sodium restriction is used for treatment of mild edema or prevention of edema when the mild restriction is ineffective. It allows 1,000 mg of sodium per day. This means that only ¼ tsp. of salt per day may be used, and no salt is used in cooking. The allowed salt may be added at the table or will be contained in 1 slice of bread and 2 tsp. of regular salted butter. Otherwise, bread should be saltfree and sweet (unsalted) butter must be used.

3. *Strict* sodium restriction is used for patients who have edema and congestive heart failure (see p. 311) despite medication and a less restrictive diet. It allows 500 mg of sodium per day. No salt is used in cooking or added at the table. Processed foods with added salt or other sodium compounds are omitted, and the amount of milk must be limited.

4. *Severe* sodium restriction may be necessary for some patients with severe cardiovascular disease. It allows only 250 mg of sodium per day. In addition to the restrictions of the 500-mg sodium diet, it requires the substitution of low-sodium milk (7 mg of sodium per 8-oz. serving) for regular milk (120 mg of sodium per 8-oz. serving). Animal protein foods tend to be relatively high in sodium, and so their use must be limited. The use of low-sodium milk is necessary to provide adequate protein in the diet without exceeding the sodium restriction. Low-sodium milk is available fresh in many communities from local dairies. It can be used as is, flavored with other foods, or used in cooking. A powdered product, Lonalac, also is available. Other foods that are restricted are the same as those limited for patients with renal disease (see Chapter 7).

Pamphlets describing various sodium-restricted diets are available for patients from the American Heart Association. They give information on various levels of sodium restriction combined with 1,200-calorie, 1,800-calorie, and unrestricted calorie content.

The level of sodium restriction and the meal pattern should ideally be planned in cooperation with the patient. If the diet is individually tailored, especially for nonhospitalized patients, the patient's compliance with the diet may improve. It sometimes is helpful also to approach a sodium restriction in stages to give the patient time to adjust to the use of less salt. This procedure requires close cooperation between the nutritional care specialist and the physician so that drug dosage and dietary sodium can be adjusted simultaneously.

There is some evidence that hypertensive patients have a reduced taste sensitivity to salt. The patients will need advice on meal planning and methods of food preparation in order to make the diet acceptable. A number of books and pamphlets containing recipes are available. This is an opportunity for the nutritional care specialist to show initiative and imagination in developing new recipes, instructing the patient on the use of alternative herbs and spices, and helping the patient to adapt recipes for favorite foods to the new diet. Cooking classes for patients sometimes are effective. Patients should be given a list of sources of any special products needed, such as low-sodium milk and bread.

Weight Reduction

Weight reduction alone is effective in reducing mildly elevated blood pressure in some patients; however, not all patients experience reduced blood pressure when weight is lost. In addition, permanent weight reduction is extremely difficult to achieve (see Chapter 15), making weight reduction a somewhat unrealistic approach to the control of hypertension.

The mechanism by which weight loss reduces blood pressure is not clear. Contributing factors may be the reduced sodium content of reduced calorie diets and changes in endocrine relationships and metabolism during weight reduction. Weight reduction generally is considered to be at least beneficial to the obese hypertensive if it can be achieved. Procedures for planning diets for weight reduction are given in Chapter 15.

Drugs

With the development of potent and safer antihypertensive drugs, less emphasis has been placed on severe sodium restriction. The drugs used may vary depending on the severity of the hypertension, which often is expressed as mild, moderate, or severe, although the distinctions are blurred.

If mild hypertension does not respond to sodium restriction, weight loss, and reduction of tension, drug therapy usually is begun with diuretics (Table 8-3). The mechanisms of their effects are not entirely clear. Some suggested modes of action are (1) reduction in blood volume, (2) alteration of sodium and water content of the muscle in the arterial wall, (3) decreased vascular response to epinephrine and norepinephrine, and (4) a vasodilator effect.[20] Overall, diuretics increase fluid loss, thereby reducing the blood pressure and decreasing the work load of the heart. Their long-term safety is unknown.

Thiazides are adequate treatment for approximately two-thirds of hypertensive patients. If potassium loss becomes a problem, potassium-sparing diuretics may be used. The side effects of these agents and recommendations for nutritional care of patients taking them are listed in Table 8-3.

Initial drug therapy for moderately hypertensive individuals is the same as for mild hypertensives but will be successful in a smaller percentage of cases. Drug treatment of individuals with severe hypertension also usually begins with a thiazide as basic therapy, supplemented with more potent antihypertensive drugs. These more potent drugs can be classified as *sympathetic blocking agents* or *peripheral vasodilators.* Some examples are presented in Table 8-3. Methyldopa and clonidine hydrochloride have a number of side effects. Propranolol hydrochloride, a beta-adrenergic receptor blocking agent, is an effective antihypertensive with fewer side effects.

If diuretics plus sympathetic blocking drugs do not control the hypertension, peripheral vasodilators (hydralazine, prazosin hydrochloride, or minoxidil) may be prescribed in addition. Minoxidil causes fluid retention when chronically administered without a diuretic. *Hirsutism* (abnormal

Table 8-3. Antihypertensive and Diuretic Drugs

Generic Name	Proprietary Name	Primary Use	Type of Action	Nutrition-Related Side Effects	Nutritional Care
Diuretics					
Thiazides		Control of hypertension	$\downarrow$Reabsorption of sodium in loop of Henle and distal tubule	$\uparrow$Potassium excretion; hypokalemia; $\uparrow$serum calcium; $\downarrow$calcium excretion; nausea, vomiting; diarrhea; orthostatic hypotension following alcohol intake; hyperglycemia	Take with meals; use high-potassium foods; avoid excess water; avoid alcohol
Bendroflumethiazide	Naturetin				
Benzthiazide	Aquatag; Exna				
Chlorothiazide	Diuril				
Cyclothiazide	Anhydron				
Hydrochlorothiazide	Esidrix; HydroDIURIL; Oretic				
Hydroflumethiazide	Saluron				
Methyclothiazide	Enduron				
Polythiazide	Renese				
Trichlormethiazide	Metahydrin; Naqua				
Related sulfonamides		Control of hypertension	$\downarrow$Sodium reabsorption	Hypokalemia	Use high-potassium foods
Chlorthalidone	Hygroton				
Metolazone	Zaroxolyn				
Quinethazone	Hydromox				
Loop diuretics		Edema control in renal disease	$\downarrow$Sodium reabsorption in loop of Henle	Hypokalemia; gastrointestinal disturbances; $\uparrow$calcium excretion; nausea, vomiting, diarrhea	Use high-potassium foods; avoid excess water; take with meals
Ethacrynic acid	Edecrin				
Furosemide	Lasix				
Potassium-sparing diuretics		Control of hypertension; treatment of liver disease with ascites	Spironolactone inhibits aldosterone action and thus inhibits sodium-potassium exchange in tubule. Triamterene inhibits sodium-potassium exchange by effect on tubule	Hyperkalemia; nausea, vomiting with triamterene	Avoid excess potassium-containing foods; avoid salt substitutes with potassium; avoid excess water; take with meals
Spironolactone	Aldactone				
Triamterene	Dyrenium				
Adrenergic blocking agents					
Central-acting agents		Antihypertensive	Stimulation of alpha-receptors in brain for depressor effect on sympathetic nervous system; increase glomerular filtration	Dry mouth; gastrointestinal disturbance; nausea; alcohol is synergistic	Take with meals; use alcohol with caution
Clonidine hydrochloride	Catapres				
Methyldopa	Aldomet				
Rauwolfia alkaloids		Antihypertensive	Reduce catecholamine	Increase gastric	Take with meals

alkaloids					
Ganglion blocking drugs: Trimethaphan camsylate	Arfonad	Antihypertensive (Used in emergencies only. Has many side effects.)	Inhibit adrenergic impulses to heart, arterioles, and venules	Paralytic ileus; fluid intolerance	
Postganglionic nerve blockers		Antihypertensive	Depletion of catecholamine at nerve ending	Constipation (?); diarrhea (?); paralytic ileus (rare); acid indigestion; exacerbates peptic ulcer; alcohol potentiates effect	Avoid highly spiced foods if necessary; avoid alcohol
Bethanidine sulfate					
Bretylium tosylate	Bretylol				
Guanethidine sulfate	Ismelin				
Alpha-adrenergic receptor inhibitors		Antihypertensive in pheochromocytoma, catecholamine excess. Rarely used.	Block alpha-receptors and reduce total peripheral resistance	Postural hypotension	
Phenoxybenzamine Hydrochloride (PO)	Dibenzyline				
Prazosin hydrochloride	Minipress				
Phentolamine (IV)	Regitine				
Beta-adrenergic receptor inhibitors		Antihypertensive	Blunt catecholamine effect; mode of action not understood	Nausea; epigastric distress; alcohol is synergistic; diarrhea	Use alcohol with caution
Acebutolol					
Atenolol					
Metoprolol	Lopressor				
Propranolol hydrochloride	Inderal				
Timolol maleate					
Vasodilators					
Direct smooth-muscle dilators		Antihypertensive in combination with diuretics	↓Peripheral resistance		
Diazoxide	Hyperstat			Hyperglycemia, sodium retention	
Hydralazine hydrochloride	Apresoline			Anorexia, nausea, vomiting, diarrhea	
Minoxidil	Loniten			Hirsutism	Vitamin E supplementations (?)
Nitroprusside				Nausea, vomiting	
Alpha-adrenergic receptor inhibitors (see under Adrenergic blocking agents)					As for diuretics

Compiled from Kaplan, N.M., Frohlich, E.D., Hollifield, J.W., et al., Pharmacologic approaches to hypertension management. In J.C. Hunt, T. Cooper, E.D. Frohlich, et al., Eds., *Hypertension Update: Mechanisms, Epidemiology, Evaluation, Management.* Bloomfield, N.J.: Health Learning Systems, 1980; Williams, G.H., Jagger, P.I., and Braunwald, E., Hypertensive vascular disease. In K.J. Isselbacher, R.D. Adams, E. Braunwald, et al., Eds., *Harrison's Principles of Internal Medicine,* 9th ed. New York: McGraw-Hill, 1980; Dollery, C.T., Arterial hypertension. In P.B. Beeson, W. McDermott, and J.B. Wyngaarden, Eds., *Cecil Textbook of Medicine,* 15th ed. Philadelphia: W.B. Saunders, 1979; and Freitag, J.J., Hypertension. In J.J. Freitag and L.W. Miller, Eds., *Manual of Medical Therapeutics,* 23rd ed. Boston: Little, Brown, 1980.

IV = intravenously; PO = orally.

hairiness) is a common side effect of minoxidil; therefore, the drug is used mostly for men. Supplementation with vitamin E has been reported to be helpful. The nutritional care specialist should be familiar with and alert to identifying the side effects of antihypertensive drugs.

Potassium

The hypertensive patient receiving diuretic medication, especially if the patient's diet is high in sodium, may be at risk of developing a potassium deficiency. The concentration of potassium in the extracellular fluid affects the excitability of the myocardium in which conduction and rhythm can be greatly affected. In hyperkalemia, myocardial fibers become less excitable and the heart may stop in diastole. In hypokalemia, cardiac arrest occurs in systole. Hyperkalemia may be rapidly fatal, whereas hypokalemia has a slower effect.

Patients should be instructed to be alert to symptoms of potassium deficiency—anorexia, malaise, and muscle weakness. Patients at risk may be instructed to increase their intake of potassium-rich foods, that is, fruits and vegetables. Meat and milk are useful as sources of potassium but only insofar as they are allowable within the patient's sodium-restricted diet. Most salt substitutes are largely potassium salts, but these are not very acceptable to many patients.

The physician will monitor serum potassium in these patients and may change the diuretic from a thiazide or furosemide to a potassium-sparing diuretic. Under these circumstances, a high-potassium diet is inappropriate.

It is possible to prescribe a potassium supplement as a medication. However, these materials are irritants to the mucosal lining of the stomach and intestine and increase the risk of ulceration. Other possible side effects are nausea, vomiting, and diarrhea. The medication is unpleasant tasting also, thereby increasing the likelihood that the patient will not take it.

Some evidence has linked a low-potassium diet with hypertension.[21,22] The interrelationship with sodium excess is unknown. Toxic materials such as lead and cadmium have also been associated with hypertension.

HYPERLIPIDEMIA

There is a high correlation between increased serum lipid concentrations, especially cholesterol, and the incidence of certain forms of cardiovascular disease. Lipids in high concentrations will deposit in arterial walls, promoting atherosclerosis and its various consequences. The absorption of dietary lipids is described in Chapter 6.

Classification of Lipoproteins

Lipids are not soluble in water and must be complexed with protein for transport in the blood. Plasma lipids, primarily triglycerides and cholesteryl esters, are carried in the blood as lipoproteins. *Lipoproteins* are very large molecules containing a core of cholesteryl esters and triglycerides with a membranelike coat composed of unesterified cholesterol, phospholipid, and protein. The protein components are known as *apolipoproteins* or *apoproteins* and are identified by a lettering and numbering system. Those believed to be of major importance are Apo A-I and A-II, Apo B, Apo C-I, C-II, and C-III, Apo D, and Apo E. The structures of these molecules are not known in all cases, but they range in molecular weight from 5,700 to 75,000. They are distributed among the lipoproteins in a relatively consistent fashion. Their location in the lipoproteins and indications of special functions are given in Table 8-4. Apo A-I is synthesized primarily in the intestine, and the liver synthesizes Apo B, C, and E.

Table 8-4. Apoproteins of Lipoproteins

Apoprotein	Location	Notes on Function
A-I	HDL, chylomicrons, intestinal VLDL	Activates LCAT
A-II	HDL	
B	VLDL, IDL, LDL, chylomicrons, chylomicron remnants	
C-I	HDL, VLDL, chylomicron remnants	Activates LCAT (?)
C-II	HDL, VLDL, chylomicrons	Activates extrahepatic lipoprotein lipase
C-III	HDL, VLDL, chylomicrons	
D	HDL fraction	Catalyzes cholesteryl ester transfer among lipoproteins
E	HDL, VLDL, chylomicrons, chylomicron remnants	

HDL = high-density lipoprotein; VLDL = very-low-density lipoprotein; LCAT = lecithin-cholesterol acetyltransferase; IDL = intermediate-density lipoprotein; LDL = low-density lipoprotein.

There are five classes of lipoproteins, each of which contains triglycerides, cholesterol, and phospholipid in different proportions. Each class consists of particles of characteristic lipid and protein composition that gives it a specific size and density. Density increases and size decreases as the proportion of protein increases. The five classes are, in order of size and density, *chylomicrons* (the largest, containing the largest proportion of lipid and the least protein), *very-low-density lipoproteins* (*VLDLs*), *intermediate-density lipoproteins* (*IDLs*), *low-density lipoproteins* (*LDLs*), and *high-density lipoproteins* (*HDLs*). High-density lipoprotein is the smallest, containing the most proteins. The properties of the lipoproteins are summarized in Table 8-5.

In the laboratory, the lipoproteins are separated with an ultracentrifuge or by electrophoresis. In the ultracentrifuge, chylomicrons have the fastest flotation rates, and HDLs, the slowest. In electrophoresis, lipoprotein migration is related to that of the plasma proteins. Chylomicrons remain at the origin. Very-low-density lipoproteins migrate beyond the beta-globulins and therefore are referred to as *pre-beta-lipoproteins.* Low-density lipoproteins migrate along with the beta-globulins and thus are called beta-lipoproteins. High-density lipoproteins migrate with alpha-globulins and are referred to as alpha-lipoproteins. Intermediate-density lipoproteins migrate to a point intermediate between VLDLs and LDLs. In normal plasma of the fasting human, the approximate proportions of these lipoproteins are as follows: LDL, 50 percent; HDL, 35 percent; and VLDL, 15 percent. The major apoproteins contained in each are indicated in Table 8-5.

Cholesterol

Of the components of the lipoproteins, cholesterol has been found by epidemiologic studies to be especially related to the incidence of cardiovascular disease. Therefore, its metabolism has been studied extensively. Cholesterol in the blood is derived either by absorption from the intestine or from endogenous synthesis, believed to occur primarily in the liver. A normal adult synthesizes 9 to 13 mg of cholesterol per kilogram of body weight per day.[23] Cholesterol in the intestine can be from the diet or it can arrive in the intestine carried in the bile. Dietary cholesterol averages 400 to 700 mg/day, all from animal foods, whereas biliary cholesterol equals approximately 750 to 1,250 mg. There probably is some de novo cholesterol synthesis in the intestine as well, but this is thought to be insignificant.

Cholesterol is absorbed with the chylomicrons from the intestine (see Chapter 6), but

Table 8-5. Major Classes of Plasma Lipoprotein

Lipoprotein Class	Density (g/ml)	Electrophoretic Mobility	Size (nm)	Composition (%)				Major Apoproteins	Origin
				Protein	Triglycerides	Total Cholesterol	Phospholipids		
Chylomicrons	<0.95	Origin	75–1,000	1–2	80–95	2–5	3–6	A-I, B, C-I, C-II, C-III, E	Intestine
VLDL	0.95–1.006	Pre-beta	30–80	5–10	40–80	10–40	15–20	A-II (intestinal VLDL), B, C-I, C-II, C-III, E	Liver; intestine
IDL	1.006–1.019	Beta	25–30	15	35	7	17	B	VLDL catabolism
LDL	1.019–1.063	Beta	19–25	25	10	45	20	B	IDL catabolism
HDL	1.063–1.210	Alpha	4–10	45–50	1–5	20	30	A-I, A-II, C-I, C-II, C-III, D (in subfraction), E	Intestine; other (?)

VLDL = very-low-density lipoprotein; IDL = intermediate-density lipoprotein; LDL = low-density lipoprotein; HDL = high-density lipoprotein.

only approximately 40 percent of the cholesterol from bile or diet that appears in the intestinal lumen is absorbed.[24] Cholesterol secreted into the intestine by the liver is excreted primarily in the feces. Little cholesterol is excreted by any other route.

A number of factors affect the proportion of cholesterol absorbed. Before cholesterol can be absorbed, it must be solubilized in the form of micelles (see Chapter 6). If the cholesterol in food is in crystalline form rather than dissolved in oil or solubilized as it is in egg yolk, the proportion absorbed is reduced. With a high-fat diet, more micelles are formed, allowing more cholesterol to be solubilized and absorbed. Plant foods contain beta-sitosterol, campesterol, and stigmasterol, which inhibit cholesterol absorption from the intestine. Their possible usefulness in lowering serum cholesterol is under investigation.

The factors controlling cholesterol synthesis also are important. Dietary cholesterol provides feedback regulation. The remnant remaining after triglyceride is removed from the chylomicron provides the most potent inhibition. It is not known whether other plasma lipoproteins or the cholesterol newly synthesized in the liver can inhibit further cholesterol synthesis. By balancing cholesterol absorption and synthesis, the cholesterol pool can theoretically be maintained within a very narrow range. Caloric intake also influences cholesterol synthesis. Excess calorie intake, whether from carbohydrate, alcohol, or protein, results in increased synthesis of triglyceride, and sometimes of cholesterol, by the liver.

The cholesterol in the liver can be used in any of three ways:

1. Of the total cholesterol, 200 to 400 mg/day may be used to form the bile acids and enter the enterohepatic circulation. This process occurs only in the liver.
2. In the normal adult, 800 to 1,200 mg/day may be secreted unchanged into the bile.
3. Cholesterol may be secreted into plasma lipoproteins.

Lipoprotein and Cholesterol Metabolism

The lipoproteins are a transport system that carries triglycerides and cholesteryl esters (cholesterol esterified to a long-chain fatty acid). Triglycerides are carried primarily to adipose cells for storage and to muscle cells for oxidation. Cholesteryl esters are carried to all body cells for use in the structure of plasma membranes, to the cells of certain endocrine glands for synthesis of steroid hormones, and to the liver for synthesis of bile acids. Before cholesteryl esters can be used for these purposes, they must be hydrolyzed to produce unesterified cholesterol.

Triglycerides and cholesteryl esters are carried in the core of the lipoprotein particle and are surrounded by a monolayer of phospholipid, along with a small amount of unesterified cholesterol and apolipoprotein. By interaction with enzymes and cell surface receptors, the apolipoprotein determines where each lipoprotein is metabolized.

Lipoprotein transport can be divided into two phases.[25] The *exogenous system* transports the lipid obtained from the intestine either from the diet or recycled in the enterohepatic circulation, and the *endogenous system* transports the lipid synthesized in the liver.

Exogenous Transport System

The exogenous system (Fig. 8-7) transports chylomicrons formed in the intestine, absorbed into the lymph, and carried to the blood (see Chapter 6). The chylomicrons bind to *lipoprotein lipase,* an enzyme that is present on the luminal surface of capillary endothelial cells in muscle and adipose tissue. The chylomicron contains Apo C-II which activates lipoprotein lipase, freeing the fatty acids and glycerol. As the triglyceride is removed, the chylomicron shrinks in

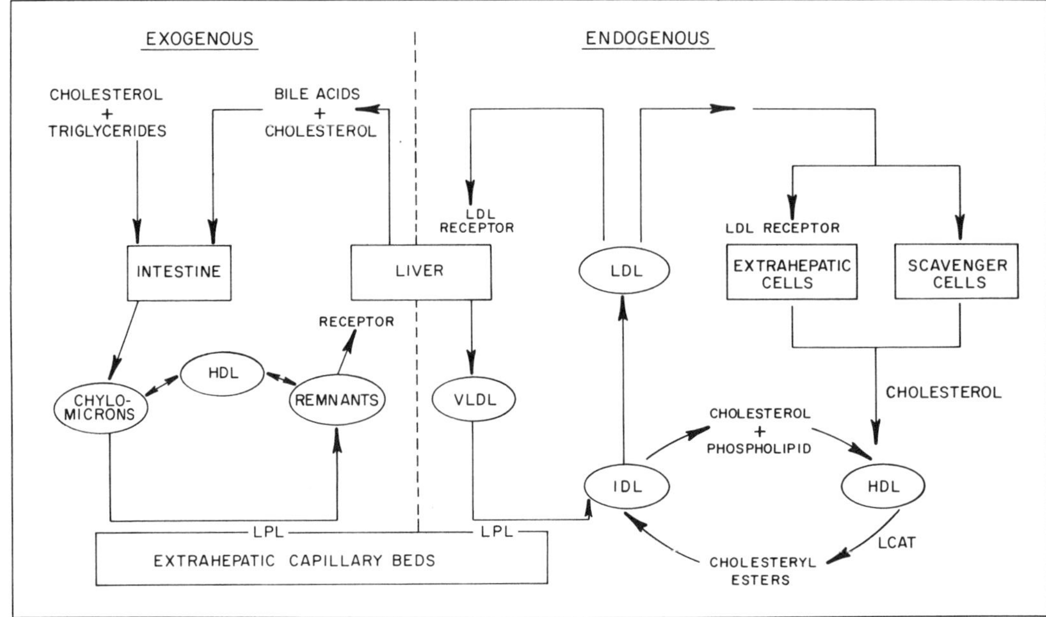

Figure 8-7. Model for lipoprotein transport in humans, illustrating the division between the exogenous and endogenous cycles. Both cycles begin with the secretion of triglyceride-rich particles (chylomicrons and very-low-density lipoproteins [VLDL]) that are converted to cholesterol-rich particles (chylomicron remnants, intermediate-density lipoproteins [IDL], and low-density-lipoproteins [LDL]) through interaction with lipoprotein lipase (LPL). HDL = high-density lipoproteins; LCAT = lecithin-cholesterol acyltransferase. (Reprinted with permission from Brown, M.S., Kovanen, P.T., and Goldstein, J.L., Regulation of plasma cholesterol by lipoprotein receptors. Science *212:629, 1981. Copyright 1981 by the American Association for the Advancement of Science.)*

size and some of the surface phospholipid and free cholesterol becomes excessive. These excess materials are transferred to HDLs.

The remaining particle, called a *chylomicron remnant,* contains cholesteryl ester, Apo B, and Apo E. It is carried to the liver where it binds to receptor cells and is taken up by endocytosis. Within the liver cell, the remnant is degraded by lysosomes. The liver uses cholesterol to form bile acid or secretes it into the bile as free cholesterol. All of this occurs very quickly, so that plasma cholesterol does not increase following a meal.

Endogenous Transport System

The liver synthesizes triglycerides from excess carbohydrate and fat and then forms, with Apo B and Apo E, a lipoprotein particle, VLDL, in order to transport the triglyceride to the adipose cells. The intestine also is a source of some VLDLs. Very-low-density lipoprotein particles also contain cholesterol. This cholesterol is obtained from the diet and from previously formed recycled cholesterol if it is available. Otherwise, the activity of the limiting enzyme, *3-hydroxymethylglutaryl coenzyme A reductase* is increased and the liver synthesizes additional cholesterol.

The VLDLs carried to the capillaries also interacts with lipoprotein lipase, as do chylomicrons. As VLDL size decreases, the excess surface material is again transferred to HDLs. The particle that evolves from a VLDL is smaller and denser: it is an IDL. Thus, an IDL is a VLDL remnant.

The excess cholesterol that has been transferred to HDLs is esterified by the action of the enzyme *lecithin-cholesterol acyltransferase* (*LCAT*) via the following reaction:

$$\text{Free cholesterol} + \text{lecithin} \xrightarrow{\text{LCAT}} \text{cholesteryl ester} + [\text{lecithin} - \text{one fatty acid}]$$

The newly formed cholesterol ester then is transferred, possibly by the action of Apo D, back to the IDL, which now has a core composed mostly of cholesteryl ester rather than triglyceride and a membrane of Apo B. The IDL is released from the capillary wall into the circulation. It next undergoes reactions that remove the remaining triglyceride and all of the apoprotein *except* Apo B, producing an LDL. The site of this conversion is unclear but may be in the liver *sinusoids* (large capillarylike structures).[25]

The LDL, consisting mostly of cholesteryl ester and Apo B, is the particle that delivers cholesterol to the tissues where the Apo B of the LDL binds to receptors ("coated pits") on the cell surface of extrahepatic tissues.[25] Its uptake by the cells apparently is regulated by the number of binding sites on the cell membranes which, in turn, are regulated by the cell's need for cholesterol.[26] The LDL is internalized and carried to the lysosomes of the cells, which degrade the Apo B to its component amino acids. The cholesteryl esters are hydrolyzed to free cholesterol by the action of *acid lipase* and used for membrane formation or hormone synthesis.

Alternatively, LDLs can be degraded by macrophages if LDL concentrations are high. Macrophages can become overloaded with cholesteryl esters at very high serum concentrations, forming *foam cells.* Normally, in a steady state, the uptake and excretion of cholesterol from extrahepatic cells are equal. Cholesterol, resulting from membrane turnover or cell death, is absorbed onto the HDL, esterified, and transferred to VLDL or IDL and thence to LDL, as described previously for the exogenous transport system.

In humans, the triglyceride-carrying particles—that is, the chylomicron remnants, VLDL, and IDL—contain Apo E. These are taken up intact by the liver, which apparently has receptors for Apo B but which also has a high affinity for Apo E (*B,E receptors*). Again, apolipoproteins are hydrolyzed to amino acids and the cholesteryl esters are hydrolyzed to free cholesterol.

In Fig. 8-7, two fairly separate pathways of the endogenous transport system are indicated, but there are three points at which they interact. These points make it possible for the exogenous triglyceride and cholesterol to influence endogenous lipid and lipoprotein metabolism.[25] Both pathways include (1) lipoprotein lipase for delivery of lipids to the peripheral cells, (2) HDLs to accept phospholipid and cholesterol from chylomicron remnants or IDLs, and (3) lipoprotein receptors with some affinities in common.

High-Density Lipoproteins

High-density lipoproteins are the smallest and densest of the lipoproteins, consisting of approximately 50 percent each of protein and lipid with a high proportion of cholesterol. Precursor HDL particles (*nascent HDLs*) are secreted by the liver, intestine, and possibly other tissues. As it matures, nascent HDLs acquire additional cholesteryl esters by the action of LCAT, as described earlier. High-density lipoproteins have been proposed as the vehicle by which cholesterol is transported to the liver.[27]

Recently a subpopulation, known as HDL_c, has been identified that may be significant in understanding the relationship between lipoprotein metabolism and cardiovascular disease. This subpopulation contains a larger amount of Apo E than does normal HDL and has a higher cholesterol content. It may share receptor sites on the endothelial cells with the Apo B of LDLs and may participate with LDLs in the pathogenesis of cardiovascular disease.[28]

Effects of Diet on Serum Lipids and Lipoproteins

A number of dietary factors influence plasma levels of lipids and lipoproteins, although the mechanisms are not entirely clear. The dietary factors fall into two categories, the quantity and nature of the lipids themselves and factors contributing to calorie excess. Knowledge of these factors is important when it becomes desirable to alter plasma lipoprotein concentrations in patients.

Sterols and Fats

Evidence indicates that excessive dietary cholesterol and fat contribute to elevated plasma cholesterol, chiefly in the form of LDLs.[29] They also increase the concentration of HDL_c and decrease normal HDLs. The cholesterol content of VLDL or its remnants also increases, particularly in people with hypertriglyceridemia, so that VLDL migrates with the beta rather than the pre-beta fraction in electrophoresis. The particle then is called beta-VLDL. There are two mechanisms by which it is proposed that hypercholesterolemia occurs as a result of increased dietary cholesterol. Cholesterol in chylomicron remnants is taken up by the liver and resecreted in VLDLs, ultimately forming more LDLs.[25] The increased LDL-cholesterol uptake might then repress B,E receptors.[30] Alternatively, hepatic cholesterol synthesis is not reduced sufficiently or synthesis of cholesterol into bile is not increased sufficiently to compensate for the increased hepatic uptake of cholesterol.[31] Chylomicrons are formed in proportion to the amount of dietary fat. Remnant formation also is increased in proportion.

The *kind of fat* in the diet, as well as the amount, can have a considerable influence on serum lipids. The fats in the diet may be divided into three classes according to the degree of saturation of their fatty acids:

1. Long-chain saturated fatty acids have no double bonds. They may be synthesized in the body from acetate and thus are not essential nutrients. They tend to cause a rise in plasma LDLs and cholesterol. The specific saturated fatty acids in the diet may be important, since all saturated fats do not seem to have the same effect on serum lipids. Myristic acid (fourteen carbons), found especially in coconut oil, and palmitic acid (sixteen carbons), found in large amounts in butterfat, beef fat, lard, and chicken fat, seem to be most hypercholesterolemic. Fish oil, corn oil, and soybean oil also seem to contain appreciable amounts of palmitic acid. Stearic acid (eighteen carbons) and the short-chain and medium-chain fatty acids have little effect.

2. Monounsaturated fatty acids are represented in foods almost solely by oleic acid. It has one unsaturated double bond at the $\omega 9$ (read "omega-9") position—that is, the double bond is between the ninth and tenth carbon atoms, counting from the end of the chain with the methyl group. Oleic acid can also be synthesized from acetate. It apparently has no effect on plasma cholesterol or total lipid concentration.

3. Polyunsaturated fatty acids cannot be synthesized in the body. They are essential as prostaglandin precursors and as components of cell membranes. They must be obtained from dietary sources and therefore are the essential fatty acids. The polyunsaturated fatty acids can be further subdivided into the $\omega 6$ and $\omega 3$ fatty acids. *Linoleic acid* (eighteen carbons, two double bonds) and *arachidonic acid* (twenty carbons, four double bonds) are the major examples of the $\omega 6$ type. Arachidonic acid is synthesized from linoleic in the liver. The major $\omega 3$ fatty acid is *linolenic acid* (eighteen carbons, three double bonds). Both $\omega 3$ and $\omega 6$ fatty acids lower plasma cholesterol and LDLs. The $\omega 6$ poly-

Table 8-6. Fatty Acid Content of Selected Fats and Oils

Type of Fat	Saturated Fats (%)	Unsaturated Fats (%) Oleic Acid	Unsaturated Fats (%) Linoleic Acid
Animal fats			
Butterfat	55	32	3
Beef	53	41	2
Pork (lard)	38	46	7
Chicken	40	36	14
Egg	35	50	Trace
Vegetable oils			
Margarine, stick	17	59	25
Margarine, soft	18	36	36
Corn	14	28	55
Peanut	21	50	28
Cottonseed	28	21	50
Soybean	14	21	50
Safflower	7	17	71
Olive	14	75	7
Palm	48	38	9
Coconut	92	6	1
Sesame	15	40	40
Sunflower	10	21	64

unsaturated fatty acids are involved in lipid transport, whereas ω3 fatty acids lower plasma triglycerides, especially VLDL.

The relative amounts of polyunsaturated fatty acids and saturated fats in the diet often are expressed as the *P/S ratio.* If a fat has a P/S ratio of 2 or more—that is, 2 g of polyunsaturated fatty acid for each gram of saturated fat—it lowers serum cholesterol, but the mechanism is not understood entirely. A diet with a high P/S ratio increases cholesterol excretion in some way.[32] It may stimulate formation of bile acids. In addition, linoleic acid in large quantities alters the lipoprotein fatty acid composition,[33] possibly decreasing their lipid-carrying capacity and reducing serum cholesterol.[34] Other possibilities include an increased rate of metabolism of cholesteryl esters of polyunsaturated fatty acids, thereby increasing the rate of excretion. On the other hand, addition of saturated fat has, on a per gram basis, twice as much effect of raising serum cholesterol and increasing the concentration of LDLs. If it is substituted in the diet for polyunsaturated fatty acids, it also may increase VLDLs. Saturated fatty acids cause the formation of smaller VLDL particles, which contain a larger proportion of cholesterol. The effect of saturated fat may be related primarily to a reduced rate of LDL catabolism. Havel and Kane[35] suggest that the increased saturation of LDL-lipids or changes in the fatty acid composition of the associated membrane influences the interaction of LDLs with B,E receptors.

Oils that contain polyunsaturated fatty acids and that are claimed to be useful in lowering plasma cholesterol concentration are cottonseed, corn, and soybean oils. Coconut oil, olive oil, and animal fats, including butterfat, are low in unsaturated fatty acids and are not useful for this purpose. Some typical values are given in Table 8-6.

Excess Calories

Excessive calorie intake increases plasma lipid levels and VLDL synthesis, regardless of the source of the calories. Triglycerides and cholesterol are increased, while HDL-cholesterol is decreased. Three mechanisms may contribute to this change: (1) increased substrate is provided for triglyceride synthesis and VLDL formation in the liver; (2) VLDL clearance is reduced; and (3) the sensitivity of adipose cells to insulin is reduced, leading to decreased lipoprotein lipase activity and reduced clearing of lipid from the plasma. In contrast, reduction of calorie intake by the obese patient causes a reduction of plasma triglyceride and cholesterol and an increase in HDL-cholesterol.

Carbohydrate

High-carbohydrate diets increase plasma triglyceride, probably by increasing hepatic synthesis.[36] However, it now appears that this is a short-term effect and that increasing carbohydrate, particularly starch, lowers plasma cholesterol and fat over the long term.[34,37]

Large quantities of *sucrose* may be hyperlipidemic in a few people but have little effect in most; the mechanism is unknown.[35] *Fructose* also is hyperlipidemic compared to glucose or starch. The mechanism is unknown but may be related to the fact that fructose goes directly to the liver and increases VLDLs. It also does not stimulate insulin release.

Fiber in the diet is reputed to lower plasma lipid in animals, but the effect in humans is equivocal. It may function (1) by increasing bulk in the diet and thus decreasing total energy intake or fat intake, (2) by increasing intestinal tract transit time, or (3) by decreasing the consumption of fat-containing and cholesterol-containing foods. On the whole, fiber is reported to have little effect on human plasma lipid levels.[37] Pectin may be an exception; it may bind bile acids and increase excretion.[35]

Alcohol

The effect of alcohol on serum lipids and lipoproteins depends on the amount and duration of intake. Alcohol may impair removal of plasma triglycerides.[38,39] Alcohol intake is associated with hypertriglyceridemia,[40] but the effect is transient except in individuals with genetic hypertriglyceridemia.[31,41] Paradoxically, ethanol intake also is associated with increased HDL levels.[42,43] The effect seems to vary with the individual and may be the consequence of the increased caloric intake, increasing the synthesis of lipoproteins high in triglycerides.[44,45]

Lecithin

Lecithin, which is derived from soybeans, has been publicized extensively as a remedy for hypercholesterolemia. It actually has little effect.[31]

Protein

Although animal experiments have indicated that casein from milk is hypercholesterolemic and that increased consumption of vegetable protein may decrease serum cholesterol,[31] a wide range of protein intakes has been found to have no effect on blood lipids in humans.

The Hyperlipoproteinemias

The term *hyperlipidemia,* or *hyperlipemia,* refers to conditions in which serum concentrations of cholesterol or triglyceride are elevated. More specific terms are *hypercholesterolemia* (elevated serum cholesterol) *hypertriglyceridemia* (elevated fasting serum triglycerides), and *hyperchylomicronemia* (elevated fasting serum chylomicrons). *Hyperlipoproteinemia* (HLP) also is a more specific term. It refers to conditions in which the serum concentration of one or more of the classes of lipoproteins is elevated. The hyperlipoproteinemias are of interest because they often are associated with serious coronary heart disease and increased mortality.

Classification and Clinical Features

Hyperlipoproteinemia may be classified as primary or secondary. *Primary HLP* arises from environmental or genetic factors that affect lipid or lipoprotein metabolism directly, whereas *secondary HLP* arises as a result of another disease such as diabetes, nephrosis, myxedema, or obstructive liver disease. It may also arise from excess calorie or alcohol intake. The lipoprotein patterns in the secondary conditions are similar to those seen in one of the primary disorders.

Five types of primary HLP have been described, and their clinical features are summarized in Table 8-7. They are distinguished by the differences in the pattern of lipoproteins in the serum. For most purposes of clinical diagnosis, the appearance of a sample of serum stored 18 hours at 4°C. or determinations of serum cholesterol and

Table 8-7. Features of the Primary Hyperlipoproteinemias

Features	Type I	Type II	Type III	Type IV	Type V
Incidence	Very rare	Common	Uncommon	Common	Uncommon
Composition of serum lipid					
Cholesterol	NL to +	+	+	NL to +	++
Triglyceride	+++	Type IIa NL or type IIb ++	++ or +++	++ or +++	+++
Clinical features	Eruptive xanthomas; abdominal pain; lipemia retinalis	Premature atherosclerosis; xanthelasmas; xanthomas; premature corneal arcus	Atherosclerosis of coronary and peripheral blood vessels; premature xanthomas; planar xanthoma	Premature coronary blood vessel disease; abnormal glucose tolerance; hyperuricemia	Hepatosplenomegaly; abdominal pain; eruptive xanthomas; hyperglycemia; hyperuricemia; lipemia retinalis
Age of detection	Early childhood	Early childhood (if severe)	Early adulthood	Adulthood	Early adulthood
Possible mechanism	Lipoprotein lipase deficiency	Decreased catabolism of beta-lipoprotein; congenital absence of low-density lipoprotein receptors in type IIa	Unknown	Excess endogenous glyceride synthesis or deficient glyceride clearance (?)	Unknown

NL = normal; +, ++, +++ = relative amount of increase.

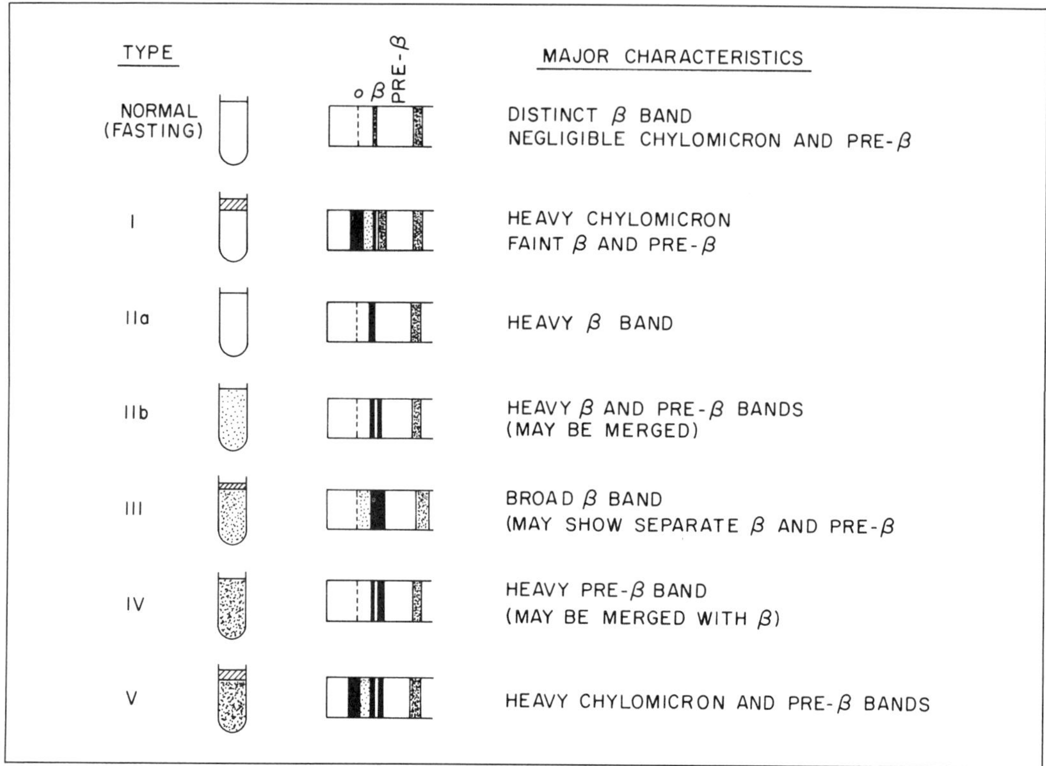

Figure 8-8. Comparison of the typical appearance of refrigerated serum and serum electrophoretic patterns from healthy subjects and hyperlipidemic subjects (types I through V). In refrigerated samples (left), white areas indicate clear serum; hatched areas represent creamy layer of chylomicrons; speckled areas indicate a turbid layer of increased pre-beta lipoprotein. On electrophoretic patterns, 0 is the origin and the lipoproteins migrate from origin to the right. Depth of shading indicates relative quantities.

triglyceride levels are practical and useful. The relationship of these tests to the classifications of HLP and lipoprotein alterations are given in Fig. 8-8 and Table 8-5. Determinations of lipoprotein classes by ultracentrifugation or electrophoresis are too time-consuming and expensive for most clinical situations.

Type I Hyperlipoproteinemia. Type I HLP results from the absence of lipoprotein lipase (or postheparin lipolytic activity) in the capillaries, so that the patient is unable to clear chylomicrons from the plasma. The condition is characterized by chylomicronemia. Lipoprotein lipase requires Apo C-II for activation and is inhibited by a high salt concentration. Primary type I HLP is a rare genetic, recessive trait that usually is detected in early childhood (see Chapter 10 for a review of genetics, if necessary). A similar blood lipid pattern sometimes occurs secondary to diabetic acidosis (see Chapter 9), myxedema (thyroid deficiency), or *dysglobulinemia* (abnormality of serum globulins). Presenting symptoms include eruptive xanthomas (lipid deposits mostly containing cholesteryl esters), abdominal pain, and *lipemia retinalis* (a high level of lipids in the blood, manifested by a milky appearance of the veins and arteries of the retina).

Since the serum has a high level of chylomicrons and these consist primarily of triglycerides, the blood has a significantly increased triglyceride concentration. Cholesterol may be normal or somewhat elevated. The electrophoretic pattern indicates a heavy band at the origin, since chylomicrons do not migrate. The pre-beta (VLDLs) and beta (IDLs and LDLs) bands are faint. If serum is stored under refrigeration, the chylomicrons can be seen as a creamy layer that rises to the top of the sample.

Type II Hyperlipoproteinemia. Type II HLP is the consequence of decreased catabolism of beta-lipoprotein (LDL). Type II HLP has been subdivided into type IIa (*hyperbetalipoproteinemia*), in which LDL alone is elevated, and type IIb, in which both VLDLs and LDLs are increased. In either case, serum cholesterol is elevated, usually to 300 to 600 mg/dl. In type IIb, serum triglycerides will also be increased.

The primary condition is apparently genetic in origin and is fairly common. It varies in severity and can be detected in childhood if severe. Type II HLP can also be produced secondary to nephrosis or hypothyroidism. Presenting symptoms include xanthelasma, xanthomas, premature *corneal arcus* (an opaque line partially encircling the margin of the cornea as a result of lipid deposits), and premature *atherosclerosis* (degeneration and hardening of the walls of the arteries, related to thickening of the tunica intima).

Electrophoresis of the serum shows a heavy beta (LDL) band. Type IIb gives a heavy pre-beta (VLDL) band in addition. The appearance of the serum is clear for type IIa and may be faintly turbid for type IIb.

Primary type IIa HLP occurs in a group of genetic disorders known as *familial hypercholesterolemia.* Apparently, it is inherited as a dominant trait and occurs in approximately 1 in 500 people. Affected individuals have a high incidence of premature and severe atherosclerosis. There appears to be a defect in uptake and degradation of LDLs in peripheral tissues caused by dysfunction of LDL receptors.[46]

Primary type IIb HLP is called *familial combined hyperlipemia.* Low-density lipoprotein receptor function is normal. Nevertheless, LDLs and VLDLs are elevated, but VLDL particles usually are smaller than normal. Affected individuals usually are overweight. Moderately obese patients have hypercholesterolemia, whereas more obese individuals tend to have hypertriglyceridemia.

Type III Hyperlipoproteinemia. Type III HLP is a fairly uncommon condition which is detected in early adulthood. It apparently is due to a defect in the catabolism of remnants of chylomicrons and VLDLs in the liver. Evidence indicates that a genetic mutation controlling Apo E structure causes the production of chylomicron remnants and IDLs that cannot bind in normal fashion to hepatic receptors.[47–49]

Low-density lipoproteins are elevated and there are increased and abnormal VLDLs. The abnormal VLDLs contain an increased amount of Apo E, and particles that have a density similar to VLDLs but are high in cholesterol accumulate. The ratio of triglyceride to cholesterol falls with the increase in cholesterol. It may be 3.3 : 1 or less (normal is 5 : 1). Both cholesterol and triglyceride are increased and may be in the range of 350 to 1,000 mg/dl. Their concentrations generally are almost equal. The electrophoretic pattern shows a heavy broad band in the beta (LDL) and pre-beta (VLDL) position. There is an abnormal lipoprotein (*floating beta-lipoprotein*) in the VLDL fraction when serum is ultracentrifuged. These materials cause a broad band in the beta position. Thus, type III HLP is sometimes called *broad beta disease.* It is also known as *familial dysbetalipoproteinemia* or *remnant removal disease.*

The refrigerated stored serum usually is turbid and sometimes there is a faint creamy layer of chylomicrons on top. Presenting symptoms include premature xanthomas, plantar and palmar xanthomas (xanthomas on the bottom of the feet and palms of the hand), and premature atherosclerosis.

Type IV Hyperlipoproteinemia. Type IV HLP (*endogenous hypertriglyceridemia, hyperprebetalipoproteinemia,* or *familial hypertriacylglycerolemia*) is the most common type of

HLP, appearing in 15 to 25 percent of the population. The stated incidence varies with the definition of normal that is used. Type IV HLP is the type most commonly seen secondary to diabetes mellitus (see Chapter 9). It might be the consequence either of excessive endogenous triglyceride synthesis or of deficient clearance, but the mechanism is unknown. It may be due to an abnormality in the liver at an insulin-sensitive site. As a consequence, there is excess triglyceride that appears in the plasma in enlarged, triglyceride-enriched VLDL particles. The condition is detected in adulthood, usually presenting with abnormal glucose tolerance (see Chapter 9), premature coronary artery disease, and hyperuricemia. It seems to be exacerbated by obesity, alcohol intake, the use of progestational hormones, and perhaps by intake of excess simple carbohydrates.

On electrophoresis, the pre-beta band (VLDL) is increased. Very-low-density lipoprotein is high in triglycerides. Type IV HLP thus is characterized by elevated triglycerides, in the 400- to 1,000-mg/dl range. Cholesterol usually is present in VLDLs in a triglyceride-cholesterol ratio of 5:1. When triglyceride levels are very high in type IV HLP, serum cholesterol is also likely to be elevated. Otherwise, it is normal. The general appearance of the serum is turbid with no visible overlying chylomicron layer.

Type V Hyperlipoproteinemia. Type V HLP is an uncommon disorder that probably is genetic in origin. It may not be related to cardiovascular disease. It is detected in adults and presents with eruptive xanthomas, *hepatosplenomegaly* (enlarged liver and spleen), abdominal pain, lipemia retinalis, and elevated blood levels of glucose and uric acid.

The serum contains elevated amounts of chylomicrons after fasting and elevated VLDLs; thus, the electrophoretic pattern shows a heavy chylomicron band at the origin and a heavy pre-beta band. The serum also contains increased amounts of triglycerides from exogenous sources in the chylomicrons and endogenous sources in VLDLs. Plasma triglycerides measure 1,000 to 6,000 mg/dl. Serum triglyceride-cholesterol ratios may be greater than 5:1, with serum cholesterol elevated or normal. The serum appears turbid with an overlying creamy layer. Lipoprotein lipase activity is low in these patients.

Lipoproteins, Cholesterol, and Atherosclerosis

Atherosclerosis is promoted if chylomicron remnants, IDLs, and LDLs are elevated in the plasma, but the mechanism is unknown. Since chylomicron remnants, IDLs, and LDLs carry cholesteryl esters, it follows that plasma cholesterol concentrations will be elevated at the same time. Elevated VLDLs or chylomicrons apparently are not associated with increased risk of atherosclerosis, and a normal HDL level is associated with a decreased risk.[26,35,50,51] Elevated HDL_c, however, may increase the risk.[28]

The serum concentrations of cholesterol-containing lipoproteins are increased by a number of nondietary as well as dietary factors. Genetics is involved. In addition, cigarette smoking, hypertension, and diabetes mellitus increase the risk of atheroslerosis, as do local factors affecting the arterial wall.

Because the causes of hypercholesterolemia and its consequences are multifactorial, there is a great deal of confusion concerning the most effective approaches to treatment. Recommendations for prevention have been particularly controversial. Another area of uncertainty concerns the circumstances under which definite attempts at therapy should begin. There are no specific concentrations of serum cholesterol or triglyceride that have clearly been defined as the lower limit of abnormal. Rather, these values occur in the population as a continuous variable. The upper limit of serum cholesterol level sometimes is defined as 200 to 250 mg/dl and sometimes as 300 mg/dl. As serum cholesterol increases further, the need for therapy becomes clearer. Generally, a serum cholesterol or triglyceride level higher than 300 mg/dl is considered to require treatment.

Management of Hyperlipoproteinemias

The management of HLP may involve diet and drugs, but nutritional management is currently of primary importance. Severe hypertriglyceridemias with chylomicronemia can lead to pancreatitis, but pancreatitis does not occur if triglycerides are reduced below 1,000 mg/dl. Elevated concentrations of lipoproteins containing Apo B and Apo E (VLDLs, chylomicron remnants, and LDLs), must be treated to prevent atherosclerosis and coronary heart disease.[35]

Nutritional Management. It has been the practice to recommend somewhat different nutritional management for each type of HLP. In type I, a low-fat intake, 25 to 35 g/day, and abstinence from alcohol is recommended, since the patient's ability to clear fat from the serum is defective. Type IIa is characterized by high serum cholesterol. Therefore, a low-cholesterol diet, with increased polyunsaturated fat and limited alcohol intake, has been recommended. In type IIb, in which both cholesterol and triglycerides are increased, recommendations in addition to those for type IIa include maintenance of the patient's ideal body weight, limitation of carbohydrate to 40 percent of calories, and maintenance of normal fat intake at 40 percent of calories. The same diet has been recommended for type III. In type IV, it is necessary to reduce triglyceride synthesis. Therefore, the recommended diet includes maintenance of ideal body weight, limitation of carbohydrate to 35 to 40 percent of calories, limitation of alcohol intake, and increased polyunsaturated fat intake. Cholesterol is not limited. In type V, maintenance of ideal body weight, high protein (21 to 24 percent of calories), normal carbohydrate (48 to 53 percent of calories), and reduced fat (25 to 30 percent of calories) are recommended. Other recommendations include limiting cholesterol intake to 300 to 500 mg/day and eliminating alcohol. These recommendations are summarized in Table 8-8.

Based on information revealed in recent years, it now is suggested that a single diet may be used for the treatment of most cases of HLP regardless of the specific type. This *unified diet* also is useful for patients in whom the specific type of HLP is unknown (for example, if HLP typing is not possible). The American Heart Association is reported to be preparing a statement recommending a diet restricted in saturated fat and cholesterol plus attainment and maintenance of ideal body weight for all individuals whose plasma cholesterol level exceeds 240 mg/dl.[35] The Association also is recommending that people with triglyceride levels in excess of 300 mg/dl be treated.

The proposed diet is to be achieved in three steps, based on the assumption that patient compliance will be improved if diet modifications are made gradually. The steps are summarized in Table 8-9. In phase 1, 30 to 35 percent of calories are fat and 300 mg of cholesterol per day are allowed. This diet restricts the use of red meat and fat-containing milk products. It eliminates the use of egg yolk, butterfat, lard, and organ meats, and substitutes egg white, skim milk, soft margarine, and vegetable oils. Phase 2 allows 30 percent of calories as fat and 200 to 250 mg of cholesterol per day. It includes a maximum of 8 oz. of meat per day, restricts the use of cheese, and further reduces fat intake. In phase 3, 20 to 25 percent of calories are fat and 100 mg of cholesterol are allowed. This diet requires that meats be used only as a "condiment," with a maximum of 3 to 4 oz./day, and the emphasis is on fish and poultry. Cheese is eliminated, except for low-cholesterol cheese. The diet in this phase is composed primarily of cereals, legumes, fruits, and vegetables.[25,31]

There is no recommendation for an increase in polyunsaturated fatty acids, although others have suggested that saturated

Table 8-8. Recommended Nutritional Management of the Primary Hyperlipoproteinemias[a]

Type	Kilocalories	Fat	Polyunsaturated Fat[b]	Cholesterol	Protein	Carbohydrate	Alcohol	Summary
I	Not restricted	25–35 g	Not limited	Not limited	Not limited	Not limited	None allowed	25–35 g fat; no alcohol
IIa	Not restricted	Limit saturated fat	Increase P/S ratio	As low as possible	Not limited	Not limited	Moderate	Low cholesterol; increase P/S ratio
IIb	Achieve and maintain ideal weight	Limit to 40% of calories	Limit saturated fat; increase P/S ratio	Limit to <300 mg	Increase to 20% of calories	Limit to 40% of calories; restrict concentrated sweets	2 servings per day maximum	Low cholesterol; protein, 20%; fat, 40% or less; carbohydrate, 40%; restrict concentrated sweets
III	Achieve and maintain ideal weight	Limit to 40% of calories	Increase P/S ratio	Limit to <300 mg	Increase to 20% of calories	Limit to 40% of calories; restrict concentrated sweets	2 servings per day maximum	Low cholesterol; protein, 20%; fat, 40% or less; carbohydrate, 40%; restrict concentrated sweets
IV	Achieve and maintain ideal weight	Limit saturated fat	Increase P/S ratio	Limit to 300–500 mg	Not limited	Limit to 35–40% of calories; restrict concentrated sweets	2 servings per day maximum	Decrease cholesterol; limit carbohydrate to 45% of calories; restrict concentrated sweets
V	Achieve and maintain ideal weight	25–30% of calories	Increase P/S ratio	Limit to 300–500 mg	Not limited	50% of calories; restrict concentrated sweets	None allowed	Decrease cholesterol; fat, 30% or less; carbohydrate, 50%; restrict concentrated sweets

Based on information from Frederickson, D.S., Bonnell, M., Levy, R.K., and Ernst, N. *Dietary Management of Hyperlipoproteinemia.* DHEW Publication no. (NIH) 75-110.

Table 8-9. Proposed Unified Diet for the Nutritional Management of the Primary Hyperlipoproteinemias

Unified Diet	Kilocalories	Fat	Cholesterol	Carbohydrate	Summary
Phase I	Achieve and maintain ideal weight	Limit to 30–35% of calories	300 mg	Increase complex carbohydrate	*For all phases:* restrict fat; limit cholesterol; increase complex carbohydrate
Phase II	Achieve and maintain ideal weight	Limit to 30% of calories	200–250 mg	Increase complex carbohydrate	
Phase III	Achieve and maintain ideal weight	Limit to 20–25% of calories	100 mg	Increase complex carbohydrate	

Based on information from Connor, W.E., and Connor, S.L. The dietary treatment of hyperlipidemia. *Med. Clin. North Am.* 66:485, 1982.

fat should constitute only 50 percent of the fat calories.[31] Increased polyunsaturated fatty acids have been associated with an incidence of gallstones, and a few controversial studies have indicated that they can promote cancer in animals. In addition, added polyunsaturated fatty acids can present difficulty in weight control.

To reduce the fat content of the diet, it is necessary to increase the carbohydrate. It is recommended that this be in the form of complex carbohydrate; thus, the fiber content of the diet would be increased.

Although it appears simple in concept, the unified diet will be controversial. In addition, implementation is likely to be difficult. For many people, it represents a radical change in current diet practices. Many patients would require careful instruction in menu planning to assure adequate intake of protein containing all essential amino acids.

Drug Treatment. Drug treatment may be indicated for those HLP patients in whom diet is ineffective after 3 months. Specific indications are increased LDL with a cholesterol level in excess of 300 mg/dl or a triglyceride level higher than 500 mg/dl.[35] The drugs commonly used for treatment of HLP and their nutrition-related side effects are given in Table 8-10. In some patients, drugs are used in combination.

ATHEROSCLEROSIS

Atherosclerosis is a disease of the tunica intima of the large and medium-sized arteries, characterized by localized fatty deposits and thickening of the arterial wall. The fat deposits distort the arteries and make them rigid. The arteries most commonly affected are the aorta, the iliac and femoral arteries (to the legs), and the coronary and cerebral arteries. *Arteriosclerosis* is a more general term encompassing several arterial diseases that have common characteristics including degeneration, thickening, and hardening (*sclerosis*) of the arterial wall. Thus, atherosclerosis is a form of arteriosclerosis. There are other forms that are classified in various ways. One useful classification gives three types. *Hypertensive arteriosclerosis* consists of a progressive increase in muscle and elastic tissue as a consequence of hypertension. *Arteriolosclerosis,* affecting mainly the arterioles, is also seen in chronic hypertension. *Mönckeberg's arteriosclerosis* results from focal calcification of peripheral arteries.

Early lesions of atherosclerosis are asymptomatic. Later, as they develop further, they interfere with the circulation and then cause systemic effects. The specific consequence varies with the site of the lesions. When the lesions occur in the coronary blood vessels, the result is ischemic heart disease. These

Table 8-10. Drug Treatment of the Hyperlipoproteinemias and Related Nutritional Care

Drug	Effect	Possible Nutrition-Related Side Effects and Contraindications	Nutritional Management
Bile acid–binding resins: cholestyramine (Questran; Cuemid); colestipol hydrochloride (Colestid)	Reduce serum cholesterol; bind bile acids and prevent reabsorption; increase production of bile acids, cholesterol synthesis, and LDL catabolism. Depend on ability to increase LDL receptors; therefore, not useful in congenital absence of LDL receptors (homozygous type IIa)	Constipation; sometimes nausea, vomiting, anorexia; steatorrhea and diarrhea (rare); fat-soluble vitamin deficiency (rare); intrinsic factor bound; decreased folate and calcium absorption	Increase fiber in the diet; mix drug with applesauce; lower dose if severe side effects occur. Monitor for mineral and vitamin deficiency. Supplement if necessary with water-soluble forms
Clofibrate (Atromid-S)	Increases VLDL clearance by increasing LPL activity; inhibits cholesterol synthesis; increases cholesterol excretion; decreases serum triglyceride and cholesterol	Stomatitis, gastritis, flatulence, decreased taste perception, malabsorption; hepatic dysfunction (rare); cholelithiasis (?)	See Chapters 5 and 6
Probucol (Lorelco)	Reduces serum cholesterol; mechanism unknown	Nausea, vomiting, flatulence, abdominal pain, diarrhea	See Chapter 6
Nicotinic acid (aluminum nicotinate [Nicobid and Nicolar])	Decreases VLDL and LDL; inhibits VLDL production; inhibits cholesterol synthesis and increases excretion; inhibits HDL catabolism	Cutaneous flushing; decreased carbohydrate tolerance; nausea	
Dextrothyroxine (Choloxin)	Reduces plasma lipids; increases fecal excretion of cholesterol	Weight loss	
β-Sitosterol	Reduces plasma lipids; inhibits cholesterol absorption from intestine	Mild laxative effect	
Neomycin	Reduces plasma lipids; inhibits cholesterol absorption from intestine	Enterocolitis; malabsorption	See Chapter 6

LDL = low-density lipoprotein; VLDL = very-low-density lipoprotein; LPL = lipoprotein lipase; HDL = high-density lipoprotein.

lesions may lead to coronary occlusion (*myocardial infarction* or *MI*). Lesions in the blood vessels in or to the brain lead to a *cerebrovascular accident* (CVA), also known as *stroke syndrome* or *apoplexy*. The sclerotic lesion can interfere with circulation to other organs and structures, such as the legs, kidneys, and pancreas. Other consequences include *arrhythmias* and *congestive heart failure*.

The Lesion

The lesion in atherosclerosis is called an *atheroma*. It can vary greatly with the pa-

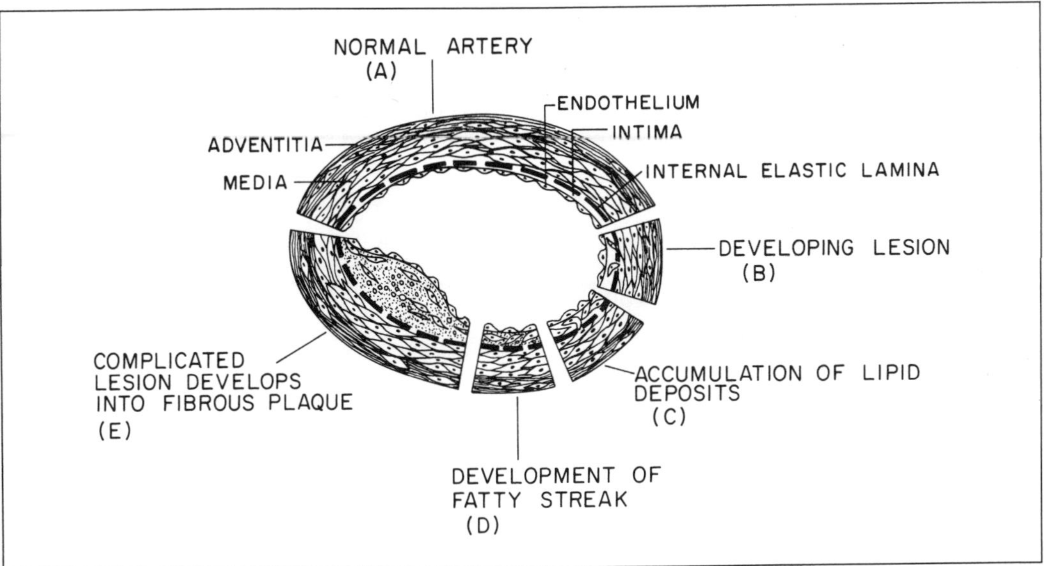

Figure 8-9. A series of possible stages in the development of the various lesions of atherosclerosis. At (A), there is a normal muscular artery and its component layers: the tunica intima bounded by endothelium and internal elastic lamina, the tunica media, and the tunica externa (adventitia). In children and young adults, the intima is thin and contains only an occasional smooth muscle cell; with age, it slowly and uniformly increases in thickness and cell content. Note that there are no fibroblasts present in either the intima or the media of mammalian arteries; fibroblasts are found only in the adventitia. (B) The first phase of a developing lesion in atherosclerosis; a focal thickening of the intima consists of an increase in smooth muscle cells and extracellular matrix. Smooth muscle cells are shown proliferating within the intima; two are in the process of migrating through fenestrae of the internal elastic lamina. Subsequent to or possibly concomitant with intimal smooth muscle proliferation, accumulation of intercellular lipid deposits (C) or extracellular lipid (D) or both occur, resulting in a fatty streak, the second stage (D). A fibrous plaque (E), the third stage, may result from continued accumulation of a connective tissue cap covering increased numbers of smooth muscle cells laden with lipids, extracellular lipid, and cell debris overlying a deeper extracellular pool of lipid. A complicated lesion may form as a result of continuing cell degeneration, ingress of blood constituents, and calcification superimposed on the elements present in the fibrous plaque. (Reprinted with permission from Ross, R., and Glomset, J.A., Atherosclerosis and the arterial smooth muscle cell. Science *180:1333, 1973. Copyright 1973 by the American Association for the Advancement of Science.)*

tient's age and sex and with the location in the body.

An early change in arterial structure consists of a slight thickening of the arterial wall, sometimes called *juvenile intimal thickening.* These early "lesions" may be normal adaptations and unrelated to pathologic processes; therefore, the term *lesion* may be a misnomer.

There are three types or stages of lesions that are considered to be classic representations of the atherosclerotic process: the fatty streak, the fibrous plaque, and the complicated lesion (Fig. 8-9). Lesions progress slowly from one stage to another on an individual basis, so that lesions in all three stages of development can coexist in the same person. Three classic lesions will be described, but it must be recognized that they are not sharply separated. Intermediate stages and, possibly, lesions that are regressing may be seen.

The lesions are believed to be the consequence of an injury to the localized areas of artery wall, leading to increased permeability to circulating macromolecules and thickening of the subendothelium. Some cells, possibly smooth muscle and connective tissue cells, proliferate. Some have an altered metabolism and acquire cholesterol-rich vacuoles, and others become necrotic. There is some repair of the lesions with collagen and elastin formation, but this may contribute to the pathologic process.

Fatty Streaks

Fatty streaks consist of flat deposits of lipids, primarily in the smooth muscle cells of the intima. These fatty streaks are known as *foam cells* but are not to be confused with macrophages that have taken up lipids in the blood. Some lipid also is deposited extracellularly in the intima. The lipid is believed to be derived from the lipoproteins, thus establishing the relationship between hyperlipidemia and atherosclerosis.

Fibrous Plaques

Fibrous plaques are more severe, permanent lesions than are fatty streaks, consisting of a capsule of lipid-containing smooth muscle cells that have proliferated along with connective tissue covering a core of necrotic cell debris and extracellular lipid. The composition of the lipid suggests that it originates in the lipoproteins. Fibrous plaques tend to protrude into the lumen of the blood vessel, reducing the size of the lumen.

Complicated Lesions

Complicated lesions develop as breaks occur in the endothelial surface of fibrous plaques. Clots then may form on this surface. Small blood vessels that have penetrated large plaques, increasing their size, may hemorrhage, with consequent thrombus formation and enlargement of the total size of the lesion. The lipid-rich core may increase in size and become necrotic while the surrounding smooth muscle cells proliferate further. Pools of lipid in the tunica media can become calcified, with loss of elasticity of the artery. If the media becomes thinner or atrophied, an *aneurysm* (sac caused by local dilation of the artery wall) can develop.

Pathogenesis

Three mechanisms for the formation of atheromas have been postulated. They are cell injury, transformation of smooth muscle cells, and lipid accumulation.

It has been proposed that atheromatous lesions arise from fibrin deposition on an injured intima. The injury may be mechanical (including the effects of hypertension), biochemical, or immunologic. The injury may consist of actual physical injury or may consist of functional changes, such as changes in cell membrane permeability. It is possible that blood platelets accumulate at the site of the injury and, in continuous or repeated injury, interact with subepithelial tissue, promoting migration into the intima from the media and proliferation of smooth muscle cells.

In the *transformation* or *monoclonal* hypothesis, the atheroma is proposed to originate from the transformation of smooth muscle cells by a mutagen. It has been suggested that the plaques are neoplastic (consisting of new cells) and not hyperplastic (from enlargement of existing cells). Lipids and the use of tobacco, for example, could contribute to atherosclerosis by carrying a mutagen to smooth muscle cells.

In a third hypothesis, serum cholesterol, especially LDL-cholesterol, is postulated to be the main cause of atherosclerosis, because high levels of LDL are taken up by smooth muscle cells and since cholesteryl oleate accumulates in the extracellular space.[26] According to this hypothesis, the lipid accumulation would lead to cell death, with accumulation of its contained lipids plus cell debris.

It seems clear that the pathogenesis of atherosclerosis does involve cell injury, lipids, platelets, and smooth muscle proliferation. Further research may define the process and interaction of these factors as a combination of all three of the proposed mechanisms.

Etiology

The etiology of atherosclerosis is unknown but is believed to be multifactorial. A number of characteristics of those who have complications of atherosclerosis, such as myocardial infarction and CVA, have been identified. These characteristics have been termed *risk factors,* and it has been assumed that the presence of risk factors increases the severity of the disease and its associated mortality. In addition, it seems logical to suppose that removal of risk factors would reduce the morbidity and death rates; however, good evidence to this effect is lacking.

The three most important risk factors for development of atherosclerosis, indicated by epidemiologic studies, are hypertension, hypercholesterolemia, and cigarette smoking. Other risk factors include obesity, lack of physical activity, diabetes mellitus, hypertriglyceridemia, and a family history of the disease, indicating a genetic predisposition. Stress and a tense, striving, overconscientious personality are considered risk factors, too. The risk factors are considered to have a synergistic relationship, so that the presence of multiple risks increases geometrically the probability of symptomatic disease. Most of the evidence relating risk factors to atherosclerotic disease is epidemiologic and therefore consists primarily of statistical evidence for probability of an association. Such evidence does not establish unequivocally a cause-and-effect relationship between a given risk factor and atherosclerotic disease.

The most consistent associations have been found with uncontrollable factors—*age, sex,* and *race.*[52,53] The incidence and extent of the disease increase with age. They also are more severe in men than in premenopausal women in the white population, but cigarette smoking and the use of estrogens for birth control significantly increase the risk for women. There is no prevalence based on gender among blacks in the United States. Various racial and ethnic groups in the United States—blacks, whites, and some Oriental groups—have been compared with Africans, black and white Central and South Americans, and equivalent populations in Oriental countries. A higher incidence of symptomatic atherosclerosis is seen in the group in the United States, suggesting that environment may be more important than race.

Atherosclerosis has been associated with hypercholesterolemia, increased LDL-cholesterol, and decreased HDL-cholesterol.[54,55] The epidemiologic evidence relating atherosclerotic disease to diet, however, is contradictory in some respects and so has been controversial. Associations of atherosclerotic disease with fat, cholesterol, carbohydrate, fiber, protein, and hard drinking water have been suggested by a variety of epidemiologic studies,[56,57] but the results of many studies are conflicting.

Studies of population groups generally have shown that in some countries in which large amounts of foods containing cholesterol and saturated fats are consumed, there is a higher incidence of atherosclerosis than is the case in countries where the diet is lower in fat.[58] However, there are exceptions, including Swedes and Eskimos.

In the United States, a few groups were identified whose diets are lower in total and saturated fat and in cholesterol. Their serum cholesterol levels were lower than that seen in a similar group from the general population.[53] In other studies in the population at large, there was no relationship between dietary and serum cholesterol.[59,60]

The results of studies of the effects of altered lipid intake in small populations in clinical research units were similarly contradictory. In addition, large-scale trials in large cities in several countries failed to demonstrate that lowering serum cholesterol with diet or drugs prevented coronary artery disease.

Prevention

As a consequence of these seeming contradictions, there has been disagreement on the advisability of recommending diet changes to the general population. Two reports that do so are based on the assumption that the evidence is sufficient to warrant diet modification in view of the seriousness of the disease.[61,62] The recommended diet, commonly called the "prudent diet," contains less than 300 mg of cholesterol per day, fat to provide no more than 30 to 35 percent of total energy, a P/S ratio of 1 or more, and an increase in complex carbohydrate accompanied by a decrease in simple sugars. The changes in the average diet in the United States that have been suggested to achieve the prudent diet are as follows:

1. Substitute skim milk for whole milk and milk products (except for young children).
2. Increase the use of chicken and fish while decreasing consumption of other meats; reduce the number of eggs eaten to a maximum of three per week.
3. Increase the intake of fruits and vegetables.
4. Use whole grain rather than refined cereals.
5. Reduce the use of sugar and fat; reduce saturated fats and substitute monounsaturated and polyunsaturated fat.
6. Reduce sodium intake.

A more recent statement from the American Heart Association makes some changes in these recommendations:[63]

1. Reduce total fat in the diet to no more than 30 percent of total energy, including saturated fat reduced from 17 percent to 10 percent, and polyunsaturated fats reduced to 10 percent or less.
2. Increase carbohydrate from 45 percent to 55 percent of total energy, primarily in the form of complex carbohydrate.
3. Reduce cholesterol intake to less than 300 mg/day from present levels of 450 to 500 mg/day.
4. Adjust total energy intake to achieve and maintain desirable body weight.
5. Reduce sodium intake (no specific amount of sodium is stated).

Clearly, this diet is less restrictive than the unified diet recommended for treatment of existing hyperlipoproteinemia.

Others do not feel that mass intervention is justified but suggest that diet changes be prescribed for those individuals who show evidence of hyperlipoproteinemia.[64]

ISCHEMIC HEART DISEASE

Ischemic heart disease (*IHD*), also known as *coronary artery disease, coronary heart disease, coronary occlusion, atherosclerotic heart disease,* and *coronary thrombosis,* is the commonest form of heart disease in individuals older than 40 years and is a leading cause of sudden death. It is a condition in which the oxygen supply to the myocardium is inadequate. It usually is the result of pathologic changes in the coronary arteries whereby the coronary circulation can no longer meet the metabolic requirements of the heart.

Ischemic heart disease is most often the result of atheromatous lesions in the coronary circulation. However, it also can result from hypertrophy of the cardiac muscle such as would occur in *aortic stenosis* (narrowing of the aorta or of the opening of the heart to the aorta). In addition, it can occur owing to a defect in oxygen binding by hemoglobin, but this is rare.

Risk Factors

A number of risk factors have been associated with an increased incidence of IHD.

Those considered most important are hypertension, hypercholesterolemia, and cigarette smoking, as in atherosclerosis. Other risk factors include obesity, physical inactivity, genetic predisposition, diabetes mellitus, hyperuricemia, and electrocardiogram abnormalities.

Specifically, serum cholesterol levels in excess of 250 mg/dl have been associated with a higher incidence of IHD. Hypertension in excess of 160/95 mm Hg is believed to exacerbate IHD, particularly in the presence of hyperlipidemia. It is thought that the increased blood pressure causes an abnormal lipoprotein transport, increasing the uptake of lipid into the intima. Cigarette smoking may cause hypoxia from inhaled carbon monoxide, which then leads to hyperlipidemia.

Although these risk factors are believed to increase the incidence of IHD when present, there is no proof that removing them reduces the mortality. Initial findings of a recently completed Multiple Risk Factor Intervention Trial (MRFIT) suggest that the reduction of risk factors is not effective.

Ischemic heart disease can be divided into two categories, angina pectoris and myocardial infarction. They differ in degree and in the rate of onset.

Angina Pectoris

Angina pectoris is characterized by *precordial* pain (pain in the region over the heart and stomach), which may radiate to the neck, jaw, back, abdomen, and arms. The pain is precipitated by factors that increase the oxygen requirement of the heart, which may include exercise, smoking, eating, anxiety, and exposure to cold. It usually occurs only after at least 50 to 75 percent of the cross-section of a coronary artery is blocked. During an acute attack of angina pectoris, in addition to the pain, patients are pale and sweating. Pulse rate and blood pressure rise.

Management is based on control of the oxygen requirements of the myocardium and reduction of precipitating environmental factors. Rest may be required for the acute phase, but some patients with stable angina will profit from a carefully prescribed and supervised exercise program. Exercise may reduce the heart rate at a given work load and increase the amount of work that can be done before the onset of angina.

There is no unequivocal evidence that coronary atherosclerosis will regress if treated in humans, but it does so in animal experiments. Therefore, diet modification as indicated for atherosclerosis is appropriate for angina patients. Patients should reach and maintain their ideal body weight or be slightly underweight.

Drug therapy includes, for acute attacks, the use of *nitroglycerin* or *isosorbide dinitrate* (Isordil), which cause vasodilation. Some patients with angina associated with hypertension or heart failure are given *digitalis* and *diuretics.* Nutrition-related side effects of diuretics are given in Table 8-3. *Beta-adrenergic receptor blocking agents* may be given to counteract the increased heart rate and contractility that accompany nitroglycerin use. *Propranolol hydrochloride* (Inderal), used for this purpose, affects also the smooth muscle receptors in organs other than the heart, including the gastrointestinal tract. Possible side effects include nausea, diarrhea, and sodium retention. The patient's diet should be modified as indicated by these side effects.

Myocardial Infarction

Clinical Manifestations and Diagnosis

In *myocardial infarction* (*coronary infarction, coronary thrombosis,* or *heart attack*), the ischemia becomes so severe that the cardiac muscle cells become necrotic. There is very little communication between the major coronary arteries, and narrowing of any one can result in an insufficient blood supply to the portion of the heart muscle that it perfuses. If the blood vessel becomes occluded, the affected cells will die because of lack of blood supply. The amount of necrotic tissue (the size of the infarct) and the consequences depend on the location of the occlusion. Death can result if, for example, the blood supply to a major portion of the left ventricle is occluded.

Prior to an infarction, patients frequently have nonspecific symptoms such as fatigue, malaise, insomnia, and flatulence. Angina pectoris usually worsens. The principal symptom of an infarction is precordial pain which the patient may mistake for severe angina or indigestion.

The electrocardiogram is especially helpful in locating the site of the lesion in myocardial infarction. Coronary angiography sometimes is used also to diagnose myocardial infarction.

When cells become necrotic, some enzymes are released and increase in concentration in the serum. Laboratory determination of serum glutamic oxaloacetic transaminase (SGOT), lactic dehydrogenase (LDH), and creatine phosphokinase (CPK) are useful. These enzymes also rise in diseases of other organs involving necrosis but are used to confirm myocardial infarction and to estimate the prognosis. A greater increase in circulating levels of these enzymes indicates greater myocardial damage and a less hopeful prognosis.

Clinical Course

Approximately 25 percent of the first episodes of myocardial infarction result in medically unattended deaths. Most additional deaths occur in the first 24 hours. The immediate objective of management is to recognize and treat arrhythmias, shock, and heart failure. The close monitoring of patients that is required has resulted in the establishment of special units for the care of these patients and others with life-threatening acute cardiovascular disease. These units commonly are known as *coronary care units* (CCU). Approximately 65 percent of patients who survive a myocardial infarction and reach the hospital have an uncomplicated convalescence.

Management

The primary objectives when the patient is admitted are to prevent death from cardiac arrest or arrhythmia, to increase the oxygen in the blood, and to reduce pain. The surviving patient usually is kept at complete bed rest for at least 10 days to reduce the work of the heart. Many patients return to normal activity after a convalescence of several months. Those with extensive myocardial damage may progress to cardiac failure.

In nutritional care of patients with myocardial infarction, decisions must be made on when to begin feeding and on the size, frequency, consistency, and temperature of the meals. Factors that must be considered in addition to the diagnosis of myocardial infarction include the use of medications such as digitalis and morphine sulfate, as well as the effects of complications such as nausea, pain, heart failure, or uncontrolled arrhythmias. Nausea may be a side effect of the morphine.

The hypoxia, pain, and anxiety accompanying a myocardial infarction activate the sympathetic nervous system. Epinephrine, norepinephrine, and cortisol are produced in larger quantities. The splanchnic circulation, which receives approximately 25 percent of the cardiac output in a resting individual, is constricted. Although there is some disagreement on this point, it seems logical to reduce the need for increased splanchnic circulation. To this end, the following guidelines have been recommended for nutritional care of patients in intensive care:

1. The patient generally is not fed orally until he or she is stable. When oral feeding is begun, a liquid diet sometimes is recommended[65,66] for at least the first 24 hours for patients with nausea, pain, or hypoxia, to reduce vomiting and possible aspiration pneumonia and to avoid gagging and possible vasovagal response which might produce arrhythmia or cardiac arrest.[65,66]
2. A few days of undernutrition with 800 to 1,200 kcal/day are suggested immediately following the attack.[67]

3. Gradually, caloric intake is increased to a maximum of 1,800 kcal.[66]
4. Small, frequent feedings that are soft and low in roughage are used to avoid abdominal distension.
5. Moderate fluid restriction is instituted if necessary to limit total volume.[66]

Higher energy intakes may be given to those patients who do not require weight reduction once they no longer need intensive care.

Little evidence is available concerning the effects of temperature extremes in food. There is evidence both for and against the restriction of the use of very cold foods.[68,69] Some cardiologists recommend the avoidance of either very hot or very cold foods.[66]

The use of caffeine and other methylxanthines (see Appendix I) also is controversial. Methylxanthines decrease calcium binding at the cell membrane, affecting the action potential and possibly causing ventricular fibrillation. In addition, they stimulate the release of catecholamines from the adrenal medulla. Catecholamines may mobilize free fatty acids, possibly causing arrhythmias. Under these circumstances, methylxanthines may be restricted until later in convalescence.[70]

Other procedures recommended in the nutritional care of the myocardial infarction patient include avoidance of flatulence-causing foods and the use of a diet reduced in cholesterol. Sodium restriction may be provided if the patient shows signs of congestive heart failure (see the next section) or pulmonary edema.[65] The risks of indiscriminate use of sodium restriction, as listed by Goldberger,[71] include (1) the danger of precipitating shock by reducing the circulating blood volume; (2) excessive sodium loss, since many myocardial infarction patients have disturbances of renal tubular function; and (3) the risk of sodium deficiency in the vomiting patient with myocardial infarction who has lost sodium in the vomitus. Sodium restriction may be used for certain patients for whom it is specifically indicated, but it is not a routine procedure.[66]

Long-term management will require adequate energy intake to maintain ideal body weight. In addition, the patient may require sodium restriction, a fat-controlled diet, or both.

CONGESTIVE HEART FAILURE

Congestive heart failure (*CHF*) occurs when the heart fails as a pump and cannot deliver an adequate amount of oxygenated blood to body tissues. A failure to deliver enough oxygen (*cardiac decompensation*) may occur at first only during exercise. As the condition worsens, decompensation occurs during normal activity and with meals and, eventually, during bed rest.

It may be caused by a primary disease of the myocardium or by a disease that affects other cardiac structures, such as the valves, conduction system, endocardium, or pericardium, and then involves the myocardium secondarily. Congestive heart failure also can occur secondary to diseases outside of the heart that cause a great increase in the work load of the heart.

Pathogenesis

Congestive heart failure may occur by three mechanisms.[72] One of these is a *decrease in the number of contractile units.* Myocardial infarction is an example in which heart muscle is destroyed and replaced by scar tissue. Second, there may be a decrease in the *quality of contractile units* (ability to contract). This occurs in *cardiomyopathies* (disorders of heart muscle of unknown cause). Last, the heart may be presented with an *excessive work load.* This increased work load may be a *pressure overload* or a *volume overload.* A pressure overload, also known as *excess afterload,* occurs when the heart must pump blood against an increased pressure. In systemic hypertension or aortic stenosis, the left ventricle is presented with an increased work load to maintain the necessary blood flow. The right ventricle receives a pressure overload in pulmonic or mitral stenosis. A volume overload can occur, for example, when the mitral and aortic valves do not close properly in diastole and blood that has been pumped out regurgitates back into the ventricle. It then has to be pumped out again on the next systole, increasing the total amount of blood that the heart must pump. Other conditions add to the work load of the heart, sometimes by increasing tissue need beyond the capacity of even a normal heart.

In some people, the heart can be damaged but it adjusts to the need (*compensated failure*) by enlarging or increasing the rate,[73] thus increasing output toward normal.[74] If a condition that increases the work load is superimposed, it may precipitate CHF. Some of these precipitating factors are fever, anemia, pregnancy, pulmonary embolism, thyrotoxicosis, or myocardial infarction. Sometimes CHF can be precipitated simply by excess sodium intake.

Congestive heart failure is divided into *left ventricular heart failure* and *right ventricular heart failure,* owing to the double pump structure of the heart. In right ventricular heart failure, there is decreased venous return to the heart and congestion (edema) of peripheral tissues. In left ventricular heart failure, there is pulmonary congestion. As congestion of the lungs becomes chronic, compliance and elasticity of the lungs are decreased.[75] Consequently, there is an increase in energy expenditure by the lungs.[76] Eventually, the failure of one side of the heart affects the other and both will fail. Sometimes CHF also is categorized as *backward* versus *forward failure, systolic* versus *diastolic failure,* or *high-output* versus *low-output failure.* Many of these types of failure are the basis for theories explaining salt and water retention. Nevertheless, a thorough explanation of these mechanisms is not yet available.

Salt and Water Retention

In heart failure, blood stagnates in the venous system returning blood to the heart, and venous pressure increases. Fluid diffuses from the blood vessels into surrounding tissues. The reduced cardiac output reduces the renal blood supply and renal blood pressure. This initiates the renin-angiotensin-aldosterone response described previously, causing sodium and water retention. Vasopressin may also be released and stimulates water reabsorption. Other factors probably are involved and may be very important. The net effect of sodium and water retention is edema and congestion in the peripheral tissues.

In moderate failure, the retained fluid increases blood flow to the heart, priming the heart to pump more blood. As failure progresses, the amount of blood increases and stretches the heart muscle so it becomes overstretched, weakens further, and eventually fails completely.

Clinical Manifestations

The signs and symptoms of CHF vary with the degree of congestion and the organs involved. The most common symptom of heart failure is *dyspnea* (respiratory distress). It may occur at first only during activity but steadily worsens until the patient is breathless even at rest. Patients also develop *orthopnea* (dyspnea when recumbent) as the failure progresses. This sensation is relieved when the patient is upright, so that the patient sleeps partly propped up on pillows or bolt upright.

Other symptoms include anorexia, nausea, a feeling of fullness, abdominal pain, malabsorption, enlarged liver, and liver tenderness, related to failure of adequate circulation to the abdominal organs. Patients may be constipated. Decreased blood supply to the brain can result in mental confusion, memory loss, anxiety, insomnia, and headache. Pallor, cool extremities, and sweating also are seen. Additional findings include pulmonary edema, fluid accumulation in the chest cavity (*hydrothorax, pleural effusion*), *ascites* (fluid accumulation in the abdominal cavity), and *cardiac edema.* Edema appears almost invariably in the legs in ambulatory patients and in the sacral region in recumbent patients.

In advanced CHF, patients may become severely malnourished, a condition known as *cardiac cachexia.* There are a number of mechanisms by which this occurs, including: (1) increased metabolic rate consequent to the enlarged heart and the increased work of breathing; (2) anorexia, nausea, vomiting; (3) malabsorption; and (4) occasionally, protein-losing enteropathy.[77]

Management

In the management of CHF, elimination of the basic cause and precipitating factors are essential if possible. In addition, the work load of the heart must be reduced. Reduction of work load is accomplished by providing oxygen, by decreasing physical activity, by diet, and with drugs.

Nutritional Care

In order to reduce fluid retention, the hospitalized patient in severe cardiac failure usually is given a diet containing 500 mg of sodium per day or less. A higher sodium level in the diet may be tolerated in moderate failure. Some patients may tolerate as much as 1,000 mg. The need for fluid restriction is an individual matter. For some patients, fluid intake need not be restricted if the patient complies with the sodium restriction. For others, a relatively severe fluid restriction may be necessary. For some it may be necessary to eliminate highly liquid foods such as some fruits.

Potassium balance must be carefully observed. Patients receiving diuretics may require potassium supplements. Calories should be low for several reasons. Obesity must be eliminated. In addition, restricting food intake will decrease the work of the heart. Feedings should be small and frequent, and vitamin and mineral deficiencies should be avoided. Sometimes discomfort is reduced if the diet is bland and low in residue. Patients should be instructed to eat slowly. Coffee is a stimulant and can cause increased heart rate and arrhythmias. Thus, there is controversy concerning its inclusion in the diet.

Drugs

A number of drugs are used in the treatment of cardiac failure, some of which have side effects of nutritional significance. Drugs are used to increase contractility of the myocardium. Digitalis often is used, but its exact mode of action is unknown. Hypokalemia predisposes the patients to digitalis toxicity and must be prevented. Symptoms of toxicity include anorexia, nausea, vomiting, abdominal discomfort, hallucinations, depression, drowsiness, and cardiac arrhythmias.

Reduction of congestive symptoms is achieved by the use of diuretics in addition to the sodium-restricted diet. Available diuretics and nutritional side effects are given in Table 8-3. In addition, vasodilators may be used. One of these, hydralazine, binds vitamin B_6 and increases its excretion and so may promote vitamin B_6 deficiency.

CEREBROVASCULAR DISEASE

Cardiovascular diseases sometimes affect the brain. The effects may take several forms. Some patients have *transient ischemic attacks* (*TIAs*) in which the blood supply to the brain is temporarily inadequate. The symptoms vary with the arteries involved, the area of the brain they perfuse, and the amount of collateral circulation. Treatment of a TIA includes cessation of smoking, treatment of hypertension, and drugs. Nutritional care usually is aimed at lowering the blood pressure and consists of some degree of sodium restriction. Diet modification for atherosclerosis may be added.

A *cerebrovascular accident* (*CVA* or *stroke syndrome*) often is the consequence of occlusion of the cerebral blood supply from atherosclerosis (*atherothrombotic brain infarct*).

Cerebrovascular accidents may be caused by a hemorrhage of an artery in the brain, most often precipitated by hypertension. In some patients, an aneurysm, which may be congenital, is the cause of a CVA.

The consequences of a CVA vary depending on the area of the brain involved. Those effects that influence the patient's ability to obtain and prepare food, to feed himself or herself, or even to swallow are of particular relevance to the function of the nutritional care specialist. Since these patients may be left with permanent handicaps, their care is discussed in more detail in Chapter 16.

PERIPHERAL VASCULAR ATHEROSCLEROTIC OCCLUSIVE DISEASE

Peripheral vascular atherosclerotic occlusive disease (*PVAOD*) is a general term referring to conditions that result from occlusion of peripheral arteries. The typical patient is a man more than 50 years of age who is hypertensive and smokes. If the condition involves the legs, as when femoral arteries are occluded, the patient develops *intermittent claudication.* The legs are comfortable at rest, but there is pain and weakness when walking. This worsens until walking is impossible, but subsides with rest. If the occlusion becomes total, the leg can become gangrenous and then must be amputated.

Patients should stop smoking. Formerly, a *sympathectomy* (transection of some portion of the sympathetic nervous system) to cause vasodilation was an accepted treatment. Some patients now are treated surgically by an endarterectomy in which the thickened tunica intima of the affected arteries is excised. Portions of affected arteries may also be removed and replaced with an artificial substitute.

Nutritional care of these patients includes the diet for prevention of further atherosclerotic disease. Care of surgical patients is described in Chapter 12.

CARDIAC CACHEXIA

Clinical Manifestations and Pathogenesis

Some patients with cardiac disease develop a condition known as *cardiac cachexia.* In this condition, there is progressive and extreme loss of both fat and lean tissue in a patient with prolonged myocardial insufficiency.[78] It occurs, for example, in many patients with congestive heart failure. Cachexia also occurs in other conditions (see Chapters 12 and 13). The metabolic basis of cachexia, however, varies with its origin. The cardiac patient with cachexia has cardiomegaly, increased basal metabolic rate, and elevated sympathetic tone, in contrast to starvation cachexia in which there is a decrease in the size of the heart, decreased sympathetic tone, and decreased basal metabolic rate.

The development of techniques for cardiac surgery has created a new group of patients with cardiac cachexia. In these patients, postoperative complications can prevent the usual postoperative food intake. The incidence of *nosocomial* (hospital-induced) cardiac cachexia has been found to range from 7 percent to 53 percent in various institutions.[79–81]

Four mechanisms have been suggested to produce this condition: anorexia, increased metabolic rate, increased nutrient losses, and impaired delivery of nutrients and removal of wastes. The relative importance of these factors is unknown.[79,81]

Anorexia may be the most important mechanism according to some investigators.[79,81,82] Increased blood flow to the digestive system can result in dyspnea and cellular hypoxia.[78] Edema as well as an unpalatable sodium-restricted diet, digitalis intoxication, and opiate use can induce anorexia.[78,79,81] Another explanation for anorexia involves increased sympathetic tone and resulting elevated blood levels of epinephrine or norepinephrine, which have been shown in animal experiments to suppress food intake.

Increased metabolic rate is seen in cachectic patients in congestive heart failure. It is thought to be the consequence of increased metabolic demands of the enlarged heart, the lungs, and bone marrow, elevated body temperature, and hormone changes.[78,83,84] The demands of the bone marrow may be caused by the stimulatory effects of hypoxia on red blood cell formation. Elevation in body temperature can result from pulmonary congestion, inflammation, and the production of endogenous pyrogens (see Chapter 12).[85,86] The hormone changes are less well understood but may involve the catecholamines.

There are a number of routes of *nutrient losses.* Iatrogenic losses, especially of protein and iron, can occur when body fluids are removed to reduce edema. Diuretics can cause sodium, potassium, and zinc depletion.[79,81] Protein-losing gastroenteropathy (see Chapter 6) also can occur in congestive heart failure. The total losses by these routes can result in the depressed serum levels of albumin, hemoglobin, potassium, calcium, magnesium, zinc, and iron seen in cardiac cachexia.[79]

Impaired delivery of nutrients has been suggested as another basis for cardiac cachexia.[79] However, increased nutrient extraction rates may account for decreased nutrient concentration in the blood.[78] *Decreased waste excretion* resulting from reduced renal function may contribute to cachexia by causing anorexia and the retention of pyrogens.[78,85,86]

Treatment

Treatment of cardiac cachexia involves recompensation of the cardiac status. Restoration of body tissue then follows. Energy may be provided for maintenance to include basal energy expenditure plus 15 to 25 percent for minimal activity and another 10 to 20 percent for hypermetabolism of severe congestive heart failure. If the patient is to have major surgery, an additional 20 to 50 percent may be required. If nutritional assessment shows the patient to be depleted, an increase of 30 to 50 percent of basal energy expenditure may be indicated. A hypermetabolic, depleted, postsurgical patient would have a very large requirement.

Small frequent feedings are preferable to large meals. Large feedings may cause accumulation of carbon dioxide and respiratory failure (see Chapter 12). Aggressive treatment with parenteral nutrition may be hazardous.

Fluids may be provided at the rate of 0.5 ml/kcal/day or 1,000 to 1,500 ml/day. Protein requirements for replacement of increased losses and to compensate for malabsorption are approximately 0.8 to 1.0 g/kg. Fat malabsorption, occurring in approximately 33 percent of cardiac cachexia patients, may be modified by decreasing long-chain fats in the diet and adding medium-chain triglycerides (see Chapter 6).

Most cardiac cachexia patients are given diets in which sodium is restricted to between 500 and 2,000 mg depending on individual factors. Zinc and magnesium, depleted by diuretics, calcium and magnesium, depleted by malabsorption, and iron, depleted by blood sampling, usually are supplemented. No definitive data are available to support these practices. Therefore, supplements often are arbitrarily set at one and a half to two times the Recommended Dietary Allowances, with frequent monitoring of blood concentrations.

Vitamins also are supplemented. Fat-soluble vitamins are given to patients with fat malabsorption. Other frequent deficits are thiamine, riboflavin, folate, and ascorbic acid.

The diet may consist of six small feedings. Caffeine often is restricted. If voluntary intake is less than 1,500 kcal, the diet may be supplemented with enteral formula feeding. Magnacal, Isocal HCN, and Ensure Plus, for example, provide feedings of high caloric density. Patients whose voluntary intake is less than 500 kcal/day are fed parenterally (see Chapter 12).

RHEUMATIC HEART DISEASE

Rheumatic fever is an infection caused by group A beta-hemolytic streptococci. The disease may be self-limiting, but it can lead to *rheumatic heart disease.*

Rheumatic heart disease follows only hypertension and coronary artery disease in incidence. It affects the valves of the heart, resulting in valvular stenosis or insufficiency or both. The mitral and aortic valves are those most frequently involved. Valvular disease can also be caused by syphilis (lues), a dissecting aneurysm of the aorta, aortic atherosclerosis, and hypertension, affecting primarily the tricuspid and pulmonic valves.

In its acute stage, rheumatic fever may lead to myocarditis, pericarditis, or pulmonary embolism. Care is primarily nonnutritional. In the chronic phase, patients may have hypertension, subacute bacterial endocarditis, atherosclerotic coronary heart disease, arrhythmias, and cardiac failure.

Nutritional care requires avoidance of obesity. Sodium intake is limited to 2 to 5 g/day. Usually vitamin supplements are given as a general support measure.

CONGENITAL HEART DISEASE

Clinical Manifestations and Pathogenesis

Infants may be born with defects of the heart known collectively as *congenital heart disease.* Some of the more frequently seen defects are *coarction of the aorta, aortic stenosis,* and *ventricular septal defect* (*VSD*) in which there is an opening between the right and left ventricles. Some infants have a *transposition of the great arteries* in which the pulmonary artery arises from the left ventricle, and the aorta, above the right ventricle. *Tetralogy of Fallot* is a combination of four defects; there is VSD, pulmonary artery stenosis, and right ventricular hypertrophy, and the aorta overrides the VSD.

Approximately 20 percent of congenital heart disease cases are caused by rubella (German measles) in the mother during the first trimester of pregnancy. Other cases are assumed to be genetic or chromosomal disorders, since congenital heart disease occurs with high frequency in patients with Turner's syndrome, Down's syndrome, Marfan's syndrome, Hurler's syndrome, Friedreich's ataxia, and glycogen storage diseases (see Chapter 10). Some drugs taken during pregnancy, some collagen diseases in pregnancy, and other environmental factors also are possible causes.

The effects of congenital anomalies of the heart vary with the type of defect present. Some patients are cyanotic or are in frank failure. Pulmonary hypertension is seen in some. Growth failure is a common finding. The mechanisms causing growth failure are not completely clear. Poor intake probably is a contributing factor, along with nutrient losses, abnormalities of metabolism, tissue hypoxia, and frequent respiratory infections. The patient also may have an increased metabolic rate.

Nutritional Management

It has been suggested that the reduced intake seen in infants may be a protective mechanism that spares the heart. For normal growth rate, however, 30 to 60 percent additional calories above normal requirements may be needed. The normal infant usually requires approximately 100 kcal/kg of body weight. Thus, the infant with congenital heart disease may need as much as 160 kcal/kg. The child should be in the best possible nutritional condition when surgical correction is undertaken, often at 12 to 15 months of age.

An infant formula may be prepared based on the following: The normal infant formula contains 20 kcal/oz. In order to increase caloric density without increasing renal solute load, sources of calories such as MCT Oil, Polycose, or Karo syrup may be added to a formula such as Enfamil, SMA Infant Formula, or Similac PM 60/40 to provide 30 kcal/oz. Formulas containing most fat as butterfat are not recommended because they are less digestible.[87]

The fluid requirement must be met, and special care must be taken in this regard. Usual total fluid volumes are based on the need for 100 to 120 ml of fluid per kilogram of body weight in infants and 60 to 80 ml/kg in children.

It is important to avoid excessive increases in the renal solute load. Renal solute load is a function of the content of protein (1 g = 4 mOsm), sodium, potassium, and chloride (1 mEq = 1 mOsm). Renal solute load of the recommended formulas at standard dilution is approximately 90 mOsm/L.

Excessive sodium intake should be avoided, but special low-sodium formulas usually are not necessary. Those commercial baby foods that still contain added sodium should not be used. Because the infant may not be able to digest starch, cereals and other starches may be omitted.[87] Vitamin and mineral supplements are necessary, since these infants often have nutrient malabsorption accompanied by increased need.[87]

HEART DISEASE AND ALCOHOLISM

Some alcoholic patients are susceptible to the development of heart disease, whereas others develop liver disease (see Chapter 11). The most common form of alcoholic heart disease consists of cardiomegaly and failure with arrhythmia. Another consists of cardiomegaly, failure, and electrocardiogram abnormalities. The third, *thiamine-responsive beriberi* or *cardiac beriberi,* responds to thiamine supplementation. Abstinence from alcohol is necessary for all three forms of alcohol-related heart disease, in addition to the usual procedures for patients in heart failure.

PICKWICKIAN SYNDROME

Pickwickian syndrome results from extreme obesity. It consists of *cyanosis* (a bluish discoloration of the skin due to insufficient oxygen), *hypoxemia* (low blood oxygen), *hypercapnia* (high blood carbon dioxide) and *secondary polycythemia* (increased numbers of red blood cells). The total lung capacity is reduced because of the obesity. The patient has right ventricular heart failure with reduced alveolar ventilation. Nutritional management consists of restricted food intake for weight reduction.

Case Study: Acute Myocardial Infarction

Phase 1. Mr. J.R.W., a white 52-year-old man measuring 5 ft 10 in. and weighing 180 lb., has been under the supervision of a physician for several years for essential hypertension. He has been taking a thiazide diuretic and was advised to reduce his sodium intake to 2,000 mg/day. He did reduce the amount of salt he used but did not follow the diet completely. After approximately 9 months, he developed a feeling of fatigue and was quite weak. His serum potassium was 3.4 mg/dl, and he was referred to a nutritional care specialist for counseling on a low-sodium diet and advice on methods of increasing his potassium intake.

Phase 2. Mr. W.'s latest physical examination showed that his blood cholesterol was 330 mg/dl and his fasting blood glucose was 125 mg/dl. Fasting triglycerides were 285 mg/dl. His blood pressure was 135/85. He stated that he "usually" took his antihypertensive medication. Body weight was up to 195 lb. At this time, the patient stated that his father had died of a heart attack at the age of 57 and that his mother has hypertension. He was diagnosed as having type IV hyperlipidemia, essential hypertension, and moderate obesity and was advised to stop smoking and to lose 30 lb. He was also referred to a nutritional counselor for advice on diet for the hyperlipidemia.

Phase 3. On a hot day in the summer, Mr. W. was mowing his lawn when he began to feel a "crushing" pain in his chest. At first, he complained of indigestion. However, when the pain continued, he called his doctor.

An electrocardiogram taken in the emergency room of the hospital was abnormal. The patient was also having trouble breathing and was sweating profusely. He was transferred to the cardiac care unit and a tentative diagnosis of acute myocardial infarction was made. Results of the blood tests showed the following:

Cholesterol	340 mg/dl
SGOT	50 units/L
CPK	187 units/L
LDH	93 units/L

Exercises

1. What is the function of the diuretic in the management of essential hypertension?
2. Why was the patient advised to reduce his sodium intake?
3. Describe the mechanism by which the potassium deficiency was produced.
4. What foods are high in potassium?
5. Discuss the relative merits and disadvantage of a high-potassium diet and potassium supplement for this patient.
6. What is the patient's ideal body weight?
7. Discuss the significance of each laboratory test result given.
8. What factors in this patient's history are risk factors for myocardial infarction?
9. What diet would you recommend for this patient during phase 2? Give the rationale.
10. Describe the lesion of atherosclerosis.
11. What are the clinical manifestations of ischemic heart disease?
12. What is the difference between angina pectoris and myocardial infarction?
13. Describe the sequence of diets you would recommend for this patient while he is in the cardiac care unit, assuming he makes an uneventful recovery.
14. What diet might be recommended when this patient is discharged from the hospital? Give the rationale.
15. The patient also was given the following medications: reserpine; clofibrate; hydrochlorothiazide. What is the mode of action and purpose of each?

References

1. Ross, R., and Glomsett, J.A. Atherosclerosis and the arterial smooth muscle cell. *Science* 180:1332, 1980.
2. Carretero, O.A., and Scicli, A.G. The renal kallikrein-kinin system in human and experimental hypertension. *Klin. Wochenschr.* (Suppl. 1) 56:113, 1978.
3. Abe, K. The kinins and prostaglandins in hypertension. *Clin. Endocrinol. Metab.* 10:577, 1981.
4. Erdos, E.G. Angiotensin I converting enzyme. *Circ. Res.* 36:247, 1975.
5. Lote, C. J. *Principles of Renal Physiology.* London: Croom and Helm, 1982.
6. Atlas, S.A., Sealey, J.E., and Laragh, J.H. Dependency of acid and cryoactivation of inactive plasma renin on prior activation of a neutral serine protease. *Kidney Int.* 12:495, 1977.
7. Aiken, J.W., and Vane, J.R. Intrarenal prostaglandin release attenuates the renal vasoconstrictor activity of angiotensin. *J. Pharm. Exp. Ther.* 184:678, 1973.
8. McGiff, J.C., Itskovits, H.D., and Terragno, N.A. The actions of bradykinin and eledoisin in the canine isolated kidney: Relationships to prostaglandins. *Clin. Sci. Mol. Med.* 49:125, 1975.
9. Pickering, G. Hypertension: Definitions, natural histories and consequences. *Am. J. Med.* 52:570, 1972.
10. Rudnick, M.R., Basil, C.P., and Narins, R.G. Diagnostic approaches to hypertension. In B.M. Brenner and H. Stein, Eds., *Contemporary Issues in Nephrology,* vol. 8. *Hypertension.* New York: Churchill Livingstone, 1981, p. 270.
11. van der Werf, T. *Cardiovascular Pathophysiology.* Oxford: Oxford University Press, 1980.
12. U.S. Department of Health, Education and Welfare. *Blood Pressure of Persons 6–74 Years of Age in the United States. Advance Data. Vital and Heath Statistics of the National Center for Health Statistics.* Washington, D.C.: Government Printing Office, 1976.
13. Stamler, J. Hypertension: Aspects of risk. In J.C. Hunt, T. Cooper, E.D. Frohlich, et al., Eds., *Hypertension Update: Mechanisms, Epidemiology, Evaluation, Management.* Bloomfield, N.J.: Health Learning Systems, 1980.
14. Meneely, G.R., Tucker, R.G., Darby, W.J., and Auerbach, S.H. Chronic sodium chloride toxicity in the albino rat: II. Occurrence of

hypertension and of a syndrome of edema and renal failure. *J. Exp. Med.* 98:71, 1953.
15. Dahl, L.K. Effects of chronic excess salt feeding: Induction of self-sustaining hypertension in rats. *J. Exp. Med.* 114:231, 1961.
16. Dahl, L.K. Salt and hypertension. *Am. J. Clin. Nutr.* 25:231, 1972.
17. American Academy of Pediatrics, Committee on Nutrition. Salt intake and eating patterns of infants and children in relation to blood pressure. *Pediatrics* 53:115, 1974.
18. Fries, E.D. Salt, volume and the prevention of hypertension. *Circulation* 53:589, 1976.
19. Morgan, T., Adam, W., Gillies, A., et al. Hypertension treated by salt restriction. *Lancet* 1:227, 1978.
20. Onesti, G. Antihypertensives and their modes of action. *Drug Therapy* 8:35, 1978.
21. Beevers, D.G., Hawthorne, V.M., and Padfield, P.L. Salt and blood pressure in Scotland. *Br. Med. J.* 281:641, 1980.
22. Grim, C.E., Luft, F.C., Miller, J.Z., et al. Racial differences in blood pressure in Evans County, Georgia: Relationship to sodium and potassium intake and plasma renin activity. *J. Chronic Dis.* 33:87, 1980.
23. Grundy, S.M. Dietary fats and sterols. In R.I. Levy, B.M. Rifkind, B.H. Dennis, and N. Ernst, Eds., *Nutrition, Lipids and Coronary Heart Disease.* New York: Raven Press, 1979.
24. Grundy, S.M., Ahrens, E.H., and Davignon, J. The interactions of cholesterol absorption and cholesterol synthesis in man. *J. Lipid Res.* 10:304, 1969.
25. Brown, M.S., Kovanen, P.T., and Goldstein, J.L. Regulation of plasma cholesterol by lipoprotein receptors. *Science* 212:628, 1981.
26. Goldstein, J.L., and Brown, M.S. The low-density lipoprotein pathway and its relation to atherosclerosis. *Annu. Rev. Biochem.* 46:897, 1977.
27. Stein, Y., Stein, O., and Gorey, R. Metabolism and metabolic role of serum high density lipoproteins. In A.M. Gotto, Jr., N.E. Miller, and M.F. Oliver, Eds., *High Density Lipoproteins and Atherosclerosis.* New York: Elsevier/North-Holland Biomedical Press, 1978.
28. Mahley, R.W. Alterations in plasma lipoproteins induced by cholesterol feeding in animals including man. In J.M. Dietschy, A.M. Gotto, Jr., and J. A. Antko, Eds., *Disturbances in Lipids and Lipoprotein Metabolism.* Baltimore: Williams and Wilkins, 1978.
29. Connor, W.E., and Connor, S.L. Dietary treatment of hyperlipidemia. In B.M. Rifkind and R.I. Levy, Eds., *Hyperlipidemia: Diagnosis and Therapy.* New York: Grune and Stratton, 1977.
30. Havel, R.J. Dietary regulation of plasma lipoprotein metabolism in humans. *Proceedings of the 1981 U.S.-Italy Joint Symposium on Nutrition and Cardiovascular Disease, Rome.* Washington, D.C.: National Institutes of Health. In press.
31. Connor, W.E., and Connor, S.L. The dietary treatment of hyperlipidemia. *Med. Clin. North Am.* 66:485, 1982.
32. Grundy, S.M. Effects of polyunsaturated fats on lipid metabolism in patients with hypertriglyceridemia. *J. Clin. Invest.* 55:269, 1975.
33. Spritz, N., and Mishkel, M.A. Effects of dietary fats on plasma lipids and lipoproteins: An hypothesis for the lipid-lowering effect of unsaturated fatty acids. *J. Clin. Invest.* 48:78, 1969.
34. Weinsier, R.L., Seeman, A., Herrera, M.G., et al. High and low carbohydrate diets in diabetes. Studies of effects on diabetic control, insulin secretion and blood lipids. *Ann. Intern. Med.* 80:332, 1974.
35. Havel, R.J., and Kane, J.P. Therapy of hyperlipidemia states. *Annu. Rev. Med.* 33:417, 1982.
36. Melish, J., Le, N.A., Ginsberg, H., et al. Dissociation of apoprotein B and triglyceride production in very-low-density lipoproteins. *Am. J. Physiol.* 239:354, 1980.
37. Kay, R.M. Effects of dietary fibre on serum lipid levels and fecal bile acid excretion. *Can. Med. Assoc. J.* 123:1213, 1980.
38. Bouchier, I.A., and Dawson, A.M. The effect of ethanol on the plasma free fatty acids in man. *Clin. Sci.* 26:47, 1964.
39. Ginsberg, H., Olefsky, J., Farquhar, J.W., and Reaven, G.M. Moderate ethanol ingestion and plasma triglyceride levels—a study of normal and hypertriglyceridemic persons. *Ann. Intern. Med.* 80:143, 1974.
40. Jones, D.P., Losowsky, M.S., Davidson, C.S., and Lieber, C.S. Effects of ethanol on plasma lipids in man. *J. Lab. Clin. Med.* 62:675, 1963.
41. Belfraze, P., Berg, B., Hagerstrand, I., et al. Alterations in lipid metabolism in healthy volunteers during long-term ethanol intake. *Eur. J. Clin. Invest.* 1:129, 1977.
42. Castelli, W.P., Gordon, T., Hjortland, M.C., et al. Alcohol and blood lipids. *Lancet* 2:153, 1977.
43. St. Leger, A.S., Cochrance, A.L., and Moore, F. Factors associated with cardiac mortality in developed countries, with particular reference to the consumption of wine. *Lancet* 1:1017, 1979.
44. Fry, M.M., Spector, A.A., Connor, S.J., and

Connor, W.E. Intensification of hypertriglyceridemia by either alcohol or carbohydrate. *Am. J. Clin. Nutr.* 26:798, 1973.

45. Kudzma, A.J., and Schonfeld, G. Alcoholic hyperlipidemia: Induction by alcohol but not by carbohydrate. *J. Lab. Clin. Med.* 77:384, 1970.
46. Brown, M.S., and Goldstein, J.L. Familial hypercholesterolemia: Model for genetic receptor disease. *Harvey Lect.* 73:163, 1979.
47. Utermann, G., Hees, M., and Steinmert, A. Polymorphism of apolipoprotein E and occurrence of dysbetalipoproteinaemia in man. *Nature* 269:604, 1977.
48. Havel, R.J., Chao, Y.-S., Windler, E.E., et al. Isoprotein specificity in the hepatic uptake of apolipoprotein E and the pathogenesis of familial dysbetalipoproteinemia. *Proc. Natl. Acad. Sci. U.S.A.* 77:4349, 1980.
49. Gregg, R.E., Zech, E.J., Schaefer, E.J., and Brewer, H.B., Jr. Type III hyperlipoproteinemia: Defective metabolism of an abnormal apolipoprotein E. *Science* 211:584, 1981.
50. Zilversmit, D.B. Atherogenesis: A postprandial phenomenon. *Circulation* 60:473, 1979.
51. Miller, G.J. High density lipoproteins and atherosclerosis. *Annu. Rev. Med.* 31:97, 1980.
52. Antonis, A., and Behrson, I. The influences of diet on serum-triglycerides in South African white and Bantu prisoners. *Lancet* 1:3, 1961.
53. Stamler, J.F. Population studies. In R.I. Levy, B.M. Rifkind, B.H. Dennis, and N. Ernst, Eds., *Nutrition, Lipids and Coronary Heart Disease.* New York: Raven Press, 1979.
54. Miller, N.E. Plasma lipoproteins, lipid transport and atherosclerosis—recent developments. *J. Clin. Pathol.* 32:639, 1979.
55. Gordon, T., Castelli, W.P., Hjortland, M.C., et al. High density lipoprotein as a protective factor against coronary heart disease—The Framingham study. *Am. J. Med.* 62:707, 1977.
56. Keys, A. Coronary heart disease—The global picture. *Atherosclerosis* 22:149, 1975.
57. Olson, R.E. Is there an optimum diet for the prevention of coronary heart disease? In R.I. Levy, B.M. Rifkind, B.H. Dennis, and N. Ernst, Eds., *Nutrition, Lipids and Coronary Heart Disease.* New York: Raven Press, 1979.
58. Blackburn, H. Diet and mass hyperlipidemia: Public health considerations—A point of view. In R.I. Levy, B.M. Rifkind, B.H. Dennis, and N. Ernst, Eds., *Nutrition, Lipids and Coronary Heart Disease.* New York: Raven Press, 1979.
59. Kannel, W.B., and Gordon, T. *An Epidemiological Investigation of Cardiovascular Disease. The Framingham Diet Study: Diet and the Regulation of Serum Cholesterol.* D.H.E.W. Report, Section 24. Washington, D.C.: Government Printing Office, 1970.
60. Nichols, A.B., Ravenscroft, C., Lanphier, D.E., and Ostrander, L.D. Daily nutritional intake and serum lipid levels. The Tecumseh study. *Am. J. Clin. Nutr.* 29:1384, 1976.
61. U.S. Senate, Select Committee on Nutrition and Human Needs. *Dietary Goals for the United States,* 2nd ed. Washington, D.C.: Government Printing Office, 1977.
62. American Heart Association. *Diet and Coronary Heart Disease.* Circular 71-003-B. Dallas: American Heart Association, 1978.
63. Grundy, S.M., Bilheimer, D., Blackburn, H., et al. Rationale of the diet-heart statement of the American Heart Association. *Circulation* 65:839A, 1982.
64. National Academy of Sciences Food and Nutrition Board. *Toward Healthful Diets.* Washington, D.C.: National Research Council, 1980.
65. Hemzacek, K.I. Dietary protocol for the patient who has suffered a myocardial infarction. *J. Am. Diet. Assoc.* 72:182, 1978.
66. Christakis, G., and Winston, M. Nutritional therapy in acute myocardial infarction. *J. Am. Diet. Assoc.* 62:233, 1973.
67. Dack, S. The diet of cardiac patients. In A. Luisada, Ed., *Cardiology—An Encyclopedia of the Cardiovascular System.* New York: McGraw-Hill, 1959.
68. Alexander, S. Effect of cold on the cardiovascular system. *Practitioner* 213:785, 1974.
69. Neill, W., Duncan, D., Kloster, F., and Mahler, D. Response of coronary circulation to cutaneous cold. *Am. J. Med.* 56:471, 1974.
70. Gould, L., Venkatamaran, K., Goswami, M., and Gomprecht, R. The cardiac effects of coffee. *Angiology* 24:455, 1973.
71. Goldberger, E. Dangers of a low-sodium diet in the treatment of acute myocardial infarction. *Am. J. Cardiol.* 8:300, 1961.
72. Hurst, J.W., Logue, R.B., Schlant, R.C., and Wenger, N.K., Eds. *The Heart, Arteries and Veins,* 3rd ed. New York: McGraw-Hill, 1974.
73. Goss, R.J. Adaptive growth of the heart. In N. Alpert, Ed., *Cardiac Hypertrophy.* New York: Academic, 1971.
74. Spann, J.F. Cardiac muscle performance in ventricular hypertrophy and congestive heart failure. In N. Alpert, Ed., *Cardiac Hypertrophy.* New York: Academic, 1971.
75. Sahn, S.H., and Levine, I. Pulmonary nodules associated with mitral stenosis. *Arch. Intern. Med.* 85:483, 1950.

76. McIlroy, M.B. Dyspnea and the work of breathing in diseases of the heart and lungs. *Prog. Cardiovasc. Dis.* 1:284, 1959.
77. Braunwald, E. Heart failure. In K.J. Isselbacher, R.D. Adams, E. Braunwald, et al., Eds., *Harrison's Principles of Internal Medicine,* 9th ed. New York: McGraw-Hill, 1980.
78. Pittman, J.G., and Cohen, P. *The Pathogenesis of Cardiac Cachexia.* New York: Grune and Stratton, 1965.
79. Heymsfield, S., Smith, J., Redd, S., and Witworth, H.B., Jr. Nutritional support in cardiac cachexia. *Surg. Clin. North Am.* 61:635, 1981.
80. Cohen, I.T., Greecher, C.P., and Trescher, B.A. Cardiac cachexia in the cancer patient. *J.P.E.N.* 5:577, 1981.
81. Blackburn, G., Gibbons, G.W., Bothe, A., et al. Nutritional support in cardiac cachexia. *J. Thorac. Cardiovasc. Surg.* 73:489, 1977.
82. Buchanan, N. Gastrointestinal absorption studies in cardiac cachexia. *Intensive Care Med.* 3:89, 1977.
83. Pool, P.E. Energy stores and energy utilization in the myocardium in hypertrophy and heart failure. In N. Alpert, Ed., *Cardiac Hypertrophy.* New York: Academic, 1971.
84. Olson, R.E. Myocardial metabolism in congestive heart failure. *J. Chronic Dis.* 9:442, 1959.
85. Cohn, A.E., and Steele, J.M. Unexplained fever in heart failure. *J. Clin. Invest.* 13:853, 1934.
86. Bondy, P.K., Cohn, G.L., Herrmann, W., and Crispell, K.R. The possible relationship of etiocholanolone to periodic fever. *Yale J. Biol. Med.* 30:395, 1958.
87. Fomon, S.J., Ziegler, E.E., and O'Donnell, A.M. Infant feed in health and disease. In S.J. Fomon, Ed., *Infant Nutrition,* 2nd ed. Philadelphia: W.B. Saunders, 1974.

Bibliography

Committee on Sodium-Restricted Diets, Food and Nutrition Board. *Sodium-Restricted Diets and the Use of Diuretics.* Washington, D.C.: National Academy of Sciences, 1979.

Heller, L.J., and Mohrman, D.E. *Cardiovascular Physiology.* New York: McGraw-Hill, 1981.

Hunt, J.C., Cooper, T., Frohlich, E.D., et al., Eds. *Hypertension Update: Mechanisms, Epidemiology, Evaluation, Management.* Bloomfield, N.J.: Health Learning Systems, 1980.

Jensen, D. *The Principles of Physiology,* 2nd ed. New York: Appleton-Century-Crofts, 1980.

Lamb, J.F., Ingram, C.G., Johnston, I.A., and Pitman, R.M. *Essentials of Physiology.* Oxford: Blackwell Scientific, 1980.

Miller, N.E., and Lewis, B., Eds. *Lipoproteins, Atherosclerosis and Coronary Heart Disease.* Amsterdam: Elsevier/North-Holland Biomedical Press, 1981.

Rushmer, R.F. *Organ Physiology. Structure and Function of the Cardiovascular System,* 2nd ed. Philadelphia: W.B. Saunders, 1976.

Stanbury, J.B., Wyngaarden, J.B., Frederickson, D.S., et al., Eds. *The Metabolic Basis of Inherited Disease,* 5th ed. New York: McGraw-Hill, 1983.

Sources of Current Information

American Heart Journal
American Journal of Cardiology
Angiology
Atherosclerosis
Circulation
Circulation Research
Heart and Lung
Journal of Chronic Diseases
Journal of Clinical Investigation
Journal of Lipid Research
Journal of Thoracic and Cardiovascular Surgery
Kidney International
Progress in Cardiovascular Diseases

V. Metabolic Disorders

9. Diabetes Mellitus, Hypoglycemia, and Other Endocrine Disorders

Frances J. Zeman, Ph.D., and Robert J. Hansen, Ph.D.

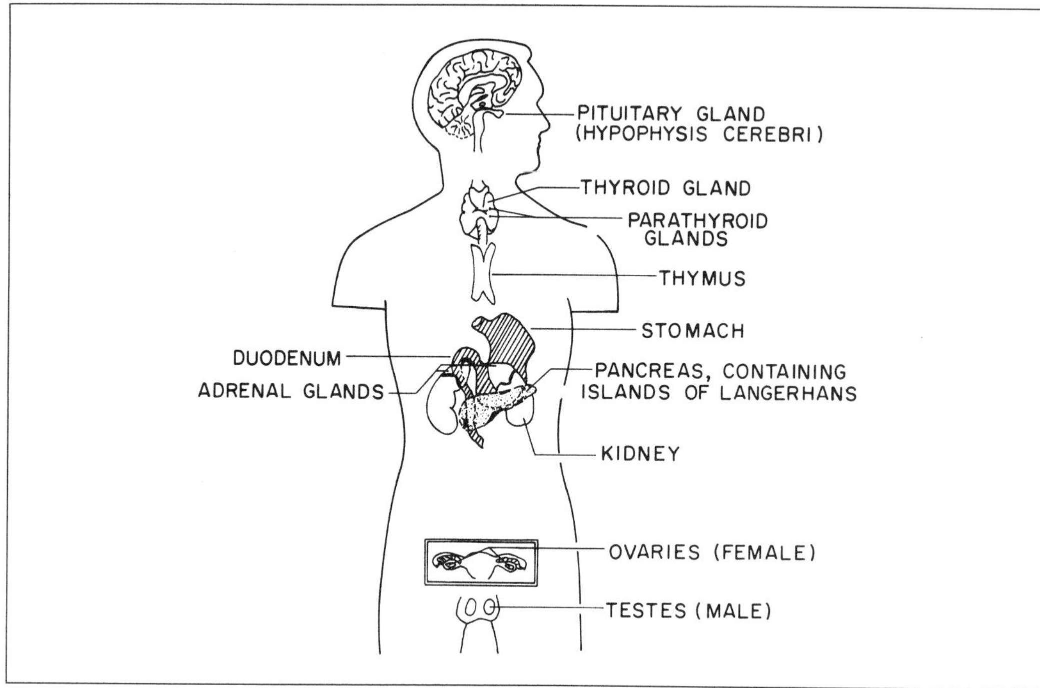

Figure 9-1. Major components of the endocrine system. (Modified with permission from Dean, W.B., Farrar, G.E., Jr., and Zoldos, A.J., Basic Concepts of Anatomy and Physiology. *Philadelphia: J.B. Lippincott, 1966, p. 265.)*

The *ductless glands* throughout the body make up the *endocrine system,* the major components of which are shown in Fig. 9-1. There are also other endocrine tissues distributed in nonendocrine organs in the body—for example, in the gastrin-secreting cells in the stomach. Endocrine glands secrete *hormones* which, along with the nervous system, control body functions. These hormones enter directly into the blood and are carried to and influence their *target organs.* The primary effects of hormones are (1) control of growth and maturation, (2) control of metabolism, (3) control of reproduction, or (4) integration of the physiologic response to stress. We are not certain that all existing hormones have been identified. We are also uncertain of the effects of many hormones that are known or of how those effects are achieved.

Secretion of some hormones is controlled by the nervous system, whereas secretion of others occurs rhythmically or in response to the blood level of some specific substances such as glucose, sodium, calcium, water, or another hormone. Many hormones, in turn, influence nervous system function. In disease, the amount of a hormone secreted may increase or decrease, so that the effects of the hormone are increased or decreased, but hormones do not develop new effects in disease.

In this chapter, those endocrine abnormalities in which nutritional care is important will be described. The main focus will be on diabetes mellitus, because of the number of patients involved and the importance of diet in its treatment.

DIABETES MELLITUS

Diabetes mellitus is a heterogeneous group of diseases of the endocrine system with common symptoms. It is characterized by a failure of control of energy production. It is unrelated to diabetes insipidus, a rare disease of the pituitary glands. When the term *diabetes* is used alone, as it will be in this chapter, it always refers to *diabetes mellitus.*

In diabetes mellitus, the cells metabolize glucose ineffectively, with secondary effects on lipid and protein metabolism. The disease is characterized by *hyperglycemia* (elevated blood glucose concentration) that is the result of an absolute or relative deficiency of insulin. It is generally believed that the observed hyperglycemia is also the consequence of the hypersecretion of glucagon, glucocorticoids, and growth hormone, although this theory has met with some disagreement.[1-3] Diabetes also is characterized by the premature development of generalized vascular disease, especially in the small blood vessels.

It is estimated that approximately 3 percent of middle-aged adults and 6.4 percent of adults in the 65- to 75-year age group are diabetic, but many are not aware of their disease. In addition, approximately 0.4 percent of young adults and 0.5 percent of school-age children are diabetic, but the disease is rare in pre-school-age children.

In the patient population of an acute care hospital, diabetic patients are found in greater number than any other group requiring a therapeutic diet. On the basis of numbers alone, diabetes would be an important problem for nutritional care specialists.

The public health significance of the disease is increased by the fact that it can have serious long-term consequences such as blindness, cardiovascular disease, renal failure, and amputations. Although some diabetics have a normal life span, the average life expectancy is half of normal when onset of the disease is in childhood and two-thirds of normal in adult-onset disease.

Classification

The forms of diabetes are classified on the basis of age of onset, severity, and on the cause when it is known.

Primary Diabetes

Most patients have *primary* or *essential diabetes*—that is, the condition apparently occurs spontaneously, not secondarily to some other defined disease state. Primary diabetes occurs in two forms. Approximately 5 to 10 percent of the patients have *type 1 diabetes,* also known as *insulin-dependent, ketosis-prone, growth-onset,* or *juvenile-onset diabetes.* The typical patient is a child or adolescent at the time of onset and is underweight, but some type 1 diabetics are adults at onset. The disease appears suddenly with severe symptoms but, after the development of the disease, there sometimes is a short period of partial remission. Later, the diabetes worsens and becomes progressively more severe. In the fully developed disease, little or no insulin is produced. Type 1 diabetes varies in the extent to which it can be controlled. The blood glucose in some patients is reasonably constant with treatment by diet, insulin, and exercise. In others, there are dangerous variations in blood glucose concentrations for unknown reasons, and these are seriously disruptive to the patient's life. This condition is known as *brittle diabetes.*

Type 2 diabetes is known also as *ketosis-resistant, non-insulin-dependent, maturity-onset,* or *adult-onset diabetes.* In the United States and similarly developed affluent societies, 75 to 90 percent of diabetic patients have this type. The ability of the pancreas to produce and secrete insulin in the type 2 patient is decreased or delayed but is not absent. In addition, the patient is considered to be insulin-resistant—that is, there is a decreased effectiveness of a given amount of insulin. The insulin deficiency is then relative rather than absolute. The onset of the disease is insidious and may be unnoticed for a long period.

The classification of a patient as type 1 (insulin-dependent) or type 2 (non-insulin-dependent) is subject to alterations. Some patients have a stable, mild form of diabetes similar to type 2, but the hyperglycemia does not respond to other treatment and insulin must be used. The patient then is classified as *type 2, insulin-dependent.* In some patients with non-insulin-dependent type 2 diabetes, the disease suddenly becomes more severe. The reason for this change is not always apparent, but sometimes the diabetes worsens temporarily with superimposed stresses, such as infection, injury, or pregnancy, and then reverts to the milder form when the stress is removed.

Secondary Diabetes

Diabetes secondary to other conditions is classifed as *type 3.* It can result from pancreatitis, cancer of the pancreas, or surgical removal of the pancreas for any reason, from liver disease, and from chronic administration of some drugs. It also is seen in *hemochromatosis* (excessive iron absorption), *acromegaly* (abnormal growth of face, hands, and feet from overproduction of growth hormone), *pheochromocytoma* (tumor of the adrenal medulla), and *Cushing's syndrome* (overactivity of the adrenal cortex). Glucocorticoids, adrenocorticotropic hormone (ACTH), glucagon, estrogen, vasopressin, and other hormones have a diabetogenic effect whether *endogenous* (produced in the body) or *exogenous* (administered as a medication). Type 3 diabetes can be reversed if the primary cause is removed soon enough. *Type 4* diabetes is associated with at least thirty other congenital metabolic disorders.

Etiology

Primary diabetes is believed to be a genetic disease that becomes evident at varying intervals after birth. The specific nature of the genetic inheritance is unknown but is complex.

The genetic pattern, related to certain HLA antigens, appears to transmit a predisposition to diabetes, rather than the disease itself, with variations in penetrance that are dependent on environmental and other genetic factors.[4] The specific environmental factors affecting penetrance are generally unknown. At one time, it was believed that racial factors, attributable to genetics, were responsible for some of the variation in the incidence of diabetes in different societies, but more recent evidence indicates that economic, social, and cultural factors are more important than race.[5] Viral infections injuring the beta cells[6–10] and autoimmune reactions[11–16] are thought to be important in type 1 diabetes.

In type 2 diabetes, there is no known association with the HLA system nor are viral factors thought to be involved.[4,17] In general, the environmental factors are classified as those that increase the demand for insulin, antagonize the action of insulin, or suppress insulin production. The primary defect may lie in the islet cells or in the target cells. Various theories suggest that, if the defect is in the pancreas, there may be an inadequate number of islets of Langerhans or the islets may be degenerating; they may be unable to recognize a stimulus to secrete or to respond to the stimulus by transmitting the message, or the defect may directly affect the synthesis, storage, or release of insulin. Alternatively, in the target cells, there may be a deficiency of glucose receptors or insulin receptors, abnormal response to hormones antagonistic to insulin, abnormal cellular response to insulin, or an antibody response which has an antiinsulin effect.[18]

Obesity is evidently the most important factor in type 2 diabetes. In the United States, approximately 75 percent of type 2 diabetics are reported to be obese, whereas in countries where obesity is uncommon, diabetes is rare.[19] Another major factor is believed to be exercise. Decreased exercise may increase the penetrance of the gene directly, or it may do so indirectly by contributing to the causes of obesity. Weight loss in obese patients usually causes a reduction in the severity of the disease and may allow it to subside altogether.

Much discussion has centered around the role of specific nutrients in impairing glucose tolerance or damaging the pancreas, apart from obesity. Deficiencies of protein, chromium, zinc, or iron have been implicated in both processes.[20] Epidemiologic and experimental studies have failed to show a relationship between carbohydrate intake and diabetes.[21-27] High sucrose intake has been proposed as a factor in genetically predisposed persons.[28-31] Fat has been similarly implicated.[20,24,32] It remains uncertain whether high levels of sucrose and fat directly affect the beta cells or whether they simply add to the risk of obesity.

The extent to which nutritional factors affect the incidence of type 1 diabetes in the lean patient is unknown. There are significant differences among different societies which may or may not relate to customary sucrose intake.

In the middle and late 1970s, many researchers proposed that increased dietary fiber intake had positive effects in the diabetic patient.[33] Feeding diets rich in natural fibers or adding fibers such as guar gum, pectin, or wheat bran to the diet results in a decrease in fasting blood glucose,[34-37] urinary glucose excretion,[34,35] daily insulin requirement,[34] and blood cholesterol and triglycerides,[33] and in improved glucose tolerance.[37] In general, non-insulin-dependent, adult-onset diabetics respond best to these high-carbohydrate, low-fat, high-fiber diets.[33,37] More research is required before the effects of high-carbohydrate, high-fiber diets are documented and understood completely. Nonetheless, many physicians currently are advocating such diets to their patients and many of these patients thus are able to postpone the time when they require insulin or oral hypoglycemic medications as part of their treatment. Anderson's group[38] has published a report on the composition and fiber content of many foods commonly used in diets for diabetics. To date, no serious nutritional side effects have been documented following long-term consumption of such diets. Certain of the fibers, especially guar gum and pectin, are poorly tolerated by some individuals and may preclude their use for some patients.

Pathology

Anatomic Changes

No pancreatic lesion is pathognomonic for diabetes mellitus. In approximately 40 percent of the patients, there are no observable anatomic changes. Degranulation of B cells, hyalinization, leukocyte infiltration, hydropic changes, and fibrosis of the pancreas have been seen in some patients at autopsy, but these conditions also occur in nondiabetics.

Metabolic Alterations

Endogenous Insulin. The normal pancreas consists of an exocrine organ, described in Chapter 6, and an endocrine tissue, the islets of Langerhans, scattered throughout. There are approximately 2 million islets which make up approximately 1 percent of the weight of the pancreas. The islets of Langerhans contain alpha cells, which produce *glucagon,* beta cells, producing *insulin,* and delta cells, producing *somatostatin.*

Insulin is a polypeptide synthesized in the form of *proinsulin.* The structure of porcine proinsulin is shown in Fig. 9-2; human insulin is similar in structure, with some differences in the amino acid sequence. Proinsulin is converted to active insulin by proteolysis which removes the C (connecting) *peptide* to produce a molecule consisting of two chains, the A chain and B chain, connected by disulfide bonds. The C peptide is inactive, but it remains in the *beta granules* in which insulin is stored in the islets and is released along with the insulin in equimolar quantities. Approximately 250 units of insulin are stored in

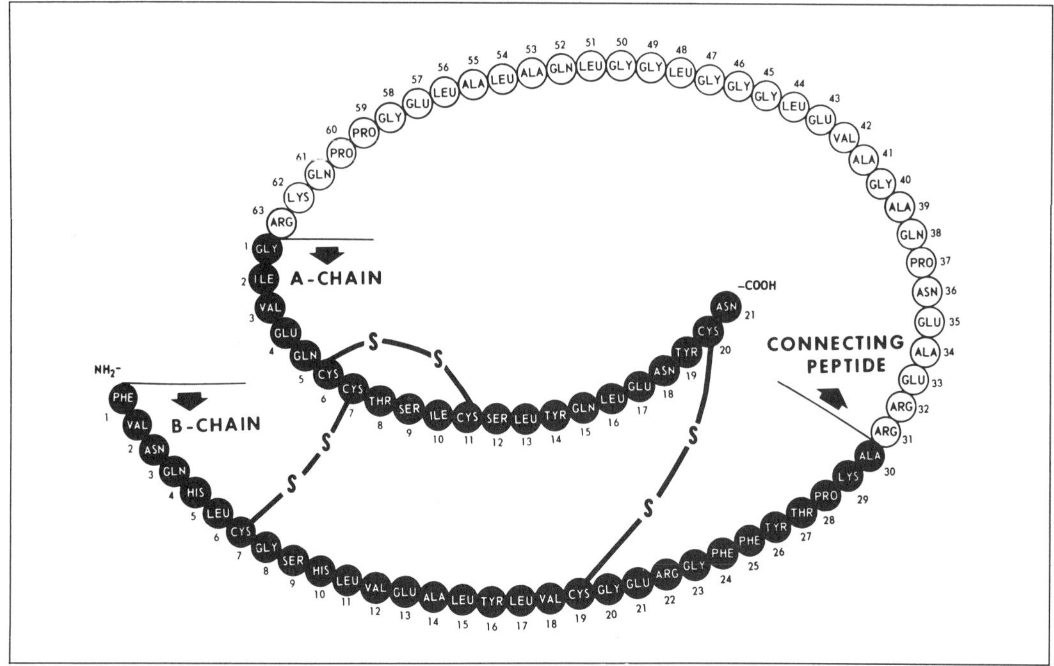

Figure 9-2. Proinsulin molecule and insulin structure: Primary structure of porcine proinsulin. The insulin sequence is represented by amino acids (dark circles). Connecting peptides are indicated by light circles. Human insulin is similar in structure but the amino acid sequence differs some. (From Shaw, W.N., and Chance, R.R., Effect of porcine proinsulin in vitro on adipose tissue and diaphragm of the normal rat. Diabetes *18:738, 1968; modified in* Diabetes *21:461, 1972. Reproduced with permission of the American Diabetes Association, Inc.*)

the human pancreas, of which 20 percent or so is secreted each day by *emiocytosis* (the opposite of pinocytosis). Calcium is required for insulin release.

The stimuli to insulin production have been studied extensively and include the hormones glucagon, gastric inhibitory peptide, gastrin, and pancreozymin, as well as dietary glucose and amino acids. In addition, increased serum calcium, acetylcholine, and the administration of sulfonylurea drugs stimulate insulin production. These factors may stimulate the release of stored insulin, a reaction that may occur within seconds, or they may stimulate the synthesis of insulin for release, a process that may require 15 minutes to 2 hours. The response of insulin release to stimulation may thus be biphasic. The half-life of free insulin in blood is 7 to 15 minutes. Insulin is degraded by *glutathione insulin transhydrogenase,* primarily in the liver, kidney, and muscle.[39]

Insulin is the major anabolic hormone secreted in response to feeding. With the secretion of insulin, youngsters can grow, increasing their protein content and storing excess energy as glycogen or triglycerides. If individuals lose the capacity to produce and release insulin, their response to feeding cannot be normal. Indeed, diabetic patients behave metabolically as if they were starved, even though they are consuming greater than normal amounts of food. The specific manner or mechanism by which insulin accomplishes its functions is not known, since no unifying hypothesis proposed thus far satisfactorily explains all the changes observed. We are limited by our present

Table 9-1. Metabolic Actions of Insulin, Glucagon, Cortisol, and Growth Hormone

Action	Insulin	Glucagon	Cortisol	Growth Hormone
Blood glucose level	↓	↑	↑	↑
Glucose uptake (M, A)	↑	NE	↓	↓
Glucose utilization (M, A, L)	↑	NE	↓	↓
Glycogenolysis (M, A, L)	↓	↑	↓	NE
Glycogen deposition (M, A, L)	↑	↓	↑	NE
Glycolytic enzyme levels (A, L)	↑	↓	↑	?
Gluconeogenesis (L)	↓	↑	↑	?
Lipolysis (A)	↓	↑	↑	↑
Lipogenesis (A, L)	↑	↓	↓	↓
Protein synthesis: (L)	↑	NE	↑	↑
(M, A)	↑	NE	↓	↑
Amino acid uptake: (L)	NE	↑	↑	↑
(M, A)	↑	NE	↓	↑
Protein degradation: (L)	↓	?	?	?
(M, A)	↓	NE	↑	?
Ureagenesis (L)	↓	↑	↑	↑
Ketogenesis (L)	↓	↑	↑	↑

M = muscle; A = adipose tissue; NE = no effect; L = liver; ↑ = the process is enhanced; ↓ = process is decreased.

knowledge to considering the effects of insulin action or the results of its absence.

To understand better the altered metabolism observed in diabetics, it is necessary to consider some of insulin's actions. Although there are many target cells of insulin, we will consider mainly insulin's effects on the liver, skeletal muscle, and adipose tissue. In general, insulin (1) promotes glucose utilization in tissues and reduces the output of glucose from the liver via glycogenolysis and gluconeogenesis; (2) promotes triglyceride storage in adipose tissue and fatty acid synthesis in liver lipogenesis and reduces lipolysis in adipose tissue and ketogenesis in the liver; (3) promotes amino acid uptake into muscle and adipose tissue and reduces amino acid catabolism and ureagenesis in the liver; and (4) promotes protein synthesis in muscle, in adipose tissue, and, to a smaller extent, in the liver and reduces protein degradation in all three tissues (Table 9-1).

The most commonly observed action of insulin, lowering blood glucose, is due to three primary actions of insulin: (1) increased transport and utilization of glucose peripherally, mainly in skeletal muscle, (2) reduced gluconeogenesis in the liver, and (3) reduced loss of amino acids, major glucose precursors, from peripheral tissues.

In addition to understanding what insulin is doing, it also is necessary to understand the functions of glucagon, adrenal glucocorticoids, and growth hormone, which will loosely be called *catabolic hormones.* These three hormones are antagonistic to almost every action of insulin. According to the definition of diabetes mellitus presented at the beginning of this chapter, the disease is a state caused initially by the absence of insulin but intensified by the hypersecretion of the catabolic hormones. Indeed, if the hypersecretion of the catabolic hormones is prevented in some way, many of the symptoms of the diabetic patient are reduced. The diabetic, then, is in hormonal imbalance: insufficient circulating insulin coupled with high circulating levels of the catabolic hormones leading to major effects on carbohydrate, lipid, and protein metabolism.

Carbohydrate Metabolism. In describing carbohydrate metabolism, the use of glucose, gluconeogenesis, and glycogen metabolism must be considered.

Glucose utilization. The studies of Levine and Goldstein[40] were the first to demonstrate clearly that insulin stimulated the transport of glucose and some other sugars into skeletal muscle. Subsequent work has shown that insulin also stimulates glucose transport into adipose tissue, fibroblasts, and some white blood cells, but not into liver, intestinal cells, renal tubules, blood vessels, pancreatic islets, the lens of the eye, or cells of the nervous system. In the absence of insulin, the rate of entry of glucose into insulin-sensitive cells is inadequate.

In addition to stimulating glucose transport, insulin enhances the rate of glucose use in the same tissues and also in the liver. Insulin enhances the activities of many enzymes in glycolysis, in the tricarboxylic acid (TCA) cycle, in fatty acid synthesis, and in glycogen synthesis. Some of the enzymes—pyruvate kinase, pyruvate dehydrogenase, and acetylcoenzyme A (acetyl-CoA) carboxylase—exist in an inactive (phosphorylated) form, and the action of insulin appears to lead to their conversion to the active (unphosphorylated) form. The net result of the changes due to the presence of insulin is that more glucose is converted to carbon dioxide, fatty acids, lactate, and glycogen than when cells do not have insulin present. This results in a lowering of blood glucose concentration.

In insulin deficiency, then, one of the striking symptoms of diabetes mellitus is hyperglycemia. This hyperglycemia is a consequence of reduced peripheral uptake and utilization of glucose and the increased production of glucose by the liver (Fig. 9-3).

Gluconeogenesis. Insulin tends to decrease gluconeogenesis by decreasing the activities of enzymes in the gluconeogenic pathway. These enzymes include pyruvate carboxylase, phosphoenolpyruvate carboxykinase, fructose-1,6-bisphosphatase, and glucose-6-phosphatase. In insulin deficiency and in the presence of glucagon and adrenal glucocorticoids, the production of glucose from glucose precursors such as lactic acid and some amino acids is increased considerably and contributes to the hyperglycemia when the effect of insulin on these enzymes is removed (see Fig. 9-3).

Glycogen metabolism. During the postabsorptive state, glycogen in the liver is metabolized to glucose to maintain blood glucose levels. Insulin promotes glycogen formation and reduces glucose release, whereas glucagon increases glycogen breakdown and promotes glucose release. The two controlled enzymes are glycogen synthase and glycogen phosphorylase (see Fig. 9-3). If the liver is exposed to high glucagon levels, phosphorylase becomes more active, and synthase, less active. Glycogen is broken down and the liver puts glucose into the blood, raising the blood glucose level. If blood insulin is high, phosphorylase becomes less active, synthase becomes more active, and glycogen is synthesized, thereby decreasing the blood glucose level.

In normal individuals, insulin and glucagon are secreted as needed, but in untreated diabetic patients, there is a lack of insulin and an excess of glucagon. Liver glycogen content is very low in these diabetics and, even though the patient may be eating excess food, little glucose is converted to glycogen in the liver. Instead, glucose remains in the blood, again contributing to hyperglycemia.

In skeletal muscle, insulin has effects on glycogen metabolism similar to those observed in the liver. In the diabetic patient, then, little muscle glycogen is synthesized, also contributing to hyperglycemia.

Lipid Metabolism. Insulin has important effects on synthesis of fatty acids, on triglyceride breakdown, and on the production and utilization of ketone bodies.

Fatty acid synthesis and storage. In addition to promoting glucose utilization, insulin

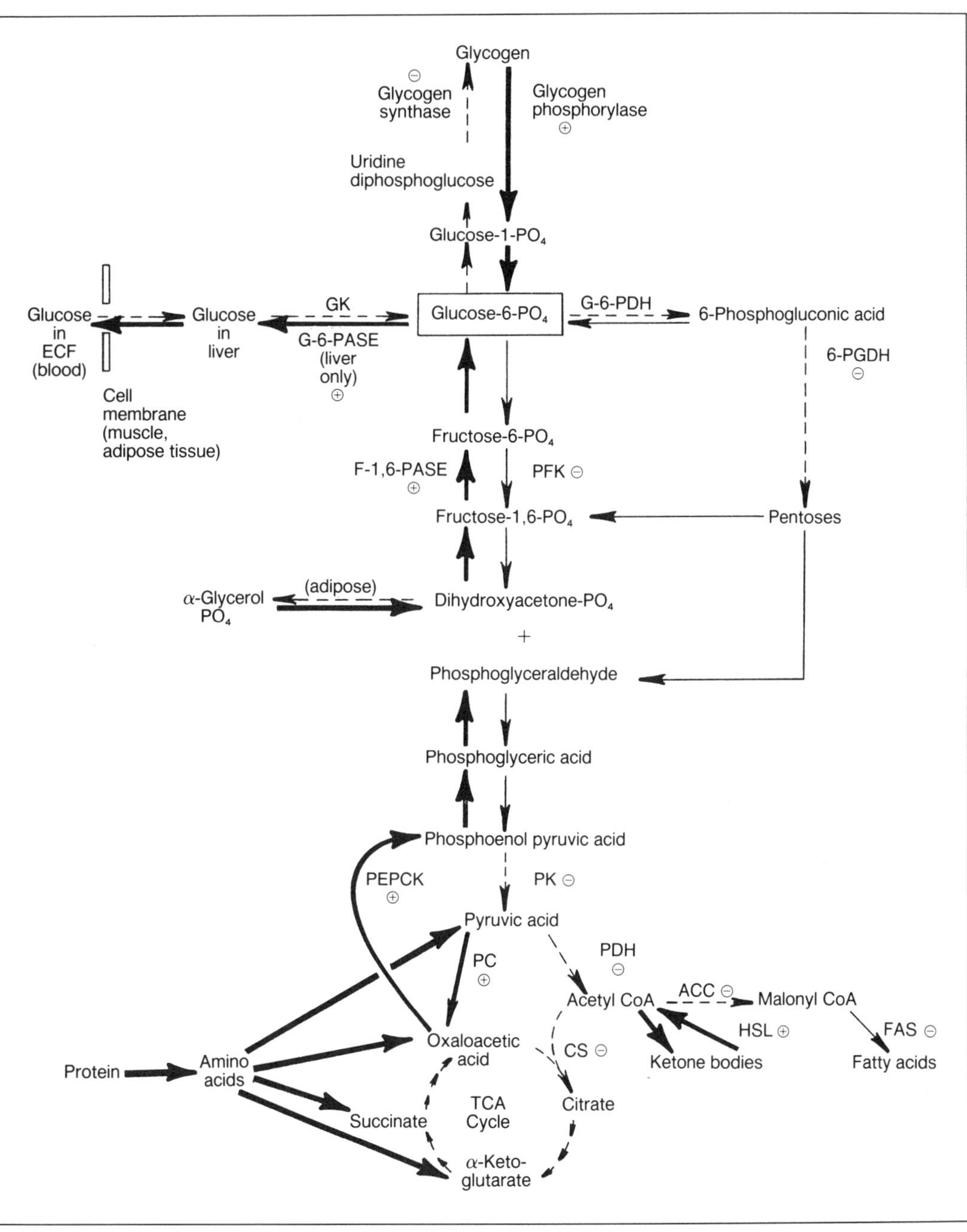

Figure 9-3. Outline of the effects of diabetes mellitus on carbohydrate metabolism. Heavy arrows indicate pathways that are accentuated by the disease, and dashed arrows indicate that the pathway is diminished. Effects of insulin deficiency on enzymes are indicated by + (increase) or − (decrease). GK = glucokinase; HK = hexokinase; G-6-PASE = glucose-6-phosphatase; G-6-PDH = glucose-6-phosphate dehydrogenase; 6-PGDH = 6-phosphogluconate dehydrogenase; PFK = phosphofructokinase; F-1,6-PASE = fructose-1,6-bisphosphatase; PK = pyruvate kinase; PEPCK = phosphoenolypyruvate carboxykinase; PDH = pyruvic dehydrogenase; PC = pyruvate carboxylase; ACC = acetyl-CoA carboxylase; FAS = fatty acid synthetase; CS = citrate synthase; ECF = extracellular fluid; TCA = tricarboxylic acid; HSL = hormone-sensitive lipase.

promotes the synthesis of fatty acids and their storage as triglycerides. In humans, most of the fatty acids appear to be synthesized in the liver, transported in the blood as very-low-density lipoproteins (VLDLs), and stored in adipose tissue. Insulin has effects on all aspects of this system.

In the liver, insulin stimulates conversion of glucose and precursors such as lactate and amino acids to acetyl-CoA by making pyruvate dehydrogenase, pyruvate kinase, phosphofructokinase, and glucokinase more active. It also stimulates the synthesis of fatty acids from acetyl-CoA by increasing the activities of acetyl-CoA carboxylase and fatty acid synthase. The net effect of insulin, then, is to promote fatty acid synthesis, whereas insulin deficiency reduces synthesis (see Fig. 9-3).

Synthesized fatty acids are esterified with glycerol to form triglycerides. These are combined with phospholipids, apolipoproteins, and cholesterol to form VLDL and are secreted into the blood. Although very little data are available on this point, it appears that insulin is necessary for the synthesis of one or more apolipoproteins. In insulin deficiency with a deficit of available apolipoproteins, synthesis and secretion of VLDL is reduced and abnormally large amounts of triglyceride accumulate in the liver, resulting in a fatty liver.

In the adipose tissue, when VLDLs as well as chylomicrons from intestinal absorption of triglycerides reach the tissue, *lipoprotein lipase* hydrolyzes the ester bonds in the triglycerides, thereby releasing glycerol and fatty acids. This enzyme is found in large amounts in the capillary beds of the adipose tissue when blood insulin levels are high, but occurs in lower amounts when the ratio of insulin to glucagon changes to favor glucagon. Under the latter circumstances, fatty acids in the blood are not released to enter the adipose tissue cells.

Normally, fatty acids enter the adipose tissue and again are incorporated into triglycerides for storage. In order to produce these triglycerides, glycerol in the form of alpha-glycerol phosphate (α-GP) is necessary. Adipose tissue has little glycerol kinase, the enzyme necessary for its production; therefore, the glycerol released from the VLDL cannot be used. Instead, most of the required α-GP is derived from glucose by glycolysis to triose phosphate (see Fig. 9-3).

When insulin deficiency occurs, glucose transport into adipose tissue cells is reduced, leading to diminished supplies of intracellular glucose. Reduced formation of α-GP results, with a consequent decrease in triglyceride synthesis and an elevation in blood lipid levels (*lipemia*).

In addition to lipoprotein lipase in the capillary bed, adipose tissue contains *intracellular triglyceride lipases* that convert stored triglycerides into glycerol and fatty acids. There are two of these lipases. One has a relatively low activity that is uncontrolled so that there is always some triglyceride breakdown (*lipolysis*). At the same time, there is a continuous need for some glucose to provide enough α-GP for reesterification of those fatty acids. The other lipase is hormone-sensitive and can be highly active. *Hormone-sensitive lipase* is activated by glucagon, epinephrine, ACTH, adrenal glucocorticoids, and growth hormone. Conversely, hormone-sensitive lipase is converted to the inactive form by insulin, thereby reducing the rate of lipolysis. As with glycogen metabolism, it is clear that the ratio of insulin to catabolic hormone is important. Storage of triglyceride is promoted by insulin, whereas lipolysis and reduced triglyceride storage occurs when the catabolic hormones prevail. As lipolysis increases when insulin is insufficient, the need for an α-GP from glucose increases. The rate of breakdown of triglycerides exceeds the ability of the adipose cell to obtain sufficient α-GP from glucose to reesterify the fatty acids, and so nonesterified fatty acids (NEFA) are released into the blood in large quantities.

Fatty acid utilization and ketone body formation. Nonesterified fatty acids are transported in the blood and used for energy by many tissues, such as cardiac muscle and well-oxygenated skeletal muscle. Increased availability of NEFA may be considered both a blessing and a curse. On the one hand, in the presence of adequate oxygen, peripheral cells such as skeletal muscle are able to use NEFA for energy, thereby requiring less glucose to be metabolized. In most tissues that use NEFA for energy, oxidation of fatty acids is carried to completion—that is, to carbon dioxide and water.

On the other hand, in the liver, metabolism can proceed as in other tissues but, if more acetyl-CoA accumulates than can be used to form citrate for the TCA cycle, a different fate for acetyl-CoA is possible. Instead, it is converted to the ketone bodies—acetoacetic acid, beta-hydroxybutyric acid, and acetone—by pathways shown in Fig. 9-4.

Normally, the production of ketone bodies is fairly small for two reasons. In the presence of insulin, lipolysis is inhibited, thereby decreasing substrate for ketone body formation. There also is a more direct control in the liver cell. *Malonyl-CoA* is a metabolite in the lipogenesis pathway (see Fig. 9-3). This pathway is activated by insulin and depressed in its absence. Malonyl-CoA, produced in the presence of insulin, inhibits the transport of fatty acids into mitochondria and thus prevents their metabolism to ketone bodies.

Some ketone bodies always are present in the blood. Acetoacetic acid, in the presence of oxygen, can be used by any tissue containing the enzyme acetoacetate succinyl-CoA transferase, as shown in Fig. 9-4. The liver, however, does not possess this enzyme and, therefore, produces ketone bodies for use by the rest of the body but not for itself.

Although the brain is not able to use NEFA for its energy needs owing to the blood-brain barrier, the brain readily uses ketone bodies. In prolonged starvation, the brain may obtain as much as 30 to 40 percent of its energy needs from ketone bodies.

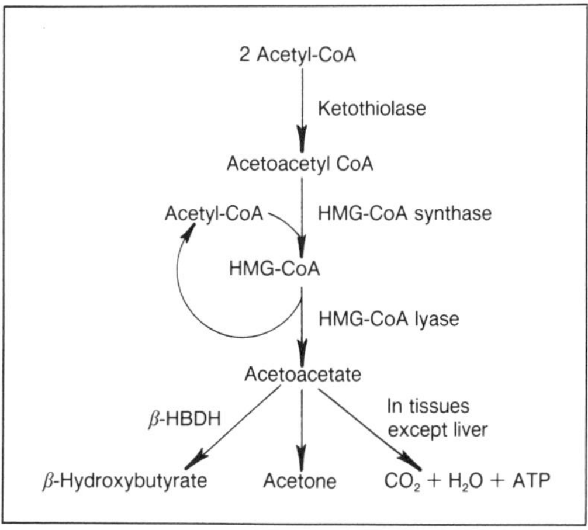

Figure 9-4. Formation of ketone bodies. HMG = hydroxymethyglutaryl; β-HBDH = β-hydroxybutyrate dehydrogenase.

Normally, the production and use of ketone bodies are well matched in quantity, but in starvation and in diabetes, when fatty acid catabolism is increased and fatty acid synthesis is depressed, malonyl-CoA levels drop and NEFA more readily enter the mitochondria and are metabolized. The liver thus is provided with vastly more acetyl-CoA than it can use for its own energy needs. The only remaining outlet for the liver is to convert acetyl-CoA into ketone bodies. The use of ketone bodies cannot keep pace with their production under these circumstances, and they accumulate in the blood and are excreted in the urine.

Development of ketoacidosis. Of the ketone bodies, acetone is produced in the smallest quantity. It is volatile and may be excreted from the lungs. A fruity odor to the breath may result from the excretion of acetone and, perhaps, of some acetoacetate by this route.

When acetoacetic and beta-hydroxybutyric acids are produced by the liver (see Fig. 9-4), they are in acid form. In the blood, the ketone bodies dissociate into hydrogen ions and their negatively charged ions. These anions, acetoacetate and beta-hydroxybutyrate, are excreted in the urine. To maintain electrical neutrality, a *fixed base* (monovalent cation) must be excreted for each ketone anion. The most prevalent cation in the body is sodium, but the normal kidney can conserve sodium efficiently, excreting potassium and ammonium ions in its place. In insulin deficiency, the production of ketone bodies can overwhelm the system, causing depletion of important cations, including sodium, from the body.

In addition, the body must deal with the hydrogen ion derived from ionization of the ketone bodies. The hydrogen ion in the blood is buffered at first by bicarbonate ion and other buffer systems. The lung and kidney excrete excess hydrogen ion as a normal metabolic product. In the uncontrolled diabetic, more hydrogen ion is produced and the system again is overwhelmed. Blood pH drops, stimulating the respiratory system to excrete more carbon dioxide, resulting from the following reaction:

$$H^+ + HCO_3^- \leftrightarrows H_2CO_3 \leftrightarrows H_2O + CO_2$$

Thus, blood bicarbonate drops and the blood has less buffer with which to deal with the acidosis. Respiration deepens, then becomes more labored. If this is insufficient to correct the pH, there is a deep, gasping respiration.

Since the kidney does not produce urine with a pH of less than 4.5 to 5.0, there is a limit to the hydrogen ion which can be excreted. Continued production of acidic ketone bodies overwhelms the kidney's ability to conserve base, and the body becomes deficient in total fixed base. The inability of the kidney to deal with all the hydrogen ion produced and the loss of bicarbonate from the blood results in a drop in blood pH to dangerously low levels.

Loss of body fat. Those who have observed patients with type 1 diabetes are struck by the fact that they are very thin with virtually no body fat. As we discussed earlier, in order to store triglycerides, it is necessary to produce more triglycerides than are being degraded by the triglyceride lipases. Recall that in the diabetic there is little or no insulin available to inactivate hormone-sensitive lipase and to promote glucose uptake and use by the fat cells, and there are high blood levels of most of the hormones that activate hormone-sensitive lipase and inhibit glucose uptake and use. Chronic activated lipolysis, therefore, leads to marked depletion of adipose tissue depots and weight loss.

Amino Acid and Protein Metabolism. Insulin is necessary for normal growth, development, and maintenance. Following the ingestion of a meal, insulin release is stimulated by absorbed glucose and amino acids. Insulin promotes amino acid transport into muscle and adipose tissue cells, promotes protein synthesis in the liver, muscle, and adipose tissue, and inhibits protein degradation in all three tissues (see Table 9-1). The mechanism of insulin's actions on these processes is not yet known in full detail. As with carbohydrate and lipid metabolism, insulin enhances uptake and synthesis and decreases degradation. Amino acids are incorporated into the functional protein of the cell (Fig. 9-5).

Insulin does not have the same effect on all proteins but is selective in its actions; in the presence of insulin, a definite profile of proteins is affected. This is comparable to insulin's actions on carbohydrate metabolism, in which the amounts of some enzymes are increased by insulin whereas the amounts of other enzymes are decreased.

In the diabetic, the anabolic actions of insulin on amino acid and protein metabolism are missing, and the catabolic processes promoted by the catabolic hormones are enhanced. Amino acid uptake into muscle is depressed, whereas amino acid uptake into the liver is accelerated. Synthesis of major classes of proteins, such as myosin, actin,

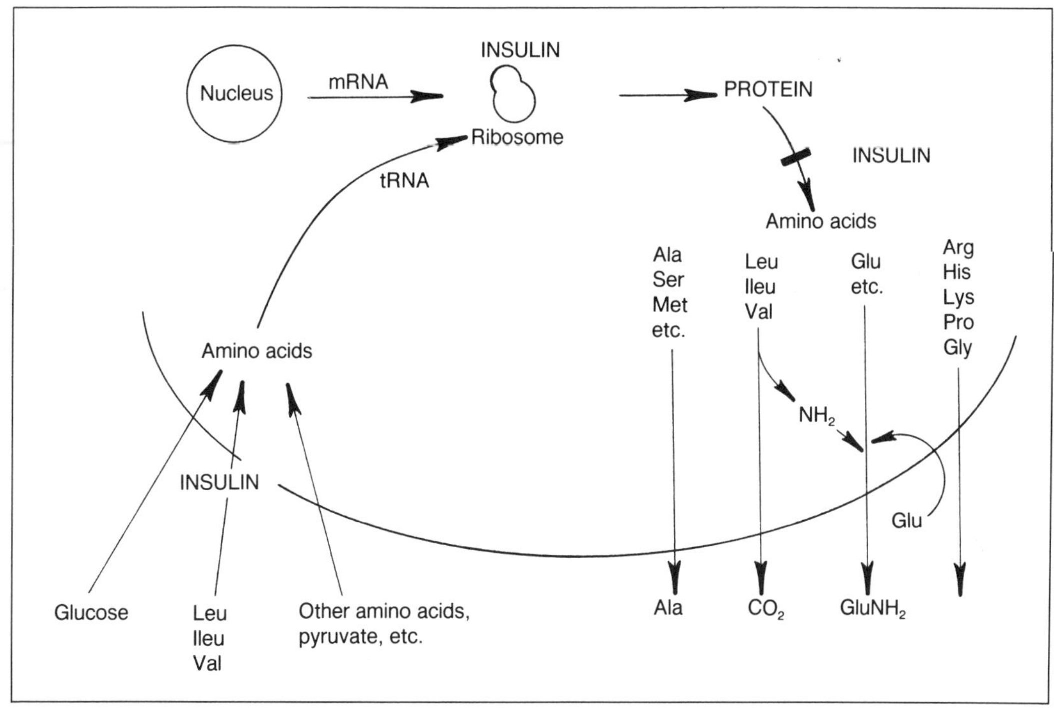

Figure 9-5. Muscle protein metabolism. mRNA = messenger RNA; tRNA = transfer RNA. (From Cahill, G.F., The physiology of insulin in man. Diabetes *20:792, 1971. Reproduced with permission from the American Diabetes Association, Inc.)*

cells, net intracellular charge decreases. Potassium ion is lost from the cell and excreted in the urine along with the ketone body anions.

glycolytic enzymes, and enzymes in the lipogenic pathway, is depressed, whereas degradation of many of these same proteins is accelerated, thus providing a greater blood concentration of many amino acids. In the liver, enzymes that degrade amino acids are increased in activity, so more amino acids are catabolized. More glucose is made by the liver from the carbon skeletons of the amino acids, and more ammonia and urea are produced by amino acid catabolism and the urea cycle. Even though the untreated diabetic is eating, he or she is in negative nitrogen balance. Lean body mass (muscle) decreases, with progressive weakness and weight loss. Blood proteins such as albumin decrease and, with loss of protein from the

Pathogenesis of Clinical Manifestations

Having reviewed the biochemical alterations seen in diabetes, we can summarize the sequence of development of clinical manifestations in logical steps. First there is *hyperglycemia* resulting from the metabolic alterations just described. Kidney tubule cells have a limited capacity to reabsorb glucose. When blood glucose levels exceed this *renal threshold* (160 to 200 mg/dl), the tubules reach their *tubular maximum* for glucose (Tm_G), approximately 350 mg/min. Additional glucose cannot be reabsorbed, and glucose is excreted in the urine (*glycosuria*). Glucose in the urine has osmotic activity, and additional water remains in the urine, causing increased urine volume (*polyuria*). Glucose osmotic activity in the extracellular fluid also causes the withdrawal of water from the cells. The resulting fluid loss causes dehydration which, in turn, causes thirst, stimulating an increase in water intake (*polydipsia*). Other symptoms of dehydration, when it is severe, include dry skin, sunken, soft eyeballs, decreased size of the tongue, decreased blood volume, and increased plasma protein concentration. Decreased protein synthesis and increased gluconeogenesis lead to loss of muscle protein and weight loss. The glucose and ketone bodies in the urine represent a loss of energy, also causing weight loss and a perception by the diabetic that more food must be ingested. Thus, the patient develops an increased appetite (*polyphagia*). These, then, are the classic symptoms of diabetes: polyuria, polydipsia, and polyphagia. The increased food intake provides additional carbohydrate, contributing to an even higher hyperglycemia.

Lipemia occurs as the result of two factors. The first is decreased lipoprotein lipase activity, resulting in reduced removal of chylomicrons and VLDLs from the blood following a meal. The second is increased release of NEFA from adipose tissue triglyceride stores. The liver takes up NEFA at a rate proportional to their concentration and metabolizes them to acetyl-CoA. Decreased lipogenesis and the limited metabolism of acetyl-CoA in the citric acid cycle causes acetyl-CoA to be diverted to the most readily available pathway—ketone body formation. The body has a limited capacity to metabolize ketone bodies as an energy source. Excess ketone bodies accumulate in the blood (*ketonemia*) and are excreted in the urine (*ketonuria*). The presence of increased amounts of ketone bodies in the tissue and body fluids is known as *ketosis.*

Of the ketone bodies, acetone is volatile and can be excreted by the lungs. Acetoacetic acid and beta-hydroxybutyric acid ionize, increasing the hydrogen ion concentration in blood. As blood pH drops, respiration is stimulated (*hyperpnea*) to excrete carbon dioxide and becomes progressively more labored (*dyspnea*) and, eventually, deep and gasping (*Kussmaul respiration*).

The kidney also excretes excess acid. As long as respiratory and renal mechanisms compensate for the increased acid production, blood pH is controlled. This is known as *compensated metabolic acidosis.* Eventually, in the uncontrolled diabetic, these mechanisms are inadequate and blood pH falls. Sodium, potassium, and bicarbonate ion are lost as respiratory and renal compensatory mechanisms are overwhelmed (*decompensated metabolic acidosis*). The patient now is *ketoacidotic.*

Brain function becomes affected. The patient becomes progressively more lethargic, stuporous, and, eventually, comatose. There are two theories regarding the cause of *diabetic coma:* decreased nerve irritability as hydrogen ion concentration increases, or dehydration leading to circulatory failure and hypotension, reducing oxygen and energy-producing substrates to the brain. Permanent brain damage can occur if the condition persists for more than 24 hours. The patient dies if blood pH continues to fall and dehydration, shock, and renal failure are not corrected.

Complications of Diabetes

The complications of diabetes may be classified as acute or chronic. A few are minor in significance, but many can be life-threatening.

Acute Complications. The acute complications are those that can be reversed quickly with the adjustment of the blood glucose level. They comprise situations in which blood glucose is either abnormally high or abnormally low.

Hypoglycemia. Hypoglycemia in the diabetic is known also as an *insulin reaction* or *insulin shock.* It occurs when blood glucose concentrations become subnormal. Many other circumstances, unrelated to diabetes, can cause hypoglycemia, too. These are described later in the section on hypoglycemia (p. 371).

In insulin-treated diabetic patients, hypoglycemia can occur for a variety of reasons. Among these are (1) failure to eat the prescribed diet, (2) delayed meals following an insulin injection, (3) vomiting, (4) diarrhea, (5) a sudden increase in severe exercise, (6) an error in insulin dosage, causing an overdose, (7) weight loss without a concomitant decrease in insulin dosage, and (8) renal insufficiency with decreased renal clearance of insulin.

As the blood glucose concentration falls, the patient begins to feel hungry and weak and may become mentally confused and emotionally unstable. As the condition progresses, the patient perspires and has a cold, clammy skin. The central nervous system symptoms become more severe with blurred vision and loss of coordination and orientation. Further progression produces incontinence, paralysis, unconsciousness, and convulsions. The mental symptoms arise from the lack of glucose for brain metabolism. Severe hypoglycemia can be fatal.

The time required for the development of the symptoms is very short, so treatment must be prompt. There is danger of permanent brain damage if the reaction is severe and lasts more than 6 hours. Repeated severe reactions, even of shorter duration, also can cause brain damage.

Mild reactions can be treated with a quick source of carbohydrate given by mouth. Fruit juice often is used. Other usable items include candy, sugar, honey, molasses, corn syrup, or any other source that can be absorbed quickly. For more severe reactions, injected glucagon may be given along with oral glucose sources to raise the blood glucose level. For unconscious or convulsive patients, glucose may be given intravenously.

Rebound hyperglycemia (the *Somogyi effect*) sometimes follows an episode of insulin-induced hypoglycemia, which has stimulated the release of glucagon and other antiinsulin hormones. These hormones stimulate glycogenolysis and gluconeogenesis, causing an elevation in blood glucose.

The Somogyi effect occurs most often in type 1 diabetes. It may follow severe exercise but sometimes occurs during the night. It is treated by a 25 to 30 percent reduction in the insulin dose.

Ketosis and ketoacidotic coma. Ketoacidosis and coma account for the deaths of 1 to 3 percent of all diabetics. Of those treated for ketoacidosis, 10 to 15 percent die; therefore, prevention is very important.

Ketoacidosis is directly opposed to insulin reaction. It can occur in undiagnosed, untreated insulin-dependent diabetes, produced as a result of the metabolic alterations previously described. However, 90 percent of cases of ketoacidosis involve known diabetics who are being treated. In these patients, the causes include (1) a decrease or omission of insulin dose or error in the type of insulin, (2) failure to follow the diet, with overeating, (3) sudden withdrawal of insulin when starting hypoglycemic agents, and (4) infections, trauma, or other stresses that cause the diabetes to become more severe. Even a well-controlled diabetic can become acidotic during infection, since he or she becomes more insulin-resistant. In ketoacidosis, glucagon or glucocorticoids tend to be elevated.

Ketoacidosis may develop slowly or rapidly. In juvenile diabetics, a rapid onset of days or even hours is possible, particularly if there is an infection. In a child, symptoms that can be observed by an adult include:

Fatigue, weakness, listlessness
Vomiting (sometimes)
Fruity odor to the breath
Kussmaul respiration and coma in 12 to 24 hours

In an adult, symptoms are the same as those in the child but usually develop more slowly. The patient may be extremely drowsy but still able to be aroused, rather than being comatose. In both children and adults, comatose or semicomatose states extending for more than 24 hours can result in irreversible brain damage and death.

The condition varies in severity. One useful classification is the following:

	Serum Bicarbonate
Phase 3: Ketosis	20 mEq/L
Phase 2: Ketoacidosis	11–20 mEq/L
Phase 1: Diabetic coma	10 mEq/L

	Serum pH
Phase 3: Ketosis	7.4
Phase 2: Ketoacidosis	7.2–7.4
Phase 1: Diabetic coma	7.2

	Acidosis
Phase 3: Ketosis	None
Phase 2: Ketoacidosis	Moderate
Phase 1: Diabetic coma	Severe

Phases 1 and 2, in particular, are serious medical emergencies. If confused or comatose, the patient is not given food; therefore, treatment is not dietary. In general, treatment consists of large doses of insulin plus intravenous fluid and electrolyte replacement. The blood and urine levels must be monitored closely and treatment must be adjusted as indicated. In addition, artificial plasma expanders sometimes are added to the intravenous fluids to treat the hypotension and shock resulting from dehydration. Blood or plasma transfusions can be used or *dextran,* a glucose polysaccharide with 1,6 linkage, may be added. As the blood glucose level falls, 5% glucose is added to guard against hypoglycemia.

When the patient is fully mentally alert, oral feeding may begin. A common procedure includes the following steps:

1. Use small amounts of fluids to test for nausea and vomiting. Do not feed orally until vomiting stops.
2. Progress to a liquid diet with milk, fruit juice, and broth to provide potassium and phosphate. Milk and fruit juice also provide glucose.
3. Progress to a full liquid to soft to regular diabetic diet as tolerated. The diabetes is regulated with regular insulin.
4. When the patient is fully controlled with regular insulin, a partial shift to some longer-acting insulin may be undertaken and the diet adjusted accordingly.

Hyperosmolar nonketotic coma. In some ways, hyperosmolar nonketotic coma is similar to ketoacidotic coma, but they differ in important respects. Hyperglycemia in hyperosmolar nonketotic coma can reach extreme levels, 900 to 3,000 mg/dl, but ketonemia is very mild or absent and acidosis does not develop. The typical patient is more than 50 years old and has mild type 2 diabetes. Many are undiagnosed until the development of an unrelated illness or trauma precipitates the coma. Some examples of precipitating factors are pancreatitis, myocardial infarction, infection, cerebrovascular accident, renal failure, burns, and gastroenteritis. This superimposed stress causes the diabetes to become more severe. Sometimes, the condition is precipitated by the excessive use of diuretics. It also can occur spontaneously.

In the pathogenesis of this condition, increased blood glucose levels develop with increasing severity of the diabetes. Glycosuria and fluid loss occur by the mechanisms already described (see p. 337). The patient may compensate with increased fluid intake at first, but this becomes insufficient and the patient becomes dehydrated. The water loss exceeds the glucose loss, and the serum becomes hyperosmolar (350 mOsm or more, compared to a normal value of 285 to 300 mOsm/L). The patient becomes more unresponsive to thirst, which causes further dehydration, greater osmolarity, and so on in a vicious circle. However, the patient does not become acidotic, since these patients do have some insulin which is sufficient to prevent massive fatty acid release but not enough to stimulate entry of glucose into peripheral cells.

Once the patient is in a coma, mortality is 40 to 70 percent. Therefore, early treatment before the condition becomes severe is essential. The major features of treatment are insulin administration, potassium replacement, and hypotonic fluid replacement. The hypotonic fluid must be given slowly or the patient may die of cerebral edema when the fluid enters brain cells containing high concentrations of osmotically active glucose.

Other problems. There are several minor complications related to insulin administration which are not easily classified as either acute or chronic. Although they are less serious than the specifically acute or chronic problems, they may be of great concern to the patient; therefore, nutritional care specialists should be aware of them. Some patients may develop *lipomas* (or *lipohypertrophy*), lumpy fat deposits, at the sites of repeated insulin injections. Treatment consists of changing injection sites. Most patients are instructed to do this when they are taught to give themselves insulin. Other patients have *lipoatrophy* (loss of fat around injection sites), producing a depressed area. This is presumed to be the effect of contaminants in the insulin and is less common when purer insulins are used. No diet modification is required; alteration of the fat content of the diet is not effective.

Chronic Complications. Very few diabetic patients experience the acute complications, whereas almost all have chronic complications. Good control has been found to delay the onset and reduce the severity of these complications. It is not known whether they can be prevented altogether or whether they are inevitable if the disease exists for a sufficiently long period.

Metabolic lesions. No single metabolic abnormality accounts for all of the chronic complications. In some cases, the pathogenesis is unknown, although some of the aberrations in metabolism are understood at least partially. They involve the redirection of glucose metabolism from insulin-sensitive to insulin-insensitive pathways.

One of these is the *sorbitol (polyol) pathway.* In cells that do not require insulin for entry of glucose, the intracellular glucose is equal to the glucose levels in the plasma. In the hyperglycemic patient, then, glucose concentration in these cells is high. The excess glucose is converted to sorbitol and fructose in the cell. Although glucose has freely entered these cells, sorbitol and fructose cannot readily leave, even if the hyperglycemia subsides. They can accumulate in the cells at concentrations far above normal (twenty times normal for sorbitol and ten times normal for fructose), and remain in the cell until metabolized. The exact mechanism by which sorbitol accumulation contributes to the etiology of complications is not understood entirely. One line of reasoning suggests that the hypertonicity consequent to sorbitol accumulation causes an influx of sodium ion and water and a loss of potassium ion. This then is followed by a decrease in amino acid and ATP concentration and a loss of small peptides, such as glutathione, which participate in cellular metabolism. Alternatively, the damage may be the consequence of reduction of the oxygen-carrying capacity of erythrocytes. In cells other than erythrocytes, in glycolysis, a kinase catalyzes the conversion of 1,3-diphosphoglycerate (1,3-DPG) to 3-phosphoglycerate. In erythrocytes, a different enzyme, *diphosphoglyceromutase,* catalyzes conversion of the 1,3-DPG to 2,3-DPG. The affinity of hemoglobin for oxygen is decreased when 2,3-DPG combines with hemoglobin and oxygen is more easily released for use by peripheral tissues. When sorbitol accumulates, it may displace 2,3-DPG and reduce the release of oxygen to the tissues. It must be recognized that the lowering of blood pH in impending acidosis may be the major mechanism for changes in oxygen release.

A second metabolic alteration leading to chronic complications involves *glycoprotein formation.* Glycoproteins are proteins bound to small polysaccharide groups. In their normal formation, a polypeptide chain is formed on a rough endoplasmic reticulum, is *glycosylated* (carbohydrates are attached) in smooth endoplasmic reticulum, and eventually is secreted. In the diabetic, there is increased synthesis of glycoproteins. Some changes in amino acid sequences have also been found, so that the glycoproteins formed may be abnormal. Glycoproteins make up the basement membrane and, in the diabetic, the basement membranes are thickened and may be abnormal. This has particular significance in renal function, leading to an increased incidence of renal disease in diabetic patients.

A third possible lesion may involve *mucopolysaccharide formation.* Mucopolysaccharides have larger proportions of carbohydrates than do glycoproteins. The greater amount of glucose available to their synthetic pathways may cause alterations in their structure. Abnormal mucopolysaccharide structures have been seen in the aorta, kidneys, skin, and retinas of diabetics. Clinical complications also occur in these tissues, but it has not been proved that they are related to abnormal mucopolysaccharides. However, the simultaneous occurrence does suggest that there is a relationship.

The biochemical lesions just described occur most frequently in blood vessels, nerves, kidneys, and eyes of diabetic patients. The consequences of these pathologic alterations seriously impair the general health and shorten the life expectancy of the patient.

Anatomic and physiologic lesions. Angiopathy (abnormalities of the blood vessels) accounts for 80 percent of diabetic deaths. It may be subdivided into *macroangiopathy* (disease in large blood vessels) and *microangiopathy* (disease in small blood vessels).

Disease in the large arteries of diabetics is morphologically identical to that found in the general population except that it occurs earlier, progresses more rapidly, and is more severe. It leads to cerebrovascular accidents, myocardial infarctions, senility, congestive heart failure, and other complications of cardiovascular disease. One consequence of macroangiopathy deserves special mention in a discussion of diabetes. Severe atherosclerosis in large vessels can occlude the vessels and reduce the circulation to a body part. This occurs particularly in the legs and feet of diabetics. The patients may complain first of pain, coldness, and fatigue in the affected limbs. The limbs become ischemic. In severe cases, wounds and infections do not heal because of poor blood supply. Ulcers and gangrene develop easily (review Chapter 1, if necessary), and amputations are frequent. For this reason, care of the feet is an important aspect of proper treatment of the diabetic patient.

Microangiopathy is found in 8 percent of normal subjects, 53 percent of prediabetics, and 98 percent of overt diabetics. Since it often occurs before the onset of overt diabetes, it may be the basis for diagnosis. Its manifestations include sclerosis of the arterioles and dilation of the venules with stasis of the blood in the venules. The basement membranes around the capillaries thicken, contributing to the loss of circulation to the limbs and to the susceptibility to infection. It also contributes in important ways to the complications that may occur in the kidney and eyes.

Nephropathy (kidney disease) is responsible for only 10 percent of all deaths but accounts for 50 to 60 percent of deaths of type 1 diabetics. It progresses without symptoms until renal failure is far advanced.

Neuropathy (lesions of the nerves) can take many forms. It is less likely to be life-threatening than are angiopathy and nephropathy but can be very distressing to the patient. As in the case of microangiopathy, symptoms sometimes occur prior to the diagnosis of diabetes. Significant nerve damage is more likely to occur in the poorly controlled diabetic. If the diabetes then is controlled and the blood glucose concentration is lowered, the progress of the neuropathy can be arrested but not entirely reversed.

The metabolic lesions that occur in the nerves may involve carbohydrate, lipid, or protein metabolic pathways, but they are not understood entirely. The sorbitol pathway may be involved, since sorbitol and fructose do occur in peripheral nerves. Other metabolic aberrations apparently reduce the rate of conversion of glucose to carbon dioxide or fatty acid.

Lipid metabolism of peripheral nerves is generally affected, resulting in differences in the fatty acid composition and abnormalities in the formation of fatty acids, cholesterol, glycolipids, and myelin. The formation of the protein in myelin is reduced. Inositol metabolism may also be involved.

Neuropathies may occur in either the sensory or motor nerves or both. They may affect one nerve or many and they may be one-sided or occur on both sides of the body. Some recovery occurs with control of the diabetes, but it can take months. Depending on the nerves involved, symptoms may include pain, weakness, numbness, and loss of one's sense of physical position.

Neuropathies in the autonomic nervous system can be disabling and, occasionally, fatal. Some of the clinical manifestations include disorders in the cardiovascular system, bladder disturbances, abnormalities of eye control, and impotence in men. Of particular interest to nutritional care specialists are the gastrointestinal disturbances, including diarrhea, constipation, incontinence, atony of the esophagus, nausea, vomiting, gastric motor disorders, pancreatic enzyme insufficiency, and gallstones, among others.[41] Celiac disease is associated with diabetes in an unusually large number of cases.[41] Nutritional care for patients with these conditions is described in Chapter 6. Riddle[42] reports that the gastrointestinal symptoms may be caused by hypoglycemia in some patients whose insulin dosage should be reduced.

Retinopathy (disease of the retina) in the diabetic is a common cause of blindness. Patients may complain of blurred vision, double vision, halos, and pain in the eyes. Sometimes these occur prior to the diagnosis of diabetes. Reduction of blood glucose and blood lipids by controlling the diabetes acts as a preventive or at least delays the advance of the disease.

Diagnosis of Diabetes Mellitus

Mild type 2 diabetes may be asymptomatic and can exist undetected for many years. Its existence sometimes is first suspected when vascular lesions are seen in the eye, or it may be detected fortuitously during a case-finding survey of the population or during a routine physical examination. The major diagnostic tests that have been in use for many years have focused on the effects of diabetes on blood glucose concentration. There are several of these tests.

In the measurement of *fasting blood glucose* (FBS), the glucose concentration is determined in blood or plasma from a patient following an 8-hour fast, usually overnight. Normal FBS is 60 to 100 mg/dl in patients up to age 50. Thereafter, it increases approximately 1 percent per year. Sometimes plasma levels are used in place of whole blood. The relationship can be calculated with the formula: $1.15 \times$ blood glucose $+ 6 =$ plasma glucose.[4] If FBS is greater than 250 mg/dl of blood or 285 mg/dl of plasma, a diagnosis of diabetes mellitus can be made. Fasting blood glucose is increased in patients under mental, emotional, or physical stress. As a result, values are not considered truly abnormal unless they exceed 130 mg/dl of blood or 150 mg/dl of plasma.

The *glucose tolerance test* (GTT) is more definitive and is of particular value for use with those patients whose FBS is somewhat high but not extreme. It is based on the assumption that a normal person can remove a specified glucose load from the blood within a defined period. Prior to the test, the patient's diet should contain at least 150 g of carbohydrate per day. Usually, this is achieved with the patient's normal diet and no special preparation is required. On the day of the test, blood for the FBS and a urine sample are obtained. In a typical procedure, the patient then is given a drink, usually containing 1.75 g of glucose per kilogram of body weight in a 15 to 25% solution flavored with lemon juice or cola. The drink must be

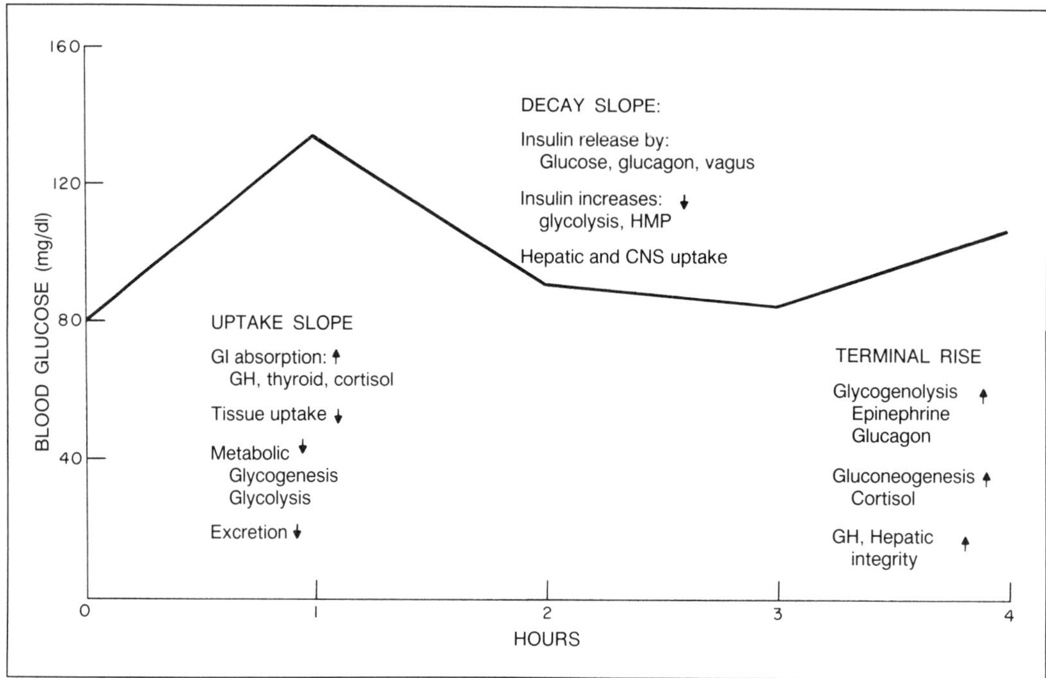

Figure 9-6. Metabolic processes in the normal oral glucose tolerance test. Processes involved in the different phases of the curve are presented. Thick arrows indicate directions of changes in blood glucose levels. HMP = hexose monophosphate (Shunt); GH = growth hormone. (Reprinted with permission from Bacchus, H., Rational Management of Diabetes. *Copyright © 1977, University Park Press, Baltimore.)*

Figure 9-7. Normal and diabetic glucose tolerance curves.

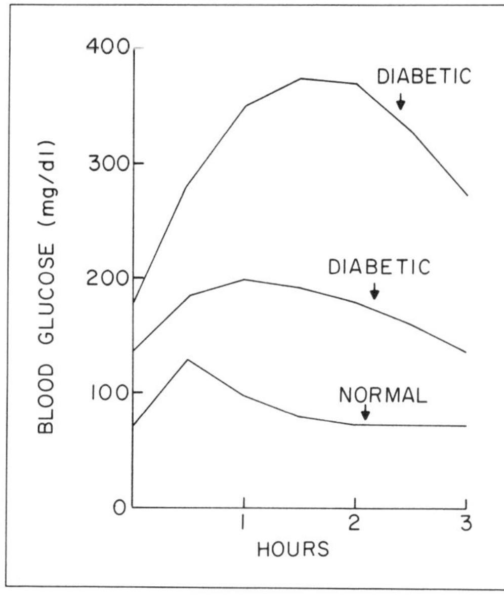

ingested within 10 to 15 minutes. The glucose content of hourly blood and urine samples is determined. A typical normal curve with affecting factors is shown in Fig. 9-6. Figure 9-7 shows a comparison between the normal and diabetic curves.

In a *cortisone glucose tolerance test,* the GTT is preceded by two doses of cortisone to mimic the effect of stress. The test applies only if the patient is younger than 45 years of age, not pregnant, and has no other diseases.

Characteristic abnormalities in the glucose tolerance curve that are indicative of diabetes are (1) increased maximum blood glucose concentration, (2) delayed return to normal blood glucose concentration, and (3)

Table 9-2. Criteria for Diagnosis of Chemical Diabetes by Oral Glucose Tolerance Test[a]

	Time of Testing	Blood Glucose (mg/dl)	Plasma Glucose (mg/dl)
Fajans and Conn[b] (1.75 g/kg of ideal body weight)	60 min.	>160	>185
	90 min.	>140	>160
	120 min.	>120	>140
	All three values should be abnormal for diagnosis		
U.S. Public Health Service—Wilkerson (100 g to all subjects)	*Fasting*	>110 = 1 point	>130 = 1 point
	60 min.	>170 = ½ point	>195 = ½ point
	120 min.	>120 = ½ point	>165 = ½ point
	180 min.	>110 = 1 point	>130 = 1 point
	Total of 2 points needed for diagnosis		
Summation of glucose levels	At time of glucose ingestion and after 1, 2, and 3 hours	>500	>600
	Abnormal values needed for diagnosis		

Reprinted with permission from Bacchus, H., *Rational Management of Diabetes.* Copyright © 1977, University Park Press, Baltimore. P. 78.

[a] These values apply to patients between 15 and 50 years of age.

[b] The Fajans-Conn criteria are similar to those for diagnosis of diabetes in childhood. Note also that the Fajans criteria are readily applicable to the first trimester of pregnancy and, with modifications, to the second and third trimesters.

late hypoglycemia, usually in 3 to 5 hours. The specific criteria used to define abnormalities vary. Some typical values are shown in Table 9-2, but it is important to remember that many drugs and other illnesses can affect glucose tolerance.

More recently, additional diagnostic tests have become available. The amount of insulin in the blood is very small, and for many years assays were impossible. The recent development of radioimmunossay techniques has increased the use of measurement of *blood insulin levels.*

The C peptide, released when proinsulin is converted to active insulin, can be used to measure endogenous insulin secretion even when the patient is receiving exogenous insulin in treatment. The diabetic patient who has no endogenous insulin will have no C peptide. The test is known as the *C peptide chain assay.*[43]

Hemoglobin A_{1c}, or *glycosylated hemoglobin,* forms 5 percent of the total hemoglobin (Hb) in the normal person. It is formed slowly throughout the life of the mature red blood cell by a reaction between the major adult hemoglobin, HbA, and glucose. In hyperglycemia, the rate of formation of HbA_{1c} increases, and levels may reach 15 percent in uncontrolled diabetes mellitus.[44] The reaction is nearly irreversible so that a high HbA_{1c} concentration will fall only as cells die and are replaced by new cells, but will not fall with a temporary decrease in the blood glucose level. The HbA_{1c} concentration, then, reflects the average degree of diabetic control over a period of 2 to 3 months[45] and can be used as a check on the patient's long-term adherence to the diet.

Progressive Development of Diabetes

Since primary diabetes is inherited, at least the predisposition is believed to exist in the newborn infant. For convenience, the process of development of the clinical manifestations of diabetes mellitus has been divided into four stages.

Prediabetes, or *diabetes premellitus,* usually is diagnosed only in retrospect. There is no decrease in glucose tolerance, but insulin secretion in response to glucose or amino acids is delayed or decreased,[46-48] and there may be some changes in the blood vessels in the eye. Prediabetic women may have a history of miscarriages, exceptionally large infants, or toxemia of pregnancy. Children whose parents are both diabetic or the identical twin of a diabetic are assumed to be prediabetic.

Subclinical diabetes exists in patients showing some sporadic carbohydrate intolerance.[49] The FBS and GTT are normal, but the cortisone glucose tolerance test is abnormal.

Latent or *chemical diabetes* is diagnosed in those patients who usually have a normal FBS but whose glucose tolerance is abnormal. They may have no symptoms of diabetes. Type 2 diabetes frequently falls into this category.

In *overt diabetes,* both the FBS and GTT are abnormal and the patient also has glycosuria and the classic symptoms of polydipsia, polyuria, and polyphagia.

Treatment

Since there is no cure for diabetes, the patient must learn to live with the disease. The overall objectives of treatment are to prolong life and to improve the quality of life as much as possible. Specifically, the treatment is directed toward:

1. Relieving the symptoms and enabling the patient to live a relatively normal life
2. Decreasing the severity of the disease by improving the body's ability to metabolize glucose and correcting faulty metabolism so that glucose tolerance is improved and insulin resistance is decreased
3. Preventing or correcting complications
4. Assuring adequate nutrition

These objectives are accomplished by control of the metabolic changes. Control may be measured in various ways. Most commonly, it is measured by the maintenance of blood glucose concentration within normal limits. Other criteria which sometimes are used include absence of symptoms, of glycosuria, or of hyperlipidemia, normal blood ketoacids, or normal measurements of function of the eye, kidney, or nervous system. It now is generally accepted that careful control of blood glucose levels prevents or delays many of the chronic complications of diabetes.[50,51]

The successful treatment of the diabetic patient is complex and requires the cooperation of the physician, nurse, nutritional care specialist, and other members of the health care team, but most of all it requires the whole-hearted cooperation of the patient. It commonly is said that, in the final analysis, the diabetic patient is self-treated.

There are four major facets of diabetic care: (1) control of the dietary intake to decrease clinical manifestations while providing for nutritional needs, (2) hypoglycemic drugs, (3) exercise, and (4) education. In addition, the general hygiene and emotional well-being of the patient often must receive attention.

Hypoglycemic Drugs

The *hypoglycemic* or *antidiabetic drugs* are those that lower the blood glucose concentration. Some diabetics do not receive these drugs but are treated by diet alone. Others receive either insulin or one of the sulfonylurea drugs.

Insulin. Insulin is given to approximately 25 percent of diabetic patients. Its use is indicated in diabetic children, all patients with sudden onset, and underweight diabetics, since these conditions are suggestive of type 1 diabetes. In addition, even if a diabetic has not been treated with insulin previously, it usually is indicated when certain complications such as ketosis, fevers, infections, surgery, burns, or pregnancy occur.

Since insulin is a protein, it would be digested if taken by mouth and therefore must be given parenterally, usually by subcutaneous injection. The most readily available insulins are a mixture of pork and beef insulin and contain impurities that are sometimes the cause of allergic reactions. Insulins prepared solely from either beef or pork are available on special order if needed. Insulins available in the United States are single-peak insulins, which are 98 percent pure. Monocomponent insulins, distributed in Europe, are 99 percent pure; they may be obtained if the physician makes an inquiry to the manufacturer.

Insulin is available in vials containing 100 units/ml. Each milligram of pure insulin equals 24 units. Some U-40 and U-80 insulin (40 units and 80 units/ml, respectively) still is available but is being phased out. There are a number of types of insulin available (Table 9-3), classified as rapid-acting, intermediate-acting, or long-acting.[52] Protamine and globin are proteins which, when combined with insulin, slow its rate of absorption. Insulin Lente (insulin zinc suspension) is manufactured by a process that produces very large crystals, thus slowing its absorption. It contains zinc but no modifying protein. Insulin Lente is a mixture of seven parts of Ultralente with three parts of Semilente insulin. The properties of the insulins listed in Table 9-3 should be studied carefully. It is essential that nutritional care specialists be familiar with the speed of onset and duration of action of each of the available insulins, since this information is important in diet planning.

Rapid-acting insulin is used when diabetes is being controlled, in the newly diagnosed diabetic, or following a ketotic episode. It also is used daily by many diabetics to control blood glucose early in the day.

If only regular insulin is used, an injection is required before each meal. To reduce the number of injections, a longer-acting and a rapid-acting insulin often are used in combination. They are mixed in the syringe by the patient just before administration. It is not possible to mix them in advance of their use, since they interact and their properties change. A common procedure is to mix the rapid-acting insulin for its effect during the morning with an intermediate-acting insulin the activity of which occurs primarily after the noon and evening meals. Commonly used combinations are regular insulin plus either NPH or Lente insulin. When these combinations are used, it may be possible to control diabetes with only one insulin injection per day, but two or more injections per day provide better control in many patients.

The type of insulin given is important, since the distribution of meals must be planned so there is enough glucose in the blood to prevent hypoglycemia when the insulin reaches its peak action. Patients receiving intermediate-acting insulin often require an afternoon snack in addition to the usual three meals. Long-acting insulins are used much less frequently, but those patients who do use them generally require a snack in the evening to prevent hypoglycemia during the night.

The amount of insulin prescribed by the physician is determined somewhat by trial and error, although there are some general guidelines. The amount prescribed is affected by the diet, the patient's own insulin production (if any), the patient's activity, body weight, the effects of other hormones, and the existence of complications.

Sulfonylureas. The sulfonylurea compounds are taken orally and so they often are called *oral hypoglycemic agents.* Those available are described in Table 9-4. The second-generation compounds, developed most recently, are more potent. Tolbutamide and chlorpropamide are those most frequently used in the United States. They may be given to almost 50 percent of diabetic patients, but serious questions have been raised concerning their value, since no long-term benefits of their use over other methods have been documented.[53] As a result, there is now greater emphasis on dietary control and, if necessary, the use of insulin.

Sulfonylurea drugs stimulate the release of preformed insulin from the pancreas when they are first given and therefore are

Table 9-3. Types and Characteristics of Commercial Insulin Preparations

Types of Insulin	Animal Source	Time of Onset (hours after subcutaneous injection)	Action Peak (hours after subcutaneous injection)	Duration (hours)	Appearance	Buffer[a]	Modifiers
Rapid-acting							
Regular (RI)	Beef, pork, or both	½–1	3–4	6	Clear		
Semilente (prompt insulin zinc suspension)	Beef	½–¾	5–7	12–18	Cloudy	Acetate	Zinc
Intermediate-acting							
Globin zinc	Beef, pork, or both	½–1	7–11	24–28	Clear		Globin
NPH (isophane or neutral protamine Hagedorn)	Beef, pork, or both	2–4	7–11	24–28	Cloudy	Phosphate	Protamine
Lente (insulin zinc suspension)	Beef	1–1½	11–18	28–32	Cloudy	Acetate	Zinc
Long-acting							
Protamine zinc[b] (PZI)	Beef, pork, or both	6–8	10–18	24–72	Cloudy	Phosphate	Protamine
Ultralente (extended insulin zinc suspension)[b]	Beef	5–8	22–26	36+	Cloudy	Acetate	Zinc
Combinations							
Regular + NPH		½–1	2–12	18–32		Phosphate	Protamine
Regular + Lente		1	2–12	18–32		Acetate	Zinc
Semilente + Lente		1	2–10	24–28		Acetate	Zinc
Semilente + Ultralente		1	2–24	36+		Acetate	Zinc

[a] Insulins with different buffers should not be used in combination.

[b] There is little indication for use of these insulins.

Table 9-4. Sulfonylurea Compounds

Drug[a]	Dosage Range (mg)	Tablet Size (mg)
First-generation compounds		
Tolbutamide (Orinase)	500–3,000	500
Chlorpropamide (Diabinese)	100–500	100, 250
Tolazamide (Tolinase)	100–750	100, 250
Acetohexamide (Dymelor)	500–1,500	250, 500
Second-generation compounds		
Glibenclamide	2.5–20	5
Glipizide	2.5–45	5
Glibornuride	12.5–100	12.5

[a] In order of frequency of use.

unsuitable for type 1 diabetes. It has been suggested that their primary mode of action during prolonged use may be to alter cell membranes and increase their responsiveness to insulin, possibly by increasing the number of receptors.[54] A summary of actions outside of the pancreas is given in Table 9-5. Since they act by stimulating formation or release of insulin, they have no effect in the type 1 diabetic who has no endogenous insulin production. They are usable in type 2 diabetes and in prediabetes and latent diabetes in an attempt to delay onset of overt disease.

Table 9-5. Extrapancreatic Effects of Sulfonylurea Drugs

Related to antidiabetes effects
Increased insulin stimulation of carbohydrate transport in skeletal muscle
Increased insulin action on the liver
Decreased triglyceride lipase in liver and adipose tissue
Decreased ketosis
Decreased glucose output from liver
Decreased lipolysis in adipose tissue
Increased uptake and oxidation of glucose in adipose tissue
Side effects
Activation of adenylate cyclase
Decreased adenosine 3′,5′ monophosphate diesterase
Altered rate of amino acid incorporation into protein
Decreased transaminase activity
Reduced intestinal glucose absorption
Decreased insulinases
Increased cardiac contractility
Decreased platelet aggregation

There are some advantages to the use of sulfonylureas. First, they are taken orally in tablet form rather than by injection, so patient acceptance is high. They may be given to the type 2 diabetic who, because of lack of understanding, poor eyesight, or other reasons, cannot safely administer his or her own insulin. There is less danger of hypoglycemia with sulfonylurea use than with insulin use. To the extent that sulfonylureas stimulate insulin production and release by normal pathways, they correct the existing deficiency rather than provide a replacement. Finally, these drugs also provide less potential for allergic reactions since they are not foreign proteins.

Their disadvantages also are important considerations and, in recent years, have been the basis for the reduction in their use in favor of dietary control with or without insulin. One study has indicated that tolbutamide was associated with an increase in the incidence and severity of cardiovascular disease,[54] but the plan of the study and the conclusions have been hotly disputed.[55]

Minor side effects occur in 3.2 percent of patients given tolbutamide and 6 percent of those receiving chlorpropamide.[56,57] They include rash, nausea, vomiting, heartburn, and alcohol intolerance. The major side effects—liver toxicity, blood dyscrasias, hypothyroidism, and hyponatremia (low serum sodium)—occur in approximately 1 percent of users, particularly in those using chlorpropamide. A major problem from the point of view of the nutritional care specialist is that oral drug treatment is so easy that many patients feel that diet is unimportant.

Nutritional Care

The best diet for the treatment of diabetes mellitus has always been a matter of controversy. Broadly speaking, the difference of opinion centers around the amount of control of hyperglycemia that is necessary and how it is to be achieved.

All diabetologists agree that control of significant hyperglycemia is desirable. They also agree that hyperglycemia is preferable to hypoglycemia. On the other hand, experts disagree on the amount of risk of hypoglycemia that is acceptable when aggressively treating high blood glucose levels.

A large body of evidence indicates that even moderate hyperglycemia has a detrimental effect on the incidence of complications and on resistance to infection, but the level of hyperglycemia that has long-term harmful effects has not been firmly established.[58-61] Thus, the recommendations for dietary control, especially for the type 1 diabetic, vary from the strict diet, attempting to control blood glucose levels within very narrow limits, to a more liberal and flexible diet, allowing a higher blood glucose concentration with greater fluctuation. It often is claimed that the strict diet is ineffective, but this may be true because many patients do not adhere to the prescribed strict diet, not because the diet is inherently ineffective.[62]

There is no controversy on the effectiveness of calorie restriction for the overweight maturity-onset diabetic. Weight reduction controls the disease and may reverse it altogether, with significant clinical benefits.[62-64] Under these circumstances, successful diet therapy in diabetes justifies a great effort on the part of the health care team.

In summary, the emphasis in type 1 diabetics is on consistency of intake in order to keep blood glucose levels under control. In the obese diabetic (type 2), emphasis is on calorie restriction. The planning process is the same in either case and will be described in some detail.

Determining the Diet Prescription. The responsibility for determining the diet prescription is basically the physician's but sometimes is delegated to the nutritional care specialist. In general, the procedure involves first estimating the total calorie need, then partitioning the calories among the various nutrients, and finally distributing the calories among the daily meals.

Estimate total calorie need. There are several methods for estimating total calorie need. For lean diabetics, the calculation is based on ideal body weight. In a typical approach, 25 to 30 kcal/kg of ideal body weight are used for a basic figure which is adjusted within a range of ±20 percent to allow for variations in activity. An alternative method allows 10 kcal/lb. of ideal body weight. To this is added an increment of 30, 50, or 100 percent for sedentary, moderate, or strenuous activity. The true criterion of adequate calories is achievement and maintenance of ideal body weight; therefore, the caloric level may be readjusted at intervals as needed.

For children, a common calculation is based on 1,000 kcal for the first year plus 100 kcal for each additional year up to age 13 or 14. For children, adequate growth and maintenance of normal weight for height are the criteria. The allowance must be increased for adolescents. The calorie allowance for a large, active, growing adolescent boy may be as high as 4,000 kcal. Sufficient energy must be provided for growth and development; hence, the emphasis is on *consistency* of intake rather than on restriction of intake.

For the obese diabetic, the diet should be reduced in calories to achieve weight loss. Frequently, approximately 20 kcal/kg of ideal body weight are prescribed. Increased exercise is helpful, of course. If and when body weight approaches ideal, the energy content in the diet can be increased to maintenance level. Usually, these diets are at least 1,000 kcal in order that other nutrients can be provided in sufficient amounts.

Partition the calories. After total energy need has been determined, the relative amounts of protein, fat, and carbohydrates must be decided. Control can be achieved with various amounts of carbohydrate. For many years, the common practice consisted of providing 40 percent of the energy from carbohydrate, 40 percent from fat, and 20 percent from protein. An 1,800-kcal diet would thus contain 180 g of carbohydrate, 80 g of fat, and 90 g of protein. Carbohydrate was limited to reduce the insulin dosage. When it became evident that diabetics are prone to early severe cardiovascular disease, a diet with less fat and more carbohydrate was recommended.[65] It was found that insulin need is more closely related to energy intake then to carbohydrate intake and that diets high in carbohydrate are tolerated well.[62] The increase in insulin dosage as a result of increased carbohydrate in the diet is not as great as had been expected.

Common calorie distributions now frequently recommended are 50 percent carbohydrate, 30 percent fat, and 20 percent protein. The 1,800-kcal diet would then consist of 225 g of carbohydrate, 60 g of fat, and 90 g of protein. Protein sometimes is only 15 percent or a minimum of 65 g, with an increased proportion of carbohydrate, to reduce food cost for the patient, but common current practice is to provide 80 to 100 g of protein. This level allows for replacement of nitrogen losses in ketosis should it occur. Protein also provides less glucose than does carbohydrate and therefore has less effect on the blood glucose level.

Both of the systems just described are currently in use. Knowledge of the patient's serum cholesterol and triglyceride levels and the degree of glycemic control (HbA_{1c}) should be considered in decisions on distribution of calories. Since the second system, including more carbohydrate and limited fat, is recommended most often, it will be used in the examples that follow.

Distribute the nutrients among meals. Once the calories are partitioned among the nutrients, the nutrients must be distributed among the daily meals. The amount of insulin and the rate and duration of its action affect the manner in which the nutrients must be distributed. The division is made primarily on the basis of the carbohydrate content. For those patients who are controlled by diet alone, by oral hypoglycemic agents, or with fast-acting insulin given before each meal, the carbohydrate usually is divided into three equal parts, one-third for each meal. This distributes the carbohydrate evenly and avoids sharp variations in blood glucose. If, however, the patient's FBS tends to be high, less carbohydrate is given at breakfast. The division may be one-fifth for breakfast and two-fifths for each of the other two meals.

When a longer-acting insulin is given, its peak activity may be at other than a usual meal time. For good control, it is important that carbohydrate be available when insulin activity is high,[66] and so a snack is given at that time. The patient taking NPH insulin, which reaches peak activity in late afternoon, may have an afternoon snack near 3:30 or 4:00 P.M. The carbohydrate in the diet of a patient receiving protamine zinc insulin, for example, may be divided as follows: one-sixth for breakfast, two-sixths at noon and evening meals, and one-sixth at approximately 8:00 P.M. since peak activity is during the night. This latter snack is called the *HS* (hour of sleep, or *hora somni*) feeding in many hospitals. Again, the true test is the degree of control that is achieved. Other divisions are possible, if necessary, to achieve this control. Very brittle diabetics, for example, sometimes are given five or even six meals and snacks per day with multiple insulin injections.

The distribution may also be varied to abide by the wishes of the patient, with insulin dosage adjusted as necessary. A patient who prefers a small breakfast and larger dinner, for example, might be given less regular insulin and more intermediate-acting insulin.

Sometimes protein is divided in a similar manner to carbohydrate. The more liberal and current approach is simply to ensure that some protein in the form of milk, meat, or a meat substitute is included in each meal or snack and otherwise to conform to the patient's wishes. Fat exchanges usually are distributed according to the preferences of the patient.

The Diabetic Meal Plan. The written prescription for a diabetic diet, which might read, "Diabetic diet, C-225, P-90, F-60, divide 1/6, 2/6, 1/6, 2/6,"* is not understandable to the patient. An important function of the nutritional care specialist is to translate this prescription into terms meaningful to the patient. Since diabetes is a chronic disease, it also is important that the diet plan be one that is acceptable for use over a long period.

In order to provide for variety and flexibility in meal planning, the American Diabetes Association, the American Dietetic Association, and the U.S. Public Health Service have sponsored an *exchange system* of diet planning which is usable for any category of diabetes.[67] The nutrient contents of the ADA diabetic exchanges are provided in Table 9-6, and their use is described in detail. It is essential that the nutritional care specialist know the values in these exchange lists (Tables 9-6 through 9-13)** and use them with ease. They provide an example of a method of diet planning that is useful in the nutritional care not only of diabetics, but also of patients with hypoglycemia and for weight reduction. With different exchange lists, this method may also be used to plan diets with controlled sodium, potassium, and other nutrients.

An exchange list for the diabetic diet consists of a group of foods that have a similar, although not necessarily identical, content of protein, fat, and carbohydrate and that have a similar function in meal planning. It allows the substitution of foods of approximately equal composition and provides for a variety of foods along with consistency of nutrient intake.

The specific foods included in the exchange lists emphasize starch rather than simpler carbohydrates. Starch seems to cause a smaller peak in blood glucose than does an equicaloric amount of dietary glucose and has greater satiety value.[68] The lists also emphasize the use of polyunsaturated rather than saturated fats. The foods in the exchange lists that are particularly useful for planning diabetic diets limited in total fat or in saturated fat, particularly as a precaution against cardiovascular disease, are indicated in bold type.

Some patients continue to use an earlier version of the exchange lists from the same source. The major differences between the two series of lists are:

1. One milk exchange in the new series refers to skim milk rather than whole milk.
2. The new series has one group of vegetables in the exchange, whereas the previous version contained two subgroups, the A vegetables and the B vegetables. Both versions list some high-carbohydrate vegetables as substitutes for bread.
3. The newer list has three subgroups of meat exchanges divided according to fat content, in contrast to averaging all meat,

* One-sixth for breakfast, two-sixths for lunch, one-sixth in a midafternoon snack, and two-sixths for dinner.

** The exchange lists are based on material in the *Exchange Lists for Meal Planning* prepared by Committees of the American Diabetes Association, Inc., and the American Dietetic Association in cooperation with the National Institute of Arthritis, Metabolism, and Digestive Diseases and the National Heart and Lung Institute, National Institutes of Health, Public Health Service, U.S. Department of Health, Education and Welfare. Tables 9-6 through 9-11 are reprinted with permission of the American Diabetes Association, Inc.

Table 9-6. Composition of Exchange Foods

ADA Exchange List Number	Exchange Food	Approximate Measure	Weight (g)	Composition per Exchange: Carbohydrate (g)	Protein (g)	Fat (g)
1	Milk	1 c.	240	12	8	Trace
2	Vegetable	½ c.	100	5	2	
3	Fruit	Varies	Varies	10		
4	Bread	1 slice (other items vary)	25	15	2	
5	Meats and meat substitutes	1 oz.	30		7	3–8
6	Fat	1 tsp. (other items vary)	5			5

Table 9-7. List 1: Milk Exchanges, Including Nonfat, Low-Fat, and Whole Milk

This list shows the kinds and amounts of milk products to use for one milk exchange. Those that appear in bold type are nonfat. Low-fat and whole milk contain saturated fat. One exchange of milk contains 12 g of carbohydrate, 8 g of protein, a trace of fat, and 80 calories.

Type	Amount (cups)
Nonfat Fortified Milk	
Skim or nonfat milk	1
Powdered (nonfat dry, before adding liquid)	⅓
Canned, evaporated skim milk	½
Buttermilk made from skim milk	1
Yogurt made from skim milk (plain, unflavored)	1
Low-fat fortified milk	
1% fat fortified milk (omit one-half fat exchange)	1
2% fat fortified milk (omit one fat exchange)	1
Yogurt made from 2% fortified milk (plain, unflavored) (omit one fat exchange)	1
Whole milk (omit two fat exchanges)	
Whole milk	1
Canned, evaporated whole milk	½
Buttermilk made from whole milk	1
Yogurt made from whole milk (plain, unflavored)	1

Table 9-8. List 2: Vegetable Exchanges

This list shows the kinds of vegetables to use for one vegetable exchange. One exchange is ½ cup. One exchange of vegetables contains approximately 5 g of carbohydrate, 2 g of protein, and 25 calories. All vegetables listed are nonfat.

Asparagus
Bean sprouts
Beets
Broccoli
Brussels sprouts
Cabbage
Carrots
Cauliflower
Celery
Cucumbers
Eggplant
Green pepper
Greens
  Beet
  Chard
  Collards
  Dandelion
  Kale
  Mustard
  Spinach
  Turnip
Mushrooms
Okra
Onions
Rhubarb
Rutabaga
Sauerkraut
String beans, green or yellow
Summer squash
Tomato juice
Tomatoes
Turnips
Vegetable juice cocktail
Zucchini

The following **raw vegetables** may be used as desired:

Chicory
Chinese cabbage
Endive
Escarole
Lettuce
Parsley
Radishes
Watercress

Starchy vegetables are found in the Bread Exchange list (Table 9-10).

Table 9-9. List 3: Fruit Exchanges

This list shows the kinds and amounts of fruits to use for one fruit exchange. One exchange of fruit contains 10 g of carbohydrate and 40 calories. All fruits listed are nonfat.

Fruit	Amount	Fruit	Amount
Apple	1 small	**Grape juice**	1/4 c.
Apple juice	1/3 c.	**Grapes**	12
Applesauce (unsweetened)	1/2 c.	**Mango**	1/2 small
Apricots, fresh	2 medium	**Melon**	
Apricots, dried	4 halves	**Cantaloupe**	1/4 small
Banana	1/2 small	**Honeydew**	1/8 medium
Berries		**Watermelon**	1 c.
Blackberries	1/2 c.	**Nectarine**	1 small
Blueberries	1/2 c.	**Orange**	1 small
Cranberries	Use as desired if no sugar is added	**Orange juice**	1/2 c.
		Papaya	1/4 c.
		Peach	1 medium
Raspberries	1/2 c.	**Pear**	1 small
Strawberries	3/4 c.	**Persimmon, native**	1 medium
Cherries	10 large	**Pineapple**	1/2 c.
Cider	1/3 c.	**Pineapple juice**	1/3 c.
Dates	2	**Plums**	2 medium
Figs, fresh	1	**Prune juice**	1/4 c.
Figs, dried	1	**Prunes**	2 medium
Grapefruit	1/2	**Raisins**	2 tablespoons
Grapefruit juice	1/2 c.	**Tangerine**	1 medium

Table 9-10. List 4: Bread Exchanges, Including Bread, Cereal, and Starchy Vegetables

This list shows the kinds and amounts of bread, cereals, starchy vegetables, and prepared foods to use for one bread exchange. Those that appear in bold type are low-fat. One exchange of bread contains 15 g of carbohydrate, 2 g of protein, and 70 calories.

Food	Amount	Food	Amount
Bread		**Grits (cooked)**	1/2 c.
White (including French and Italian)	1 slice	**Rice or barley (cooked)**	1/2 c.
		Pasta (cooked): spaghetti, noodles, macaroni	1/2 c.
Whole wheat	1 slice		
Rye or pumpernickel	1 slice	**Popcorn (popped, no fat added, large kernel)**	3 c.
Raisin	1 slice		
Bagel, small	1/2	**Cornmeal (dry)**	2 tbsp.
English muffin, small	1/2	**Flour**	2 1/2 tbsp.
Plain roll, bread	1	**Wheat germ**	1/4 c.
Frankfurter roll	1/2	Crackers	
Hamburger bun	1/2	**Arrowroot**	3
Dried bread crumbs	3 tbsp.	**Graham, 2 1/2-in. square**	2
Tortilla, 6-in.	1	**Matzo, 4 in. × 6 in.**	1/2
Cereal		**Oyster**	20
Bran flakes	1/2 c.	**Pretzels, 3 1/8 in. long × 1/8-in. diameter**	25
Other ready-to-eat unsweetened cereal	3/4 c.		
		Rye wafers, 2 in. × 3 1/2 in.	3
Puffed cereal (unfrosted)	1 c.	**Saltines**	6
Cereal (cooked)	1/2 c.	**Soda, 2 1/2-in. square**	4

Table 9-10. List 4: Bread Exchanges, Including Bread, Cereal, and Starchy Vegetables (continued)

Food	Amount	Food	Amount
Dried beans, peas, and lentils		Corn bread, 2 in. × 2 in. × 1 in. (omit one fat exchange)	1
Beans, peas, lentils (dried and cooked)	½ c.	Corn muffin, 2-in. diameter (omit one fat exchange)	1
Baked beans, no pork (canned)	¼ c.	Crackers, round butter type (omit one fat exchange)	5
Starchy vegetables		Muffin, plain small (omit one fat exchange)	1
Corn	⅓ c.	Potatoes, French fried, length 2 in. to 3½ in. (omit one fat exchange)	8
Corn on cob	1 small	Potato or corn chips (omit two fat exchanges)	15
Lima beans	½ c.	Pancake, 5 in. × ½ in. (omit one fat exchange)	1
Parsnips	⅔ c.	Waffle, 5 in. × ½ in. (omit one fat exchange)	1
Peas, green (canned or frozen)	½ c.		
Potato, white	1 small		
Potato (mashed)	½ c.		
Pumpkin	¾ c.		
Winter squash, acorn or butternut	½ c.		
Yam or sweet potato	¼ c.		
Prepared foods			
Biscuit, 2-in. diameter (omit one fat exchange)	1		

Table 9-11. List 5: Meat Exchanges, Including Lean, Medium-Fat, and High-Fat Meats

Meat	Type or Cut	Amount
Lean Meat[a]		
Beef	**Baby beef (very lean), chipped beef, chuck, flank steak, tenderloin, plate ribs, plate skirt steak, round (bottom, top), all cuts rump, spare ribs, tripe**	1 oz.
Lamb	**Leg, rib, sirloin, loin (roast and chops), shank, shoulder**	1 oz.
Pork	**Leg (whole rump, center shank), ham, smoked (center slices)**	1 oz.
Veal	**Leg, loin, rib, shank, shoulder, cutlets**	1 oz.
Poultry	**Meat** without skin **of chicken, turkey, cornish hen, guinea hen, pheasant**	1 oz.
Fish	**Any fresh or frozen**	1 oz.
	Canned salmon, tuna, mackerel, crab, and lobster	¼ c.
	Clams, oysters, scallops, shrimp	5, or 1 oz.
	Sardines (drained)	3
Cheeses containing less than 5% butterfat		1 oz.
Cottage cheese, dry and 2% butterfat		¼ c.
Dried beans and peas (omit one bread exchange)		½ c.
Medium-fat meat[b]		
Beef	Ground (15% fat), corned beef (canned), rib eye, round (ground commercial)	1 oz.
Pork	Loin (all cuts tenderloin), shoulder arm [picnic], shoulder blade, Boston butt, Canadian bacon, boiled ham	1 oz.

[a] This list shows the kinds and amounts of lean meat and other protein-rich foods to use for one low-fat meat exchange. One exchange of lean meat (1 oz.) contains 7 g of protein, 3 g of fat, and 55 calories. To plan a diet low in saturated fat, select only those exchanges that appear in bold type. *Trim off all visible fat.*

[b] This list shows the kinds and amounts of medium-fat meat and other protein-rich foods to use for one medium-fat meat exchange. One exchange of medium-fat meat (1 oz.) contains 7 g of protein, 5 g of fat, and 75 calories (or one lean meat exchange + one-half fat exchange. *Trim off all visible fat.*

(continued)

Table 9-11. List 5: Meat Exchanges, Including Lean, Medium-Fat, and High-Fat Meats (continued)

Meat	Type or Cut	Amount
Liver, heart, kidney, and sweetbreads (these are high in cholesterol)		1 oz.
Cottage cheese, creamed		1/4 c.
Cheese	Mozzarella, ricotta, farmer's cheese, Neufchâtel, Parmesan	1 oz. 3 tbsp.
Egg (high in cholesterol)		1
Peanut butter (omit two additional fat exchanges)		2 tbsp.
High-fat meat[c]		
Beef	Brisket, corned beef (brisket), ground beef (more than 20% fat), hamburger (commercial), chuck (ground, commercial), roasts (rib), steaks (club and rib)	1 oz.
Lamb	Breast	1 oz.
Pork	Spare ribs, loin (back ribs), pork (ground), country style ham, deviled ham	1 oz.
Veal	Breast	1 oz.
Poultry	Capon, duck (domestic), goose	1 oz.
Cheese	Cheddar types	1 oz.
Cold cuts		4 1/2-in. × 1/8-in. slice
Frankfurter		1 small

[c] This list shows the kinds and amounts of high-fat meat and other protein to use for one high-fat meat exchange. One exchange of high-fat meat (1 oz.) contains 7 g of protein, 8 g of fat, and 100 calories (or one lean meat exchange + one fat exchange). *Trim off all visible fat.*

Table 9-12. List 6: Fat Exchanges

This list shows the kinds and amounts of fat containing foods to use for one fat exchange. To plan a diet low in saturated fat, select only those exchanges that appear in bold type. They are polyunsaturated. One exchange of fat contains 5 g of fat and 45 calories.

Food	Amount	Food	Amount
Margarine, soft, tub or stick[a]	1 tsp.	Butter	1 tsp.
Avocado (4-in. diameter)[b]	1/8	Bacon fat	1 tsp.
Oil: corn, cottonseed, safflower, soy, sunflower	1 tsp.	Bacon crisp	1 strip
		Cream	
Oil, olive[b]	1 tsp.	Light	2 tbsp.
Oil, peanut[b]	1 tsp.	Sour	2 tbsp.
Olives[b]	5 small	Heavy	1 tbsp.
Almonds[b]	10 whole	Cream cheese	1 tbsp.
Pecans[b]	2 large whole	French dressing[c]	1 tbsp.
Peanuts[b]		Italian dressing[c]	1 tbsp.
Spanish	20 whole	Lard	1 tsp.
Virginia	10 whole	Mayonnaise[c]	1 tsp.
Walnuts	6 small	Salad dressing, mayonnaise type[c]	2 tsp.
Nuts, other[b]	6 small	Salt pork	3/4-in. cube
Margarine, regular stick	1 tsp.		

[a] Made with corn, cottonseed, safflower, soy, or sunflower oil only.

[b] Fat content is primarily monounsaturated.

[c] Can be used on fat-modified diet if made with corn, cottonseed, safflower, soy, or sunflower oil.

Table 9-13. Free Foods: Use as Desired

These foods have no appreciable protein, fat, or carbohydrate content if used in usual quantities.

Coffee	**Chili powder**	**Mustard**	**Saccharin and other noncaloric sweeteners**
Tea	**Cinnamon**	**Nutmeg**	**Vinegar**
Bouillon, without fat	**Garlic**	**Onion seasoning**	**Pickles (sour or unsweetened dill)**
Gelatin, unsweetened	**Horseradish**	**Parsley seasoning**	
Rennet tablets	**Lemon, lime**	**Pepper, red or black**	
Celery salt	**Mint**		

Table 9-14. Sample Calculation of a Diabetic Meal Plan Using Exchange Lists

Diet Prescription: Calories, 1,800; P-90; F-60; C-225
Divide 1/6, 2/6, 1/6, 2/6 with 4 P.M. feeding.

ADA Exchange List Number	Exchange Group	Number of Exchanges	Carbohydrate (g)	Protein (g)	Fat (g)
1	Milk	2	24	16	
2	Vegetable	2	10	4	
3	Fruit	4	40		
Subtotal			(74)		
4	Bread				
	(225 − 74) ÷ 15≅	10	150	20	
Subtotal				(40)	
5	Meat				
	(90 − 40) ÷ 7≅	7		49	21
6	Fat				
	(60 − 21) ÷ 5≅	8			40
Total			224	89	61

fish, poultry, egg, and cheeses into one category.

Some institutions make other changes in the lists, although most are very similar. It is important, when instructing patients, to know which exchange lists they have been using.

For each diabetic diet, a meal plan is calculated in terms of exchange lists. A sample calculation is shown in Table 9-14. The steps in this calculation are as follows, using the values from Table 9-6 for examples:

1. Estimate the number of milk, fruit, and vegetable exchanges that will fit into the meal plan. To some extent, this is a trial-and-error process, but the following are useful guides, *subject to patient preferences:*

   Milk: A minimum of two exchanges for adults to a maximum of one exchange for each feeding. Quantities for children and adolescents are adjusted for age.
   Fruits: A minimum of three exchanges, one for each regular meal, to a maximum of one for each feeding.
   Vegetables: Two exchanges, one for inclusion at noon and one at the evening meal.

2. Total the carbohydrate provided in the milk, fruit, and vegetable exchanges (74) and subtract this total from the amount prescribed (225); (225 − 74 = 151).
3. Divide the result by the amount of carbohydrate in one bread exchange to find the number of bread exchanges needed (151 ÷ 15 = 10).
4. Total the protein in the milk, vegetable, and bread exchanges (40) and subtract this total from the amount prescribed (90); (90 − 40 = 50).
5. Divide the result by the amount of protein in one meat exchange (7) to find the number of meat exchanges needed (50 ÷ 7 = 7).
6. Subtract the fat in the meat (21) from the amount prescribed (60); (60 − 21 = 39).
7. Divide the result by the amount of fat in one fat exchange (5) to find the number of fat exchanges needed (39 ÷ 5 = 8).

When the number of exchanges from each list necessary to meet the diet prescription is determined, the exchanges are distributed among the meals. An example of that process is shown in Table 9-14. The patient is given this meal plan along with the exchange lists for planning variety into his or her meals and is instructed in their use. The

Table 9-15. Diabetic Meal Plan Incorporating Exchanges

Meal Distribution: 225 ÷ 6 = 37. Therefore: 37, 75, 37, 75.

	Breakfast		Lunch		Snack		Dinner	
Exchange	No. of Servings	Carbohydrates (g)	No. of Servings	Carbohydrates (g)	No. of Servings	Carbohydrates (g)	No. of Servings	Carbohydrates (g)
Milk	1	12			1	12		
Fruit	1	10	1	10	1	10	1	10
Vegetable			1	5			1	5
Bread	1	15	4	60	1	15	4	60
Meat	1		3				3	
Fat	2		3				3	
Total		37		75		37		75

use of a meal plan with the exchange lists eliminates the need for daily calculation of the diet. It also provides the consistency of intake required by the type 1 diabetic and the limitation of calories for the type 2 diabetic.

Planning Daily Menus. The use of the exchange system makes it possible to provide variety in meals. Some foods are essentially free of protein, fat, or carbohydrate and patients may add these to the planned diet at will. These "free" foods are listed in Table 9-13. Using the meal plan calculated in Table 9-15, two days' menus are given in Table 9-16 as examples. Patients should not be encouraged to make exchanges *between* lists but only *within* lists; for example, two vegetables should not be substituted for one fruit exchange or three vegetables for one bread exchange.

For some patients, six exchange lists are too complex to manipulate satisfactorily, and so simplified systems have been devised. One example has three exchanges:

2 oz. of meat with 14 g of protein, 10 g of fat
Fruits and vegetables with 2 g of protein, 5 g of carbohydrate
"Starches" with 2 g of protein and 15 g of carbohydrate

Milk is included in the meat exchange list, and fat is stated as a total per day to be distributed as desired.

Weighed, measured, and unmeasured diets. At one time, it was thought necessary to weigh all foods for diabetic patients very carefully on a gram scale, but weighing is no longer believed to be necessary. Instead, a *measured diet* is recommended in which common household equipment, measuring spoons and measuring cups, are used. Since many cuts of meat do not lend themselves to this type of measure, meat portions sometimes still are weighed. Alternatively, the patient may be taught to estimate closely the portion size of meats, using food models. Few practitioners recommend the *unmeasured diet.* For the great majority of diabetics, the measured diet is the method of choice.

Some patients refuse to follow any diet; others are not sufficiently motivated to lose weight. The nutritional care specialist must be prepared to encounter these patients and to be nonjudgmental. If food intake is relatively consistent on a day-to-day basis and if hypoglycemic agents can be adjusted accordingly, a reasonable degree of control may be possible. Essentially, the patient is choosing to risk the effects of poorer control in order to suffer less disruption of his or her current life-style.

Foods not recommended. Although some foods are poor choices for a diabetic diet, very few are absolutely forbidden to the diabetic patient. In general, *concentrated sources of simple carbohydrates,* such as candies, cakes with icings, and other sweetened

Table 9-16. Sample Diabetic Menus

Menu 1		Menu 2	
Breakfast	Exchange Value	Exchange Value	*Breakfast*
¼ cantaloupe	1 fruit	1 fruit	½ c. orange juice
1 egg, poached	1 lean meat + ½ fat	1 lean meat + ½ fat	1 soft-cooked egg
1 slice wheat toast	1 bread	1 bread	1 slice raisin toast
1½ tsp. margarine	1½ fat	1½ fat	1½ tsp. margarine
1 c. skim milk	1 milk	1 milk	1 c. skim milk
Coffee or tea, black	Free	Free	Coffee or tea, black
Lunch			*Lunch*
		1 vegetable	½ c. vegetable juice cocktail
		2 bread	6 rye wafers
Spaghetti with meat sauce			Sandwich
1 c. cooked spaghetti	2 bread	2 bread	1 hamburger bun
3 oz. lean ground beef	3 meat + 1½ fat	3 meat	3 oz. sliced chicken
½ c. tomatoes	1 vegetable	3 fat	3 tsp. mayonnaise
Herbs and garlic	Free	Free	Lettuce
2 slices Italian bread	2 bread		
1½ tsp. margarine	1½ fat		
Sour pickles	Free	Free	Cranberry garnish, sweetened with saccharine
½ c. diced pineapple	1 fruit	1 fruit	1 medium peach
Iced tea with lemon	Free	Free	Coffee or tea, black
Snack			*Snack*
1 c. plain skim milk yogurt	1 milk	1 milk	1 c. skim milk
2 graham crackers	1 bread	1 bread	3 arrowroot crackers
1 small orange	1 fruit	1 fruit	2 medium plums
Dinner			*Dinner*
Broth	Free		
6 saltines	1 bread		
3 oz. baked red snapper	3 meat	3 meat	3 oz. sliced leg of lamb
½ c. mashed potatoes	1 bread	2 bread	2 small potatoes
		1 bread	½ c. green peas
½ c. green beans	1 vegetable	1 vegetable	Sliced tomato salad
		1 fat	1 tbsp. French dressing
1 plain roll	1 bread	1 bread	1 plain roll
3 tsp. margarine	3 fat	2 fat	2 tsp. margarine
¾ c. strawberries	1 fruit	1 fruit	4 apricot halves
on one 2-in. biscuit	1 bread		
Coffee or tea, black	Free	Free	Coffee or tea, black

baked goods, are strongly discouraged since they tend to cause rapid changes in blood glucose concentrations. Some sugars also may raise serum triglycerides. Under special circumstances—the birthday of a diabetic child, for example—a small serving of birthday cake or other treat is allowed in the meal pattern if the patient or parent is knowledgeable of substitution procedures.

Mixtures of indefinite composition also are discouraged because of difficulty in fitting these items into the meal plan. As a result, the diabetic patient is not able to use many commercially prepared convenience foods such as stews, casseroles, and breaded and fried products. However, equivalent dishes can be made in the home where their composition can be controlled. A beef stew, for example, can be made from diced beef (meat and fat exchanges) and onions and carrots (vegetable exchange) or other vegetables. Thickening can be provided with flour (bread exchange), and herbs and spices are free. Other recipes are contained in recipe books for diabetics. The exchange equivalents usually are given with the recipes.

Some manufacturers of canned soups and other convenience foods have made lists of the exchange values of the products. The nutritional care specialist should keep a library of such lists on hand for the patient who wishes to have a favorite food allowed occasionally in his or her diet. To make such allowances generally improves compliance with the diet. Since food values change with changes in manufacturing processes, it is necessary to keep the information current.

Special foods for diabetic diets. Some special foods are available for use in diabetic diets. Most foods labeled as "diabetic" or "dietetic" are unnecessary for the diabetic patient, and many are very expensive. In addition, the patient often believes that they are free foods which can be added to the meal plan at will. In fact, they often contain appreciable, but unspecified, amounts of carbohydrate. Their use should be discouraged with the exception of *unsweetened canned fruits.* These have an important place in the diet of the diabetic patient, particularly in those parts of the country and during those seasons when fresh fruits are limited in variety.

The use of *diabetic candy* should normally be discouraged for several reasons. Diabetic candies usually are not calorie-free. Also, with their use, diabetics may develop a taste for sweets and then may substitute the candies for foods of greater nutritive value. It is the opinion of some diabetologists, however, that their limited use for children on very special occasions can be justified.

Alternative sweeteners. Sweeteners that may serve as an acceptable alternative to sucrose are important to some diabetic patients. There are a number of these categorized according to their kilocalorie content. One group is kilocalorie-free or nearly so, and the other contains an appreciable kilocalorie content.

Of the kilocalorie-free sweeteners, *saccharin* has been used for the longest period. It is 300 to 350 times as sweet as sucrose but leaves a bitter aftertaste and therefore is unacceptable to some patients. The use of saccharin is controversial, since it was reported to be *carcinogenic* (cancer-causing), but it has not been withdrawn from use because of public protests at attempts to do so.

Some patients are very attached to sweetened coffee, tea, and soft drinks and may find saccharin an acceptable substitute for sugar, but it cannot be used as a sugar substitute in baking. Also, it may be added to foods, such as rhubarb or cranberries, only after cooking, or it will develop a bitter taste.

Cyclamates are more acceptable in flavor and are thirty times sweeter than sucrose. They were banned by the U.S. Food and Drug Administration because they were reported to be carcinogenic in animals[68] but are approved for use in Canada and some European countries.

Aspartame, 200 times as sweet as sucrose, is made from a combination of phenylalanine and aspartic acid. It has recently been approved for use in the United States.[69] Aspartame provides a small number of kilocalories and may soon appear in breakfast cereals, chewing gum, powdered beverages, whipped toppings, puddings, gelatin, and as a tabletop sweetener. The first products are beginning to appear on the market. It is unstable in soft drinks and is not yet used for that purpose. There is some controversy concerning the risk of brain tumors and of possible danger to the fetus if used during pregnancy.[69]

Other products of potential use are being developed, but it is unlikely that any will be approved for sale soon.

Some *carbohydrate* and *polyol sweeteners* with appreciable kilocalorie contents have been approved as substitutes for sucrose and glucose. All must be calculated into the diet if they are to be used. Usually, it is advisable to discourage their use.

Fructose sometimes is suggested as a sweetener, since it is 70 percent sweeter than

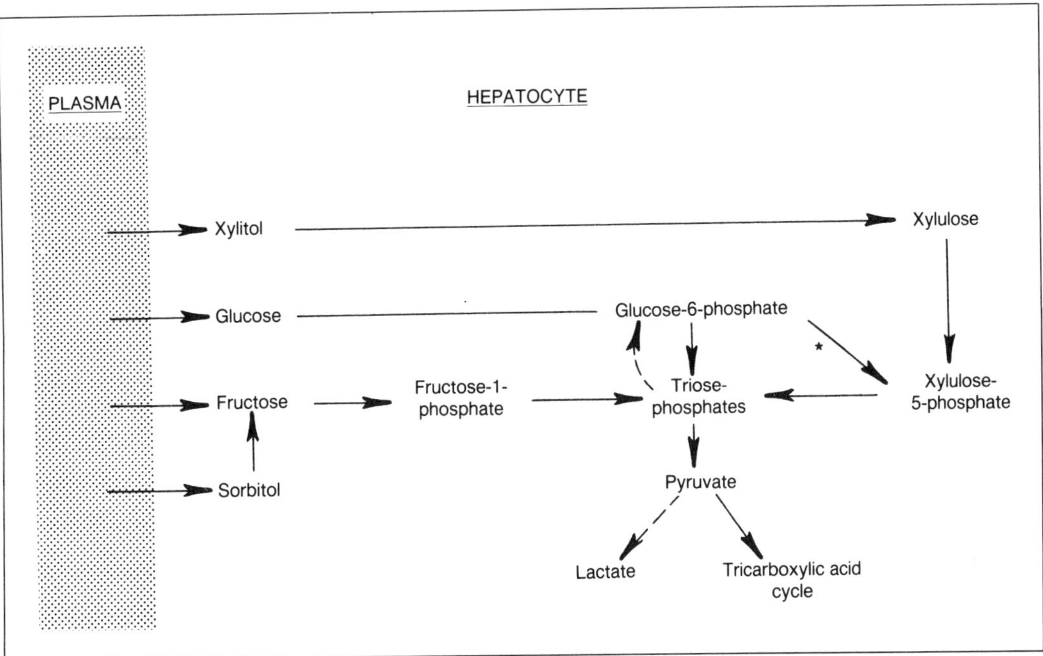

Figure 9-8. Normal metabolic pathways for cellular utilization of glucose, fructose, sorbitol, and xylitol (solid lines). With a significant increase in the triose pool, such as after the intravenous administration of fructose or xylitol, lactate production increases; with insulin deficiency, as in untreated diabetes, trioses are converted into glucose-6-phosphate and can lead to further hyperglycemia (dashed lines). (The asterisk indicates the hexose monophosphate shunt.) (From Brunzell, J.D., Use of fructose, xylitol or sorbitol as a sweetener in diabetes. Diabetes Care *1:223, 1978. Reproduced with permission from the American Diabetes Association, Inc.)*

sugar and can thus be used in small quantities.[70] When fructose is absorbed, it is metabolized by the liver. Insulin is not required for its entry into hepatic cells nor for the steps in its metabolism to trioses. The trioses can then enter the glycolytic pathway or be used to synthesize glucose and triglycerides, regulated primarily by insulin (Fig. 9-8). In nondiabetic individuals and in well-controlled diabetics receiving sufficient insulin, most of the glucose formed from fructose is stored as glycogen and has little effect on blood glucose concentration. If, however, the patient is severely deficient in insulin, the glucose is released and plasma glucose rises. In patients who are mildly insulin-deficient or who have insulin-independent (type 2) diabetes, the rise is less than that resulting from intake of an equivalent amount of sucrose, glucose, and sometimes starch.[71,72] These results are seen over the short term. Long-term effects are unknown. The wisdom of the use of fructose by diabetics is questionable at the present time, but the matter probably deserves further investigation.

High-fructose corn sweetener is a related product composed of "corn sugar" (primarily glucose) and fructose. One formulation contains 90 percent fructose. The remainder is predominantly glucose. Since it is perceived as being sweeter than sucrose, it may be used in smaller quantities. Its appreciable kilocalorie content, however, makes it unsuitable for use in diabetic diets.

Some *sugar alcohol* or *polyol sweeteners* have been approved for use in foods, but their kilocalorie content makes them of questionable value for diabetics. Their metabolic pathways are shown in Fig. 9-8.

Sorbitol is an alcohol produced by reduction of glucose or fructose and is widely used as a sweetening agent. It provides 4 kcal/g but is only 50 to 70 percent as sweet as sucrose. It is poorly absorbed from the gastrointestinal tract and thus may cause an osmotic diarrhea if amounts in excess of 30 to 50 g/day are used. It is metabolized to fructose (see Fig. 9-8) and is not involved in complications of diabetes related to sorbitol accumulation.[73] Diabetic children tolerate sorbitol well with no glycosuria or change in the blood glucose concentration.[74]

Xylitol is oxidized to trioses in the liver (see Fig. 9-8). Like sorbitol, it can cause diarrhea. In addition, it is very expensive. It has the same caloric value and is a little sweeter than sugar, but rarely causes a rise in blood glucose greater than 5 mg/dl.

There are no major differences in the effects of fructose, sorbitol, and xylitol. Fructose and xylitol are sweeter; both sorbitol and xylitol can cause diarrhea. All three are equal to glucose and sucrose in caloric density; therefore, their use by the obese diabetic is questionable. The use of fructose by treated diabetics of normal weight is being investigated.

Alcoholic beverages. The consumption of alcoholic beverages must be considered for some patients. Diabetic patients taking oral hypoglycemic agents have reduced alcohol tolerance and experience palpitation and flushing after alcohol. The real danger of alcohol ingestion by diabetics is that hypoglycemia may be precipitated in insulin-dependent patients if they are fasting. The hypoglycemia may be unrecognized and untreated, since symptoms are similar to those of intoxication. Furthermore, alcohol provides 7 kcal/g of alcohol but does not provide essential nutrients. The use of alcoholic beverages should therefore be discouraged. If it becomes clear, however, that the patient intends to drink occasionally, it is best to instruct him or her in the procedure for substituting alcoholic beverages in the meal plan. Most hospital diet manuals contain a list of the common alcoholic beverages and mixed drinks along with their exchange values. Most can be substituted for an appropriate number of fat exchanges. Some also contain carbohydrate and require substitution for a bread exchange. Some common substitutions are as follows:[75]

Alcoholic Beverage	*Exchanges*
12 oz. beer	1 bread, 2 fat
1½ oz. 80-proof liquor	3 fat
3½ oz. dry wine, 12 percent	1½ fat

Vitamin and Mineral Supplements. Some patients inquire about their need for vitamin and mineral supplements. With few exceptions, they are not needed by the patient with uncomplicated diabetes who adheres to the prescribed diet. Occasionally, a financially very poor patient is given a diet with minimum protein levels to reduce cost; such a patient may profit from iron and calcium supplements. Very obese patients on severely calorie-restricted diets also may require supplements. If the patient has diarrhea secondary to neuropathy or pancreatitis, supplements may be necessary. Supplements of thiamine and vitamin B_{12} have been tried in the treatment of neuropathy and were found to be ineffective.

Other Considerations in Nutritional Care. In addition to the items already described, there are a number of other considerations in the nutritional care of the diabetic patient, since the diabetic diet must become a permanent part of the patient's life. Compliance will be improved if the diet is compatible with the patient's previous habits and preferences. Under these circumstances, the diet must be tailor-made for each patient. Some of the factors that must be considered are:

1. *Financial resources:* Many diabetic patients are elderly and living on small fixed incomes. Some are on public aid. The existence of diabetes causes additional expense.
2. *Local markets and availability of food:* It is especially necessary to ascertain that unsweetened canned fruit is available.

3. *Social life of the patient:* Instruction should be given, if necessary, on the limited use of alcohol and the substitution of snack foods into the meal plan.
4. *Work situation and type of activities:* The patient's working hours and level of activity from day to day, or even within a day, must be considered. Also important is how meals generally are provided (e.g., whether lunch is carried to work or purchased there).
5. *Family group and the home:* If someone other than the patient prepares meals, that person should be instructed along with the patient. The facilities available for food preparation must also be considered.
6. *Meal habits of the family:* The diet should be compatible with the number, time, and size of family meals. Necessary changes in insulin dosage or time of injection must be discussed with the physician.
7. *Ethnic food habits, food preferences, and dislikes:* If a patient usually eats certain foods that are not included on the exchange lists, these foods should be added. Various lists of Japanese, Chinese, Mexican, and Jewish foods are available for this purpose from state and local dietetic associations. If a patient adamantly refuses to eat the foods in one of the exchange lists, the diet must be planned without it. Some examples which may be encountered are the lactose-intolerant patient, the vegetarian patient, and the patient who refuses to eat vegetables.
8. *Possible mechanical difficulties:* This consideration most often involves the condition of the patient's teeth. Occasionally, the diabetic diet must be combined with nutritional care for patients with pathologic conditions of the head and neck (see Chapter 5) if the patient has infection, trauma, or surgery in this area.
9. *Pathologic conditions in addition to diabetes:* Many patients have other conditions that require diet modifications. These must be combined with the diabetic diet and the exchange lists must be altered accordingly. Also important is whether the patient has a handicap that intereferes with shopping for food or meal preparation.
10. *Intelligence, education, eyesight, and language difficulties and the psychological response of the patient* are important factors in instructing the patient.

Adjustments for Exercise. Adjustments must also be made in the diabetic diet for exercise. Exercise is considered an important part of the treatment of diabetes. It has the same positive effects as in the nondiabetic population. In diabetics, it is particularly important for its effects in prevention of obesity, prevention of intravascular blood clotting, and normalization of blood lipids.

Insulin is required for glucose uptake by resting muscle, but much smaller amounts are required by the working muscle.[76] Therefore, regular moderate exercise, such as a walk following meals, often is recommended to reduce the amplitude of the rise in blood glucose.

If the sedentary patient indulges in sudden, intense physical activity, an increase in carbohydrate intake often is necessary to prevent hypoglycemia. Usually 10 to 15 g of carbohydrate per hour of moderate exercise or 20 to 30 g per hour of vigorous exercise is an adequate supplement.[61] Urine or blood testing following sporadic bouts of exercise is desirable. If exercise is increased on a regular basis, the patient may require less insulin. Glucose tolerance improves with increased insulin sensitivity.[77,78] Although some insulin is required for membrane transport, glucose metabolism for energy production requires much less insulin than does the storage of glucose as glycogen or triglyceride.

If regular exercise is decreased, the insulin-dependent diabetic needs to decrease the energy intake; otherwise, hyperglycemia and weight gain will ensue. Insulin dosage should *not* be increased as an alternative to calorie reduction to control the hyperglycemia.

In contrast to the well-regulated diabetic, in the patient with hyperglycemia and ketonemia, exercise makes the diabetes worse, since exercise increases the secretion of the insulin antagonists glucagon and growth hormone.[79,80] It therefore is important that an exercise program and nutritional care go hand in hand.

Adjustments for Missed Meals or Reduced Appetite. Other problems which arise occasionally are missed meals or episodes of reduced appetite. The patient at home may suffer minor illnesses that reduce appetite and may experience delays in meals for reasons such as social occasions. Carbohydrates should be carried by the patient for use on these occasions; hard candies are useful.

In the hospital, if a patient receiving insulin misses or refuses to eat part of a meal, a common practice is to attempt to replace the food with one of equivalent value within a 3-hour period. If this cannot be accomplished, replacement of as much of the carbohydrate as possible should be attempted; the protein and fat usually are not replaced. Fruit juices, regular soft drinks, candy, sweetened gelatin, or sweetened tea are used for the purpose of replacing the carbohydrate. If this, too, is impossible, the physician is notified and the patient is carefully observed for signs of hypoglycemia. In an emergency, glucose can be given intravenously. If food intake is reduced for longer periods, the prescribed calories and insulin may be reduced temporarily. Replacement is *not* necessary for patients who are controlled by diet alone.

In some illnesses, especially infections, the patient becomes more insulin-resistant. Even though food intake is decreased, blood glucose may rise. Thus, it is important that the insulin dosage be continued. Patients should be carefully instructed that they should not eliminate their insulin if they are not well enough to eat, since they may actually need more insulin when ill. The diabetic diet can be planned as a liquid diet if necessary. This may be a useful procedure in case of sore throats, tooth extractions, or similar events.

In the patient with chronic complications or other accompanying pathologic conditions, other diet modifications may be combined with the diabetic diet. In the patient with advanced nephropathy, for example, diets appropriate for chronic renal failure may be planned in combination with the diabetic diet. Since the diabetic diet is very flexible, there are few diets with which it cannot be combined.

Self-Management

Insulin-dependent diabetic patients who are alert and intelligent may be taught self-management and may alter their regimen to control their blood glucose levels when necessary. Nutritional care specialists must be familiar with the procedures involved so that they can participate in the education of the patient.

To manage their own care, patients must have an indication of their blood glucose status. Although direct measurement of blood glucose seems the logical approach, urine testing for glucose has been the method of choice for many years. It has several advantages. Obtaining the urine is easy, painless, and noninvasive, and testing methods are simple and inexpensive.

The test materials consist of the necessary chemicals in a tablet or impregnated on a stick or tape. There are several forms available: Diastix, Clinistix, Clinitest (a tablet), and Tes-Tape. All measure glucose in the urine, although Clinitest also gives a positive reaction to galactose, lactose, fructose, or maltose in the urine. A large amount of ascorbic acid in the urine may interfere with any of the tests.

The tests involve the development of a color which then is compared with a series of colored standards. Diabetics are taught to test their urine one or more times per day. For some, four times per day—before each meal and at bedtime—is recommended.

There are limitations to urine testing. It gives no indication of levels of blood glucose less than that of the patient's renal threshold. Thus, if the renal threshold is 180 mg/dl, the test will be negative at any value below that level, even though the blood glucose still may be above normal. Urine testing, of course, also gives no warning of impending hypoglycemia.

When these tests show an abnormal result, or when feeling ill, the patient may also test for ketone bodies. Keto-Diastix will measure both glucose and ketones. Ketostix and Acetest may also be used.

Blood glucose testing has been difficult for patients because of difficulties in obtaining blood and because of complex testing methods, but some new developments may have provided partial solutions to these problems.[81] Single-use lancets are available in order to prick fingers to obtain blood. The blood can be put on Dextrostix or a reagent strip, either of which must be read in a meter, but the cost of the meter is beyond the means of many diabetics. New development may eventually lower the cost of these systems. An alternative product, Chemstrip bG, can be interpreted by comparison with color samples on the side of the bottle. Better patient compliance has been reported for patients who monitor their blood glucose.[82,83]

Very recently, a method for patient monitoring of HbA_{1c} has been developed.[84] The method is relatively complex but was reported to be effective in reinforcing patient education.

At the same time as the urine or blood is tested, patients keep a record so that adjustments can be made to respond to any pattern of hypoglycemia or hyperglycemia that develops. These records are of use in self-management and also by members of the health care team. A spill of glucose in the urine at a given time each day, for example, might indicate to the nutritional care specialist the need to redistribute the meal plan to make the immediately preceding meal smaller. Alternatively, the physician might wish to increase or redivide the insulin prescription.

Emotional Problems in the Diabetic Patient

The emotional state of the patient may have a profound effect on his or her ability to be educated in self-care and on the control of the diabetes. Sometimes, the first duty of the nutritional care specialist is to calm fear in the patient or parents. This must be done before any meaningful instruction can occur. Some examples of problems that may be encountered are:

- The emotionally upset patient who is hyperglycemic from stresses such as family or job problems
- The child who tries to control parents by refusing to eat
- The adolescent who refuses to adhere to any treatment plan in order to assert independence

The counseling skills of the nutritional care specialist are important in these and similar situations.

Education of the Patient

The health care team cannot control diabetes without the cooperation of the patient, and, to be able to participate fully in his or her own care, the patient must be well informed and well motivated. Unfortunately, patient education has been, and often still is, seriously neglected. It should begin as soon as the disease is diagnosed and should continue throughout the life of the patient. In addition, those people closely associated with the diabetic must be taught, including the parents of child patients, the families of all patients, teachers, and associates at work and at recreation.

The list of items that must be taught to the diabetic patient and members of the family is long. Those items needed by all patients are:

The basic concepts of the disease and methods for controlling it
Principles of dietary management, including procedures for following the meal plan, the use of exchange lists, diet during minor illnesses, adjustments for changes in exercise
Urine testing—why it is important, how to do it, how to interpret results, and record keeping
Knowledge of acute complications—how to prevent them and how to recognize them
Knowledge of chronic complications—how to recognize them and what therapy to institute
Personal hygiene
Exercise
Social problems, including employment, licenses, and insurance

In addition, some patients will need to know about the following, depending on the nature of their particular disease, the therapy used, and their other needs:

How to use insulin, including the kind of insulin, dose, syringe care, prevention of infection, adjustment of the dose in special situations, and its relation to urine testing
The type, dose, and possible complications of oral hypoglycemic agents
Family planning; genetic counseling
Camp and school
Community resources and other sources of information
Effects of other medications on diabetic control

It should be obvious that effective patient education requires the effort of the entire health care team. It also requires individualization. There is no packaged program that can be applied to all patients, but there are many helpful teaching aids. Among them are pamphlets (used almost invariably), programmed teaching machines, demonstrations, food models, slides, and movies. Although individual instruction is important, diabetic patients can productively be taught in classes in ambulatory care centers and in hospitals. Bed patients, as well as ambulatory patients, may be gathered for class, complete with wheelchairs and stretchers if necessary. The patients often profit from association with other diabetics. Nutritional care specialists should be familiar with the teaching materials available for both individual and class use and should be expert in applying them and aware of their limitations.

Other information is available to diabetic patients. Many patients subscribe to a magazine published six times yearly.[85] In some communities, there are local diabetes associations with groups for professionals and groups for patients. There are also books available for patients, giving information on the disease in general. A recent recipe book includes the most recent revision of the exchange values.[75]

The Diabetic Child

Approximately 4 percent of diabetics are children, or more than 100,000 in the United States alone. Important precipitating factors are infection, trauma, and possibly puberty. Obesity is not common. Peak ages of onset are 13 years for boys and 10 years for girls.[4] The syndrome is the typical type 1 diabetes with sudden onset and temporary remission of weeks or months, followed by the onset of overt diabetes which usually becomes total in 2 to 6 years. Since no insulin is produced in the typical child patient, insulin is essential in treatment. Strict diet control often is considered preferable for prevention of acute and chronic complications.[4] However, there are those who suggest that the variation in activity and varying growth rates in children require that the child's appetite serve as the primary guide to food intake.

This does not mean, however, that all control should be abandoned. At the very least, commercial influences, such as advertisements on television, and social influences on food intake should be minimized.

General recommendations for an unmeasured diet for the diabetic child are as follows:[86,87]

1. The child should eat something at each meal, plus one or two small snacks as necessary. The foods on the exchange lists should be used as a guide to meal planning.
2. Concentrated sugar should be used only during vigorous athletic events and for treating hypoglycemia.
3. Meals should be provided at approximately the same time each day.
4. The child's appetite should determine the amount eaten, but meals must not be omitted.
5. Since the child is at risk of developing hypertension and cardiovascular disease, salt and cholesterol intake should be reduced.

Management of emotional and behavioral problems is important in the care of diabetic children and adolescents. Emotional problems also may appear in the parents. Sometimes the patients fail to cooperate in, or even reject, treatment. In adolescents seeking independence, management often is rejected since it is equated with dependence. At puberty, insulin and nutrition requirements are changing rapidly, adding further to the instability.

The rationale of management should be explained as soon as the child is capable of understanding, and responsibility for care should be transferred to the patient as soon as possible. Very young children can collect their urine samples, bring their insulin from its storage place, and select the injection site. Later, they can test their own urine. Most children can learn to give their own insulin at 7 to 8 years of age. Teenagers should learn self-management.

Group therapy often is helpful in managing the diabetic child. In many areas, summer camp sessions for diabetic children and adolescents are available and have been found to be very effective in promoting knowledge of the disease, greater independence in self-care, and improved social adjustment.

Diabetes and Pregnancy

Diabetic women can become pregnant, although there is a decrease in fertility if the diabetes is not controlled well. When pregnancy does occur, diabetes and pregnancy have a detrimental effect on each other. The pregnancy increases the severity of the diabetes, and the diabetes affects the growth of the fetus and placenta and increases the incidence of complications. Nevertheless, 95 percent of such pregnancies can be successful *if the diabetes is controlled well.*

Effects of Pregnancy on Diabetes

Some women with existing type 1 or type 2 overt diabetes become pregnant. In other patients, diabetes first appears in overt form during pregnancy. Four categories of diabetes in pregnancy have been recognized. Diabetes that first appears at approximately 5 months' gestation and disappears after delivery is known as *gestational diabetes.* It will reappear in subsequent pregnancies, usually in more severe form in each succeeding one. The other three categories are *pregestational* and include (1) latent diabetes that becomes overt during pregnancy, (2) subtotal diabetes that becomes exacerbated, and (3) the precipitation of permanent diabetes with severe ketoacidosis.

In a healthy, nondiabetic pregnancy, there are some metabolic changes that are *diabetogenic*—that is, they tend to increase blood glucose levels. The placenta produces *human chorionic somatomammotropin* (HCS), also known as *human placental lactogen.*[88] It is believed to be the major diabetogenic factor.[4] Human placental lactogen increases maternal lipolysis, increasing the circulating levels of free fatty acids and ketones. Their antiinsulin effects cause a decrease of entry of glucose into adipose tissue and muscle and an increase in circulating glucose.

In addition, *insulinase* is produced by the placenta during the second and third trimesters of pregnancy. It degrades insulin, but recent studies suggest that placental insulinase degrades insulin only in the fetus and not in the mother.[89,90] Since maternal and fetal glucose are interchangeable, there nevertheless may be an effect on maternal glucose levels.[4]

Plasma total cortisol levels, primarily bound to globulin, also are elevated during pregnancy, although free cortisol concentration is normal. The increase in cortisol-binding globulin (CBG) is thought to result from increased estrogen activity. When progesterone levels increase later in pregnancy, they compete for CBG and free cortisol is released, stimulating gluconeogenesis with a consequent increase in blood glucose.

The additive effects of these factors vary with the duration of the pregnancy. In the diabetic mother, sensitivity to insulin seems to increase in the first trimester and the diabetes becomes less severe, possibly owing to reduced anterior pituitary function or increased glucose utilization by the products of conception.[91] There also may be a drop in the renal threshold. As a result, diabetes in some adult-onset diabetics may improve in the first trimester, but this does not occur in the type 1 diabetic.

In the remainder of the pregnancy, diabetes of either type 1 or type 2 becomes more severe, with a sudden change in the fifth month. There is an average increase in the insulin requirement of 66 percent in the third trimester. In addition, pregnancy tends to exacerbate existing or latent neuropathy, nephropathy, and retinopathy.

Effects of Diabetes on Pregnancy

Maternal deaths occur among diabetics at the same rate as in the non-diabetic population, but complications occur more frequently in diabetics, primarily *hydramnios* (excess amniotic fluid that threatens the fetus), *toxemia* (a syndrome with edema, hypertension, albuminuria, and sometimes convulsions), and *ketoacidosis*. An additional problem is an increase in abortions, miscarriages, and intrauterine deaths of the fetus. *Perinatal* (from 7 months' gestation to 1 month postnatally) survival is approximately 90 percent of all diabetic pregnancies.[92]

Even minor degrees of hypoglycemia have adverse effects on the fetus. In fetuses who live to the perinatal period, there is an increased rate of complications and postnatal deaths. Problem infants can be categorized in two groups. In pregnant women with diabetes of long duration with vascular complications, the infants may be small for their gestational age. These infants sometimes are called *intrauterine growth–retarded* (IUGR) or simply *small-for-gestational-age infants*. However, it is important to remember that other, nondiabetic conditions also may cause IUGR. Deaths of newborn infants of diabetic mothers occur primarily in these small infants. The loss is approximately 20 percent and often is related to respiratory distress or congenital anomalies.

Another group of newborn infants of uncontrolled diabetic mothers consists of those who are fat, flabby, and heavy at birth (*macrosomia*). This large size can lead to *dystocia* (difficult labor) and is assumed to contribute to the increased incidence of birth injuries.

Maternal-fetal relationships are not entirely understood in either the normal or diabetic pregnancy, but some facts seem fairly clear. Many nutrients cross the placenta in amounts dependent on their concentration in the maternal blood; therefore, maternal metabolism largely determines which nutrients reach the fetus. There are a few other influencing factors, but circulating levels of many maternal and fetal metabolites are parallel. Insulin is very important in determining the amount and makeup of the nutrient mix reaching the fetus. Ketones and glucose, for example, cross the placenta in proportion to maternal blood levels.

Maternal insulin does not cross the placenta, but the formation and function of the beta cells in the fetal pancreas may be influenced by the amount of glucose and other nutrients reaching them. Although immature alpha and beta cells do not respond to physiologic levels of glucose, increased amounts of maternal nutrients may result in developmental changes in the beta cells so that more insulin is released. This fetal hyperinsulinism can result in increased body fat and delayed maturation of the pulmonary system—hence, the macrosomia and respiratory distress previously described.

It has been suggested further that the change in available nutrients during development may have permanent effects on developing cells, especially those cells that have a limited ability to replicate. These are the cells of the brain, adipose tissue, and muscles, and perhaps the beta cells of the pancreas. High levels of glucose and ketones have been shown to be damaging to the fetus, but the limits of the change in maternal fuel metabolism that can occur without harming the fetal cells are unknown.

During gestation, the fetus uses glucose as its primary fuel, and various hormonal adaptations in the mother assure an adequate supply. Glucose is transferred across the placenta by facilitated diffusion,[93] and amino acids are transferred by active transport.[94] Typically, FBS in the pregnant woman is 55 to 65 mg/dl.[95,96] In early pregnancy, plasma glucagon and growth hormone are relatively unchanged, but plasma insulin decreases, thus promoting ketogenesis.[97] Later, human placental lactogen causes a slower disposal of glucose, acting as an antiinsulin.[98] Beta cells in the nondiabetic pregnant woman have an increased sensitivity to glucose in later pregnancy, and the maternal beta cells will produce more insulin. However, in the woman whose functional reserve is reduced, gestational diabetes results. The GTT shows a curve that is higher than normal, delayed, and prolonged.[99] The prolonged response modulates the variations in maternal blood glucose and, thus, the variations in blood glucose to which the fetus is exposed.

Nutritional Care

The objective of diabetic control in pregnancy is to create, insofar as possible, normal conditions, including (1) a low FBS, (2) avoidance of ketonemia, which is known to damage the fetus, and (3) moderation of the amplitude of variation in the blood glucose concentration.

The Antenatal Diet. The criteria for control of the blood glucose must be the normal values in the *pregnant,* nondiabetic woman. It has been recommended, for example, that FBS should be less than 90 mg/dl with a GTT showing less than 160 mg/dl at 1 hour, less than 145 mg at 2 hours, and less than 125 mg/dl at 3 hours.[92] Home blood glucose monitoring has been strongly recommended.[81]

In order to modulate the variations in blood glucose, the woman usually needs multiple doses of daily insulin during pregnancy. When a hypoglycemic drug is required, insulin is given, not an oral agent. The effects of oral agents on blood glucose levels in pregnancy and on *teratogenesis* (production of fetal deformities in utero) are not entirely clear.

The total energy content of the diet must be increased in order to provide for sufficient weight gain. A total gain of 27.5 lb. is associated with the lowest blood pressure and is considered desirable. There should be little gain in the first 3 months, with a 350- to 400-g/week gain thereafter. An underweight pregnant diabetic who does not gain sufficient weight risks hemorrhage and production of an IUGR infant. In addition, ketonemia and consequent fetal central nervous system damage can result from calorie restriction. Thus, the diet should support normal, but not excessive, weight gain, even if the patient is obese at the onset. Weight reduction in the obese patient should be undertaken only after pregnancy.

The total energy cost of pregnancy has been estimated to be 75,000 kcal. The pregnant woman has been estimated to need 38 to 50 kcal/kg or an additional 300 kcal/day.[92,100] Within this allotment, the American Diabetes Association[101] recommends 45 percent carbohydrate or at least 200 g. If the patient has glycosuria, amounts lost in excess of 30 g/day should be added to the prescribed diet. The protein accumulation in pregnancy, estimated at 925 g, is provided by an additional 30 g/day or more.[102] At least 1.3 g of protein per kilogram of body weight per day should be allowed for an adult woman, and 1.5 to 1.7 g/kg/day are recommended for the pregnant adolescent.[96] The remaining calories are provided by fat.

In order to avoid overnight fasting ketonemia, the diet should be distributed so that the patient has an evening snack containing 35 g of carbohydrate and some protein.[92] The remainder of the diet should be distributed to prevent sharp peaks in blood glucose concentration.

In the normal pregnant woman, changes in the renin-angiotensin-aldosterone system (see Chapter 8) result in sodium retention and an increase in fluid volume. This action is normal and preserves an effective blood volume; therefore, sodium in the diet should not be restricted.[93] The vitamin and mineral requirements are the same as those in the nondiabetic pregnant woman.

Diet During and After Delivery. Cesarean sections are common because of the large size of many infants born to diabetic mothers. Vaginal deliveries often are induced early but usually not before 36 weeks. Glucose is given intravenously during delivery or surgery to control blood glucose, and insulin is provided subcutaneously or intravenously.

In normal uncomplicated deliveries, patients are returned to their usual diet the same day. Patients with cesarean sections are treated in the same way as in any major surgery on diabetics (see under The Diabetic Patient in Surgery).

Management of the Newborn Infant. The infant of the diabetic mother is not itself diabetic and can be expected to develop normally, but neonatal hypoglycemia is common in the early newborn period. During pregnancy, pancreatic secretion of insulin by the fetal pancreas is stimulated. In the immediate postnatal period, when the infant is no longer receiving the mother's glucose, this high rate of insulin production results in a severe decrease in blood glucose. Insulin production eventually subsides to normal, but hypoglycemia must be guarded against in the interim. If the blood glucose level falls below 20 mg/dl, intravenous glucose is needed.

The infant may have inherited a predisposition to diabetes and should be observed at intervals throughout his or her life with this in mind.

The Diabetic Patient in Surgery

Diabetic patients require surgery for cardiovascular disease, gallbladder disease, cancer of the pancreas, and amputations somewhat more often than does the nondiabetic population. They also may require other types of surgery at the same rate as the rest of the population.

The anxiety, the anesthesia, and the surgical procedure itself are stress factors which may cause an increase in catecholamine and cortisol production. This tends to cause a reduction in diabetes control. Patients controlled with oral hypoglycemic agents are given a small dose of insulin prior to surgery. For insulin-dependent patients, the insulin dose is reduced. Patients are given intravenous glucose the day of surgery to prevent starvation ketosis. Insulin may be included in the intravenous solution.

Postoperatively, the patient is returned to the previous diet and insulin as rapidly as possible. Regular insulin often is used for faster control. The diabetic diet can be incorporated into liquid, soft, and most other diets as necessary. The principles of nutritional care of the surgery patient in general are discussed in Chapter 12 and apply equally to the patient who is diabetic.

Recent Trends in Diabetes Research

Current diabetes research is directed toward development of methods to provide insulin at more physiologic levels. Transplantation of islets or of B cells is being studied. Work also is proceeding on the further development of an artificial pancreas with a blood glucose sensor and an insulin dispenser. Other approaches include studies of the use of a somatostatin analogue to control glucagon release, the role of chromium and zinc in the disease process, and the use of immunization to control viral causes of diabetes.

HYPOGLYCEMIA

In addition to diabetes mellitus, there are many other disorders in which derangements of carbohydrate utilization occur. Hypoglycemia is a clinical manifestation of many of these disorders. Since nutritional care is important in hypoglycemia, the pathologic conditions in which it occurs are described. It is important to remember that hypoglycemia is a manifestation of disease; it is not the disease itself.

Hypoglycemia usually is defined as a blood glucose concentration lower than 45 to 50 mg/dl; however, the onset of symptoms occurs at varying levels in different individuals. In adults, symptoms usually occur when blood glucose is 40 mg/dl or less. Infants can tolerate lower levels, sometimes 30 or even 20 mg/dl.

Clinical Manifestations

The signs and symptoms of hypoglycemia vary somewhat with the rate of fall of the blood glucose level. When the rate of fall is rapid, the secretion of epinephrine is stimulated in an attempt to restore normal glucose levels. The symptoms are those that result from an increase in circulating epinephrine: sweating, weakness, hunger, and *tachycardia* (increased heart rate).

On the other hand, if blood glucose falls slowly—that is, over many hours—the major effects are on the brain, since the brain uses mainly glucose as a fuel and hypoglycemia deprives it of fuel.[103] The effects include headache, blurred vision, *diplopia* (double vision), incoherent speech, and mental confusion. If the hypoglycemia persists over a long period, there may be sensory or motor deficits in the limbs, hemiplegia, and psychiatric problems. Permanent brain damage can occur. The condition can also progress to convulsions, coma, and death.

Classification

Hypoglycemia has been categorized in many ways. One useful classification is given in Table 9-17. It differentiates between

Table 9-17. Classification of Hypoglycemia

Spontaneous hypoglycemia
Fasting
- Pancreatic beta cell tumor, functioning
- Nonpancreatic tumor associated with hypoglycemia
- Liver disease: acquired (diffuse liver disease) or congenital (glycogen storage disease, galactosemia)
- Alcoholism and poor nutrition
- Endocrinopathies: hypofunction of anterior pituitary gland, adrenal cortex, thyroid, pancreatic alpha cells

Reactive (postabsorptive)
- Functional reactive
- Reactive secondary to early diabetes
- Dumping syndrome
- Leucine sensitivity
- Hereditary fructose intolerance

Exogenous hypoglycemia (insulin or sulfonylureas)
Iatrogenic (resulting from treatment by physician or surgeon)
Factitious (artificial—may be self-administered)
Homicidal
Suicidal

exogenous hypoglycemia, resulting from administration of hypoglycemic drugs, and *spontaneous hypoglycemia,* in which the cause is endogenous. Spontaneous hypoglycemias can be divided into two groups—*reactive* or *postabsorptive,* in which the symptoms occur within 1 or 2 hours after eating, and *fasting hypoglycemia,* which occurs approximately 8 hours following the last meal. Another classification has two useful divisions—*organic,* in which there is an identifiable anatomic lesion, and *functional,* in which no recognizable anatomic lesion can be found. Some organic lesions cause fasting hypoglycemia and some cause the reactive type. Functional disorders generally are reactive.

Diagnosis

To treat hypoglycemia, it is necessary to know the etiology. Therefore, diagnostic procedures must be used not only to establish the existence of the condition, but also to pinpoint its cause. There are a number of procedures available.

Fasting blood glucose will assist in distinguishing reactive from fasting hypoglycemia. It is low in the fasting type but normal in the reactive type.

The *oral glucose tolerance test* will differentiate early diabetic from functional hypoglycemia.[104] The test must be conducted for the full 5 hours. Comparative oral glucose tolerance test curves in various hypoglycemic syndromes are shown in Fig. 9-9.

Intravenous glucose tolerance tests can confirm a diagnosis of dumping syndrome (see Chapter 5), since hypoglycemia will not occur in these patients if the glucose is not taken orally.

A *prolonged fast* of 48 to 72 hours is considered the ultimate test to detect organic hyperglycemia. A person with a functioning islet cell tumor usually develops symptoms in 24 hours, whereas a normal person can have 40 to 50 mg/dl of blood glucose within 48 hours and remain symptom-free. If no symptoms occur in 72 hours, the patient is exercised carefully and a blood sample is taken. A normal person will show a rise in blood glucose following exercise, but a patient with an islet cell tumor will have a further decrease. Symptoms also may occur at this time.

The *intravenous tolbutamide response test* sometimes is used in place of the prolonged fasts. The patient is given an intravenous dose of tolbutamide, and the blood glucose concentration is determined at intervals. Following an overnight fast, a 30-minute test can be used to aid in the diagnosis of diabetes,[105] or a 3-hour test may differentiate fasting hypoglycemia.[106]

In the *leucine sensitivity test,* a leucine load is given intravenously or orally, and blood samples are collected every 10 minutes for 1 hour. A fall to at least 40 mg of glucose per deciliter of blood indicates idiopathic sensitivity, functioning islet cell tumor, or factitious hypoglycemia due to sulfonylurea.[107]

The *fructose loading test* is conducted with a procedure similar to the GTT. Blood samples are analyzed for glucose, fructose, and phosphorus. An abnormal rise in fructose and rapid fall in glucose and serum inorganic phosphorus suggest hereditary fructose intolerance.

Serum insulin levels are used to distinguish a functioning islet cell tumor from a nonpancreatic tumor, which usually does not cause elevated insulin levels.

Circulating antibodies to insulin, if found, are useful in detecting the individual who has *factitious hypoglycemia* following self-administration of insulin.

Nutritional Care

Nutritional care of the hypoglycemic patient depends on the cause of the condition and on other treatments involved.

Fasting Hypoglycemia

In those patients whose hypoglycemia is the consequence of a tumor, the treatment of choice is, of course, the surgical removal of

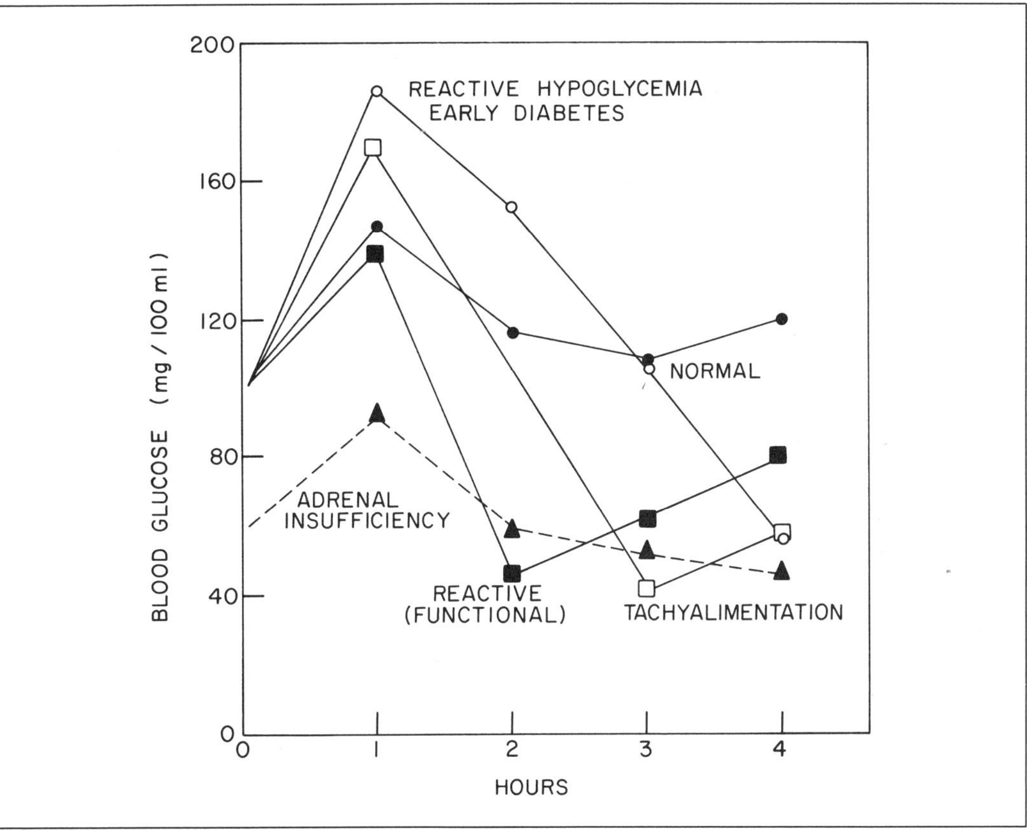

Figure 9-9. Oral glucose tolerance curves in hypoglycemic syndromes. A representative normal curve is presented for comparison. Note that in functional reactive hypoglycemia the 1-hour glucose level is lower than in the curve of tachyalimentation and in early diabetes. (Reprinted with permission from Bacchus, H., Rational Management of Diabetes. *Copyright © 1977, University Park Press, Baltimore.)*

the tumor. In *insulin-producing islet cell tumors,* the patient secretes insulin during exercise or fasting, often showing symptoms before breakfast, when meals are delayed, and sometimes as early as 2 to 3 hours following a meal. Usually, the patient will already have begun a schedule of eating at regular and frequent intervals, a process that sometimes, but not always, results in massive obesity. Frequent feeding must continue until surgical removal of the tumor. Pancreatic tumors may be difficult to find. If the surgery is unsuccessful or if the condition is inoperable, the frequent feeding must continue. The patient may be given steroid drugs. Nutritional care for patients given these drugs is discussed on page 375. If the pancreas is removed totally, the patient is diabetic and must be treated accordingly.

Nonpancreatic tumors associated with hypoglycemia are of various types and thus produce the hypoglycemic effect by more than one mechanism. When the tumor is removed, the hypoglycemia disappears. If the condition is inoperable, the diet used for functional hypoglycemia (see the next section) may be helpful in conjunction with an antihypoglycemic drug such as diazoxide. Additional aspects of nutritional care of patients with carcinoid syndrome or Zollinger-Ellison syndrome are discussed in Chapter 6. Other disorders causing hypoglycemia in association with fasting are discussed in detail elsewhere.

Reactive Hypoglycemia

There are five types of reactive hypoglycemia. In the nondiabetic population, the most common is the functional form.

Functional Reactive Hypoglycemia. Functional reactive hypoglycemia often is associated with anxiety, tension, and emotional upsets. There is some discussion as to which is cause and which is effect and whether some of the patients are actually hypoglycemic. Many seem to develop symptoms at levels tolerated well by normal persons. The glucose tolerance curve begins at normal levels and tends to be rather flat. The blood glucose then subsides to hypoglycemic levels with a spontaneous rebound.

The condition tends to be self-limiting in months or years. In the meantime, a modified diet is helpful. One diet that has been recommended is the high-protein, low-carbohydrate diet, which has the following features:[108]

Kilocalories: To maintain normal weight. The basis for estimation is the same as that described for diabetic patients.

Carbohydrate: Limited, to reduce stimulation of insulin release, to 75 to 120 g, usually at least 100 g. Free sugars are avoided.

Protein: Increased, to provide a source of glucose without stimulation of insulin release, commonly to 120 to 140 g.

Fat: To provide the remaining kilocalories.

Division into meals: Carbohydrate *and protein* are divided as equally as is feasible among multiple feedings. Some patients require as many as six equal feedings per day.

Other restrictions: Alcohol should be avoided as it interferes with gluconeogenesis. Some institutions recommend the avoidance of caffeine-containing substances (see Appendix I).

The ADA exchange lists for diabetic diets and the same calculation procedure are used to calculate the diet (see pp. 350–358). For example, assuming an 1,800-calorie diet, the distribution might be 100 g of carbohydrate, 140 g of protein, and 95 g of fat. If the patient requires six meals, the division should aim for 16 g of carbohydrate and 23 g of protein in each. Fat is distributed as desired. The patient may need calcium and riboflavin supplements, since milk often cannot be included in the diet.

An alternative approach to diet modification is based on the assumption that restriction of slowly absorbed carbohydrate, such as starch, does not relieve the symptoms. Therefore, only free sugars are restricted; the diabetic diet is used as a general guide, sometimes with division into five or six feedings.[109]

Given the variability of patient needs and responses to diet modification, the nutritional care specialist should be prepared to work with the patient to determine the modifications needed within general guidelines.

Organic Reactive Hypoglycemia. Organic reactive hyperglycemias comprise four conditions. *Dumping syndrome* is described in Chapter 5. Hypoglycemia also occurs in *early diabetes* (Fig. 9-9). *Hereditary fructose intolerance* is a congenital metabolic disorder (see Chapter 10). The remaining entity is *leucine sensitivity,* which occurs almost exclusively in infancy and is thought to be a sign of immature development. The symptoms of leucine sensitivity commonly appear first after ingestion of milk, and treatment consists of restriction of sources of leucine, including milk. The condition is self-limiting and usually disappears by 6 years of age.

THE ADRENAL CORTEX

Adrenocortical Insufficiency

Adrenocortical insufficiency may be a chronic primary disease (*Addison's disease*) or it may result secondarily from tumors, infections, pituitary hypofunction, or surgical removal.

Under these circumstances, *glucocorticoids* and *aldosterone* become deficient.

A deficiency of aldosterone causes a decrease in sodium reabsorption in the renal tubules, an increased loss of sodium, chloride, and water, potassium retention, and a decrease in blood volume and cardiac output. If untreated, the patient may enter a potentially fatal *addisonian crisis* within a few days.

A concomitant deficiency also occurs in glucocorticoid hormones, which function in carbohydrate metabolism. As a result, gluconeogenesis is depressed and blood glucose falls between meals, producing a mild hypoglycemia. The patient may also have nausea, vomiting, diarrhea, anorexia, and weight loss.

The primary treatment for most patients is hormone replacement with medications. Sometimes, increased sodium chloride is given to reduce the need for the costly drug. The patient can then be advised to eat salty foods, salt his or her food generously, and take salt tablets. Patients may carry foods with carbohydrate, protein, and salt as a precaution. Cheese and crackers or salted nuts are useful for this purpose. The patient should also strive to maintain normal weight.

Adrenocortical Hyperfunction

Cushing's syndrome is due to excessive adrenocortical activity resulting from lesions in the hypothalamus or pituitary gland, which control adrenal function, or from lesions of the adrenal gland itself. It can also result from idiopathic hyperplasia of the adrenal cortex or excess corticosteroid medication.

The excess glucocorticoid causes increased gluconeogenesis, and the patient may become protein-depleted. Blood glucose levels may rise. All patients have abnormal glucose tolerances and 20 percent develop diabetes mellitus. There are abnormal fat deposits, particularly in the face and over the clavicle. Excess aldosterone causes sodium and water retention and depletion of potassium. A high-protein, sodium-restricted diet sometimes is used for symptomatic relief; however, the main treatment is surgical resection of the adrenal glands. This procedure produces Addison's disease which is easier to treat.

Adrenocorticotropic Hormone or Glucocorticoid Therapy

Adrenocorticotropic hormone (ACTH), which stimulates glucocorticoid production, or the glucocorticoids themselves are used in the treatment of many disorders. They are given particularly for their antiinflammatory and antiimmune effects and may be used for long periods in chronic inflammatory and autoimmune disorders and in transplant patients.

Over the long term, glucocorticoids stimulate gluconeogenesis, causing negative nitrogen balance with muscle wasting. At the same time, these drugs decrease insulin sensitivity and therefore are diabetogenic. A diet containing 1 g of protein per kilogram of body weight with liberal carbohydrate for protein sparing is recommended. Given the reduced insulin sensitivity, concentrated simple carbohydrates should be avoided.

Increased hydrochloric acid secretion may cause peptic ulcer; therefore, frequent small meals may be preferable. Antacids sometimes are recommended.

Water and electrolyte changes are variable. The patients receiving the drugs as replacement therapy may need added salts and fluid, as previously noted. Others may retain sodium and fluid and lose potassium, making sodium restriction to 1,000 mg/day helpful. Potassium intake may be increased with medication or high-potassium foods.

THYROID DYSFUNCTION

The thyroid gland secretes the hormones *triiodothyronine* (T_3), *thyroxine* (T_4), and *thyrocalcitonin.* These hormones control the metabolic rate, regulating carbohydrate and lipid metabolism and stimulating oxygen metabolism. They also control or promote growth and skeletal maturation, protein anabolism, and hematopoiesis. These effects result in increased heart rate and cardiac output and also increased mental acuity.

Hyperthyroidism

Hyperthyroidism (also known as *exophthalmic goiter, thyrotoxicosis, Graves' disease,* or *Basedow's disease*) may be an autoimmune disease. It can be treated by surgical excision of the thyroid gland, antithyroid drugs, or radioactive iodine.

Until such time as the hyperthyroidism is controlled, there are some metabolic effects that require nutritional care. In particular, the patients have an increased metabolic rate. If other fuels are not available, they will metabolize body protein, with a resulting negative nitrogen balance and muscle loss. They require a high-calorie diet which may reach 5,000 kcal, depending on the severity of the condition. Protein should be provided for maintenance plus replacement of any losses, usually 1 to 2 g per kilogram of body weight. High levels of carbohydrate should also be provided for protein sparing. Fortunately, these patients usually have a ravenous appetite. Mineral and vitamin supplements may be needed in proportion to the increase in the metabolic rate. Stimulants such as beverages containing caffeine and alcoholic beverages are restricted.

Hypothyroidism

A deficiency in activity or secretion of T_3 or T_4 or both is known as *hypothyroidism, Gull's disease, myxedema* (if advanced), or *Hashimoto's thyroiditis* in women. It can be caused by inadequate iodine, increased intake of goitrogens, an inborn error of metabolism, or idiopathic atrophy of the thyroid.

Hormone replacement by medication is the main feature of treatment. Some of the clinical manifestations also suggest the need for nutritional care. The metabolic rate decreases and the patient may gain excess weight. A reduced-calorie diet then is indicated. Not all patients gain weight, since appetite may be depressed. The blood cholesterol level rises consequent to a decreased cholesterol breakdown. Reduction in dietary cholesterol may be useful. Lastly, patients often have decreased intestinal peristalsis with resulting constipation. A high-fiber diet with generous amounts of fluids is helpful.

OTHER NUTRITION-ENDOCRINE RELATIONSHIPS

Almost every step in the body's handling of nutrients is affected by one or more hormones. Conversely, a person's nutritional status can have important effects on endocrine function. Only those circumstances in which nutritional care is of particular importance were discussed in this chapter. It is not possible to describe all the interrelationships that might occur. The nutritional care specialist should, nevertheless, be alert to the need for nutritional intervention in patients with other endocrine disturbances. It also is important to realize that the nutritional deprivation that occurs as a consequence of many disorders may seriously affect endocrine function.

Case Study: Juvenile-Onset Diabetes Mellitus

Debbie T., a 13-year-old girl, was admitted to the hospital with chief complaints of weight loss, thirst, and urinary frequency. Her mother reported that the child had lost approximately 9 lb. in 4 weeks. Thirst and frequent urination were particularly noticeable for the past week.

Examination revealed the following:

Weight	90 lb.
Height	62 in.
Urine glucose	4+
Urine acetone	Positive
Blood glucose	670 mg/dl

The following was written in the patient's chart:

S: Pt. c/o thirst, urgency, generally "feels bad."
O: BS = 670 mg/dl; U/A = 4+ glucose, large acetone
A: DM
P: Give RI until stabilized. Then adjust to NPH. Diet as recommended by dietitian.

An interview by the dietitian elicited the following 24-hour recall:

Breakfast	½ c. orange juice
	¾ c. cereal with ½ banana
	½ c. milk
Lunch	½ c. tuna salad
	2 slices bread
	1 peach
	½ pint milk
Snack	12 oz. soft drink
	"A few" potato chips
Dinner	Small hamburger with catsup
	⅓ c. buttered green beans
	⅙ apple pie
Snack	12 oz. soft drink

Exercises

1. Explain the reasons for the symptoms observed.
2. Why was the patient's blood glucose level elevated?
3. If the patient had not been treated promptly, how would her disease have progressed?
4. What diet would you recommend for this patient during her hospitalization?
5. Make a diet plan and write 1 day's sample menu.
6. How should the patient's diet be adjusted when she is discharged from the hospital? (Note: She swims daily from 4:00 to 5:00 P.M.)
7. Outline the information that the patient and her parents need to know to maintain her in good health.

Case Study: Diabetes Mellitus in the Elderly*

Millie R. is a 75-year-old woman living with her 80-year-old sister, for whom she is caring. They live in a low-income urban community in a third-floor walk-up apartment. Millie comes regularly to the Medical Clinic. She complained at her most recent visit of blurred vision, symptoms of polydipsia and polyuria, and a weight loss of 6 lb. in the past 2 weeks.

On admission to the hospital, her blood glucose measured 888 mg/dl. A diagnosis of urinary tract infection and nonketotic hyperglycemia was made.

You obtain the following information from her chart:

Medical history	Hypertension, congestive heart failure, asthma
Family history	Sister has had non-insulin-dependent diabetes mellitus for 10 years
Current medications	Digoxin, furosemide (Lasix), hydrochlorothiazide, propranolol hydrochloride (Inderal), prednisone
Height	4 ft 11 in.
Weight	119 lb. (usual weight 125 lb.)
Cholesterol	380 mg/dl

* Adapted from a case study provided by Mary Ellen Collins, R.D., of Brigham and Women's Hospital, Boston, Mass.

Subjective: "I'm the thinnest I've ever been and I'm too old to lose weight. I can't be more active because my asthma kicks up. I know about diabetes. My sister has it and she eats the way I do."

On questioning, the following 24-hour recall information was obtained:

Breakfast	2 large shredded wheat biscuits
	1 c. whole milk
	1 slice toast with margarine, jelly
Snack	½ grapefruit, 1 tsp. sugar
Dinner	1 pork chop, approximately 4 oz., with fat

1 c. rice or potato with gravy
Greens with salt pork
2 slices bread with margarine
Snack ½ grapefruit, 1 tsp. sugar

Exercises

1. Explain the mechanism by which the patient's blood glucose level could become so high without producing ketosis.
2. If this patient were not treated, how would you expect her disease to progress?
3. Evaluate the patient's diet, based on the 24-hour recall.
4. What diet would you recommend for this patient?
5. Make a meal plan and write 1 day's menu.
6. Which items in her present diet would you like to replace with foods more appropriate for this patient?
7. What problems would you anticipate in instructing this patient on her diet?

References

1. Gerich, J.E., Lorenzi, M., Karam, J.H., et al. Abnormal pancreatic glucagon secretion and postprandial hyperglycemia in diabetes mellitus. *J.A.M.A.* 234:159, 1975.
2. Unger, R.H., and Orci, L. Role of glucagon in diabetes. *Arch. Intern. Med.* 137:482, 1977.
3. Felig, P., Wahren, J., Sherwin, R., and Hendler, R. Insulin, glucagon, and somatostatin in normal physiology and diabetes mellitus. *Diabetes* 25:1091, 1976.
4. Bacchus, H. *Rational Management of Diabetes.* Baltimore: University Park Press, 1977.
5. West, K.M. Epidemiological evidence linking nutritional factors to the prevalence and manifestations of diabetes. *Acta Diabetol. Lat.* (Suppl.) 9(1):405, 1972.
6. Hinden, E. Mumps followed by diabetes. *Lancet* 1:1381, 1962.
7. Craighead, J.E. The role of viruses in the pathogenesis of pancreatic disease and diabetes mellitus. *Prog. Med. Virol.* 19:161, 1975.
8. Steinke, J., and Taylor, K.W. Viruses and the etiology of diabetes. *Diabetes* 23:631, 1974.
9. Forrest, J.M., Menser, M.A., and Burgess, J.A. High frequency of diabetes mellitus in young adults with congenital rubella. *Lancet* 2:332, 1971.
10. Ross, M.E., Onodera, T., Brown, K.S., and Notkins, A.L. Virus-induced diabetes mellitus: IV. Genetic and environmental factors influencing the development of diabetes after infection with the M variant of encephalomyocarditis virus. *Diabetes* 25:190, 1976.
11. Irvine, W.J., Clarke, B.F., Scarth, L., et al. Thyroid and gastric autoimmunity in patients with diabetes mellitus. *Lancet* 2:163, 1970.
12. Whittingham, S., Mathews, J.D., Mackay, I.R., et al. Diabetes mellitus, autoimmunity and ageing. *Lancet* 1:763, 1971.
13. Bottazzo, G.F., Florin-Christensen, A., and Doniach, D. Islet-cell antibodies in diabetes mellitus with autoimmune polyendocrine deficiencies. *Lancet* 2:1279, 1974.
14. McCuish, A.C., Barnes, E.W., Irvine, W.J., and Duncan, L.J.P. Antibodies to pancreatic islet cells in insulin-dependent diabetics with coexistent autoimmune disease. *Lancet* 2:1529, 1974.
15. Lendrum, R., Walker, G., and Gamble, D.R. Islet-cell antibodies in juvenile diabetes of recent onset. *Lancet* 1:880, 1975.
16. Huang, S.W., and Maclaren, N.K. Insulin-dependent diabetes: A disease of auto-aggression. *Science* 192:64, 1976.
17. McDevitt, H.O., and Bodmer, W.F. HL-A, immune response genes, and disease. *Lancet* 1:1269, 1974.
18. Friedman, G.J. Diet in the treatment of diabetes mellitus. In R.S. Goodhart and M.E. Shils, Eds., *Modern Nutrition in Health and Disease,* 6th ed. Philadelphia: Lea and Febiger, 1980.
19. Kannel, W.B., Pearson, G., and McNamara, P.M. Obesity as a force of morbidity and mortality in adolescence. In F.P. Heald, Ed., *Adolescent Nutrition and Growth.* New York: Appleton-Century-Crofts, 1969.
20. West, K.M., Oakley, E.L., Sanders, M.E., and Rubenstein, A.H. Nutritional factors in the etiology of diabetes. In H. Keen, Ed., *Epidemiology of Diabetes.* London: World Health Organization, 1977.
21. Cohen, A.M., Bavly, S., and Posnamski, R. Change of diet of Yemenite Jews in relation to diabetes and ischaemic heart disease. *Lancet* 2:1399, 1969.

22. Campbell, G.D. Diabetes in Asians and Africans in and around Durban. *S. Afr. Med. J.* 37:1195, 1963.
23. Reid, J.M., Fullmer, S.D., Pettigrew, K.D., et al. Nutrient intake of Pima Indian women: Relationships to diabetes mellitus and gallbladder disease. *Am. J. Clin. Nutr.* 24:1281, 1971.
24. West, K.M., and Kalbfleisch, J.M. Influence of nutritional factors on prevalence of diabetes. *Diabetes* 20:99, 1971.
25. Cohen, A.M., Briller, S., and Shafrir, E. Effect of long-term sucrose feeding on the activity of some enzymes regulating glycolysis, lipogenesis and gluconeogenesis in rat liver and adipose tissue. *Biochim. Biophys. Acta* 279:129, 1972.
26. Anderson, J.W., Herman, R.H., and Zakim, D. Effect of high glucose and high sucrose diet on glucose tolerance of normal men. *Am. J. Clin. Nutr.* 26:600, 1973.
27. Brunzell, J.D., Lerner, R.L., Porte, O., and Bierman, E.L. Effect of a fat free, high carbohydrate diet on diabetic subjects with fasting hypoglycemia. *Diabetes* 23:128, 1974.
28. Caliendo, M.A. *Nutrition and Preventive Health Care.* New York: Macmillan, 1981.
29. Hildebrand, S.S., Ed. Is the risk of becoming diabetic affected by sugar consumption? *Proceedings of the Eighth International Sugar Research Foundation Conference.* Bethesda, Md.: International Sugar Research Foundation, 1974.
30. Campbell, G.O., Batchelor, E.L., and Goldberg, M.D. Sugar intake and diabetes. *Diabetes* 16:62, 1967.
31. Cohen, A.M. Environmental aspects of diabetes. *Isr. J. Med. Sci.* 8:358, 1972.
32. Himsworth, H.P. Diet and the incidence of diabetes mellitus. *Clin. Sci.* 2:117, 1935–1936.
33. Spiller, G.A., and Kay, R.M., Eds. *Medical Aspects of Dietary Fiber.* New York: Plenum, 1980.
34. Jenkins, D.J., Goff, D.V., Leeds, A.R., et al. Unabsorbable carbohydrates and diabetes: Decreased postprandial hyperglycemia. *Lancet* 2:172, 1976.
35. Jenkins, D.J., Leeds, A.R., Gassull, M.A., et al. Decrease in postprandial insulin and glucose concentrations by guar and pectin. *Ann. Intern. Med.* 86:20, 1977.
36. Miranda, P.M., and Horwitz, D.L. High-fiber diets in the treatment of diabetes mellitus. *Ann. Intern. Med.* 88:482, 1978.
37. Brunzell, J.D., Lerner, R.L., Hazzard, W.R., et al. Improved glucose tolerance with high carbohydrate feeding in mild diabetes. *N. Engl. J. Med.* 284:521, 1971.
38. Anderson, J.W., Lin, W.-J., and Ward, K. Composition of foods commonly used in diets for persons with diabetes. *Diabetes Care* 1:293, 1978.
39. Tomizawa, H.H. Mode of action of insulin-degrading enzyme of beef liver. *J. Biol. Chem.* 237:428, 1962.
40. Levine, R., and Goldstein, M.S. On the mechanism of action of insulin. *Recent Prog. Horm. Res.* 11:343, 1955.
41. Taub, S., Mariani, A., and Barkin, J.S. Gastrointestinal manifestations of diabetes mellitus. *Diabetes Care* 2:437, 1979.
42. Riddle, M.C. Relief of gastrointestinal symptoms by correcting insulin excess. *Diabetes Care* 4:296, 1981.
43. Block, M.B., Rosenfield, R.L., Mako, M.E., et al. Sequential changes in beta-cell function in insulin-treated diabetic patients assessed by C-peptide immunoreactivity. *N. Engl. J. Med.* 288:1144, 1973.
44. Koenig, R.J., and Cerami, A. Hemoglobin A_{1c} and diabetes mellitus. *Annu. Rev. Med.* 31:29, 1980.
45. Gonen, B., Rubenstein, A.H., Rockman, H., et al. Haemoglobin A_1: An indicator of the metabolic control of diabetic patients. *Lancet* 2:734, 1977.
46. Colwell, J.A., and Lein, A. Diminished insulin response to hyperglycemia in prediabetes and diabetes. *Diabetes* 16:560, 1967.
47. Floyd, J.C., Jr., Fajans, S.S., Conn, J.W., et al. Secretion of insulin induced by amino acids and glucose in diabetes mellitus. *J. Clin. Endocrinol.* 28:266, 1968.
48. Cerasi, E., and Luft, R. The prediabetic state, its nature and consequences. *Diabetes* 21(Suppl. 2):685, 1972.
49. Conn, J.W., and Fajans, S.S. The prediabetic state. A concept of dynamic resistance to a genetic diabetogenic influence. *Am. J. Med.* 31:839, 1961.
50. Job, D., Eschwege, E., Guyot, C., and Tchobroutsky, G. Effect of multiple daily insulin injections on the course of diabetic retinopathy. *Diabetes* 24(Suppl. 2):397, 1975.
51. Crofford, O. *Reports to Congress of the National Commission on Diabetes* (DHEW Publication No. (NIH) 76-1018). Washington, D.C.: Government Printing Office, 1975.
52. Levine, R., and Smith, M. Antidiabetic drugs. In Modell, W., Ed., *Drugs of Choice 1976–1977.* St. Louis: C.V. Mosby, 1976.

53. Lebovitz, H.E., and Feinglos, M.N. Sulfonylurea drugs: Mechanism of antidiabetic action and therapeutic usefulness. *Diabetes Care* 1:189, 1978.
54. University Group Diabetes Program. A study of the effects of hypoglycemia agents on vascular complications in patients with adult-onset diabetes. *Diabetes* 19(Suppl. 2):747, 1970.
55. American Diabetes Association. The UGDP controversy. *Diabetes Care* 2:1, 1979.
56. O'Donovan, C.V. Analysis of long-term experience with tolbutamide (Orinase) in the management of diabetes. *Curr. Ther. Res.* 1:69, 1959.
57. Shen, S.W., and Bressler, R. Clinical pharmacology of oral antidiabetic agents. *N. Engl. J. Med.* 296:493, 1977.
58. Bloodworth, J.M.B. Diabetes mellitus and vascular disease. *Postgrad. Med.* 53(3):84, 1973.
59. Lundbaek, K. Diabetic angiopathy. *Mod. Concepts Cardiovasc. Dis.* 43:103, 1974.
60. Marble, A., White, P., Bradley, R.F., and Krall, L.P., Eds. *Joslin's Diabetes Mellitus,* 11th ed. Philadelphia: Lea and Febiger, 1971.
61. West, K.M. Diabetes mellitus. In H.A. Schneider, C.E. Anderson, and D.B. Coursin, Eds., *Nutritional Support of Medical Practice.* New York: Harper and Row, 1977.
62. West, K.M. Diet therapy of diabetes: An analysis of failure. *Ann. Intern. Med.* 79:425, 1973.
63. Goodman, J.I., Schwartz, E.D., and Frankel, L. Group therapy of obese diabetic patients. *Diabetes* 2:280, 1953.
64. Goldberg, R.B., Bersohn, I., Joffee, B.I., et al. Hyperlipidaemia, obesity and drug misuse in a diabetic clinic. *S. Afr. Med. J.* 48:270, 1974.
65. Bierman, E.L., Albrink, M.J., Arky, R.A., et al. Special report: Principles of nutrition and dietary recommendations for patients with diabetes mellitus. *Diabetes* 20:633, 1971.
66. Pollack, H., and Dolger, H. Advantages of prozinsulin (protamine zinc insulin) therapy: Dietary suggestions and notes on the management of cases. *Ann. Intern. Med.* 12:2019, 1939.
67. Committees of the American Diabetes Association and the American Dietetic Association. *Exchange Lists for Meal Planning.* Chicago: American Dietetic Association and American Diabetes Association, in cooperation with the National Institute of Arthritis, Metabolism, and Digestive Diseases and the National Heart, Blood, and Lung Institute. U.S. Department of Health, Education and Welfare, 1976.
68. Egeberg, R.O., and Steinfeld, J.L., Frantz, I., et al. Report to the Secretary of HEW from the Medical Advisory Group on Cyclamates. *J.A.M.A.* 211:1358, 1970.
69. Smith, R.J. Aspartame approved despite risks. *Science* 213:986, 1981.
70. Brunzell, J.D. Use of fructose, xylitol or sorbitol as a sweetener in diabetes mellitus. *Diabetes Care* 1:223, 1978.
71. Brunzell, J.D. Use of fructose, sorbitol, or xylitol as a sweetener in diabetes mellitus. *J. Am. Diet. Assoc.* 73:499, 1978.
72. Bohannon, N.V., Karam, J.H., and Forsham, P.H. Advantages of fructose ingestion over sucrose and glucose in humans. *Diabetes* 27(Suppl. 2):438, 1978.
73. Gabbay, K.H. The sorbitol pathway and the complications of diabetes. *N. Engl. J. Med.* 288:831, 1973.
74. Steinke, J., Wood, F.C., Domenge, L., et al. Evolution of sorbitol in the diet of diabetic children at camp. *Diabetes* 10:218, 1961.
75. American Diabetes Association and American Dietetic Association. *Family Cookbook.* Englewood Cliffs, N.J.: Prentice-Hall, 1980.
76. Berger, M., Hagg, S., and Ruderman, N.B. Glucose metabolism in perfused skeletal muscle. *Biochem. J.* 147:231, 1975.
77. Saltin, B., Lindgarde, F., Houston, H., et al. Physical training and glucose tolerance in middle-aged men with chemical diabetes. *Diabetes* 28:30, 1978.
78. Ruderman, N.B., Ganda, O.P., and Johansen, K. The effect of physical training on glucose tolerance and plasma lipids in maturity-onset diabetes. *Diabetes* 28:89, 1978.
79. Berger, M., Berchtold, P., Cüppers, H.J., et al. Metabolic and hormonal effects of muscular exercise in juvenile type diabetes. *Diabetologia* 13:355, 1977.
80. Wahren, J., Felig, P., and Hagenfeldt, L. Physical exercise and fuel homeostasis in diabetes mellitus. *Diabetologia* 14:213, 1978.
81. Jovanovic, L., and Peterson, C.M. Is home blood glucose monitoring for you? *Diabetes Forecast* 33(4):30, 1980.
82. Peterson, C.M., Forhan, S.E., and Jones, R.L. Self-management: An approach to patients with insulin-dependent diabetes mellitus. *Diabetes Care* 3:82, 1980.
83. Schneider, J.M., Huddleston, J.F., Curet, L.B., and Menzel, D.L. Pregnancy complicating ambulatory patient management of diabetes. *Diabetes Care* 3:7, 1980.

84. McDermott, K., Cooks, M., and Peterson, C.M. Patient-determined glycosylated hemoglobin measurements: An aid to patient education. *Diabetes Care* 4:480, 1981.
85. American Diabetic Association. *Diabetes Forecast.*
86. Schmitt, B.D. An argument for the unmeasured diet in juvenile diabetes mellitus. *Clin. Pediatr.* (Phila.) 14:68, 1975.
87. Malone, J.T. Nutrition and childhood diabetes. In L.A. Barness, Ed., *Nutrition in Medical Practice.* Westport, Conn.: AVI, 1981.
88. Josimovich, J.B., Kosor, B., Boccella, L., et al. Placental lactogen in maternal serum as an index of fetal health. *Obstet. Gynecol.* 36:244, 1970.
90. Freinkel, N., and Goodner, C.J. Insulin metabolism and pregnancy. *Arch. Intern. Med.* 109:235, 1962.
91. Bellman, O., and Hartmann, E. Influence of pregnancy on the kinetics of insulin. *Am. J. Obstet. Gynecol.* 122:829, 1975.
92. Mintz, D.H., Skyler, J.S., and Chez, R.A. Diabetes mellitus and pregnancy. *Diabetes Care* 1:49, 1978.
93. Chinard, F.P., Danesino, V., Hartmann, W.L., et al. The transmission of hexoses across the placenta in the human and the rhesus monkey. *J. Physiol.* (Lond.) 132:289, 1956.
94. Young, M. Placental transport of free amino acids. In J.H.P. Jonxis, H.K.A. Visser, and J.A. Troelstra, Eds., *Metabolic Processes in the Foetus and Newborn Infant.* Baltimore: Williams and Wilkins, 1971. Pp. 97–108.
95. Gillmer, M.D.G., Beard, R.W., Brooke, F.M., and Oakley, N.W. Carbohydrate metabolism in pregnancy: I. Diurnal plasma glucose profile in normal and diabetic women. *Br. Med. J.* 3:399, 1975.
96. Gillmer, M.D.G., Oakley, N.W., Brooke, F.M., and Beard, R.W. Metabolic profiles in pregnancy. *Isr. J. Med. Sci.* 11:601, 1975.
97. Freinkel, N., Metzger, B.E., Nitzan, M., et al. 'Accelerated starvation' and mechanisms for the conservation of maternal nitrogen during pregnancy. *Isr. J. Med. Sci.* 8:426, 1972.
98. Tyson, J.E., Fiedler, A.J., Austin, K.L., and Farinholt, J. Placental lactogen and prolactin secretion in human pregnancy. In K. Moghissi and E.S.E. Hafez, Eds., *The Placenta: Biological and Clinical Aspects.* Springfield, Ill.: Charles C Thomas, 1974.
99. Freinkel, N., and Metzger, B. Some consideration of fuel economy in the fed state during late human pregnancy. In R.A. Camerini-Davalos and H.S. Cole, Eds., *Early Diabetes in Early Life.* New York: Academic, 1976.
100. Jacobson, H.N. Current concepts in nutrition: Diet in pregnancy. *N. Engl. J. Med.* 297:1051, 1977.
101. *A Guide for Professionals: The Effective Application of 'Exchange Lists for Meal Planning.'* New York and Chicago: American Diabetes Association and American Dietetic Association, 1977.
102. King, J.C. Protein metabolism in pregnancy. *Clin. Perinatol.* 2:243, 1975.
103. Lefebver, P.J., and Luyckx, A.S. Spontaneous and insulin-induced hypoglycemia. In K. Sussman and R. Metz, Eds., *Diabetes Mellitus,* 4th ed. Philadelphia: W.B. Saunders, 1975.
104. Freinkel, N., and Metzger, B.E. Oral glucose tolerance curve and hypoglycemias in the fed state. *N. Engl. J. Med.* 280:820, 1969.
105. Unger, R.H., and Madison, L.L. Comparison of response to intravenously administered sodium tolbutamide in mild diabetic and nondiabetic subjects. *J. Clin. Invest.* 37:627, 1958.
106. Fajans, S.S., Schneider, J.M., Schteingart, D.O., and Conn, J.W. The diagnostic value of sodium tolbutamide in hypoglycemic states. *J. Clin. Endocrinol. Metab.* 21:371, 1961.
107. Fajans, S.S. Leucine-induced hypoglycemia. *N. Engl. J. Med.* 272:1224, 1965.
108. Conn, J.W. The advantage of a high protein diet in the treatment of spontaneous hypoglycemia. *J. Clin. Invest.* 15:673, 1936.
109. Pemberton, C.M., and Gastineau, C.F. *Mayo Clinic Diet Manual.* Philadelphia: W.B. Saunders, 1981.

Bibliography

American Diabetes Association. Principles of nutrition and dietary recommendations for individuals with diabetes mellitus. *Diabetes Care* 2:540, 1979.

Brownlee, M., Ed. *Handbook of Diabetes Mellitus,* Vols. 1–5. New York: Garland STPM Press, 1981.

Colwell, J.A., Lopes-Virella, M., and Halushka, P.V. Pathogenesis of atherosclerosis in diabetes. *Diabetes Care* 4:131, 1981.

Fain, J.N. Mode of action of oral hypoglycemia drugs. *Fed. Proc.* 36:2712, 1977.

Freinkel, N., and Josimovich, J., Eds. American

Diabetes Association Workshop—Conference on Gestational Diabetes. *Diabetes Care* 3:399, 1980.
Jarrett, R.J. Symposium on nutrition and diabetes. *Proc. Nutr. Soc.* 40:209, 1981.
Kozak, G.P. *Clinical Diabetes Mellitus.* Philadelphia: W.B. Saunders, 1982.
Schade, D.S., Eaton, R.P., Alberti, K.G.M.M., and Johnston, D.G. *Diabetic Coma.* Albuquerque: University of New Mexico Press, 1981.
Skyler, J.S. Complications of diabetes mellitus: Relationship to metabolic dysfunction. *Diabetes Care* 2:499, 1979.
Skyler, J.S. Diabetes and exercise: Clinical implications. *Diabetes Care* 2:307, 1979.
Sussman, K., and Metz, R. *Diabetes Mellitus: Vol. IV. Diagnosis and Treatment.* New York: American Diabetes Association, 1975.
Tepperman, J. *Metabolic and Endocrine Physiology,* 4th ed. Chicago: Year Book Medical, 1980.
Traisman, H.S. *Management of Juvenile Diabetes Mellitus,* 3rd ed. St. Louis: C.V. Mosby, 1980.
Turner, M., and Thomas, B., Eds. *Nutrition and Diabetics.* London: John Libbey, 1981.
Williams, R.H. *Textbook of Endocrinology,* 5th ed. Philadelphia: W.B. Saunders, 1974.
Wood, F.C., Jr., and Bierman, E.L. New concepts in diabetic dietetics. *Nutrition Today* 7:4, 1972.

Sources of Current Information

Diabetes
Diabetes Care
Diabetologia
Journal of Clinical Endocrinology and Metabolism
Recent Progress in Hormone Research

10. Inborn Errors of Metabolism

Sushma Palmer, D.Sc., and Frances J. Zeman, Ph.D.

The diseases categorized in Chapter 1 as developmental disorders may be subdivided into three groups: disorders caused by mutations of single genes, those caused by mutations of multiple genes interacting with the environment, and those caused by chromosomal abnormalities. The diseases discussed in this chapter are known as *inborn errors of metabolism.* They are primarily those disorders in which a mutation of a single gene or a small number of related genes causes a metabolic abnormality. There are a large number of these conditions, but we will discuss here only those for which nutritional care is an essential component of management.

Because genetic aberration is the basis for inborn errors of metabolism, the fundamental concepts of genetics that are necessary for an understanding of these diseases will be explained first. Some general principles of pathophysiology and nutritional care applied to the inborn errors will then be described, followed by a description of specific disorders and their nutritional management.

FUNDAMENTALS OF GENETICS

The hereditary information in each cell is contained in its nucleus. It is necessary to understand, first, how this information is transmitted to new cells during growth in an individual.

Transmission of the Genetic Code

The hereditary information in the nucleus is contained in *chromosomes.* These consist of strands of *DNA,* the basic genetic material of all cells. DNA is a generic term that refers to many specific compounds, just as the word *protein* encompasses many compounds formed from amino acids. It now is well established that DNA molecules consist of chains of nucleotides, usually found in pairs, that are twisted around each other to form a coiled double helix. The two strands are held together by hydrogen bonds between pairs of nitrogenous bases, one on each strand, arranged so that the base, adenine, always is bonded to thymine or a similar analogue and guanine always is bonded to cytosine or a similar analogue. Thus, the nitrogenous base on one strand can serve to identify the nitrogenous base on the other. If the strands are separated, each serves as a template for the structure of the other, and two double helixes, exactly like the first, can be made from the two separated strands. This process of replication underlies the function of DNA as the hereditary material.

In the nonreplicating cell, the strands of DNA are not visible but, in preparation for cell duplication, the double helix unwinds and duplicates itself as just described. At the beginning of cell replication (called *mitosis*), the two strands become visible under the microscope. The formations seen at the beginning of mitosis, the chromosomes, contain the DNA strands. Following duplication of the DNA, each chromosome will consist of two identical strands (*chromatids*) joined at a point called the *centromere.* When the cell replicates, the centromere divides so that one chromatid becomes a new chromosome in each of the daughter cell nuclei, leaving each cell with the same genetic code as the original nucleus.

Every organism has a number of chromosomes characteristic of its species. There are 46 chromosomes in humans. Humans, along with other higher plants and animals, are *diploid*—that is, they inherit a complete set of 23 chromosomes from each parent. The human chromosomes, therefore, occur in pairs, known as *homologous pairs.*

Every living organism must be able to synthesize its own precise proteins. The instructions for the structure of these proteins are carried in the DNA molecules. This is the information transmitted as inherited traits. In specifying the sequence of amino acids that make up a protein, a sequence of either two or three contiguous nucleotides function as a code word or *codon* which identifies a specific amino acid. When amino acids, such as glycine, that are identified by only two nucleotides form part of the sequence, the identity of the third nucleotide becomes irrelevant. However, a third nucleotide is always present to maintain the sequence of triplets. There are also codons that specify the beginning and end of a sequence of amino acids.

The genetic code also must be transmitted from one generation to the next. In the germ cells or *gametes* (*ovum* and *sperm*), the cells divide by a special process called *meiosis* in such a way that the germ cell contains 23 chromosomes. Thus, it is called *haploid* since it has half the usual number of chromosomes. The process by which this is accomplished distinguishes meiosis from mitosis. In the first phase of meiosis, the original chromosomes replicate to create two chromatids that are joined at the centromere in the same fashion as in mitosis. However, the homologous pairs then become attached at their centromeres to form a *tetrad.* At this point, an interchange (*crossover*) can occur between the segments of 1 chromosome and the corresponding segments of the homologous chromosomes, resulting in new combinations so that the two chromatids of each chromosome are no longer identical. The chromatids of the homologous chromosomes are assorted randomly as these new chromosomes separate to form two new nuclei. This separation is the first meiotic division.

The time of the second meiotic division differs in the sperm and ovum. In the sperm, the sister chromatids separate, each forming two more nuclei with only half as many chromosomes. Since the chromatids are not identical, there are now four sperm cells, each with unique chromosomes. This process occurs prior to the fertilization of the ovum. The ovum, still containing 46 chromosomes, is fertilized after the first meiotic division by a sperm containing 23 chromosomes. The second meiotic division of the ovum occurs after fertilization and provides the 23 maternal chromosomes constituting the genetic inheritance of the new infant.

The units of heredity within the chromosomes are the *genes,* the part of the total DNA molecule that specifies the code for a given function (a structural protein or enzyme, for example). The position of a gene for a given trait is known as the *locus.* The genes for many traits exist in variant forms (*alleles*) which account for variation in a trait. Some traits have only one allele, but others have many. A simple example would be alleles for brown eyes and blue eyes. As described in Chapter 7, there are many alleles for histocompatibility. Although the general population may have many alleles for some traits, a given individual can have a maximum of two for any one trait, one from each parent.

The function of many genes, as described for DNA, is to specify the structure of a polypeptide. Genes sometimes work as a group. An *operon* is a group of structural genes which operate somewhat as a single unit and code for enzymes or other proteins. They usually lie adjacent to each other and are controlled as a unit. All cells of the body have the same genetic information. Therefore, following differentiation, much of the DNA code is silenced—that is, made nonfunctional—so that the cells can perform different functions. Thus, adjacent to the operon is an *operator gene,* which serves as an on-off switch for the operon, and a *regulator gene,* which may bind to the operator to turn it off.

Expression of the Genetic Code

Genotype and Phenotype

Each individual normally possesses two genes for each trait. If both genes for a given trait are identical, the person is *homozygous* for that trait but, if the alleles are different, the person is *heterozygous* for that trait. The genetic makeup of an individual is termed the *genotype,* and its visible expression is the *phenotype.* For example, if a person with brown eyes has one allele for brown eyes and one allele for blue eyes, these two alleles constitute the genotype, and the phenotype includes brown eyes. If a trait is expressed when it is present on only one of a pair of chromosomes, it is a *dominant* trait. If it is expressed only when present on both of the chromosomes (homozygous), it is a *recessive* trait. In the brown-eyed example used previously, there is a dominant gene for brown eyes and a recessive gene for blue eyes. Sometimes, the gene expression is intermediate between the forms of the traits specified by the allele (*incomplete dominance*) or two dominant alleles are fully expressed (*codominant*).

The relationship between genotype and phenotype is variable. Some genes have *incomplete penetrance*—that is, the allele is expressed in some individuals but not others, as in diabetes mellitus. Incomplete penetrance often is accompanied by *variable expressivity,* in which the trait may be expressed in somewhat different ways.

Some genes are *pleiotropic;* they affect several apparently unrelated aspects of the phenotype. In many cases, however, the affected aspects may indeed be related and may share some similar steps in their metabolism.

A single feature may be controlled by more than one gene pair and may also be influenced by the environment. For example, genetic effects on height sometimes are modified by diet. The expression of some genes is affected by the internal environment so that the trait is not expressed at birth but appears postnatally.

Sex-Linked Traits

An additional concept which must be understood is that of *sex-linked traits.* There are 22 homologous pairs of chromosomes known as *autosomes* present in both males and females. The twenty-third pair (*sex chromosomes*) differ in males and females. Females have 2 X chromosomes and males have 1 X chromosome and a much smaller Y chromosome. Females receive 1 X chromosome from each parent and provide an X chromosome to each offspring. Males receive an X chromosome from their mothers and a Y chromosome from their fathers. They provide an X chromosome to their daughters and a Y chromosome to their sons. Thus, it is the father who determines the sex of the child.

The Y chromosome has no genes related to traits other than those involved in sex determination, but the X chromosome carries genes affecting other functions. The expression of these genes, called *sex-linked* or *X-linked* traits, may be different in the two sexes. Thus, there are four basic modes of inheriting single gene mutations in humans: *autosomal recessive, autosomal dominant, X-linked recessive,* and *X-linked dominant.*

Males are always *hemizygous* for the genes on the X chromosome, since they have only 1 X chromosome. A sex-linked allele that is recessive in the female will be expressed in the male since there is no alternative allele. Also, a male can receive and transmit to his daughters a sex-linked trait that he received from his mother but he cannot transmit it to his sons since the sons will not receive an X chromosome from him. However, he can pass X-linked traits to his grandsons via his daughters.

Since females have 2 X chromosomes, they may be homozygous or heterozygous for sex-linked traits. If they are heterozygous for a sex-linked recessive trait, they become *carriers* who do not exhibit the trait but can transmit it to half their offspring of either sex. Daughters express sex-linked recessive traits if a male who expresses the trait (their father) mates with a female homozygote (their mother). They may or may not express the trait if the mother is a carrier (heterozygote).

Mutations

Genes usually are very stable, but they can undergo *mutation,* an inheritable change in structure, so that a different allele is formed. We do not know all the causes of mutations nor can we generally identify the cause of a specific mutation. We do know that X-radiation, ionizing radiation, and some chemicals are among their causes. The significance of these will be discussed further in Chapter 13.

Mutations causing disorders of interest to nutritionists may be subdivided into two categories: chromosomal aberrations and point mutations. *Point mutations* involve only a small number of nucleotide pairs in the DNA molecule. The change may consist of insertion, deletion, or substitution of a base pair. Since the code for the amino acid structure of a polypeptide consists of sets of nucleotides, these shifts sometimes lead to the production of a new polypeptide. If the code for an amino acid is identified by the first two nucleotides, there is no effect of a mutational change in the third. This is known as a *silent mutation.* Many mutations are this type.

Approximately one-fourth of all mutations involving a substitution do cause changes in amino acid sequence (*missense mutations*). The severity of the effect depends on the function of the polypeptide whose structure has been altered. Initially, it was believed that one gene contained the code for one enzyme. Subsequently, it was found that this is not precisely accurate. Therefore, the concept has been changed to *"one gene, one polypeptide."* If an enzyme contains more than one chain, each of which is specified by a different gene, mutations of any of these genes have the potential to alter the activity of that enzyme. On the other hand, if a single chain has more than one active site and catalyzes more than one metabolic reaction, a single mutation would affect more than one enzyme action. Missense mutations may thus have effects of varying severity. The conditions discussed in this chapter are, in many cases, the consequences of this type of mutation, but are less severe than those that cause prenatal death.

In other cases, known as *no-sense mutations,* the codon for an amino acid might be mutated to a "stop" signal. Under these circumstances, the synthesis is stopped before the chain is completed, usually resulting in the complete absence of a trait (or enzyme). Deletion or insertion of a base also will cause a no-sense mutation because it will cause a shift in the whole sequence of triplets. No-sense mutations are, however, relatively rare.

Some conditions occur with a frequency that suggests they are the result of a combination of multiple gene mutations and environmental effects. Diabetes mellitus (Chapter 9) and cleft palate (Chapter 16) have been included in this category.

It is important to know the frequency with which a point mutation will be expressed in succeeding generations. This is particularly important when the mutation results in an adverse effect such as an inborn error of metabolism. When each parent carries an autosomal recessive trait, the probability that the trait will be expressed is the same for *each* pregnancy. Let us assume, as an example, that the mode of inheritance of an inborn error of metabolism from a given pair of parents carries the probability that there will be one affected child (homozygote), two carriers (heterozygotes), and one child who does not carry the trait. The probability that the child from the first pregnancy will have the disease is one in four. If the first child is a homozygote—that is, has the disease—there is no guarantee that the next three offspring from successive pregnancies will include one normal child and two carriers. Rather, in the second pregnancy (and all others), the probability that the child will be a homozygote is still one in four.

Chromosomal Abnormalities

Chromosomal abnormalities can have many effects because they affect many genes. They are of two general types: variations in the normal number of chromosomes or gross structural abnormalities of individual chromosomes. A fragment of a chromosome can become attached to another chromosome and thus become *translocated.* Sometimes a piece of a chromosome is *deleted.* Some deletion syndromes result in conditions described elsewhere in this book. They include cleft palate, low birth weight, seizures, failure to thrive (see Chapter 16), and congenital heart disease (see Chapter 8).[1] A third type of chromosomal abnormality is an *inversion* in which two breaks occur in the structure of a chromosome. The free piece then is realigned after a 180-degree reversal of its orientation. Chromosomal abnormalities may lead to fetal death, various congenital malformations (most of which are associated with mental retardation), and, in some cases, to neoplasia.[1]

INTRODUCTION TO INBORN ERRORS OF METABOLISM

The concept that an abnormal gene could impair metabolism and produce a pathologic condition called an *inborn error of metabolism* was first introduced by Garrod[2] in 1908. These inborn errors of metabolism now are known to cause defects of structural proteins, transport proteins, functioning proteins, and proteins that regulate gene expression or gene repair.

In most of the conditions described in this chapter, there is a block in a metabolic pathway caused by a mutation in a single gene. Because one gene is supposed to control the synthesis of one polypeptide, a change in the gene structure could result in a change in the structure of that polypeptide and a consequent change in the activity of the protein product. The protein product may be an enzyme and the condition is classified as an *enzyme defect.* More recently, *defects in transport* have also been recognized as a form of inborn error.

Pathophysiology

The pathophysiologic consequences of the product of a mutant gene depend on the normal metabolic role of the affected pathway. In general, the causes of pathophysiologic effects are categorized as follows:[1]

Abnormal Enzyme Function in Major Metabolic Pathways

The generalized diagram of a metabolic pathway in Fig. 10-1 illustrates the means by which a disorder may be produced. If we assume that the mutant gene product is an abnormal enzyme with reduced or absent activity resulting in a metabolic block in the major pathway, the consequences of such a metabolic block may include accumulation of a precursor to toxic levels, deficiency of an end product, production of toxic products from a normally minor pathway, and overproduction of intermediate products through loss of feedback control.

Accumulation of a Precursor to Toxic Levels. The most commonly described inborn error of metabolism is the accumulation of a precursor to toxic levels. If we assume, in Fig. 10-1, that enzyme cd is missing and there is a block in the metabolic step from product C to product D, the immediate precursor, product C, or more remote precursors, A or B, might increase in concentration in body

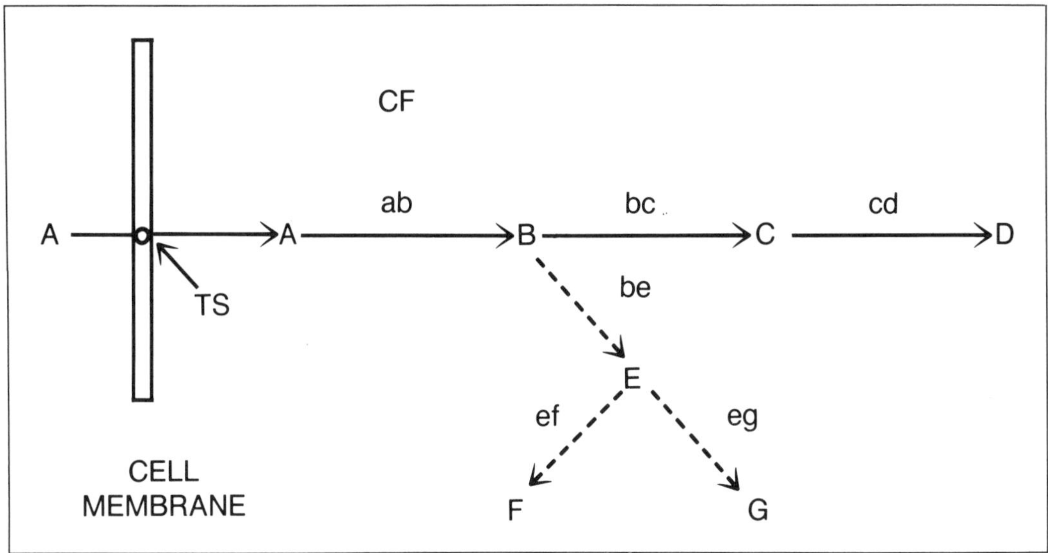

Figure 10-1. A model metabolic pathway. Substrates and metabolic products are indicated in capital letters. Enzymes are represented by lowercase letters corresponding to the substrate and product at their site of action. Solid arrows indicate the major pathway, and hatched arrows, the minor pathways. CF = cofactor; TS = transport system.

tissues. The means by which the toxic effects are produced frequently are unclear. If a substance that accumulates is relatively insoluble and difficult to excrete, it may be stored, producing one of the inborn errors known as *storage diseases.*

Deficiency of End Product. Sometimes a pathologic condition occurs because an essential end product is reduced in concentration. In our model (Fig. 10-1), if product D is essential and there is no alternative pathway, a block at enzyme ab, bc, or cd would result in a deficiency of product D.

Production of Toxic By-Products from a Normally Minor Pathway. In some disorders, the precursor in the major pathway is not the immediate cause of the disease. Instead, a minor pathway may become more active, as a consequence of precursor accumulation, and produce large quantities of a material normally present in minute quantities. In Fig. 10-1, let us assume that there is a block at bc or cd and product B accumulates. The pathways B → E → F, B → E → G, or both, might then become more active and possibly produce pathlogic consequences.

Overproduction of Intermediate Products Through Loss of Feedback Control. A pathologic condition may result from a loss of feedback regulation when an essential end product is missing. For example, if it is assumed that product D in Fig. 10-1 is a hormone the release of which is controlled by another hormone, the absence of feedback control from product D might cause overproduction of the controlling hormone, with consequent pathologic effects.

Defective Plasma Membrane Transport

The transport of essential substances from outside to inside the cell is compromised in some inborn errors. There is some evidence, primarily in microbes, of the existence of permeases. Errors in permease activity might result in transport defects. In humans, most transport defects have been identified in the kidney tubules or intestinal absorptive cells, leading to decreased intestinal absorption, increased renal excretion, or both. Malfunction of the transport system (see Fig. 10-1) could lead to a deficiency of any of the products, A, B, C or D.

Reduced Coenzyme Production or Binding

Disorders related to reduced coenzyme production or binding have been called *vitamin-dependent inborn errors* or *vitamin dependency syndromes.* Theoretically, a very large number of disorders is possible. However, very few are understood completely. It has been suggested that defects in production or binding of cofactors might result from (1) failure to transport the vitamin into certain cells, (2) failure to produce the coenzyme from the vitamin, or (3) failure to bind the cofactor to the apoenzyme to form the active enzyme.[1] In some cases, vitamins or coenzymes in larger than normal quantities may stabilize and increase the activity or concentrations of affected enzymes and prevent the adverse effects which would otherwise result from a metabolic block. Because cofactors function with many apoenzymes, their defects affect many reactions and thereby alter many functions.

Deficiency or Abnormality of Circulating Proteins

A variety of protein materials that circulate in blood cause disease when their concentration or structure and function are altered. Very few of these diseases are amenable to dietary manipulation.

Abnormality of Structural Protein

Genetic abnormalities of collagen-related protein have been associated with metabolic disease. Most abnormalities of this type are not amenable to specific dietary treatment; however, some cause organ dysfunction that requires nutritional care. One such abnormality of collagen-related material causes kidney failure.

Abnormalities of Enzymes that Regulate Drug Metabolism

Abnormalities of enzymes that regulate drug metabolism are expressed only if a patient is exposed to the drug in question. Generally, such disorders are not treated with diet, although a large dose of vitamin B_6 is useful in some patients receiving isoniazid.

Clinical Manifestations

Some inborn errors of metabolism are lethal, whereas others cause varying degrees of incapacitation and still others are benign. In general, if an infant shows unexplained failure to thrive (see Chapter 16), vomiting, feeding difficulties, lethargy, coma, acidosis, jaundice, hepatomegaly, irritability, or hyperactivity, inborn errors must be considered in the differential diagnosis.

The more specific consequences of an inborn error will vary not only with the type of defect, but also with the degree of impairment. Some patients have variants of the classic disease, and the consequences of these variants differ in severity from those of the classic disease. The consequences of a metabolic disorder can sometimes be moderated by appropriate treatment, especially if the disease is diagnosed early. It is important to begin treatment early in most types of treatable inborn errors of metabolism. The central nervous system of the newborn infant is very vulnerable to damage, and many inborn errors, if untreated, can result in mental retardation. The consequences of individual disorders will be described later in this chapter. In some disorders, there is no known method of treatment.

Diagnosis

Most inborn errors of metabolism are not accompanied by pathognomonic symptoms, and thus a variety of diagnostic procedures are necessary to identify specific errors. Genetic screening (the search in the population for certain genotypes) can be used to detect certain inborn errors. In most developed countries, for example, it now is common practice to screen all neonates for phenylketonuria. Other conditions are so rare or their consequences so mild that mass screening is not considered to be cost-effective. In others, adequate screening methods are lacking.

The general types of diagnostic tests used include biochemical analysis of blood, urine, other body fluids, or tissue samples obtained by biopsy. Concentrations of normal substrates, metabolites, or products may be identified as being abnormally high or abnormally low, or the presence of unusual substrates may be detected. In other assays, enzyme activity is determined. Variants of normal proteins sometimes are identified by electrophoresis, enzyme kinetics, or alterations in such properties as response to heat, pH, substrates, inhibitors, or cofactors. Other recent methods include tissue cultures of fibroblasts, blood cells, and cells in the amniotic fluid.

These methods as well as others sometimes are used to identify heterozygote carriers. Many inborn errors are autosomal recessive traits, and the trait can be detected by diagnostic tests. If carriers can be identified, the incidence of the disease can sometimes be reduced by genetic counseling. In addition, if heterozygote carrier parents can be identified, the disease can sometimes be diagnosed before the child is born. *Amniocentesis* (sampling of cells from amniotic fluid) is used for prenatal detection of some inborn errors. This procedure carries some risk but may be necessary in families in which the trait is known to exist. The risk is especially justified in diseases in which early diagnosis and treatment can prevent severe physiologic consequences, impaired growth, and mental retardation.

Management

General Principles of Prevention and Management

The types of treatment available for inborn errors of metabolism depend to some extent on our knowledge of the pathologic processes involved. In some diseases, little is known about these processes, and management must be limited to rehabilitation or to genetic counseling to reduce incidence.

When the impaired metabolic pathway is known, other possibilities exist. It is for this group of patients that nutritional care often is important. The general types of procedures might include the following:

1. For accumulation of precursor to toxic levels: restrict source of the precursor.
2. For deficiency of end product: provide replacement.
3. For production of toxic by-product: restrict source of its precursor.
4. For diseases involving sensitivity to environmental factors (e.g., drugs): avoid exposure.
5. For deficient coenzymes: give increased quantities of the vitamin involved.

In some disorders, the specific product of a defective gene, whether an enzyme, a structural protein or a regulator, is known and influences possible treatment. For instance, if an enzyme is deficient, it might be replaced. One such disorder is cystic fibrosis of the pancreas (see Chapter 6), for which replacement of pancreatic enzymes is a common method of treatment. The number of disorders that can be treated in this way is very limited, however. If the defective gene affects regulation, replacement of the missing repressor, inducer, or inhibitor is a theoretical approach to treatment; currently, though, this is seldom possible and is the subject of ongoing research. The production of abnormal structural proteins can sometimes be prevented, or its consequences can be treated with drugs.

Another area of ongoing research involves genetic engineering to "repair" a defective gene. This approach could be applied only if the specific mutation is known. In some disorders, organ transplants are useful.

Table 10-1. Approximate Nutritive Composition of Special Dietary Products[a]

Nutrient	Lofenalac[b]	Phenyl-Free[b,c]	Product 3200 AB[b]	MSUD Diet Powder[b]	Product 3200 K[b]	Product 80056[b]
Kilocalories	454	406	460	473	464	486
Protein (g)	15	20.3	15	82	14	0
Fat (g)	18	6.8	18	20	19	22.5
Carbohydrate	60	66	60	633	60	73.5
L-Amino acids (g)						
Essential						
Isoleucine	0.75	1.08	0.86	0	0.67	0
Leucine	1.41	1.70	1.76	0	1.16	0
Lysine	1.57	1.85	1.91	0.80	0.87	0
Methionine	0.45	0.62	0.56	0.25	0.16	0
Phenylalanine	0.08	0	<0.08	0.55	0.76	0
Threonine	0.77	0.93	0.65	0.55	0.52	0
Tryptophan	0.19	0.28	0.20	0.20	0.16	0
Valine	1.20	1.24	1.38	0	0.71	0
Histidine	0.39	0.46	0.40	0.28	0.34	0
Nonessential						
Arginine	0.34	0.68	0.39	0.50	0.96	0
Alanine	0.64		0.76	0.45	0.60	0
Aspartate	1.34	5.15	1.60	1.14	1.72	0
Cystine	0.025	0.34	0.042	0.25	0.107	0
Glutamate	3.78	1.85	4.31	2.09	2.76	0
Glycine	0.35	3.30	0.40	0.60	0.59	0
Proline	1.13		1.13	0.90	0.68	0
Serine	1.02		[illegible]	[illegible]		

Vitamin D (IU)	284	406	284	[illegible]	[illegible]	
Vitamin E (IU)	7.1	10	7.1	7	7.2	0
Vitamin C (mg)	37	53	37	38	38	45
Thiamin (μg)	428	609	438	370	440	450
Riboflavin (μg)	714	1,015	714	440	720	540
Vitamin B_6 (μg)	290	508	290	300	360	360
Vitamin B_{12} (μg)	1.4	2.5	1.4	1.5	1.8	1.8
Niacin (μg)	5,714	8,122	5,714	5,900	5,800	7,200
Folic acid (μg)	72	100	72	74	30	90
Pantothenic acid (μg)	2,142	3,046	2,142	2,200	2,200	2,700
Choline (mg)	61	86	61	63	62	76
Biotin (μg)	36	30	36	40	22	45
Vitamin K (μg)	72	102	72	74	71	90
Inositol (mg)	72	102	22	72	73	90
Minerals						
Calcium (mg)	435	634	435	488	2,500	540
Phosphorus (mg)	326	508	326	266	1,500	300
Magnesium (mg)	51	76	51	52	300	63
Iron (mg)	8.6	12	8.6	9	50	11
Iodine (μg)	32	66	32	33	150	41
Copper (μg)	429	609	429	400	2,500	540
Manganese (mg)	0.7	1	0.7	0.7	3.5	0.9
Zinc (mg)	2.9	4.1	2.9	3	15	3.6
Sodium (mEq)	9	10	9	8	61	3
Potassium (mEq)	12	18	12	11.5	66	9
Chloride (mEq)	9	14	9	10	80	4

Modified with permission from the American Academy of Pediatrics Committee on Nutrition, Special diets for infants with inborn errors of amino acid metabolism. *Pediatrics* 57:783, 1976. Copyright © the American Academy of Pediatrics, 1976. Composition of MSUD Diet Powder obtained from Mead Johnson and Company, Evansville, Ind.

[a] Per 100 g of powder.
[b] Mead Johnson and Company.
[c] Originally 3229-A.

Table 10-2. Approximate Daily Requirements for Various Nutrients at Different Ages in Infancy and Childhood

Nutrient	Unit of Measure	0–2 Months	2–5 Months	6–12 Months	1–2 Years	2–3 Years	3–4 Years	4–6 Years	6–8 Years	8–10 Years
Calories[a]	kcal	120/kg	110/kg	100/kg	1,100	1,250	1,400	1,600	2,000	2,200
Volume (H_2O)	ml	100/kg	110/kg	100/kg	1,100	1,250	1,400	1,600	2,000	2,200
Carbohydrate[b]	g				Total kilocalories × 0.50 ÷ 4					
Protein[c]										
Infants	g/kg	1.8–2.2	1.8–2.0	1.8						
Children	g/day				25	25	30	30	35	40
Fat	g				Total kilocalories × 0.35 ÷ 9					
Sodium	mEq/kg	3	3	3	3	3	3	3	3	3
Potassium	mEq/kg	3	3	3	3	3	3	3	3	3
Calcium	mg	400	500	600	700	800	800	800	800	800
Phosphorus	mg	200	400	500	700	800	800	800	900	1,000
Magnesium	mg	40	60	70	100	150	200	200	250	250
Iron	mg	6	10	15	15	15	10	10	10	10
Iodine	μg	25	40	45	55	60	70	80	100	110
Phenylalanine										
Infants	mg/kg	47–90	47–90	25–47						
Children[d]	mg/day				200–500	200–500	200–500	200–500	200–500	200–500
Histidine	mg/kg	16–34	16–34	16–34						
Leucine										
Infants	mg/kg	76–150	76–150	76–150						
Children	mg/day				750–1,000	750–1,000	750–1,000	750–1,000	750–1,000	750–1,000
Isoleucine										
Infants	mg/kg	79–110	79–110	50–75						
Children	mg/day				500–750	500–750	500–750	500–750	500–750	500–750
Valine										
Infants	mg/kg	65–105	65–105	50–80						
Children	mg/day				400–600	400–600	400–600	400–600	400–600	400–600
Methionine[e]										
Infants	mg/kg	20–45	20–45	20–45						
Children	mg/day				400–800	400–800	400–800	400–800	400–800	400–800

Lysine										
Infants	mg/kg	90–120	90–120	90–120						
Children	mg/day				1,200–1,600	1,200–1,600	1,200–1,600	1,200–1,600	1,200–1,600	1,200–1,600
Threonine										
Infants	mg/kg	45–87	45–87	45–87						
Children	mg/day				800–1,000	800–1,000	800–1,000	800–1,000	800–1,000	800–1,000
Tryptophan										
Infants	mg/kg	13–22	13–22	13–22						
Children	mg/day				60–120	60–120	60–120	60–120	60–120	60–120
Vitamin B_1 (thiamine)	μg	200	400	500	600	600	700	800	1,000	1,100
Vitamin B_2 (riboflavin)	μg	400	500	600	600	700	800	900	1,100	1,200
Vitamin B_6 (pyridoxine)	μg	200	300	400	500	600	700	900	1,100	1,200
Vitamin B_{12}	μg	1.0	1.5	2.0	2.0	2.5	3.0	4.0	4.0	5.0
Folic acid	μg	50	50	100	100	200	200	200	200	300
Niacin	mg	5	7	8	8	8	9	11	13	15
Vitamin C	mg	35	35	35	40	40	40	40	40	40
Vitamin A	IU	1,500	1,500	1,500	2,000	2,000	2,500	2,500	3,500	3,500
Vitamin D	IU	400	400	400	400	400	400	400	400	400
Vitamin E	IU	5	5	5	10	10	10	10	15	15

Reprinted with permission from the American Academy of Pediatrics Committee on Nutrition, Special diets for infants with inborn errors of amino acid metabolism. *Pediatrics* 57:786, 1976. Copyright the American Academy of Pediatrics, 1976.

[a] The caloric requirement is increased when protein is provided as a mixture of the corresponding free L-amino acids.

[b] Minimum fraction is 50 percent of total calories; optimum value is given.

[c] Minimum fraction is 4 percent of total calories; optimum value is given.

[d] More phenylalanine (>800 mg) is required in the absence of tyrosine.

[e] More methionine is required in the absence of cyst(e)ine.

[f] More cyst(e)ine is required in the presence of a blocked transsulfuration outflow pathway for methionine metabolism.

Note: These data are compiled from National Academy of Sciences/National Research Council data on Recommended Dietary Allowances (RDA) and from amino acid data of Holt and Snyderman (Holt, L.E., and Snyderman S.E.: The amino acid requirements of infants. *J.A.M.A.* 175:100, 1961; and The amino acid requirements of children. In W.L. Nyhan, Ed., *Amino Acid Metabolism and Genetic Variation.* New York: McGraw-Hill, 1967.). These dietary RDA have the limitations of any statement of dietary requirement because of the individual variations a physician will encounter in working with a patient. This limitation is particularly true with amino acid requirements for which amounts in excess of the requirement are toxic. There is limited information on amino acid requirements of infants and children at different ages; the figures given here are in excess of the minimum requirements. Consequently, this table should be used only as a guide and should not be regarded as an authoritative statement to which individual patients must conform.

Principles of Nutritional Management

Inborn errors that respond to alterations in diet, although relatively few in number, are of particular interest to the nutritional care specialist and provide an opportunity to perform an important service. Proper nutritional management of some of these disorders is sometimes lifesaving and sometimes prevents profound mental retardation.

From the foregoing discussion, it is clear that approaches to nutritional management include (1) restriction of sources of accumulated products, or their precursors or byproducts, (2) replacement of end products, or (3) increased vitamin dosage.

In some inborn errors, it is necessary to restrict severely the intake of certain nutrients. If the adverse effect is the result of accumulation of a nonessential nutrient, such as galactose or fructose, the offending material might be eliminated from the diet. If the nutrient occurs widely in food, the patient or family will need counseling on sources of that nutrient, substitute foods, and menu planning to assure nutritional adequancy.

On the other hand, if the disease requires the restriction of an essential nutrient, the process consists of restriction of that nutrient to the level of minimum requirements and becomes more hazardous and complex. Disorders of amino acid metabolism are good examples of this type of problem. The amino acid must be provided in amounts necessary for normal growth and development and the maintenance of essential metabolic processes, but an excess must be avoided. In addition, essential end products, if deficient as a result of the metabolic block, must be provided. Thus, the patient is walking a fine line between excess and deficiency.

There are two general methods by which adequate but not excessive administration of amino acids can be achieved. In some disorders, total protein intake can be reduced to minimal levels with an increase in nonprotein energy sources. Alternatively, if natural proteins contain an excess of the offending amino acid, a semisynthetic formula with reduced amounts of the offending substrate may be used. These formulas are either protein hydrolysates from which the amino acid in question has been removed or mixtures of pure amino acids. Most of them contain added carbohydrate, fat, vitamins, and minerals to provide adequate nutrition.

The composition of the currently available formulas are given in Table 10-1. Their uses in specific diseases will be described in the section Disorders of Amino Acid Metabolism. They are particularly useful in infancy, when the brain is growing most rapidly and the diet consists almost exclusively of a liquid formula. When these formulas are used, the restricted amino acid usually is provided by measured amounts of milk combined with the special formula. When the child is old enough, solid foods are added, carefully controlling the total amount of the offending amino acid.

The length of time that a child may need such a restricted diet varies. If the primary adverse consequence is impaired myelination of the brain, the diet may be liberalized or may become unnecessary once myelination is complete. In other disorders, the diet is needed for a lifetime.

The tolerance of the patient for an offending amino acid can vary with the circumstances. In diseases in which products of amino acid metabolism tend to accumulate, the patient will have the greatest tolerance for natural protein during periods of rapid growth and when the nutritional status is optimum. In these circumstances, much protein is being used for synthesis, preventing accumulation of toxic metabolites. If, on the other hand, the use of the offending amino acid for growth is impaired by illness or lack of other essential nutrients, the load on the affected degradative pathway is increased, and a toxic metabolite is more likely to accumulate. Therefore, the maintenance of optimum nutrition is highly desirable.

The daily requirements for various nutrients in infancy and childhood are given in Table 10-2. The nutritional care specialist must be familiar with these requirements that serve as guidelines in assessing nutritional adequacy and planning diets for patients with inborn errors to assure normal growth and physical and mental development.

DISORDERS OF AMINO ACID METABOLISM

Of the inborn errors of metabolism that are amenable to nutritional management, errors of amino acid metabolism, particularly involving essential amino acids, are among those that occur most commonly. Nutritional management requires careful continuing cooperation of the nutritional care specialist and the patient, his or her family members (especially parents), teachers, and others. Failure of nutritional management of many disorders of amino acid metabolism can have devastating consequences.

The Hyperphenylalaninemias

The *hyperphenylalaninemias* are a group of disorders that manifest themselves by abnormally high blood levels of phenylalanine. One of these, *phenylketonuria* (PKU), was discovered by Fölling,[3] who found phenylpyruvic acid in the urine of two mentally retarded children. A number of variant forms of PKU have also been identified. Each of these forms involves a defect in the conversion of phenylalanine to tyrosine.

Classic Phenylketonuria

Metabolic Abnormalities. The biochemical defect in classic PKU is a deficit of liver *phenylalanine hydroxylase,* the enzyme that catalyzes the conversion of phenylalanine to tyrosine (Fig. 10-2). As a consequence, there is an accumulation of phenylalanine in body fluids. Concentrations typically exceed 50 mg/dl of blood within a few weeks after birth.

As the blood phenylalanine concentration rises, the activity of alternative pathways increases (see Fig. 10-2). The increased concentration of the substrate induces the action of phenylalanine transaminase and increases phenylpyruvic acid production. The phenylpyruvic acid then is converted to phenyllactic and phenylacetic acids and phenylacetylglutamine. These are found in increased quantities in the urine. Thus, PKU is an example of a disorder in which precursors accumulate and in which there is enhanced activity in minor metabolic pathways.

Excess phenylalanine also affects the metabolism of other amino acids. The absorption of tryptophan from the intestine is inhibited by phenylalanine. Bacterial action on the tryptophan in the intestine increases production of indoleacetic and indolelactic acids from tryptophan. These are absorbed and excreted in increased quantities in the urine. The concentration of blood serotonin, a metabolite of tryptophan, is decreased, and the excretion of 5-hydroxyindoleacetic acid, the metabolite of serotonin, is decreased secondarily.

Tyrosine becomes an essential amino acid for PKU patients, because they cannot form tyrosine from phenylalanine. In addition, tyrosine metabolism is inhibited by the presence of excess phenylalanine. The production of tyrosine metabolites, such as melanin and epinephrine, thus are reduced.

Clinical Manifestations. The phenylketonuric infant generally is considered to be mentally normal at birth. However, some effects may occur before birth. A study of a group of infants with PKU showed lower birth weights, increased numbers of premature births, and perinatal difficulties.[1] Therefore, the prenatal effects deserve further study.

The postnatal consequences of PKU have deservedly received much more attention, since the untreated disease has a devastating effect on the central nervous system. The most severe consequence is impaired mental

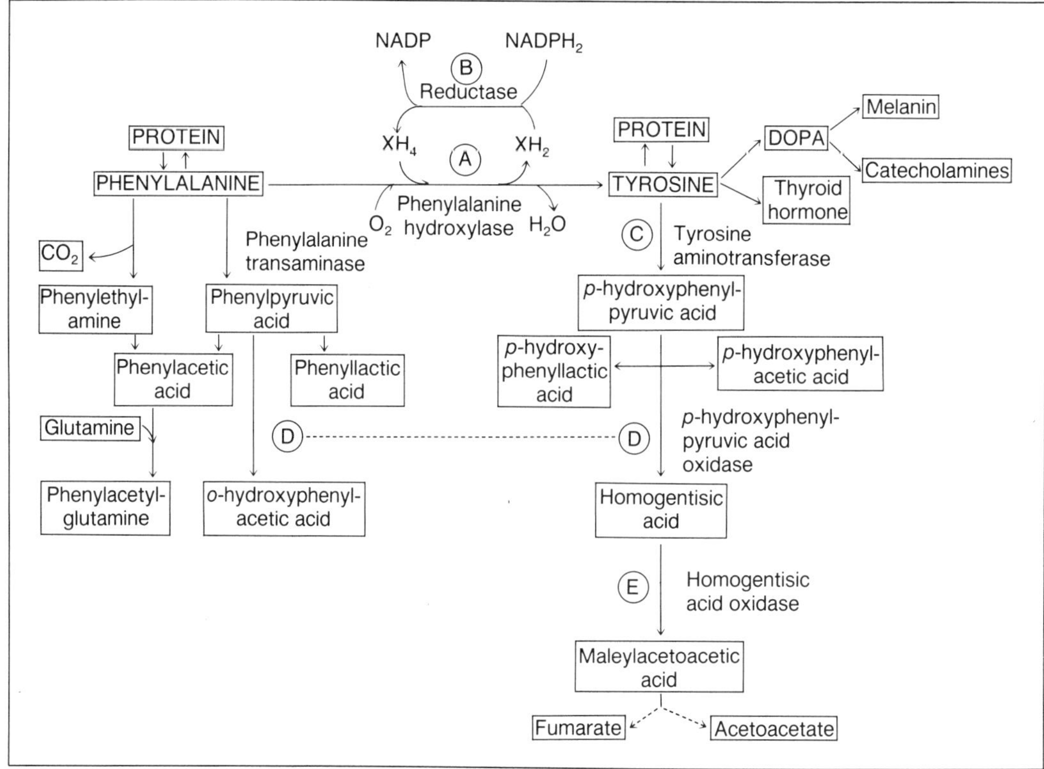

Figure 10-2. Sites of metabolic blocks in phenylalanine and tyrosine metabolism. **A.** *Phenylketonuria.* **B.** *Dihydropteridine reductase deficiency.* **C.** *Tyrosinemia, type* 2. **D.** *Neonatal tyrosinemia and hereditary* (*type* 1) *tyrosinemia.* **E.** *Alkaptonuria.*

development, and it has been estimated that an untreated phenylketonuric infant can lose 50 I.Q. points in its first year. Most untreated patients eventually have an I.Q. of about 20, and only a few have an I.Q. higher than 60 (on a scale in which normal is approximately 100). Many require institutionalization.

The effect on the brain in an untreated phenylketonuric infant becomes particularly noticeable at 4 to 6 months of age. Some behavioral and neurologic manifestations such as hyperactivity, feeding difficulties, and vomiting occur within the first 3 months but may be mistaken for other disorders. The condition progresses to listlessness, apathy, or hyperactivity. Many patients become agitated and aggressive. They may have muscle tremors and later develop an abnormal gait and posture. Approximately one in four patients has convulsions.

The cause of mental retardation in PKU is not understood. The brain is smaller, and myelination is deficient. It has been suggested that the brain damage could be the consequence of unavailability of the amino acids that are needed for protein synthesis, a deficiency of serotonin,[4] the action of phenylethylamine,[5] or other metabolic effects. It is possible that a combination of factors causes the brain damage.

The reduced production of melanin and the consequent deficiency of melanin pigment in the skin, hair, and eyes causes the child to be fairer in coloration than the rest of the family. Many phenylketonuric patients have a mousy or musty odor which has been attributed to phenylacetic acid in the urine and perspiration. Some patients have eczema of unknown origin. Other manifestations of classic PKU include *microcephaly* (a small head in proportion to body size) and reduced life expectancy, possibly related to institutionalization.

The consequences of PKU can be considerably moderated and, in some cases, entirely avoided if treatment is begun in the early postnatal period, ideally in the first 2 weeks. If this is done, the patient should grow and develop normally both mentally and physically. Failure to institute treatment in the first few weeks postnatally is likely to lead to brain damage and mental retardation. The brain damage is irreversible, but other biochemical and clinical manifestations subside to some degree if the child is treated later.

Heredity and Incidence. Phenylketonuria is inherited as an autosomal recessive trait, and classic PKU occurs in homozygotes for the trait. Therefore, the parents are assumed to be heterozygous carriers. The incidence of hyperphenylalaninemia varies. It is highest in Germany and the British Isles and lowest in Finland, Switzerland, and Sweden. Incidence in the United States is estimated to be approximately 1 in 12,500 live births.

Diagnosis and Monitoring. Because the consequences of untreated PKU are so serious, most states now require testing of neonatal infants to detect PKU. The normal infant has a serum phenylalanine level of less than 2 mg/dl. A test result of 4 mg/dl or higher must be investigated further. If serum phenylalanine is 20 mg/dl or more and serum tyrosine is normal (1 to 4 mg/dl), treatment is begun immediately.

Several types of diagnostic tests have been used. For years, a commonly used test consisted of the reaction between ferric chloride and phenylpyruvic acid in the infant's urine to form a green color. Ferric chloride (in the form of Phenistix) or 2,4-dinitrophenylhydrazine (DPNH) may be used at home to detect phenylpyruvic acid and are useful for monitoring identified cases. These tests give a general guide to the effectiveness of treatment. However, they have serious disadvantages for use in initial diagnosis, because they are not specific for phenylpyruvic acid but will react with other compounds, and some metabolites interfere with the reaction. Also, they are not sufficiently sensitive, and appreciable brain damage may occur if treatment is delayed owing to false-negative results in these tests.

More recently developed methods for measuring serum phenylalanine are preferable for diagnosis. The *Guthrie bacterial inhibition assay* uses a drop of blood obtained by heel prick and can detect phenylalanine levels greater than 4 mg/dl of whole blood. The blood on the filter paper is applied to the surface of agar containing the organism *Bacillus subtilis* and *beta-2-thienylalanine,* a phenylalanine antagonist. High levels of phenylalanine will overwhelm the action of the antagonist, allowing the organism to grow at a rate proportionate to the phenylalanine concentration. Alternatively, the blood sample can be eluted from the filter paper and the phenylalanine level measured by a photofluorometric assay.

When the screening test indicates the possibility of PKU, quantitative determinations of serum phenylalanine and its metabolites should be done promptly. High levels of phenylalanine and the presence of *o*-hydroxyphenylacetic acid in the urine are pathognomonic for PKU.

The blood phenylalanine concentration rises postnatally as the infant is fed protein containing excess phenylalanine. Thus, it is important that the test not be done too early. It is estimated that 5 percent of cases are missed because of inadequate protein feeding prior to the test.

The general criteria for diagnosing classic PKU are (1) evidence of sustained hyperphenylalaninemia with levels of phenylalanine greater than 16 mg/dl when dietary intake of phenylalanine is normal; (2) failure of plasma tyrosine to rise after loading with phenylalanine; (3) decrease in plasma phenylalanine to nearly normal levels when dietary phenylalanine is restricted to approximately 250 to 500 mg/day in infancy and childhood; and (4) presence of the heterozygote trait in the parents.

Nutritional Management. Experience in recent years has demonstrated normal mental and physical development in patients with classic PKU if they are managed properly with low-phenylalanine diets. Although there is some disagreement as to the length of time that the diet is required and a few untreated phenylketonuric individuals have normal intelligence, a large body of evidence now supports the continued use of the phenylalanine-restricted diet.

Excess phenylalanine must be avoided, but the minimum requirement must be provided in carefully measured quantities since it is an essential amino acid. Care must also be taken to assure intake of enough phenylalanine and other nutrients to avoid tissue catabolism. If the patient is undernourished and tissue is catabolized, phenylalanine is released, with possible subsequent brain damage. Therefore, the objectives of nutritional management of PKU patients are:

1. To supply an adequate diet to support normal growth rate
2. To supply sufficient phenylalanine for protein synthesis
3. To avoid excessive phenylalanine which would lead to elevated concentrations in the blood

Guidelines for approximate daily intakes of phenylalanine, protein, and energy are given in Table 10-3. Some practitioners recommend greater protein intakes than those given in Table 10-3. There are several reasons for this difference of opinion. Estimates of protein requirements for infants are approximate at best, since detailed knowledge is lacking. Protein requirements vary with the source and type of protein and are dependent on digestibility. In general, the protein requirements for breast-fed infants are believed to be lower than for formula-fed infants. Since infants with PKU usually are bottle-fed, there is some tendency to aim for a higher protein intake. Nevertheless, it must be recognized that supporting data are lacking. In addition, many infants with inborn errors of metabolism are poor feeders, and the higher intakes often are not achievable.

Table 10-3. Approximate Daily Intake of Phenylalanine, Protein, and Kilocalories in Phenylketonuria

Age (yr)	Phenylalanine (mg/kg/day)	Protein (g/kg/day)	Kilocalories (per kg/day)
0.0–0.5	50–60	2.2–2.5	110–120
0.5–1	30–50	2.0–2.5	100–120
1–3	20–30	1.8–2.0	90–100
4–6	20–25	1.5–1.8	80–90
7–10	15–25	1.2–1.5	80–85
11–14	10–15	1.0–1.2	60–70
15–18	5–15	0.8–1.2	40–60
19–22	5–10	0.8–1.0	40–50
Pregnancy	10	1.3	50

Based on data from the National Academy of Sciences, Food and Nutrition Board, *Recommended Dietary Allowances,* 9th ed. Washington, D.C.: National Academy of Sciences, 1980; and Berry, H.K., Hyperphenylalaninemias and tyrosinemias. *Clin. Perinatol.* 3:15, 1976.

Natural foods offer variety but also are sources of phenylalanine. Thus, their use is limited by the need to limit phenylalanine intake. As a consequence, a formula free of or low in phenylalanine is used to help meet the child's nutritional requirements. If too much or too little phenylalanine is present, protein metabolism may be inefficient and may interfere with normal growth and development.

Steps in planning a phenylalanine-restricted diet. Steps in planning a phenylalanine-restricted diet are described in detail and will serve as a model for planning nutritional management of other inborn errors described later in this chapter.[6,7]

Step 1: Use Table 10-3 or the Recommended Dietary Allowances (Table 10-2) to *compute the daily requirement for protein, phenylalanine, and energy.* For example, let us assume the patient is a 6-month-old infant weighing 7 kg, with a good control of serum phenylalanine and normal growth and development, with 30 mg of phenylalanine, 2.5 g of protein, and 110 kcal/kg body weight in the diet. The total daily requirements would then be:

Phenylalanine requirement: 30 mg/kg × 7 kg = 210 mg
Protein requirement: 2.5 mg/kg × 7 kg = 17.5 g
Energy requirement: 110 kcal × 7 kg = 770 kcal

Adjustments in these values must be made frequently, sometimes weekly, as the child grows.

Step 2: Calculate the amount of low-phenylalanine powdered formula required to meet 80 to 90 percent of the daily protein requirement. Most of the protein must be derived from this source, since natural foods, which may also serve as protein sources, contain too much phenylalanine.

Low-phenylalanine formulas generally available in the United States are Lofenalac for infants and Phenyl-Free for older children. The phenylalanine, protein, and energy contents of these formulas for purposes of diet calculation are included in Table 10-4. Further details of composition are contained in Table 10-1. Some new products are beginning to be sold but are not generally available. The nutritional care specialist should be alert to the appearance on the market of new products for these patients.

If Lofenalac is used in our 6-month-old, 7-kg patient, the calculation could be as follows:

Protein to be derived from Lofenalac:
80% of 17.5 = 14 g

Thus, the amount of Lofenalac needed is 14.0 g of protein divided by 1.4 g/Tbsp. or

Table 10-4. Phenylalanine, Protein, and Energy Content of Selected Food Groups

Food Group	Phenylalanine (mg)	Protein (g)	Energy (kcal)
Phenylalanine-restricted protein sources, 1 tbsp.[a]			
Lofenalac	7.5	1.4	43
Phenyl-Free	0	2.0	41
Evaporated milk, 1 oz.	104	2.1	42
Vegetables, variable serving[b]			
Strained and junior	15	0.5	20
Table	15	0.6	10
Fruits, variable serving[b]			
Strained and junior	15	0.6	150
Table and juices	15	0.6	70
Breads, crackers, cereals[b]	30	0.6	30
Miscellaneous (largely potatoes and pastas)[b]	30	0.6	32
Soups, canned, condensed[b]	15		
Fats, selected desserts[b]	5	0.1	60
Free foods (candies, carbonated beverages, sugars, starch, nondairy creams)	0	0	Variable

Modified with permission from Acosta, P.B., and Elsas, L.J., II, *Dietary Management of Inherited Metabolic Disease.* Atlanta: ACELMU Publishers, 1976, p. 14.
[a] 1 Tbsp. = 10 g = 1 measure, which is included in the container.
[b] For lists of specific foods and serving sizes, see P.B. Acosta and E. Wenz, *Diet Management of PKU for Infants and Preschool Children,* D.H.E.W. Publication No. (HSA) 78-5209, Washington, D.C.: U.S. Department of Health, Education, and Welfare, 1978.

10.0 Tbsp. (10 "measures"). A measuring device is included in the container and holds 1 Tbsp. or 10 g.

Step 3: Calculate the amount of evaporated milk to be added to provide enough phenylalanine for growth. The relevant nutritive values for evaporated milk are given in Table 10-4.

Again using our example of a 6-month-old, 7-kg infant, the amount of evaporated milk may be calculated as follows:

Phenylalanine in Lofenalac = 10 Tbsp. × 7.5 mg/Tbsp. = 75 mg
Phenylalanine to be provided from milk or other sources = 210 mg − 75 mg = 135 mg
Therefore, add 1 oz. evaporated milk × 104 mg/oz. = 104 mg

The calculated amount of milk is mixed with Lofenalac so that the child does not develop a taste for milk.

The remaining amount of phenylalanine will be provided by solid foods (see Step 5).

Step 4: Calculate the amount of fluid needed including that mixed with the Lofenalac powder. The amount varies with age and preference. Lofenalac is a concentrated source of protein and carbohydrate. Therefore, children tend to need more fluid than usual. For small infants, it may be as high as 130 to 200 ml/kg. Older children with PKU generally will demand more fluids than do nonphenylketonuric children. The extra fluid reduces the solute load excreted by the kidneys and assists in the elimination of byproducts of phenylalanine metabolism.

Let us assume that the fluid requirement of our hypothetical infant is 120 ml/kg.

Thirty ml equals approximately 1 oz. Then:

$$120 \times 7 \text{ kg} = 840 \text{ ml}$$

$$\frac{840 \text{ ml}}{30 \text{ ml/oz.}} = 28 \text{ oz. of fluid.}$$

The Lofenalac and evaporated milk are diluted and the mixture can be made up to a total volume of 28 oz. The number of formula feedings and the size appropriate for various ages are given in Appendix N. For the infant in our example, 4 bottles of 7 oz. each might be appropriate.

Step 5: Calculate the amounts of solid foods to be included in the diet. Solid foods should be introduced at the same age as for the nonphenylketonuric child. Appropriate ages at which various solid foods are given to the normal child are shown in Appendix N. Examples of the phenylalanine content of groups of foods are contained in Table 10-4. These groups may be used in a manner similar to the way the exchange lists are used for diabetic diets (see Chapter 9). Detailed lists of the contents of each solid food group with exchange lists are available in hospital diet manuals and various educational materials for patients.

The exchange lists for fruits, vegetables, breads and cereals, soups, fats, and miscellaneous items contain foods divided according to their phenylalanine content—0, 5, 15, or 30 mg per serving. The phenylalanine, protein, and energy content are listed for individual foods within each list. Serving sizes vary within each list. For example, 5 Tbsp. of strained carrots contain 0.5 g of protein and 19 kcal, and 2 Tbsp. of strained green beans contain 0.3 g of protein and 7 kcal: Despite the difference in serving size, both will provide 15 mg of phenylalanine. Serving sizes generally are small, often expressed in tablespoons, since the patient is very young. On the average, phenylalanine makes up 5 percent of the protein in breads, cereals, and fat, 3.3 percent of the protein in vegetables, and 2.6 percent of the protein in fruit. Meat, fish, and poultry are excluded, since they are too high in phenylalanine content. The parent is instructed in menu planning using the exchanges. Phenylalanine should be distributed evenly in planning meals. In addition, phenylalanine from natural foods must be offered within an hour of the time that the formula is given to ensure that all the amino acids necessary for protein synthesis are available simultaneously.

Step 6: Provide additional energy sources if needed. For example, corn syrup, honey, or sugar can be added to the formula if the formula and solid foods do not provide sufficient energy. For example, assume the kilocalorie requirement is 770 and the following energy is supplied:

Energy Source	*Kilocalories*
10 Tbsp. Lofenalac	430
1 oz. evaporated milk	42
1 serving fruit purée	150
1 serving vegetable purée	20
Total	642

The deficit is 128 kcal (770 − 642). This amount could be provided in 2 Tbsp. of corn syrup to be added to the Lofenalac.

Usually, breast-fed infants are weaned quickly and bottle-fed with Lofenalac when a diagnosis of PKU is made. Occasionally, however, a mother prefers to continue to breast-feed. A procedure for partial breast feeding of PKU infants is available for use in this situation.[8]

Human milk has 0.8 to 0.9 g/dl of protein compared to 3.3 g/dl in cow's milk. It is lower in phenylalanine and higher in nonprotein nitrogen. A mean value of 41 mg of phenylalanine per deciliter of breast milk is used for purposes of calculation. The diet is calculated to allow for a combination of breast feeding and Lofenalac feeding. The amount of breast milk ingested is determined by weighing the baby before and after feeding. The amount of breast milk the infant takes can be controlled by limiting the time allowed for breast feeding.

Making dietary adjustments for age. As the child grows older, adjustments must be made to meet increased need for nutrients for growth and development. Some general guidelines follow.

The addition of solid foods and self-feeding should begin on a normal schedule. One such schedule is:

Feed Lofenalac partly as a paste beginning at 3 to 4 months. It may be mixed with fruit or honey.

Add fruit purée at 2 to 3 months, and vegetable purée and strained cereals at 3 to 4 months.

Low-phenylalanine breads may be given at 5 to 8 months. Sources of these products are listed in Appendix M.

Add coarsely chopped foods and begin cup feeding at approximately 9 months.

Begin finger and spoon self-feeding at 10 to 12 months.

Raw foods can be given at 15 to 18 months.

Phenyl-Free is substituted for Lofenalac for the older child, to allow greater use of solid foods. Fruit juices and fruit drinks may be used to flavor Phenyl-Free. "Free" foods—that is, foods that are phenylalanine-free—may be added to provide adequate energy. These foods are forms of pure carbohydrates and fats. Excess use should be avoided to assure that other foods are not refused. In addition, a multiple vitamin and iron supplement may be needed.

Feeding problems. Feeding problems may arise as they do in nonphenylketonuric children, but are likely to be the source of great anxiety to the parents of a child with PKU. The nutritional care specialist can be very helpful in counseling such parents. Koch et al.[9] have suggested some reasons for certain common problems:

If a child is *unduly hungry,* the prescribed diet may be inadequate, or the child may be refusing the Lofenalac and solid foods do not satisfy the appetite. Possibly, the prescribed foods are being refused in order to obtain sweet foods.

Loss of appetite may occur if the child is ill or if there are too many sweet foods in the diet. Overprescription of Lofenalac may lead to reduced appetite for other foods, or there may be a phenylalanine deficiency.

Refusal of Lofenalac can result temporarily from a normal fluctuation of appetite, or there may be failure to offer Lofenalac consistently. Other causes of refusal may be the inclusion of calorie-containing beverages, or too much water added to Lofenalac, making the volume excessive. Also, the formula may be too thick and unpalatable, or the child may be manipulating the parents.

Refusal of solid foods can result from a normal fluctuation of appetite or the refusal of prescribed food to obtain sweet free foods. Possibly, Lofenalac has been overprescribed. Alternatively, the child may be manipulating the parents.

Follow-up. Frequent measurements of serum phenylalanine levels and urinary metabolites are used as guidelines to determine the effectiveness of dietary control in PKU patients. A generally used schedule for determination of blood phenylalanine levels includes twice-per-week assays in the initial adjustment period, followed by assays once per week for infants, once every 2 or 3 weeks for toddlers, and once monthly thereafter. A record of food ingested prior to blood sampling should be kept to aid in interpretation of the test results. In addition, periodic measurements of physical growth, nutritional adequacy of the diet, and psychological and neurologic evaluations are necessary to monitor the patient's progress.

The serum phenylalanine concentration usually is maintained between 3 and 7 mg/dl. Some centers permit a 3- to 10-mg/dl range. Evidence indicates that maintenance of the concentration at this slightly elevated level does not cause intellectual damage, and it reduces the danger of protein malnutrition by allowing a greater protein intake.

The diet must be continually monitored and adjustments made when control is lost. Loss of dietary control with increased serum phenylalanine may be the result of (1) prescription of more protein and phenylalanine than is needed, (2) failure to follow the diet, or (3) infection, undernutrition, or trauma that causes tissue catabolism with release of phenylalanine. If serum phenylalanine rises beyond the acceptable level, corrective measures must be taken promptly.

The diet prescription should be recalculated as necessary. In some circumstances, however, the primary need is more careful adherence to the prescribed diet, and nutritional counseling can be very important. The parents must understand the importance of the diet and the procedures for following the diet and for record keeping. They must make every effort to assure that siblings, grandparents, neighbors, and others do not feed the child foods that are not allowed. These procedures are relatively simple when the patient is fed only a bottled formula. However, the formula is fairly expensive, and many parents react unfavorably to its odor and taste. When solid foods are added, the process becomes more complicated. Planning meals and record keeping are difficult, and so parents must be instructed very thoroughly. In addition, the child's condition can place stress not only on parents but on siblings, who may resent the attention provided to the affected child.

When a child becomes ill and tissue catabolism causes a rise in serum phenylalanine, a diet lower in phenylalanine may be needed. Sometimes a phenylalanine-free diet is needed.

Problems may also arise from amino acid deficiency. A deficiency can occur as a consequence of lack of understanding of the diet by the parents; food refusal; vomiting or malabsorption, which reduces the amount of amino acid available; or inadequate intake due to an excess volume of formula or other food. A deficiency also can arise when the prescribed amount of phenylalanine is inadequate. This can occur, for example, following an illness when the amino acid requirement is increased to provide for healing or if energy intake is inadequate.

The first symptoms of a deficiency of phenylalanine are feeding difficulties, reduced rate of weight gain, and skin rash. These occur when plasma phenylalanine is less than 1 mg/dl (60 μmole/L). If the deficiency continues, gastrointestinal upsets, edema, lethargy, anemia, and bone changes ensue. The condition may progress to mental retardation, convulsions, and death.

At 3 months of age, the child can be given a "challenge" to be certain of the accuracy of the diagnosis. The child is given foods containing 180 mg of phenylalanine for each of 3 consecutive days and blood phenylalanine levels are determined. If blood phenylalanine rises quickly, the test is terminated early. In some infants, phenylalanine levels fail to rise, indicating that the child is not phenylketonuric.

Duration of Diet. The duration of currently accepted diet therapy is still a matter of controversy. Many investigators have attempted to determine the effects on development of terminating the diet at 3 to 10 years of age, and some have reported no adverse effects, but the follow-up in most cases was short.[10–12] In the United States, there is a trend toward later discontinuation. Current practice varies greatly.

Alternatives to Phenylalanine Restriction in Phenylketonuria. Methods other than dietary phenylalanine restriction have been attempted for treating PKU, but with limited success. Berry et al.[13] recently used oral supplements of valine, isoleucine, and leucine in PKU patients and reported significant reduction in the ratio of phenylalanine in the cerebrospinal fluid and serum.

Vorhees et al.[14] discuss the potential for combined administration of phenylalanine and *p*-chlorophenylalanine, the use of large amounts of neutral amino acids other than phenylalanine, and the use of alphamethylphenylalanine in combination with phenylalanine. They concluded that future research on the treatment for PKU holds considerable promise.

Variant Forms of Phenylketonuria

It is apparent that persistent elevation in phenylalanine levels postnatally is not sufficient evidence by itself for diagnosis of classic PKU. There are a number of variants of PKU (Table 10-5) which appear to have a substantially lower incidence than classic PKU. From the biochemical standpoint, as Table 10-5 shows, it is important to distinguish classic PKU from *atypical* and *transient* forms in which the enzymatic defect is similar but the effects are not as severe as in the classic disease. In these cases, plasma phenylalanine levels can be maintained within the normal range by moderate or temporary restriction of phenylalanine in the diet.

Another group of patients, approximately one-fourth of all patients with hyperphenylalaninemia, have a mild or benign disease without the clinical manifestations of classic PKU. The postnatal rise in plasma phenylalanine in these patients is slow, seldom reaching 20 mg/dl. Phenylpyruvate derivatives usually are not produced in significant amounts. Measurements of phenylalanine hydroxylase activity and oral loading tests with L-phenylalanine are used to distinguish this form of hyperphenylalaninemia from classic PKU. The need for dietary restriction varies, and surveys show that intellectual development usually is normal in untreated patients with mild hyperphenylalaninemia.[15]

In contrast, biochemical findings in *dihydropteridine reductase deficiency* are similar to those of classic PKU in the newborn period, but dietary restriction of phenylalanine is not sufficient to control the neurologic symptoms.[16] The patient has normal phenylalanine hydroxylase activity but may have a defect in biopterin metabolism. Phenylalanine hydroxylase requires a cofactor, biopterin, in an active tetrahydro form (see Fig. 10-2) as a hydrogen ion donor. Biopterin, upon releasing the hydrogen, forms an unstable dehydro compound (*quinonoid biopterin*). This compound normally is recycled by the action of the deficient enzyme.

Maternal Phenylketonuria

Some children with PKU who received proper early treatment have grown to adulthood and reproductive age. As a result, an additional complication, *maternal PKU,* has appeared in recent years.[17,18]

Table 10-5. Differential Diagnosis of Hyperphenylalaninemia

Disorder	Enzyme Affected	Mode of Inheritance	Biochemical Findings
Classic phenylketonuria	Phenylalanine hydroxylase	Autosomal recessive	Plasma phenylalanine >16 mg/dl; diet therapy with 250–500 mg phenylalanine per day needed to normalize plasma levels
Atypical phenylketonuria	Phenylalanine hydroxylase	Probably autosomal recessive	Plasma phenylalanine >16 mg/dl; responds to diet with >500 mg phenylalanine per day
Transient phenylketonuria	Phenylalanine hydroxylase	Autosomal recessive	Transient plasma phenylalanine levels >16 mg/dl; condition becomes benign or normal several months or years after birth
Benign hyperphenylalaninemia	Phenylalanine hydroxylase	Autosomal recessive	Plasma phenylalanine >16 mg/dl; clinically benign; no diet therapy needed
Phenylketonuria (dihydropteridine reductase deficiency)	Dihydropteridine reductase	Probably autosomal recessive	Resembles classic phenylketonuria but no central nervous system response to low-phenylalanine diet

Based on Rosenberg, L.E., and Scriver, C.R., Disorders of amino acid metabolism. In P.K. Bondy and L.E. Rosenberg, Eds., *Metabolic Control and Disease,* 8th ed. Philadelphia: W.B. Saunders, 1980.

A high blood phenylalanine level in the mother is toxic to the fetus and causes intrauterine growth retardation, congenital anomalies, and mental retardation. Investigators have reported variable success in treating women with PKU with a phenylalanine-restricted diet during pregnancy.[19] However, care has to be taken to avoid restriction of phenylalanine in the diet during pregnancy to the extent that microcephaly and intrauterine growth retardation would ensue. Few adult women with PKU have produced normal infants. Still unresolved is the question of whether dietary treatment begun after conception is helpful, and the outcome of treatment begun before conception has not been evaluated.[18] It is important that the adult woman who has PKU and who is contemplating pregnancy be given genetic counseling so that she understands the risks.

Disorders of Tyrosine Metabolism

Variant Forms

Several disorders of tyrosine metabolism are responsive to nutritional management. *Transient* or *neonatal tyrosinemia* occurs in approximately 0.5 percent of full-term infants and there is a greater incidence in premature infants. The condition subsides quickly in most infants but may persist in a few. In these, it generally disappears by 3 months of age, even without treatment.

A block may exist at the metabolic step requiring *p*-hydroxyphenylpyruvic acid (*p*-HPPA) oxidase (see Fig. 10-2) and possibly also at the steps requiring tyrosine transaminase and phenylalanine hydroxylase. These enzymes normally become active at birth, but some infants have an immature liver and inadequate development of these liver enzymes, thereby resulting in high blood tyrosine levels and consequent urinary excretion of *p*-hydroxyphenyllactic acid and *p*-HPPA.

The condition is exacerbated by a high-protein diet, including many infant formulas made with cow's milk which is high in tyrosine. As a consequence, a low intake of phenylalanine and tyrosine has been suggested for management. This may be accomplished temporarily by restricting the total protein content of the diet. Ascorbic acid is required for normal *p*-HPPA oxidase, and doses of 50 to 100 mg of ascorbic acid per day sometimes will correct the metabolic consequences. There is some controversy regarding the necessity for treatment because the condition generally is benign. However, retardation has been reported in some affected infants.

Hereditary tyrosinemia or *tyrosinemia type 1,* also known as *inborn hepatorenal dysfunction,* is a more serious condition in which there is a block similar to that seen in neonatal tyrosinemia (see Fig. 10-2).[20] It is an autosomal recessive trait that occurs in 1 in 50,000 to 100,000 births, and is characterized by severe impairment of liver and renal tubule function. Mental retardation may occur but is not obligatory.[21] The metabolic defect is demonstrated by tyrosyluria and accumulation of *p*-hydroxyphenyllactic and *p*-hydroxypyruvic acids. In addition, hypermethioninemia occurs in many cases, resulting from an accompanying deficiency of the methionine-activating enzyme cystathionine synthetase. Clinical manifestations in the *chronic form* include failure to thrive, progressive liver disease and renal damage, cataracts, hypoglycemia, hypotonia, rickets, hyperpigmentation, and mental retardation. Hereditary tyrosinemia may be fatal if untreated. In the *acute form,* onset is in the first 6 months of age and leads to death from liver failure in 90 percent of untreated patients.

The clinical manifestations of this condition cannot be explained on the basis of a deficit in activity of *p*-HPPA oxidase alone, although the enzyme deficit may have an effect. It has been suggested that the biochemical disorders may be secondary to another lesion and that the disease may not be an inborn error of metabolism in the generally accepted sense of the term.[22]

The diet must be tyrosine-restricted and phenylalanine-restricted since phenylalanine is a source of tyrosine. Product 3200 AB (see Table 10-1) may be used for this purpose, but it is high in methionine. Patients with high plasma methionine levels may have improved liver and renal function if methionine intake is restricted also. Frequent feedings prevent the hypoglycemia. Those patients with rickets consequent to the renal disease may improve with large doses of vitamin D.

Two other disorders of tyrosine metabolism, possibly related to tyrosine aminotransferase dysfunction, have been described. One, referred to as *tyrosinosis* (*Medes type*), is known to have occurred in one case only. It was described by Medes[23] at a time when present analytic methods were not available and is thought to represent a tyrosine aminotransferase deficit. It probably is benign, and no treatment is required. The disorder was characterized by increased blood tyrosine and increased urinary excretion of *p*-HPPA (see Fig. 10-2).

The second disorder has been called *tyrosinemia type 2, hypertyrosinemia,* or *tyrosinosis* (*Oregon variety*).[24] It is thought to represent a deficit of the soluble form of tyrosine aminotransferase which occurs in the cytosol of the liver cells as opposed to a less soluble form which exists in the mitochondria. The patients have elevated serum tyrosine, increased excretion of the phenolic acids (*o*-hydroxyphenylpyruvic, *o*-hydroxyphenyllactic, and *o*-hydroxyphenylacetic acids [see Fig. 10-2]), erythematous palmar and plantar lesions, mental retardation, and corneal ulcers. Some of the lesions respond to dietary manipulation. A diet restricted in phenylalanine and tyrosine is recommended.[25,26]

Lastly, a disorder of tyrosine metabolism that is due to a deficit of *homogentisic acid oxidase* leads to *alkaptonuria*, one of the four conditions originally described by Garrod.[2] Biochemical manifestations include lifelong homogentisic aciduria. The condition seems benign at first, but the homogentisic acid forms a dark compound of unknown composition, possibly a polymer, which accumulates in connective tissue and gives it a black color. This condition, known as *ochronosis*, is accompanied by a crippling arthritis.

Once they are established, there is no treatment for the ochronosis and the arthritis, but the use of a phenylalanine-restricted and tyrosine-restricted diet has been suggested as a possible approach to prevention. Since the diet is relatively unpalatable and alkaptonuria appears benign at first, this approach has not been tried for a sufficiently protracted period to be evaluated.

Nutritional Management

The restriction of phenylalanine and tyrosine in diets for tyrosinemias is intended to maintain plasma tyrosine between 1.5 and 6.5 mg/dl. A recommended program for monitoring includes plasma tyrosine determinations three times per week for 2 weeks following diagnosis and weekly thereafter until stabilization.[7] Plasma tyrosine, phenylalanine, and methionine then are determined monthly. A 3-day diet record should precede blood sampling to aid in interpretation of results. Growth, development, liver function, and renal tubular function should also be evaluated at intervals.

The diet is calculated by a procedure very similar to that used for PKU. The recommended intakes of tyrosine, phenylalanine, protein, and energy need to be estimated. Some currently used guidelines are contained in Table 10-6. Product 3200 AB (Mead Johnson) is used as the basis of the diet. It is a powder to which water is added. Milk is added in measured amounts to supply the necessary phenylalanine and tyrosine. Additional water to meet the fluid requirement is provided separately if necessary. As the child gets older, vegetables, fruit, and breads and cereals are calculated into the diet from exchange lists as described previously. The average content of phenylalanine and tyrosine in the food groups in the exchange lists is given in Table 10-7.

Branched-Chain Ketoaciduria

Branched-chain ketoaciduria (*BCK*) is known also as *maple syrup urine disease* (*MSUD*). In addition to the classic form of the disease, there are several genetic variants — *intermittent, intermediate*, and *thiamine-responsive.*[16]

Table 10-6. Guidelines for Daily Intake of Phenylalanine, Tyrosine, Protein, and Energy in Tyrosinemia

Age (yr)	Phenylalanine (mg/kg)	Tyrosine (mg/kg)	Protein (g)	Energy (kcal)
0–0.25	68–80	60–80	2.2–4.4/kg of body weight	120/kg
0.25–0.5	58–75	61–82	2.2–3.3/kg of body weight	115/kg
0.5–1	42	42	2.0–2.2/kg of body weight	110/kg
1–3	25–85	25–85	23	1,300
4–8	22–50	8–50	30	1,800
9–10	25	25	36	2,400
11–14	1,026 (total)	523 (total)	44	2,400–2,800

Modified with permission from Acosta, P.B., and Elsas, L.J., II, *Dietary Management of Inherited Metabolic Disease.* Atlanta: ACELMU Publishers, 1976, p. 40.
Note: The total phenylalanine and tyrosine should be considered in the prescription, since most phenylalanine is converted to tyrosine.

Table 10-7. Average Phenylalanine, Tyrosine, Protein, and Energy Content of Food Groups for Use in Phenylalanine-Restricted and Tyrosine-Restricted Diets

Food Groups	Phenylalanine (mg)	Tyrosine (mg)	Protein (g)	Energy (kcal)
Product 3200 AB				
100 g	82	21	15	458
1 Tbsp.	7	<2	1.3	5.1
Milk				
Whole, 100 ml	185	163	3.5	67
Evaporated, 100 ml	336	357	7.0	137
Vegetables[a]	15	10	0.5	10
Fruits[a]	10	5	0.4	55
Breads and cereals[a]	18	12	0.4	15
Fats[a]	4	6	0.1	90
Free foods[a]	0	0	0	Variable

Modified with permission from Acosta, P.B., and Elsas, L.J., II, *Dietary Management of Inherited Metabolic Disease.* Atlanta: ACELMU Publishers, 1976, p. 42.

[a] Serving size varies. See exchange lists for phenylalanine-restricted and tyrosine-restricted diets.

Classic BCK is an autosomal recessive disorder. It is characterized by convulsions soon after birth, a peculiar maple syrup–like odor of the urine, feeding difficulties, and a constant shrill cry. These are soon followed by neurologic symptoms including a loss of *tendon reflexes* and *Moro's reflex* (see Chapter 16). Alternating periods of hyperactivity and flaccidity commonly are seen. The patient may die during the first few weeks or months.[27] Brain damage and mental retardation commonly occur in untreated survivors in the classic disease. Its incidence is estimated to be 1 in 80,000 to 1 in 250,000 live births.

Biochemical Abnormalities

The metabolic defect in classic BCK consists of a deficiency of *branched-chain keto acid decarboxylase,* the enzyme that is necessary for oxidative decarboxylation of the branched-chain amino acids (BCAAs) leucine, isoleucine, and valine (Fig. 10-3). It is not clear yet whether there is one enzyme or three closely related enzymes under common genetic control that are responsible for the three reactions.

The affected amino acids and their keto derivatives accumulate in the plasma and urine. Keto derivatives accumulate and clinical symptoms appear when the amino acid levels exceed 1 mM in the plasma.[28] Leucine accumulates to the greatest extent, although the block affects all three amino acids.

The accumulation of the amino acids themselves, rather than their metabolites, is believed to be responsible for the mental retardation. The mechanism responsible for retardation appears to be defective myelination in the brain.[29]

Diagnosis

Homozygous BCK patients can be easily identified because of the characteristic odor of the urine that usually appears in the first week of life. A mass screening technique uses a bacterial inhibition assay, and diagnosis is confirmed by quantitative determination of the plasma levels of BCAAs, of branched-chain alpha-keto acids, and of alloisoleucine, which is a metabolite of the accumulated isoleucine.

Heterozygotes can be detected by the presence of alloisoleucine in fasting blood samples, by tolerance tests for the BCAAs, or by a test of the ability of leukocytes to metabolize leucine keto derivatives.

Variant forms of BCK are differentiated from the classic disease on the basis of the same tests. In addition, clinical features vary

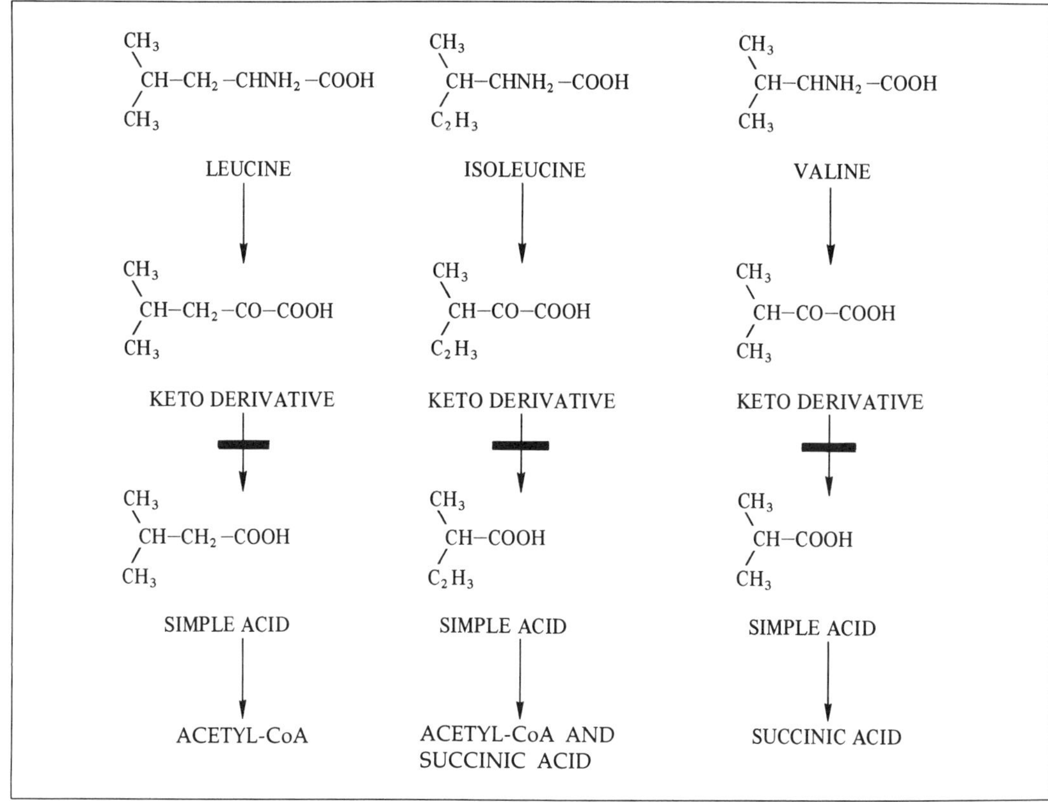

Figure 10-3. Biochemical block in branched-chain ketoaciduria. The deficiency or absence of branched-chain decarboxylase prevents oxidative decarboxylation of leucine, isoleucine, and valine, thereby preventing the formation of acetyl-CoA, acetyl-CoA and succinic acid, and succinic acid, respectively. (Reprinted with permission from Scribanu, N., and Palmer, S., Maple syrup urine disease. In S. Palmer and S. Ekvall, Eds., Pediatric Nutrition in Developmental Disorders, *1978. Courtesy of Charles C Thomas, Publisher, Springfield, Ill. P. 217.)*

somewhat. Comparison of the level of keto acid decarboxylase activity to normal controls can be useful in diagnosis.

Nutritional Care

Infants with BCK are at maximal risk in the immediate postnatal period; therefore, a restricted diet must begin as soon as a diagnosis is made.[7] Branched-chain ketoaciduria often responds well to strict dietary control begun very soon after birth.

The objectives of nutritional management in BCK are analogous to those for the management of PKU. The accumulation of abnormally high levels of the branched-chain amino acids and their metabolites in the body fluids must be prevented. At the same time, sufficient quantities of these essential amino acids must be provided in the diet to support normal growth and development. There are currently two types of formulas available for this purpose in the United States, although others may be available soon. One feeding method consists of a mixture of gelatin and crystalline amino acids as a source of protein. A commercial mixture from which the three offending amino acids have been omitted may be purchased. To this gelatin–amino acid mixture is added a sufficient amount of milk to provide the required minimal level of the BCAAs, oil, and carbohydrate to meet energy needs, plus a mineral mix, vitamins, and sufficient water to meet the fluid requirement. A product providing the vitamins, minerals, fat, and carbohydrate, Product 80056 (see Table 10-1) may be combined with the gelatin–amino acid mixture for greater convenience.

A second, more complete, formula is MSUD Diet Powder (see Table 10-1). It consists of an amino acid mixture free of BCAAs. It also includes the necessary carbohydrate, fat, vitamins, and minerals. Supplementation with a small amount of milk provides the necessary amounts of BCAAs and constitutes a complete formula.

When BCK is diagnosed, the infant is given a formula made of a mixture free of BCAAs until the serum level of BCAAs falls to normal concentrations. However, the plasma concentrations of all three BCAAs usually are not reduced simultaneously. Once each is normalized, supplements of that amino acid must be given in physiologic amounts or provided as natural foods to prevent deficiency. Leucine often falls most slowly and may require 8 to 10 days to reach normal levels.

Once the concentration of all three BCAAs in the serum is normalized, a more complete diet can be calculated. The procedures are very similar to those used for PKU patients:[7]

1. Calculate the requirements for protein, energy, isoleucine, leucine, and valine (Table 10-8).
2. Calculate the amount of milk or other foods required to provide BCAAs for normal growth (see Table 10-9). Many clinicians specifically prescribe only the leucine, which is controlled within narrow limits of 1 to 2 percent. Isoleucine and valine may vary 10 to 30 percent but should be monitored also.
3. Calculate the amount of formula required to supply *at least* the protein requirement (Table 10-9).
4. Calculate the amount of fats and carbohydrates necessary to supply the required energy, and the necessary minerals must be added separately.
5. Add water to meet fluid needs.
6. Provide vitamin supplements as required.

Solid foods should be added at normal times during growth and development. Normal ages for addition of solid foods to the

Table 10-8. Guidelines for Daily Intake of Protein, Isoleucine, Leucine, Valine, and Energy for Children with Branched-Chain Ketoaciduria

				Protein (g)		
Age (yr)	Isoleucine (mg/kg)	Leucine (mg/kg)	Valine (mg/kg)	Gelatin–Amino Acid Mixture	Pure Amino Acids	Energy (kcal)
0–0.25	70	161	93	2.2/kg	4.4/kg	120/kg
0.25–0.5	70	161	93	2.2/kg	3.3/kg	115/kg
0.5–0.75				2.0/kg	2.5/kg	110/kg
0.75–1				2.0/kg	2.5/kg	105/kg
1–3				25	25	1,300
4–6				30	30	1,800
7–10	30	45	33	35	35	2,400

Adapted with permission from Acosta, P.B., and Elsas, L.J., II, *Dietary Management of Inherited Metabolic Disease.* Atlanta: ACELMU Publishers, 1976, p. 69.

Note: There are no data available on amino acid needs from age 7 months to approximately 10 years. Plasma levels of branched-chain amino acids should be used to determine amounts to offer in the diet.

Table 10-9. Nutrient Composition of Foods for Children with Branched-Chain Ketoaciduria

Food and Serving Size	Protein (g)	Isoleucine (mg)	Leucine (mg)	Valine (mg)	Energy (kcal)
Gelatin, 100 g	85.6	1,357	2,930	2,421	342
MSUD Diet Powder, 100 g	8.2	0	0	0	473
Product 80056	0	0	0	0	490
Whole milk, 100 ml	3.5	223	344	240	67
Vegetables[a]	0.7	23	30	27	15
Fruits[a]	0.6	15	25	25	90
Breads and Cereals[a]	0.4	15	35	20	20
Fats[a]	0.1	7	10	8	70

Modified with permission from Acosta, P.B., and Elsas, L.J., II, *Dietary Management of Inherited Metabolic Disease.* Atlanta: ACELMU Publishers, 1976, p. 71.
[a] Serving size varies. See exchange lists for isoleucine-restricted, leucine-restricted, and valine-restricted diets.

infant's diet are given in Appendix N. See Table 10-9 for categories of acceptable foods and their nutritional values. These foods are grouped into four lists: vegetables, fruits, breads and cereals, and fats. Detailed exchange lists stating serving sizes that vary within the lists, are given to parents. Foods within a list can be exchanged in a manner similar to that used in planning a low-phenylalanine diet. Additional energy, if needed, can be provided with fats and pure carbohydrates.

If therapy is begun in the immediate postnatal period with a synthetic diet restricted in the amounts of BCAAs, the following results can be expected:

Mental development may be normal.
The typical odor of the urine fades as chemical control is achieved.
Hypertonicity becomes less noticeable and disappears.
Normal tendon reflexes reappear with improvement in the sucking and swallowing reflexes.
The seizures cease, followed by a return of the electroencephalogram to normal.

It is difficult to decide how rigidly the plasma amino acid levels should be controlled, but it is important to keep them within normal limits (2.5 mg/dl for valine, 0.97 mg/dl for isoleucine, and 1.58 mg/dl for leucine). An effort should be made to maintain plasma leucine between 2 and 5 mg/dl.[7] Leucine levels greater than 10 mg/dl are associated with the appearance of *ataxia* (failure of muscle coordination). A recommended schedule suggests monitoring until normal levels are reached, and then monitoring weekly until 1 year of age, twice monthly up to 3 years of age, and monthly thereafter. A 3-day diet record should be kept prior to obtaining each blood sample and submitted with the sample to assist in interpretation.

Possibly as a result of a defect in gluconeogenesis, hypoglycemia is a common complication in untreated BCK patients.[30] Another frequent complication is the onset of infections. Because they lead to a rapid breakdown of body protein and to amino acid imbalance in the plasma, they are potentially life-threatening. Several patients have died at age 10 years or later from infections or from severe acidosis, which is also a common occurrence.

As is the case with PKU, the duration of diet therapy is still a matter of much debate. Because the chief anatomic lesion in this disease is defective myelination, the necessity for dietary control may be assumed to be reduced after myelination is complete. In older, untreated patients, the degree of developmental delay appears to be less severe. Whether this represents a less severe form of the disease or some form of compensation is not clear yet.

Variant Forms

The *intermittent* form of BCK consists of attacks that are similar to classic BCK, but the biochemical findings disappear periodically. Onset may be as late as at 8 years of age and often is precipitated by an infection. An attack may be fatal. Peritoneal dialysis may be necessary during acute episodes, followed by a low-protein diet as a precaution between episodes. Mental retardation may result, but some patients are reported to have normal intelligence.

A few patients have an *intermediate* or *mild* type of the disease. Branched-chain amino acids and keto acids accumulate, but their concentrations are lower than those seen in the classic form of the disease. Mental retardation has been present in most patients described, and protein restriction was not helpful.[27]

Some patients respond to the administration of thiamine. It has been suggested that thiamine may prolong the biologic half-life of the deficient enzymes. In *thiamine-responsive BCK,* the Committee for Improvement of Hereditary Disease Management[31] recommends the administration of approximately 10 mg of thiamine per day and a moderately-low-protein diet (2 g/kg/day).

The Homocystinurias

Several different forms of *homocystinuria* are recognized. From the nutritional standpoint, the homocystinurias are important because of their relatively high frequency, which is estimated to be 1 in 35,000 to 1 in 200,000 live births for the classic form.[32] Except

Table 10-10. Comparison of Clinical and Biochemical Features in Three Forms of Homocystinuria

Feature	Cystathionine Beta-Synthetase Deficiency	Defective Cobalamin Coenzyme Synthesis	$N^{5,10}$-Methylene-tetrahydrofolate Reductase Deficiency
Mental retardation	Common	Common	Common
Growth retardation	Absent	Common	Absent
Dislocated optic lenses	Almost always	Absent	Absent
Thromboembolic disease	Common	Absent	Rare
Megaloblastic anemia	Absent	Rare	Absent
Homocystine in blood and urine	Increased	Increased	Increased
Cystathionine in blood and urine	Decreased	Normal or increased	Normal or increased
Methylmalonate in blood and urine	Normal	Increased	Increased
Serum cobalamin	Normal	Normal	Normal
Serum folate	Normal or decreased	Normal or increased	Normal or decreased
Response to vitamin	Pyridoxine	Cobalamin (vitamin B_{12})	Folate
Dietary methionine restriction	Helpful	Harmful	Harmful

From Rosenberg, L.E., and Scriver, C.R., Disorders of amino acid metabolism. In P.K. Bondy and L.E. Rosenberg, Eds., *Metabolic Control and Disease,* 8th ed. Philadelphia: W.B. Saunders, 1980, p. 695.

for PKU, they may be the most common treatable inherited disorder of amino acid metabolism.

Biochemical and Clinical Abnormalities

The biochemical and clinical features of three forms of homocystinuria are summarized in Table 10-10.

Cystathionine beta-synthetase deficiency homocystinuria, the most common form, is inherited as an autosomal recessive disorder involving a block in the metabolism of homocysteine to cystathionine (Fig. 10-4). In addition to the clinical features shown in Table 10-10, patients with this type of homocystinuria commonly have a light complexion and growth failure, but these features are not present in all cases. Homocystinurics frequently have significant skeletal abnormalities. Arterial and venous thromboses may be fatal in early adulthood. Mental retardation, apparently related to excessive homocystine, is common in untreated patients, but it progresses slowly and may not be recognized early.

Homocystinuria is characterized by severe elevation of methionine (approximately 30 mg/dl, as compared with slightly more than 0.45 mg/dl normally) and homocysteine (5 mg/dl, as compared with normally undetectable levels) in the plasma and excessive excretion of homocystine in the urine (270 mg/L as compared with normally undetectable levels).

As shown in Table 10-10, there are two other genetic defects that result in less common forms of homocystinuria. Homocystinuria accompanies any condition in which the rate of homocysteine methylation catalyzed by N^5-methyltetrahydrofolate–homocysteine methyltransferase is reduced significantly (see Fig. 10-4). This can occur from failure to form N^5-methyltetrahydrofolate, as a consequence of a reductase deficiency, thereby resulting in a decreased rate of

Figure 10-4. Sites of metabolic blocks in the homocystinurias. **A.** *Classic disease due to impaired cystathionine beta-synthetase.* **B.** *Reductase deficiency with failure to form N^5-methyltetrahydrofolate.* **C.** *Methyltransferase deficiency with failure to form methyl-B_{12}.* **D.** *Impaired cellular uptake of vitamin B_{12}.*

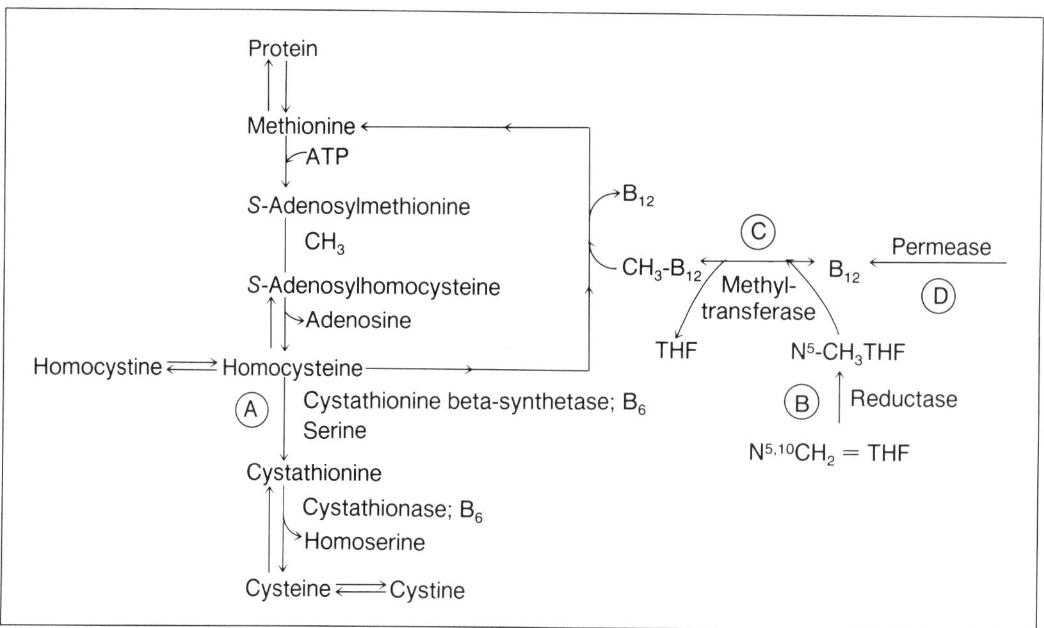

transfer, or in failure to form methyl-B_{12}, a cofactor required by N^5–methyltetrahydrofolate–homocysteine methyltransferase. This may occur in cases of vitamin B_{12} deficiency or through impaired cellular uptake or metabolism of vitamin B_{12}.

Diagnosis

For preliminary screening, the urine is tested for an excessive amount of disulfide. Quantitative determination of homocystine in fasting blood and in urine confirms the diagnosis. Urine normally contains no detectable homocystine. The concentration of methionine must be measured to determine the exact enzyme involved. An elevated methionine level indicates a deficiency of cystathionine beta-synthetase, whereas a normal or reduced methionine level suggests that another enzyme is involved.

Nutritional Management

The major objectives in the nutritional management of the form of homocystinuria due to synthetase deficiency are to reduce the intake of the precursors of homocysteine and yet to supply the dietary elements necessary for growth and development. Patients diagnosed at birth and treated since early infancy have been reported to grow normally, both physically and mentally.[32] The methionine requirement per kilogram of body weight needs to be reduced and adjusted as the child grows. General guidelines to determine the approximate amounts of methionine, protein, and energy needed are contained in Table 10-11. In older, untreated cases, dietary restriction is unable to reverse dislocated lenses, mental retardation, or other clinical features; however, it may be of assistance in preventing lethal vascular occlusions.

In newly diagnosed patients, increased doses of some vitamins can be tried first to differentiate between the types of homocystinuria. Some homocystinuric patients have been successfully treated with 250 to 500 mg of pyridoxine, suggesting that their form of homocystinuria is vitamin B_6–responsive.[33] The biochemical basis for vitamin B_6 responsiveness is not clear,[27] but vitamin B_6 is a coenzyme for cystathionine synthetase and may act by stabilizing the subunits of the mutant enzyme.

Patients with the transferase deficiency produced by cobalamin malabsorption or a defect in vitamin B_{12} metabolism are reported to respond to parenteral cobalamin administration, whereas one case with decreased N^5-methylenetetrahydrofolate reductase deficiency showed dramatic psychological improvement with folate

Table 10-11. Guidelines for Daily Intake of Methionine, Protein, and Energy in Homocystinuria due to Synthetase Deficiency

			Protein (g)		
Age (yr)	Methionine (mg/kg B.W.)	Cystine (mg/kg B.W.)	From Isomil	From Product 3200 K	Energy (kcal)
0–0.5	42	300	2.0/kg B.W.	4.4/kg B.W.	120/kg B.W.
0.5–1	20	200	1.5/kg B.W.	2.5/kg B.W.	110/kg B.W.
1–3	10–23	150	1.25/kg B.W.	25	1,300
4–6	10–18	100	1.00/kg B.W.	30	1,800
7–10	10–13	100	1.00/kg B.W.	35	2,400

Adapted with permission from Acosta, P.B., and Elsas, L.J., II, *Dietary Management of Inherited Metabolic Disease.* Atlanta: ACELMU Publishers, 1976, p. 55.
B.W. = body weight.

supplements. These forms of homocystinuria do not respond to methionine restriction.[27] Further research is needed to determine beneficial therapeutic approaches for these conditions.

A low-protein, low-methionine diet has been used successfully by some investigators to treat patients who are identified early but who do not respond to vitamin therapy.[32] In addition, supplements of cystine are necessary. The mutation prevents the production of cysteine from methionine and cysteine (or cystine) becomes an essential amino acid. In addition, foods low in methionine are also low in cystine.

The formula used, Product 3200 K (see Table 10-12), is a soy protein isolate with a small amount of added methionine. It provides 34 mg of methionine per 100 kcal or 138 mg/100 g of powder and contains fat, carbohydrate, vitamins, and minerals at levels that usually are appropriate for the infant. No vitamin supplements are needed.

Table 10-12. Nutrient Content of Commercial Formulas and Foods Used in a Methionine-Restricted Diet

Food	Total Protein (g)	Methionine (mg)	Energy (kcal)
Product 3200 K (powder), 100 g	13.9	138	464
Isomil (normal dilution), 100 ml	2.0	36	67
Milk, whole, 100 ml	3.5	85	67
Vegetables[a]			
Group 1	0.7	10	10
Group 2	1.5	10	35
Fruits[a]	0.8	5	75
Breads and cereals[a]	1.5	20	55
Fats[a]	0.1	2	65
Free foods[a]	0	0	Variable

Modified with permission from Acosta, P.B., and Elsas, L.J., II, *Dietary Management of Inherited Metabolic Disease.* Atlanta: ACELMU Publishers, 1976, p. 56.

[a] Serving size varies. See exchange lists for methionine-restricted diets.

The procedure used for calculation of the formula is similar to that used for PKU and BCK. Exchange lists are available for two subgroups of vegetables and for fruits, breads and cereals, and fats. Items from a list of selected foods are used to increase the energy content of the diet. Mean values for these food groups also are given in Table 10-12. Specific lists of the foods contained in each exchange list are available in some hospital and clinic diet manuals and in instruction materials for patients. These lists must be supplied to patients or parents.

Plasma methionine must be monitored two or three times weekly until the condition stabilizes and weekly thereafter during the first year, twice monthly until 5 years of age, and monthly thereafter. The objective of treatment is to achieve a methionine concentration of less than 1.0 mg/dl of fasting plasma. A food record of 3 days' intake immediately prior to each blood analysis is helpful in evaluation. Although dietary restriction may be difficult to maintain in older patients, there is no indication that the diet can be discontinued without considerable risk of clinical manifestations. Patients with low or normal levels of plasma methionine should not be treated with a low-methionine diet.

Other Disorders of Amino Acid Metabolism

Table 10-13 summarizes the major clinical and biochemical manifestations, principles of diagnosis, and dietary management in other inborn errors of amino acid metabolism.[34-74] Although most of these are known to be transmitted as autosomal recessive disorders and most of them are rare, it should be noted that ornithine transcarbamylase deficiency is thought to be an X-linked disorder, and that histidinemia, Hartnup disease, and cystinuria occur fairly frequently. The incidence of each is estimated to be in the general range of 1 in 10,000 to 1 in 30,000 live births.

Disorder, Inheritance, and Incidence	Enzymatic Defect	Clinical and Biochemical Findings	Diagnosis	Dietary Management
Disorders of branched-chain amino acids				
Hypervalinemia (Wada et al.,[34] Wada[35]); autosomal recessive	Valine aminotransferase? Possible defect in transamination or decarboxylation	Vomiting, lethargy, failure to thrive, mental retardation, delayed motor development, increased plasma and urinary valine	Hypervalinemia and hypervalinuria, concentration of other branched-chain acids normal	Provide nutrient intake sufficient to maintain growth[36,37] and maintain plasma valine in normal range. MSUD Diet Powder plus leucine and isoleucine. When plasma valine approaches normal (2.6 mg/dl), add milk to provide approximately 65–105 mg of valine per kilogram of body weight for maintenance of normal plasma valine in infants. Replace milk with solid foods as appropriate for age[38]
Isovaleric acidemia (Tanaka et al.[39]); autosomal recessive; 1 : 200,000	Isovaleryl-CoA dehydrogenase (converts isovaleryl-CoA to beta-methylcrotonyl-CoA)	Severe metabolic acidosis and ketosis, vomiting, lethargy, neurologic symptoms, convulsions which may be fatal; or mental retardation, offensive body odor, plasma and urinary elevation of isovaleric acid, isovalerylglycine in blood (6–30 mg/dl) and in urine[38]	Isovaleric acid in blood during acute episodes; thin-layer chromatography to detect isovalerylglycine in urine[40]	Provide adequate nutrient intake and minimal leucine needed to maintain growth and nitrogen balance; management of acidosis; low-protein diet to restrict leucine;[41] MSUD Diet Powder plus isoleucine and valine until serum isovaleric acid level approaches normal (0.6 mg/dl). Then add milk to provide approximately 76–229 mg of leucine per kilogram of body weight for infants. Replace milk with other foods as appropriate for age;[38] supplements of glycine (250 mg/kg/day) to promote isovalerate excretion and relieve clinical symptoms[42]

(continued)

Table 10-13. Diagnosis and Dietary Treatment of Selected Disorders of Amino Acid Metabolism (continued)

Disorder, Inheritance, and Incidence	Enzymatic Defect	Clinical and Biochemical Findings	Diagnosis	Dietary Management
Methylmalonic acidemias (Oberholzer et al.[43]); autosomal recessive in most cases	Two disorders: methylmalonyl-CoA mutase deficiency or defect of cobalaminocoenzyme synthesis; possible methylmalonyl-CoA racemase defect	Poor feeding, dehydration, hypotonia, intermittent apnea, persistent vomiting,[38] elevated urinary and plasma methylmalonic acid, severe ketoacidosis and hyperglycinemia in early infancy, hyperammonemia, absence of megaloblastic anemia in some. May be fatal. In milder cases, methylmalonic acid in urine up to 5 g/day (compared to <5 mg) and up to 34 mg/dl in plasma (normally undetectable)[16]	Diagnosis of unexplained ketoacidosis, elevated methylmalonic acid in urine, elimination of B_{12} deficiency (in cobalamin-responsive cases), homocystinuria, hypermethioninemia, assay of methylmalonyl-CoA mutase activity in fibroblasts to differentiate the two forms[44]	Rosenberg and Scriver[16] suggest 1,000-μg/day vitamin B_{12} injection to test for B_{12}-responsive trait. In B_{12}-responsive cases, cobalamin injection of up to 200 μg/day, starting with lower doses. Low-protein diet (0.5–1.0 g/kg/day) in non-B_{12}-responsive form;[45,46] low-methylmalonate precursor formulas also useful. Reduce valine, isoleucine, methionine, threonine. Product 80056 with the required amino acids added[38]
Propionic acidemia (ketotic hyperglycinemia (Childs et al.[47]); autosomal recessive	Propionyl-CoA carboxylase	Recurrent attacks of ketoacidosis, vomiting, seizures, electroencephalographic changes, hyperammonemia, neutropenia aggravated by infection or high-protein diet; symptoms vary in severity and death may occur in early infancy; branched-chain amino acids induce hyperglycinemia and propionate formation	Propionic acid in plasma or urine; propionicacidemia more reliable feature than hyperglycinemia since it does not occur in nonketotic hyperglycinemia;[48] confirmation by enzyme assay in leukocytes or fibroblasts[49]	Provide calories from carbohydrate; add vitamins and minerals. May use Product 80056.[38] Limit protein to control propionic acidemia and infections. Limit odd carbon chain fatty acids and cholesterol;[50] some patients respond to biotin[51] — 5 mg biotin twice daily until plasma propionate is normal. Give S-14 (Wyeth) at 0.5 g of protein per kilogram and increase until ketones are positive; then decrease to prior protein intake. Limit isoleucine, leucine, methionine, threonine, valine, which precipitate

recessive; 1:15,000		blood, urine, other tissues; impaired formation of urocanic acid; impaired speech and mental retardation in 40%; excessive imidazole pyruvic acid in urine	phy or other method, may be confused with PKU; direct or indirect evidence of histidase deficiency for confirmation	potential clinical consequences (controversial)[53,54]
Disorders of imino acid metabolism				
Hyperprolinemia, types I and II (Scriver[55]); autosomal recessive	Type I: proline oxidase; type II: pyroline-5-carboxylic acid dehydrogenase	Block in proline metabolism; clinical symptoms not well defined. *Type I:* probably benign; elevated plasma proline (<2 mM). *Type II:* probably benign; may affect brain development; hyperprolinemia usually more severe than in type I (>1.5 mM)	Plasma proline >0.45 mM considered abnormal; partition paper chromatography or more precise chemical method to detect proline in urine and plasma	Low-protein diet (approximately 6 mg/kg/day compared to normal intake of 125–300 mg/kg/day) may lower plasma proline.[56,57] Need for diet therapy questionable if condition is benign
Hyperhydroxyprolinemia (Efron et al.[58]); autosomal recessive	4-Oxoproline reductase	Probably benign; elevated plasma hydroxyproline (normal, 0.01 mM); other amino acids normal; urinary hydroxypyroline elevated; may have hyperactivity and mental retardation, but not proved	Partition paper chromatography of serum, plasma, or whole blood to detect hydroxyproline; elevated urine levels alone not definitive diagnosis	Low-hydroxyproline diet not effective in lowering hydroxyproline in body fluids.[59] Need for therapy questionable
Disorders of tryptophan metabolism				
Xanthurenic aciduria, pyridoxine-responsive (Knapp[60]); possibly X-linked	Kynureninase	Kynureninase requires pyridoxal phosphate as a coenzyme; the mutation may reduce affinity for the latter. Significant xanthurenic aciduria, sometimes with mental retardation	Significant reduction in kynureninase activity in liver biopsy in absence of pyridoxal phosphate; abnormal tryptophan loading test[61]	Favorable response to pyridoxine supplements[61]

Table 10-13. Diagnosis and Dietary Treatment of Selected Disorders of Amino Acid Metabolism (*continued*)

Disorder, Inheritance, and Incidence	Enzymatic Defect	Clinical and Biochemical Findings	Diagnosis	Dietary Management
Disorders of urea cycle				
Carbamylphosphate synthetase deficiency (Scriver and Rosenberg[27])	Carbamylphosphate synthetase 1 (CPS 1)	Hyperammonemia and lethal ammonia intoxication in first week of life (blood ammonia >1,000 mg/dl); coma soon after protein feeding; CPS 1 activity 5–15% of normal	Direct assay of enzyme in hepatic tissue; exclusion of other causes of partial reduction in CPS 1 activity	Possibly low-protein diet (1–1.5 g/kg) to control hyperammonemia and nervous system symptoms,[16] or new approach with nitrogen-free analogues of amino acids[62]
Ornithine transcarbamylase deficiency (Russell et al.[63]); X-linked	Ornithine transcarbamylase (OTC)	Ammonia in blood and CSF elevated; urinary and CSF glutamine increased; OTC activity absent or <10%; mental retardation, feeding problems, seizures, coma (more severe in men)	Deficiency of OTC in liver; other urea cycle enzymes normal; hyperammonemia; need to distinguish from orotic aciduria	Complete OTC deficiency lethal; partial deficiency responds to low-protein diet (1–1.5 g/kg).[16,64] Generous kilocalories, excess aspartate, arginine[38]
Citrullinuria (McMurray et al.[65]); autosomal recessive	Argininosuccinic acid synthetase (ASS)	Three forms. *Acute neonatal:* hyperammonemia; may be lethal; poor feeding, poor respiration, seizures. *Intermediate:* vomiting, irritability, poor growth, mental retardation. *Benign:* elevated plasma, CSF, and urinary citrulline (excretion 1.3–1.7 μg/day compared to <0.001 μg normally)	Detection of citrulline by Ninhydrin positive spot on paper chromatography and confirmation by amino acid analyzer; deficient ASS activity in liver	Low-protein diet, same as for CPS or OTC deficiency; generous kilocalories
Argininosuccinicaciduria (Allan et al.[66]); autosomal recessive	Argininosuccinase	Variable; may be severe mental retardation, seizures, liver disease, abnormal hair; argininosuccinicaciduria,	Demonstration of argininosuccinic acid (ASA) in urine by paper chromatography[16]	Early institution of low-protein diet (1 g/kg/day in four to six feedings) to control urinary ASA; possibly arginine

transport				
Hartnup disease (Baron et al.[69]); autosomal recessive; 1:26,000	Defect in intestinal absorption and renal transport of tryptophan; increased absorption of indole derivatives from gut	Pellagralike skin rash, attacks of transient cerebellar ataxia, constant aminoaciduria; symptoms may be absent in infancy. *During attacks:* unsteady gait, change in mental state; may be delirium. Elevation of indole derivatives in plasma and urine, decreased niacinamide synthesis because of reduced tryptophan absorption, mental retardation in some cases	Reduced plasma tryptophan (30% of normal), characteristic aminoaciduria, and increased fetal excretion of threonine, tyrosine, phenylalanine, histidine, and tryptophan only. On tryptophan loading: increased urinary output of indican, indoleacetic acid, and its glutamine derivatives[16]	Variable clinical picture makes evaluation of therapeutic regimens difficult. Significant improvement of skin rash with niacinamide supplements (40–250 mg/day).[16,70] High-protein diet
Cystinuria (Garrod,[2] Wollaston,[71] Scriver and Rosenberg[27]); most common IEM (with possible exception of PKU); autosomal recessive; 1:20,000 or higher	Defect in intestinal and renal transport for dibasic amino acids and cystine[72]	Aminoaciduria characterized by great excess of cystine, lysine, arginine, and ornithine; cystine excess predisposes to renal, bladder, and ureteral calculi, possibly growth retardation, and impaired cerebral function	Hexagonal flat cystine crystals in concentrated urine; detection of cystine with cyanide-nitroprusside test; confirmation by characteristic aminoaciduria; need to distinguish from homocystinuria and cystinosis	Object is to reduce urinary cystine excretion and prevent cystine calculi formation; increasing urine volume and alkalinity helpful.[73] Low-methionine, low-protein diet may lower urinary cystine excretion[74]

PKU = phenylketonuria; CSF = cerebrospinal fluid; IEM = inborn error of metabolism.

DISORDERS OF CARBOHYDRATE METABOLISM

In this section, we review the role of nutrition in the diagnosis and management of inborn errors of galactose, fructose, and glycogen metabolism. These disorders range in effect from benign to lethal. Other inherited conditions related to carbohydrate metabolism, described in other chapters, include errors of carbohydrate digestion (Chapter 6) and diabetes mellitus (Chapter 9). Nutritional care for renal calculi resulting from hyperoxaluria is described in Chapter 7.

Disorders of Galactose Metabolism

The term *galactosemia* encompasses two disorders characterized by impaired galactose metabolism.[75] They represent defects in two different enzymes that participate in the metabolism of galactose to glucose. Each of these defects has an incidence of approximately 1 in 40,000 to 1 in 100,000 live births.

Biochemical Abnormalities

The normal pathways of galactose metabolism are summarized in Fig. 10-5, which also indicates the metabolic blocks in the two forms of galactosemia. The first type is the result of a *galactokinase deficiency* which blocks the formation of galactose-1-phosphate from galactose, the first step of galactose metabolism. This metabolic error results in the accumulation of galactose in the body tissues. The increase in the concentration of galactose in the lens of the eye enhances the activity of the alternative pathway for the

Figure 10-5. Pathways of galactose metabolism. **A.** *Site of metabolic block in galactokinase deficiency.* **B.** *Site of metabolic block in transferase deficiency.*

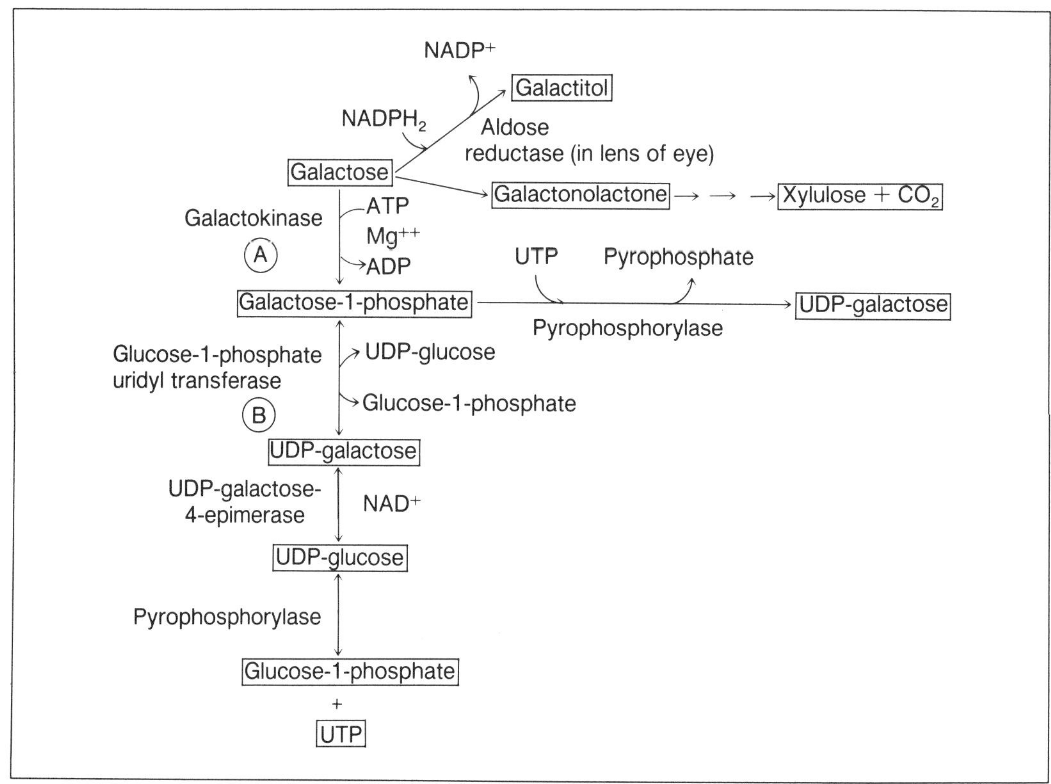

formation of galactitol (see Fig. 10-5). Galactitol is nondiffusible. It accumulates in the lens and causes cataracts.[76] In addition, galactose and galactitol are excreted in the urine.

The second type of galactosemia results from the absence of or decrease in activity of *galactose-1-phosphate uridyl transferase.* This enzyme normally catalyzes the second step of galactose metabolism in which UDP-galactose is formed from galactose-1-phosphate and UDP-glucose (see Fig. 10-5). Inactivity of this transferase leads to the accumulation of both galactose and galactose-1-phosphate in erythrocytes, liver, spleen, lens of the eye, kidney, heart, muscle, cerebral cortex, and other tissues.[77] Galactose accumulates because the excessive galactose-1-phosphate inhibits the previous step, the conversion of galactose to galactose-1-phosphate. Galactose and galactitol are excreted in the urine in galactokinase deficiency.

There also are secondary metabolic blocks. Excessive galactose-1-phosphate inhibits conversion of glucose-1-phosphate to glucose-6-phosphate, which functions in the release of glucose from liver glycogen. Glucose release is inhibited secondarily.

In addition to galactitol formation, there are two proposed alternative pathways. First, the reaction involving the oxidation of galactose to galactonic acid and xylulose operates in some patients.[78] Second, the activity of pyrophosphorylase for conversion of galactose-1-phosphate to UDP-galactose (see Fig. 10-5) is believed to be minimal and does not increase in galactosemia. Therefore, it does not provide an effective alternative pathway for galactose metabolism.

The reaction involving UDP-galactose-4-epimerase activity is reversible. As a consequence, UDP-glucose can be converted to UDP-galactose. The body thus is able to provide endogenous galactose for the formation of brain cerebrosides and complex polysaccharides. As a consequence, dietary galactose is not an essential nutrient.

Diagnosis

Transferase deficiency can be diagnosed by tests that detect reducing substances like galactose in the urine. The diagnosis is confirmed by elevated galactose levels and increased galactose-1-phosphate levels in the red blood cells. Measurements of the transferase and galactokinase provide definitive differential diagnosis. Screening tests have been developed for early diagnosis.[79,80]

Clinical Manifestations

Galactokinase deficiency, as previously described, is associated with cataract development in the first few weeks of life, but cataracts may develop in utero. There are no other clinical symptoms. Mental retardation usually is not a feature of galactokinase deficiency.

Transferase deficiency, on the other hand, is characterized by vomiting, anorexia, diarrhea, hypoglycemic attacks, jaundice, cirrhosis of the liver (see Chapter 11), and hepatomegaly (enlarged liver), as well as cataracts. The presence of renal damage is indicated by albuminuria and aminoaciduria. Mental retardation occurs in severe cases. The disease has varying degrees of severity and may express itself as no more than gastrointestinal hyperirritability in mild cases. The symptoms may appear at birth unless a galactose-free diet was used during pregnancy. In that case, the symptoms develop rapidly after milk feeding is begun, usually within 3 to 5 days. The high lactose content of milk, 7 percent in human milk and 5 percent in cow's milk, contributes significantly to the galactose load in infancy.

The mechanisms by which the toxic effects are produced in transferase deficiency are not understood completely. The secondary block of the pathway to glycolysis may be responsible for the liver cell damage. The inhibition of glucose-6-phosphatase interferes with glucose release from liver glycogen and results in hypoglycemia. Since liver and kidney damage are not seen in galactokinase deficiency, it is likely that these effects are associated with the accumulation of galactose-1-phosphate.

Mental retardation in transferase deficiency also is thought to be related to the failure to metabolize galactose-1-phosphate. Normally, the brain does not use galactose readily but does so when blood galactose levels are high. Large quantities of galactose-1-phosphate in the neurons may inhibit normal neuronal metabolism and cause brain damage.

Nutritional Management

The biochemical and clinical manifestations of both transferase deficiency and galactokinase deficiency can be well controlled by elimination of the sources of galactose from the diet, at least for the first 2 years of life.[81] Treatment has to be started early, within the first month of life, to avoid or at least arrest cataract formation. Because cataracts can form in utero, restriction of galactose during pregnancy is necessary if maternal galactosemia is suspected.[82]

Because milk and milk products contain lactose, they are omitted from the galactose-free diet in infancy. Lactose yields approximately 50 percent galactose when metabolized. Several commercial milk substitutes—Nutramigen, ProSobee, and Isomil—that are essentially free of lactose and galactose can be used. Their composition is given in Appendix L. Requirements for protein, calcium, and riboflavin, for which milk is an important dietary source, can be met adequately by using these milk substitutes. If the infant does not accept any of these products, a meat-based formula is an acceptable alternative. Recently developed milk analogues are devoid of cow's milk products and use soy protein and sodium caseinate as the source of protein. However, these products need to be supplemented with calcium or protein in the diet. Soybeans, peas, and beans contain oligosaccharides of which galactose is a constituent. Although it is assumed that these substances are not metabolized to free galactose, soy products should be used with caution unless the patient can be monitored carefully.

Examples of other foods that must be restricted are fruits and vegetables that are processed with lactose. Peas, lima beans, and sugar beets also are sources of galactose and must be eliminated. Organ meats such as liver, pancreas (sweetbreads), and brain contain galactose. Meat products containing fillers must be avoided unless it is certain that they contain no milk products. Creamed dishes need to be eliminated, and breads, cereals, and margarines must be milk-free. The labels on margarines must be read carefully to assure that the product is usable. Pure oils, lard, and hydrogenated shortening are devoid of milk, lactose, and galactose and are safe to use.[7] Desserts such as cakes, pastries, cookies, puddings, and frozen desserts also must be avoided unless they are milk-free.

The parents, and later the patient, should be carefully instructed in avoidance of milk, milk products, and any foods, drugs, or toiletries containing lactose or galactose. The nutritional care specialist must provide information on foods to avoid, instruction on reading and interpreting labels, recipes for acceptable milk-free substitutes for common foods, and information on menu planning for normal nutrition.

The objectives of the diet are to reduce erythrocyte galactose-1-phosphate to less than 3 mg/dl and urinary galactose to less than 10 mg/dl. The newly diagnosed patient is monitored weekly until normal levels are reached, then monthly throughout infancy, and four to six times per year thereafter. The nutritional care specialist should assess the diet periodically. It also is essential to monitor the progress of children on galactose-restricted diets by means of physical examination, including palpation of the liver, anthropometric measurements, and urine tests for hexitol. In addition, they should undergo wrist roentgenography for bone age, psychological evaluation, and slit-lamp examination for cataracts annually and an electroencephalogram every 2 years.[83]

Dietary control instituted early in infancy usually can prevent the development of cataracts and hypoglycemia and permit normal liver function and normal physical growth. If cataracts are present at birth, the diet may prevent their further development but may not cause them to regress. Mental development may be impaired if dietary control is inadequate. Mental deficiency, once established, is not reversed by galactose restriction. Severe restriction of galactose is agreed to be necessary during the first year of life; however, opinions differ about the required duration of dietary restriction thereafter.[84] Segal[85] contends that there is no good evidence to suggest that a relaxation of the restricted diet is warranted. However, older patients may have psychological problems associated with stringent galactose restriction, and the use of some snacks may have to be considered.

Disorders of Fructose Metabolism

Pathways of fructose metabolism and the primary metabolic blocks in fructose metabolism are shown in Fig. 10-6.

Essential Fructosuria

Essential fructosuria is an autosomal recessive trait characterized by a deficiency of

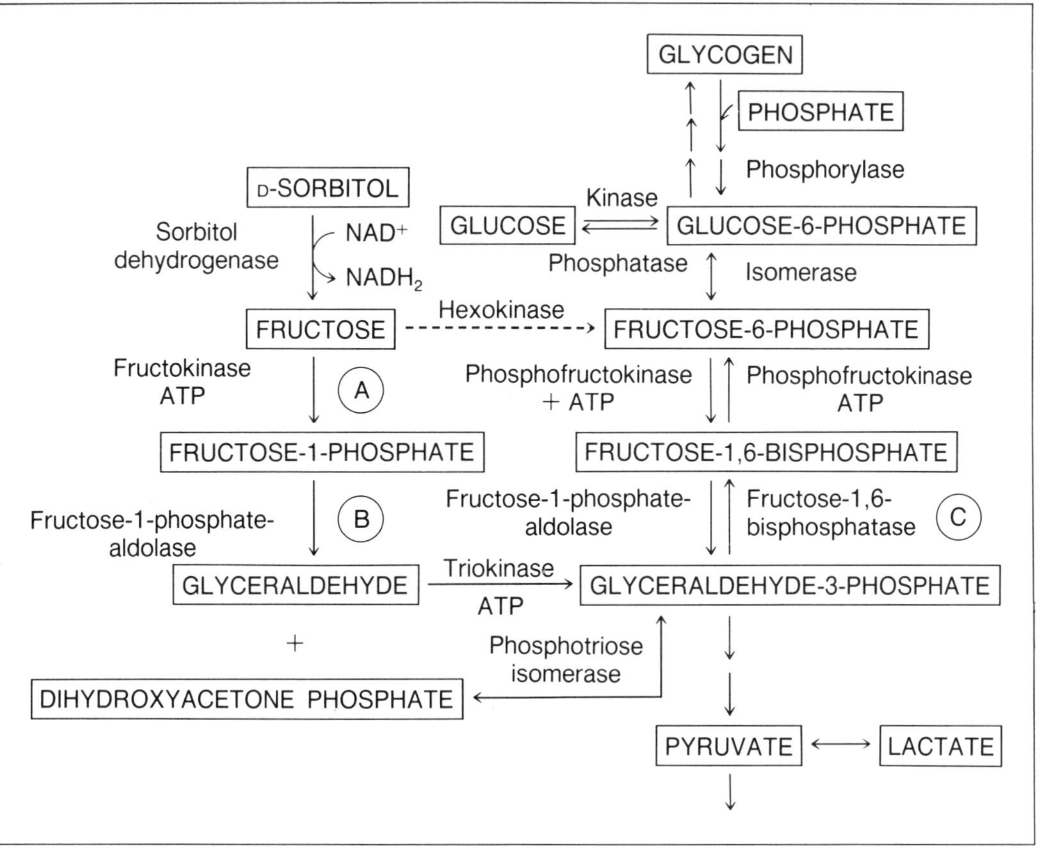

Figure 10-6. Pathways of fructose metabolism, and sites of blocks in errors of fructose metabolism. **A.** *Essential fructosuria.* **B.** *Hereditary fructose intolerance.* **C.** *Fructose-1,6-bisphosphatase deficiency.*

hepatic fructokinase. Fructose accumulates and blood fructose levels rise. Fructose is excreted in the urine when it reaches the renal threshold of 10 to 20 mg/dl. The condition is asymptomatic and does not require treatment.[86] Therefore, it will not be discussed further.

Hereditary Fructose Intolerance

Hereditary fructose intolerance has much more serious effects. It is an autosomal recessive trait characterized by a defect in *fructose-1-phosphate aldolase* (aldolase B).[87]

Biochemical Abnormalities. The enzymatic defect results in the accumulation of fructose-1-phosphate, and there is a secondary inhibition of fructokinase leading to fructosemia and fructosuria. Apparently a secondary inhibition of the metabolism of fructose-1,6-bisphosphate also occurs. The accumulation of fructose-1-phosphate and fructose-1,6-bisphosphate appears to inhibit phosphorylase in the liver, thereby reducing the release of glucose from glycogen. Gluconeogenesis also is blocked at the step involving the mutant aldolase.

The formation of fructose-1-phosphate binds and sequesters phosphate, causing hypophosphatemia. The availability of ATP apparently is decreased. The inhibition of phosphorylase, hypophosphatemia, and inhibition of gluconeogenesis all are believed to contribute to the hypoglycemia seen in this condition.[86]

Clinical Manifestations. The clinical manifestations of hereditary fructose intolerance vary with the age of the patient and the severity of the disease. The condition is manifested in infants at a later age than is galactosemia, since sources of fructose normally are fed later. When fructose is fed, some consequences are immediate and short-lived whereas others become chronic.

Immediate effects include nausea, vomiting, and various signs of hypoglycemia including sweating, trembling, and disturbances of consciousness, including coma. Laboratory analyses show mild fructosemia, fructosuria, hypophosphatemia, and aminoaciduria. Liver damage is demonstrated by hyperbilirubinemia and a rise in the serum level of hepatic enzymes. The cause of liver damage is unknown. It has been suggested that hepatocyte metabolism is damaged by the unavailability of phosphate for ATP formation, thus damaging the liver.

Chronic effects in children include failure to thrive, jaundice, hepatomegaly, dehydration, edema, ascites, and seizures. Renal damage is demonstrated by an inability to acidify the urine and by albuminuria and aminoaciduria. Death may occur from cachexia if the condition is not treated.

Later, affected children and adults develop a strong aversion to fruit and sweets. The effects on the liver and kidneys apparently are reversible. Patients generally have no dental caries. The disease does not appear to cause brain damage and intelligence is normal. Symptoms tend to decrease with age.

Diagnosis. An intravenous fructose tolerance test is used for diagnosis. Affected persons will respond with a fall in plasma glucose and inorganic phosphorus. The diagnosis can be confirmed by liver biopsy and measurement of aldolase activity.

Nutritional Management. The patient must be given a diet free of fructose. Since sucrose and sorbitol are sources of fructose, this diet must also be free of these substances. The diet requires the elimination of all fruits and fruit juices, most vegetables, and all products to which sucrose or sorbitol has been added. These include many breads and cereals, meat products that are sugar-cured or breaded, and milk drinks that are sweetened. Desserts containing sugar, honey, fruit, or fruit juice must be eliminated. (Honey contains fructose.) Desserts labeled *dietetic* may be used if they do not contain sugar, fructose, or sorbitol.

Table 10-14. Major Clinical Symptoms, Diagnosis, and Management of Glycogen Storage Diseases

Disease Type and Enzyme Defect	Clinical Manifestations	Diagnosis	Nutritional Management
Type I (von Gierke's disease; hepatorenal glycogen storage disease); glucose-6-phosphatase	Anorexia, weight loss, vomiting, enlargement of liver and kidney, failure to thrive, stunted growth, severe hypoglycemia in infancy, acidosis, hyperlipemia, hyperuricemia, and gout	Increased glycogen storage (normal structure), glucose-6-phosphatase absent in fresh liver biopsy, subnormal response to glucagon or epinephrine	Treatment is symptomatic: surgical construction of portacaval anastomosis; feeding medium-chain triglycerides, and frequent small feedings (six to eight per day) of normal diet with high-glucose feedings between meals; glucose polymers useful
Type II (Pompe's disease); α-1,4-glucosidase	Hepatomegaly, hypotonia, cardiomegaly, maybe cardiorespiratory failure and death	Muscle biopsy analysis for α-1,4-glucosidase	No known effective treatment. Low-carbohydrate, high-protein, high-fat diet attempted but not generally effective
Type III (Cori's disease); amylo-1,6-glucosidase (debranching enzyme)	Similar to type I but milder; lipids, glucose, and electrocardiogram normal; muscle wasting and weakness	Liver biopsy or leukocytes for enzyme assay; excessive storage of abnormal glycogen	Similar to type I, but a diet high in protein is recommended; give night feeding to avoid hypoglycemia
Type IV; amylo-1,4→1,6-transglucosylase (branching enzyme)	Hepatosplenomegaly, cirrhosis, ascites, liver failure, accumulation of abnormal glycogen	Absence of amylo-1,4→1,6 transglucosylase activity in leukocytes, excessive storage of abnormal glycogen	No known effective treatment
Type V (McArdle's disease); muscle phosphorylase	Weakness, cramping of muscles on exercise in young adults, failure of blood lactate to rise	Absence of phosphorylase and increased glycogen on muscle biopsy	Intravenous glucose infusions to relieve muscular pain
Type VI (Hers' disease); liver phosphorylase(?)	Hepatomegaly, normal spleen; absence of hypoglycemia, lipemia, and acidosis	Depressed liver enzyme activity, normal glucose-6-phosphatase and amylo-1,6-glucosidase, and increased liver glycogen	A high-protein diet and frequent small feedings
Type VII; muscle phosphofructokinase	Weakness and cramping of skeletal muscle on exercise	Decrease in muscle phosphofructokinase on biopsy	No dietary treatment known
Type VIII; liver phosphorylase	Hepatomegaly, cerebral degeneration	Reduction in liver phosphorylase activity	No dietary treatment known
Type IX; liver phosphorylase kinase	Hepatomegaly; no splenomegaly, hypoglycemia, or acidosis	Same as type VI, but response to large dose of glucagon normal (X-linked; men only)	No dietary treatment known
Type X; cAMP-dependent phosphorylase kinase	Hepatomegaly; skeletal muscle and heart normal	Absence of phosphorylase kinase activity, no response to glucagon	No dietary treatment known
Type O; glycogen synthetase	Hypoglycemic seizures; mental retardation	Absence or reduction in activity of glycogen synthetase	Frequent small feedings with high sugar content, high-protein feedings in between

Based on Palmer, S., Glycogen storage diseases. In S. Palmer and S. Ekvall, Eds., *Pediatric Nutrition in Developmental Disorders.* Springfield, Ill.: Charles C Thomas, 1978; and Bondy, P.K., and Rosenberg, L.E., Eds., *Metabolic Control and Disease,* 8th ed. Philadelphia: W.B. Saunders, 1980.

Patients will need ascorbic acid supplements, but the vitamin must not be sugarcoated. Patients should also be given guidance on menu planning for nutritional adequacy.

Hereditary Fructose-1,6-Bisphophatase Deficiency

Hereditary fructose-1,6-bisphosphatase deficiency is a rare disorder that is associated with hypoglycemia and lactic acidosis. The symptoms resemble those of tyrosinosis. The clinical manifestations often are precipitated by an infection, and the mortality is high. As a consequence, nutritional management is not a common approach.

Figure 10-7. Major pathways in the synthesis and degradation of glycogen in glycogen storage diseases.

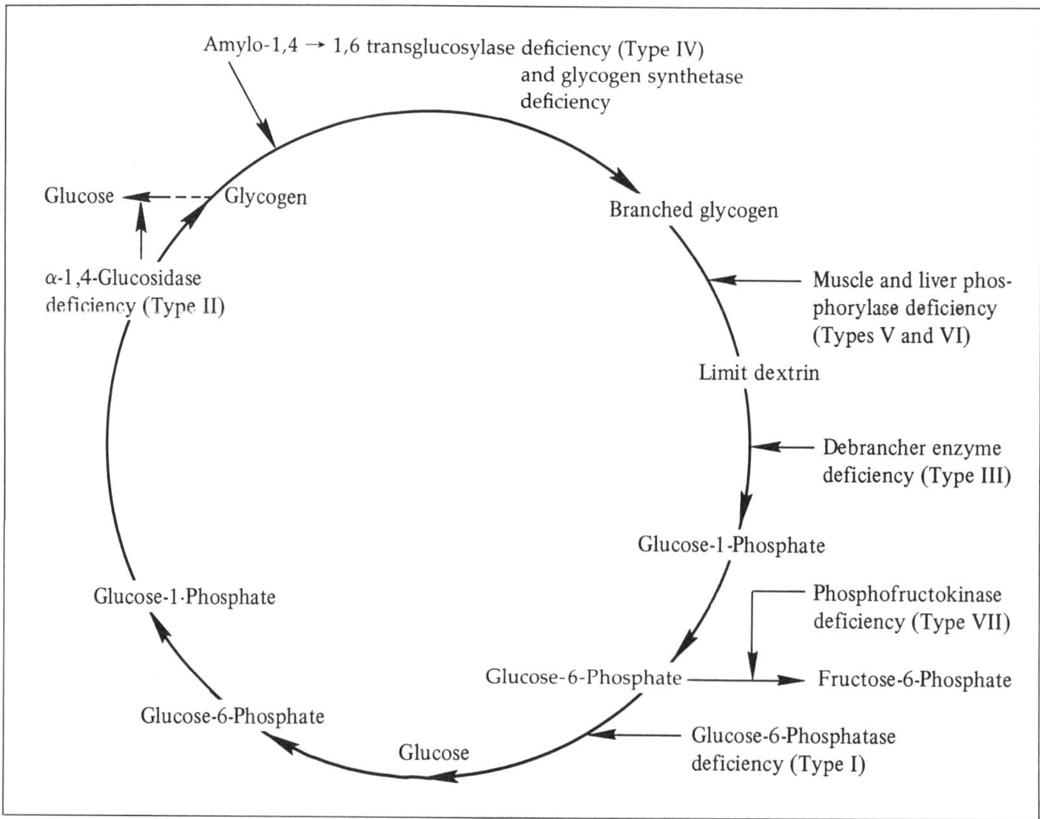

Glycogen Storage Diseases

A group of disorders known as the *glycogen storage diseases* are associated with abnormalities in glycogen metabolism. These disorders, shown in Table 10-14, are associated with the absence or reduction in activity of different enzymes involved in glycogen metabolism. The glycogen storage diseases are rare, but the exact incidence of each has not been determined yet. Not all are amenable to nutritional management but all are shown in the table to demonstrate their interrelationship.

Biochemical Abnormalities

The major pathways of glycogen metabolism and the enzymatic effects associated with various glycogen storage diseases are shown in Fig. 10-7. The predominant biochemical defect due to the enzymatic disturbance in the pathway of glycogen synthesis or degradation is the storage of excessive amounts or an abnormal form of glycogen in various body tissues, mainly in the liver. The usual human content of glycogen is less than 5 g/100 g of wet weight of liver and less than 2 g/100 g of wet weight of muscle.

The diseases of glycogen storage affect primarily either the liver or the skeletal muscle and myocardium, although other organs sometimes are involved. In the diseases with the hepatic enzymatic effect, the liver is greatly enlarged. Other symptoms are severe hypoglycemia, hypertriglyceridemia, hypercholesterolemia, and increased blood urate and lactate levels. Death in childhood is uncommon. If the disease affects the muscle primarily, it causes cramps, muscular weakness and atrophy, massive glycogen infiltration into the muscles, reduced muscular function and, in some cases, myocardial failure and death.

Diagnosis and Nutritional Management

In the glycogen storage diseases, the most reliable diagnostic test is the demonstration of the absence of or reduction in the activity of the specific enzyme. As shown in Table 10-14, differential diagnosis is necessary to distinguish between the different types of glycogen storage diseases.

The management and prognosis of these diseases varies considerably. In some instances—for example, type I—severe metabolic abnormalities eventually may lead to death, whereas in other types, such as type V, there is minimal disability. Dietary modification usually is not effective in controlling the outcome of most glycogen storage diseases, although some of the symptoms (e.g., hypoglycemia) can be relieved by specific intervention. Techniques for nutritional management are summarized in Table 10-14.

DISORDERS OF LIPID TRANSPORT

The disorders of lipid transport resulting from single gene mutations that are closely related to cardiovascular disease were discussed in Chapter 8. Another disorder in this category, abetalipoproteinemia, is described in Chapter 6. This section contains two other examples of lipid transport disorders, lecithin: cholesterol acyltransferase (LCAT) deficiency and Refsum's disease.

Familial Lecithin: Cholesterol Acyltransferase Deficiency

Familial lecithin: cholesterol acyltransferase (LCAT) deficiency is a very rare autosomal recessive disorder characterized by the absence or severe deficiency of LCAT activity in plasma. Lecithin: cholesterol acyltransferase catalyzes the formation of cholesteryl esters by promoting acyl group transfer from lecithin to the unesterified cholesterol of plasma lipoproteins. It acts directly on high-density lipoproteins and is activated by the A-I apolipoprotein (see Chapter 8). The biochemical abnormalities accompanying LCAT deficiency include anemia, abnormal plasma lipoproteins, hypertriglyceridemia, and variable plasma cholesterol levels. The anemia in LCAT deficiency is characterized by hemolysis and reduced compensatory erythropoiesis, and by the presence of abnormal erythrocytes known as *target cells* because of their appearance. In addition, foam cells appear in the bone marrow. Characteristic clinical features include corneal opacity, especially in cases with albuminuria and anemia, proteinuria that is detectable early in life, and renal insufficiency and renal failure that can develop later.[88,89]

Dietary treatment has been attempted in LCAT deficiency and is geared toward reducing the total fat content of the diet to lower the high-molecular-weight low-density lipoproteins in the plasma.[89,90] This may be of some value in protecting against kidney damage. Further research in this area is needed.

Refsum's Disease

Refsum's disease is known also as *phytanic acid storage disease.* Phytanic acid is a twenty-carbon branched chain acid that is found in some foods. The biochemical lesion consists of a failure to convert phytanic acid to alpha-hydroxyphytanic acid, the initial step in its conversion to pristanic acid (Fig. 10-8).[91] The activity of the enzyme phytanic acid alpha-hydroxylase, which catalyzes this step, is absent. Subsequent steps in the metabolism of pristanic acid by beta-oxidation are not affected.

Refsum's disease is a rare autosomal recessive disorder.[92,93] It is characterized by peripheral neuropathy, ataxia, *retinitis pigmentosa* (a progressive sclerosis, pigmentation, and atrophy of the retina leading to blindness), and disorders of the skin and bones.[91] These symptoms result from the accumulation of phytainc acid in tissues, particularly the liver and kidneys.[92] Normal human plasma contains only traces (0.3 mg/dl) of phytanic acid, but in patients with this disease, 5 to 30 percent of total fatty acids are phytanic acid.

Figure 10-8. Metabolic block in Refsum's disease.

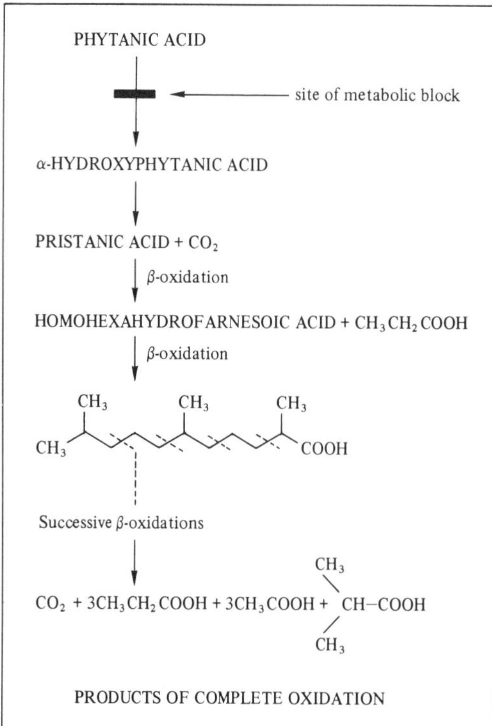

The sources of phytanic acid probably are exclusively dietary. The major dietary sources have been identified as dairy products,[94] with traces in some vegetables (e.g., squash and tomatoes) and fish oils.[95] Phytol, a component of chlorophyll which is ubiquitous in green leafy vegetables, is also a precursor of phytanic acid. However, it is present in the bound form in the chlorophyll molecule in green vegetables and, in its bound form, is not thought to be an important dietary source of phytanic acid.[96]

Several investigators have reported success in treating Refsum's disease by restricting the phytanic acid content of the diet.[91,96–98] The response of plasma phytanate to dietary treatment is associated with improvement or even regression of peripheral neuropathy.[96,97] Reducing the intake of phytanic acid from its estimated level of approximately 60 mg/day can lower plasma phytanic acid levels, but a drastic reduction to approximately 3 mg of phytanate daily is reported to be necessary for normalizing plasma phytanic acid levels.[96] Severe restriction of total caloric intake may be necessary. Therefore, careful monitoring of the diet and follow-up of patients is recommended. Therapeutic benefits are reported to be maximized if the diet therapy is initiated early.[91]

DISORDERS OF PURINE AND PYRIMIDINE METABOLISM

A number of hereditary syndromes are associated with abnormalities in purine and pyrimidine metabolism. Here we will briefly describe two such syndromes, gout and hereditary xanthinuria.

Gout

The term *gout* is used to describe a cluster of clinical symptoms associated with hyperuricemia (increased levels of uric acid in the blood). It is a form of arthritis found in a variety of hereditary disorders and in some disorders related to environmental factors. Gout is a common ailment, accounting for 4 to 5 percent of all patients with arthritis in major clinics in the United States, and with an overall incidence of 0.3 percent. It occurs much more frequently in men than women.

Biochemical Abnormalities

The hyperuricemia of gout results most commonly from a genetic defect that leads to excessive synthesis of the purine precursors of uric acid or, in other cases, from normal purine synthesis but diminished uric acid excretion.

A variety of enzymatic defects may result in excessive purine synthesis. The ones leading to hyperuricemia and gout are (1) deficiency of glucose-6-phosphatase (glycogen storage disease type I), (2) hypoxanthine-guanine phosphoribosyl transferase (HPRT) deficiency in patients with the Lesch-Nyhan syndrome, and (3) increased activity of phosphoribosylpyrophosphate synthetase. Hyperuricemia and gout also may appear in association with a number of other hereditary disorders.

Clinical Features

Clinically, gout is characterized by recurrent, paroxysmal, acute attacks due to severe inflammation in peripheral joints, followed by complete transient remission. Gradually, these episodes become more frequent and lead to chronic disability and joint destruction. The incidence of renal calculi and renal and vascular damage is exceedingly high. The clinical features are the result of urate deposits in tissues because of the limited solubility of uric acid and its salts in biologic fluids. At the low pH of the urinary tract, free acid forms calculi in the kidney and bladder, and at the high pH of the plasma, crystals of monosodium urate monohydrate are precipitated in and around the joints, tendons, *subchondral* (beneath cartilage) bones, and kidney parenchyma. Only a small percentage of hyperuricemic patients develop gouty arthritis.

Treatment

Acute attacks of gouty arthritis respond well to therapy with a variety of *antiinflammatory drugs,* and *antihyperuricemic drugs* are used for lowering plasma uric acid levels.[99] *Diet therapy* now is used only as an adjunct to drugs, although it was used more extensively before the advent of effective drugs.

Dietary restriction of foods high in purine can lower serum urate concentration, but the response to even a purine-free diet has been reported as moderate at best.[100] Nevertheless, a purine-restricted diet (in essence, a restriction of high-protein foods) containing 200 g of meat, poultry, or fish twice weekly and low in dried beans, lentils, bran, and wheat germ frequently is recommended as adjunctive therapy. Organ meats are exceedingly high in purine and may have to be eliminated.[101] High-fat diets, consumption of alcohol, and very-low-calorie diets tend to increase serum urate concentration and may provoke acute attacks of gout.[102,103] Increased consumption of fluids and maintenance of an alkaline pH in the urine also assist in the treatment of gout.[99]

Hereditary Xanthinuria

Hereditary xanthinuria results from a deficiency of xanthine oxidase and leads to excessive secretion of hypoxanthine and xanthine, the precursors of uric acid. The enzyme deficiency results in reduced formation of uric acid and consequent hypouricemia and sometimes is accompanied by hypercalciuria.

In most patients with xanthinuria, the disease has a benign course and requires no treatment. However, in patients with recurrent renal calculi, a high-fluid diet, maintenance of an alkaline pH in the urine, and dietary restriction of purine-containing foods may be beneficial.[99] (See Chapter 7 for a discussion of the nutritional care of patients with renal calculi.)

VITAMIN DEPENDENCY DISORDERS

In the last two decades, there has been increasing awareness that many inborn errors of metabolism are associated with an increase in the requirement for certain vitamins that function as coenzymes at different steps in metabolic pathways. This heterogeneous group of disorders, often referred to as *vitamin dependency syndromes,* is poorly understood. Interest in these disorders has focused chiefly on conditions involving folate, vitamin B_{12} (cobalamin), pyridoxine, and vitamin D. Hartnup disease might be considered a vitamin dependency syndrome with a transport defect or a disorder of amino acid metabolism. For convenience, it was included in Table 10-13. The vitamin dependency disorders will be described briefly, since the primary treatment is administration of vitamins.

Folate Dependency

A number of inborn errors of folate metabolism have been described recently. For example, increased folate requirement is known to occur in homocystinuria owing to $N^{5,10}$-methylenetetrahydrofolate reductase deficiency, and in inborn errors of vitamin B_{12} metabolism,[104] Lesch-Nyhan syndrome,[105] orotic aciduria, sickle cell disease (see Chapter 14), and *psoriasis* (a chronic skin disease).[106]

Vitamin B_{12} Dependency

Vitamin B_{12} (cobalamin) has been associated with several inborn errors of metabolism. It acts as a coenzyme in several reactions, particularly those involving transfer of single-carbon atoms.

The reactions of two enzymes in mammalian cells are known to require cobalamin coenzymes. One of these enzymes is *methylcobalamin-dependent homocysteine-N⁵-methyltetrahydrofolate methyltransferase,* the metabolic function of which is illustrated in Fig. 10-4 in relation to homocystinuria. The second enzyme is *adenosylcobalamin-dependent methylmalonyl-CoA mutase.* This enzyme catalyzes a step in the metabolism of propionyl-CoA to methylmalonyl-CoA and then to succinyl-CoA. Propionate is an intermediate product in the metabolism of isoleucine, valine, methionine, threonine, odd-chain fatty acids, and cholesterol. A variety of inherited defects in this metabolic pathway lead to one form or another of *methylmalonic acidemia* (MMA). Some types of MMA are not vitamin-dependent, whereas other defects involve steps in cobalamin metabolism and lead to impaired methylmalonyl-CoA mutase activity and thus to methylmalonic acidemia. These conditions respond to pharmacologic doses of cyanocobalamin. Additional abnormalities in cobalamin metabolism have also been identified and are accompanied by homocystinuria, cystathioninuria, and hypomethioninemia.[104]

Pyridoxine Dependency

Pyridoxine or *vitamin B_6* is a cofactor in approximately fifty decarboxylase and transaminase enzymes. Hunt et al.[107] were the first to report a case of intractable seizures in an infant on an apparently pyridoxine-sufficient diet. The seizures were unresponsive to anticonvulsant drugs and physiologic doses of pyridoxine; however, a massive dose of pyridoxine (10 mg) relieved the symptoms. The seizures were thought to be due to a deficiency of gamma-aminobutyric acid, a neurotransmitter, the synthesis of which requires glutamic acid decarboxylase and pyridoxal phosphate as a cofactor (see Chapter 11).[108] Additional types of vitamin B_6 dependency involve an increased requirement of the coenzyme in disorders of cystathionine synthetase (homocystinuria) and kynureninase (hyperxanthurenic aciduria).[109] Laboratory experiments also suggest that impaired vitamin B_6 function may contribute to the pathogenesis of PKU.[110] Other inborn errors that are reported to respond to high doses of pyridoxine are glycinuria, cystathioninuria, and Hartnup disease.[111]

Hereditary pyridoxine dependency usually occurs soon after birth, although some symptoms may become apparent only later. Dietary deficiency of vitamin B_6 must be ruled out in diagnosing this condition.

Pyridoxine dependency states respond promptly; however, an oral dose of up to 50 mg of pyridoxine daily may be required to achieve control.

Vitamin D-Dependent Rickets

Vitamin D-dependent rickets is an autosomal recessive trait that is responsive to large doses of vitamin D. The affected enzyme, 1-alpha-hydroxylase in the renal tubular cells, catalyzes the conversion of 25-(OH)-vitamin D_3 to 1,25-$(OH)_2D_3$. Vitamin D-dependent rickets is thought to arise from a defect in this enzyme, but this has not been confirmed.[112]

The condition responds dramatically to supplements with vitamin D and calcium. A well-balanced diet is an adjunct to therapy,[113] and the nutritional care specialist should work with parents or patients on planning for adequate nutrition.

Familial Vitamin D-Resistant Rickets

Familial vitamin D-resistant rickets (FVDRR), in contrast to vitamin D-dependent rickets, is an X-linked dominant trait with an estimated incidence of 1 in 25,000 live births. The condition is characterized by rickets in children and osteomalacia in adults. Stature may or may not be affected. The cardinal biochemical sign in FVDRR is hypophosphatemia associated with decreased tubular resorption of inorganic phosphate and a consequent increase in urinary phosphate.

The exact mechanism for the hypophosphatemia is poorly understood. The abnormality usually is attributed to a defect in renal tubular phosphate reabsorption. It is possible that there is decreased conversion of vitamin D to the biologically active form, 25-hydroxycholecalciferol. There is increased fecal excretion of vitamin D in plasma and urine. Williams and Winters[114] suggest that the primary biochemical abnormalities mentioned could be responsible for decreased intestinal absorption of calcium. The reduced calcium absorption might then lead to rickets in children, osteomalacia in adults, or secondary hyperparathyroidism with attendant hypophosphatemia and phosphaturia.

Alternatively, Albright's group[115,116] has proposed that decreased calcium absorption is the primary, not a secondary, defect in FVDRR, and that hyperparathyroidism is the secondary effect. So far, no theory has explained the disorder completely. Since the condition affects transport, it is included in those disorders classified as transport defects.

The objectives of treatment are to control the bone disease and promote growth. Current treatment consists of oral supplements of inorganic phosphate and large doses of vitamin D,[113] but the treatment is not always completely effective, especially in males.[112] The effective vitamin dose sometimes is in the toxic range, with a potential for renal damage. The nutritional care specialist should observe the patient for signs of vitamin toxicity and monitor the diet for nutritional adequacy.

DISORDERS OF MINERAL METABOLISM

Considerable attention has been directed to the etiology and treatment of *Wilson's disease,* a metabolic disease known to be due to an inherited abnormality of copper metabolism, and to *acrodermatitis enteropathica,* a disorder of zinc metabolism.

Wilson's Disease

Wilson's disease, also known as *hepatolenticular degeneration,* is an autosomal recessive disorder, although it appears to be slightly more common in males than in females. The incidence of Wilson's disease is unknown.

It is characterized by degenerative changes in the brain, cirrhosis of the liver, and *Kayser-Fleischer rings* (greenish brown pigmented rings at the outer margin of the cornea).[117] Hepatic and renal impairment, especially progressive failure in the renal tubular transfer of amino acids and other substrates, are common. Clinical symptoms rarely occur in early childhood.

The exact enzymatic defect has not been identified, but the abnormal gene product causes impaired incorporation of copper into ceruloplasmin (the blue copper-containing protein) and results in the excretion of copper in the bile. Excess copper is deposited in various tissues, particularly the liver, brain, cornea, and kidney. Serum copper and ceruloplasmin usually are decreased in Wilson's disease.[117] Urinary copper excretion is increased and serum phosphate and urate levels are decreased.

The diagnosis of Wilson's disease is based on the presence of Kayser-Fleischer rings, neurologic features, and liver disease. Positive diagnostic tests include measurement of decreased serum ceruloplasmin and copper levels and increased liver stores of copper.

The objective of treatment is to relieve the tissues of copper and prevent its reaccumulation. Wilson's disease is treated with penicillamine, a copper-chelating agent. The disease can be controlled effectively but is invariably fatal if untreated. Treatment must be continued indefinitely.

Nutritional management is an adjunct to penicillamine therapy. The patient is advised to avoid liver, nuts, mushrooms, cocoa, chocolate, and shellfish, which are high in copper content. Follow-up is essential to ensure a well-balanced diet. Oral administration of potassium sulfide to precipitate copper in the bowel in the form of insoluble copper sulfide also is helpful in preventing the reaccumulation of copper. Pyridoxine supplements are needed to prevent pyridoxine deficiency that could result from prolonged penicillamine therapy.

Acrodermatitis Enteropathica

The primary biochemical abnormality in acrodermatitis enteropathica has not been identified, although a defect in some factor responsible for the absorption or gastrointestinal transport of zinc has been hypothesized.[118] Acrodermatitis enteropathica is characterized by severe diarrhea, dermatitis of the oral, anal, and genital areas, and *alopecia* (hair loss) in early infancy, often following the change from breast milk to cow's milk. Chronic diarrhea, malabsorption, steatorrhea, and lactose intolerance are common. Ophthalmic manifestations include blepharitis, conjunctivitis, photophobia, and corneal opacities. Tremor, irritability, and occasional cerebellar ataxia occur, infections are common, and retarded growth and hypogonadism are characteristic.[118] If untreated, the condition is fatal in most cases.

Acrodermatitis enteropathica is diagnosed by the clinical picture, especially the dermatitis and gastrointestinal manifestations in younger children. In addition, the biochemical parameters of zinc deficiency — low plasma and urinary zinc levels and reduced serum alkaline phosphatase and erythrocyte zinc levels — have been reported in many patients. Another consistent biochemical finding is aberrant fatty acid metabolism with some impairment in the elongation-saturation system of fatty acid metabolism.[119]

Small daily supplements (35 mg) of zinc sulfate bring about complete relief of symptoms. The use of approximately 150 mg of oral zinc sulfate daily in divided doses is recommended to guard against intercurrent infections and to promote adequate growth during adolescence.[120–123] A diet high in zinc may be helpful as adjunctive therapy.[123]

Case Study: Phenylketonuria

Jennifer C. was 10 days old when her parents were told that the screening test for PKU was positive. Further tests showed a serum phenylalanine concentration of 35 mg/dl. The parents were instructed by the nutritionist on the use of a low-phenylalanine formula. Mrs. C. was very careful to follow the directions of the nutritionist at the clinic, and Jennifer's serum phenylalanine fell to 6 mg/dl. Jennifer liked her formula and grew at a normal rate. She also seemed to be developing normally mentally.

Several months later, the clinic staff told Jennifer's parents that they wanted to challenge the diet. As instructed by the nutritionist, Mrs. C. fed Jennifer a formula made with evaporated milk and water. At the end of 24 hours, Jennifer's serum phenylalanine level rose sharply, and the challenge was discontinued. Jennifer was returned to her low-phenylalanine diet.

As Jennifer developed, solid foods were added to her diet at the usual times for normal children. On one occasion, Jennifer had an upper respiratory infection and refused to drink all her formula. When her serum phenylalanine was determined, it had risen to 15 mg/dl. The nutritionist examined carefully the 3-day food intake record that Mrs. C. had brought to the clinic.

Exercises

1. What is the normal serum phenylalanine level in the newborn infant?
2. Why does serum phenylalanine increase in classic PKU?
3. What other metabolic alterations occur?
4. Calculate a Lofenalac formula to be given to Jennifer when she weighs 10 kg.
5. Later, Jennifer's diet prescription was altered to contain 340 mg of phenylalanine, with 120 mg of it from Lofenalac, 16 g of protein, and 800 kcal. Jennifer is capable of eating strained fruits and vegetables and infant cereals. Plan a diet for Jennifer, assuming she eats six times a day.
6. What is the purpose of the diet challenge?
7. Why did Jennifer's serum phenylalanine level rise when she had an infection? What advice would you give Jennifer's mother concerning Jennifer's diet during such a period?
8. Assuming Jennifer is 1 year old and weighs 10 kg, calculate a diet for her if she has the following: (a) branched-chain ketoaciduria; (b) tyrosinemia, type 2; and (c) synthetase deficiency homocystinuria.

References

1. Elsas, L.J., II, and Priest, J.H. Medical genetics. In W.A. Sodeman, Jr., and T.M. Sodeman, Eds., *Sodeman's Pathologic Physiology,* 6th ed. Philadelphia: W.B. Saunders, 1979.
2. Garrod, A.E. The Croonian lectures on inborn errors of metabolism. *Lancet* 2:1, 73, 142, 214, 1908.
3. Fölling, A. Uber Ausscheidung von Phenylbrenztraubensaure in den Harn als Stoffweschselanomalie in Verbindung mit Imbezillitat. *Hoppe-Seylers Z. Physiol. Chem.* 227:169, 1934.
4. Woolley, D.W., and van de Hoeven, T. Serotonin deficiency in infancy as one cause of a mental defect in phenylketonuria. *Science* 144:883, 1964.
5. Udenfriend, S. The primary enzymatic defect in phenylketonuria and how it may influence the central nervous system. In J.A. Anderson and K.F. Swaiman, Eds., *Proceedings of a Conference on Phenylketonuria and Allied Metabolic Diseases.* Washington, D.C.: U.S. Government Printing Office, 1979.
6. Acosta, P.B., and Wenz, E. *Diet Management of PKU for Infants and Preschool Children.* D.H.E.W. Publication No. (HSA) 78-5209. Washington, D.C.: U.S. Department of Health, Education, and Welfare, 1978.

7. Acosta, P.B., and Elsas, L.J., II. *Dietary Management of Inherited Metabolic Disease: Phenylketonuria, Galactosemia, Tyrosinemia, Homocystinuria, Maple Syrup Urine Disease.* Atlanta: ACELMU Publishers, 1975.
8. Ernest, A.E., McCabe, E.R.B., Neifer, M.R., and O'Flynn, M.E. *Guide to Breast Feeding the Infant with PKU.* Washington, D.C.: U.S. Government Printing Office, 1979.
9. Koch, R., Wenz, E., and Steinber, M.S. *PKU—Guide to Management.* Los Angeles: Children's Hospital of Los Angeles and California State Department of Health, 1977.
10. Berry, H.K. Hyperphenylalaninemias and tyrosinemias. *Clin. Perinatol.* 3(1):15, 1976.
11. Koff, E., Kammerer, B., Boyle, P., and Pueschel, S.M. Intelligence and phenylketonuria: Effects of diet termination. *J. Pediatr.* 94:534, 1979.
12. Farriaux, J.P., Desombre-Denys, D., Charles-Bassi, M.A., and Dhondt, J.L. Le traitement de la phénylcétonurie. Remarques à propos d'une analyse de vingt et un cas. *Sem. Hop. Paris* 57:356, 1981.
13. Berry, H.A., Bofinger, M.K., Hunt, M.M., et al. Reduction of cerebrospinal fluid phenylalanine following oral administration of valine, isoleucine and leucine. *Pediatr. Res.* In press, 1983.
14. Vorhees, V.V., Butcher, R.E., and Berry, H.K. Progress in experimental phenylketonuria: A critical review. *Neurosci. Biobehav. Rev.* 5:177, 1981.
15. Levy, H.L., Shih, V.S., Karolkewica, V., et al. Persistent mild hyperphenylalaninemia in the untreated state. A prospective study. *N. Engl. J. Med.* 285:424, 1971.
16. Rosenberg, L.E., and Scriver, C.R. Disorders of amino acid metabolism. In P.K. Bondy and L.E. Rosenberg, Eds., *Metabolic Control and Disease,* 8th ed. Philadelphia: W.B. Saunders, 1980.
17. Mabry, C.C., Nelson, T.L., and Denniston, J.C. Newly appreciated cause of mental retardation: Observation on two phenylketonuric mothers and their children. *J. Pediatr.* 63:877, 1963.
18. Lenke, R.R., and Levy, H.L. Maternal phenylketonuria and hyperphenylalaninemia. An international survey of the outcome of untreated and treated pregnancies. *N. Engl. J. Med.* 303:1202, 1980.
19. Komrower, G.M., Sardhawalla, I.B., Coutts, S.M., and Ingram, D. Management of maternal phenylketonuria: An emerging clinical problem. *Br. Med. J.* 1:1383, 1979.
20. Sakai, K., and Kitagawa, T. An atypical case of tyrosinosis (1-parahydroxyphenyllactic aciduria): I. Clinical and laboratory findings. *Jikeikai. Med. J.* 4:1, 1957.
21. Halvorsen, S., and Gjessing, L.R. Tyrosinosis. In H. Bickel, F.P. Hudson, and L.E Woolf, Eds., *Phenylketonuria and Some Other Inborn Errors of Metabolism.* Stuttgart: Georg Thieme, 1971.
22. Goldsmith, L.A., Kang, E., Bienfang, D.C., et al. Tyrosinemia with plantar and palmar keratosis and keratitis. *J. Pediatr.* 83:798, 1973.
23. Medes, G. A new error of tyrosine metabolism: Tyrosinosis. The intermediary metabolism of tyrosine and phenylalanine. *Biochem. J.* 26:917, 1932.
24. Kennaway, N.G., and Buist, N.R. Metabolic studies in a patient with hepatic cytosol tyrosine aminotransferase deficiency. *Pediatr. Res.* 5:287, 1971.
25. Buist, N.R., Kennaway, N.G., and Fellman, J.H. Disorders of tyrosine metabolism. In W.L. Nyhan, ed., *Heritable Disorders of Amino Acid Metabolism.* New York: John Wiley and Sons, 1974.
26. Llenado, M., and Ekvall, S. Tyrosinosis. In S. Palmer and S. Ekvall, Eds., *Pediatric Nutrition in Developmental Disorders.* Springfield, Ill.: Charles C Thomas, 1978.
27. Scriver, C.R., and Rosenberg, L.E. *Amino Acid Metabolism and Its Disorders.* Philadelphia: W.B. Saunders, 1973.
28. Lancaster, G., Mamer, O.A., and Scriver, C.R. Branched-chain alpha-ketoacids isolated as oxime derivatives: Relationship to the corresponding hydroxyacids and amino acids in maple syrup urine disease. *Metabolism* 23:257, 1974.
29. Bowden, J.A., Brestel, E.P., Cape, W.T., et al. α-Keto-isocaproic acid inhibition of pyruvate and α-ketoglutarate oxidative decarboxylation in rat liver slices. *Biochem. Med.* 4:69, 1970.
30. Haymond, M.M., Karl, I.W., Feign, R.D., et al. Hypoglycemia in maple syrup urine disease: Defective gluconeogenesis. *Pediatr. Res.* 7:500, 1973.
31. Committee for Improvement of Hereditary Disease Management. Management of maple syrup urine disease in Canada. *Can. Med. Assoc. J.* 115:1005, 1975.
32. Mudd, S.H., and Levy, H.L. Disorders of transsulfuration. In J.B. Stanbury, J.B. Wyngaarden, D.S. Fredrickson, et al. Eds., *The Metabolic Basis of Inherited Disease,* 5th ed. New York: McGraw-Hill, 1983.
33. Abel, E., Michell, M., and Ekvall, S. Homocystinuria. In S. Palmer and S. Ekvall, Eds., *Pediatric Nutrition in Developmental Dis-*

orders. Springfield, Ill.: Charles C Thomas, 1978.

34. Wada, Y., Tada, K., Minagawa, A., et al. Idiopathic hypervalinemia. *Tohoku J. Exp. Med.* 81:46, 1963.
35. Wada, Y. Idiopathic hypervalinemia: Valine and alpha ketoacids in blood following an oral dose of valine. *Tohoku J. Exp. Med.* 87:322, 1965.
36. Holt, L.E., Jr., Gyorgy, P., Pratt, E.L., et al. *Protein and Amino Acid Requirements in Early Life.* New York: University Press, 1960.
37. Brooks, E. Hypervalinemia. In S. Palmer and S. Ekvall, Eds., *Pediatric Nutrition in Developmental Disorders.* Springfield, Ill.: Charles C Thomas, 1978.
38. Crump, I. Inborn Errors of Metabolism: Dietary Therapy. In San Diego Pediatric Nutrition Group, *Pediatric Nutrition Manual.* San Diego: University of California Medical Center, 1981.
39. Tanaka, K., Budd, M.A., Efron, M.L., et al. Isovaleric acidemia: A new genetic defect of leucine metabolism. *Proc. Natl. Acad. Sci. U.S.A.* 56:236, 1966.
40. Ando, T., and Nyhan, W.L. A simple screening method for detecting isovalerylglycine in urine of patients with isovaleric acidemia. *Clin. Chem.* 16:420, 1970.
41. Levy, H.L., Erickson, A.M., Lott, I.T., et al. Isovaleric acidemia. Results of family study and dietary treatment. *Pediatrics* 52:83, 1973.
42. Krieger, I., and Tanaka, K. Therapeutic effects of glycine in isovaleric acidemia. *Pediatr. Res.* 10:25, 1976.
43. Oberholzer, V.G., Levin, B., Burgess, E.A., and Young, W.F. Methylmalonic aciduria, an inborn error of metabolism leading to chronic metabolic acidosis. *Arch. Dis. Child.* 42:492, 1967.
44. Willard, H.F., and Rosenberg, L.E. Inborn errors of cobalamin metabolism: Effect of cobalamin supplementation in culture on methylmalonyl CoA mutase activity in normal and mutant human fibroblasts. *Biochem. Genet.* 17:57, 1979.
45. Palmer, S., Ekvall, S., and Umali, M. Methylmalonic aciduria. In S. Palmer and S. Ekvall, Eds., *Pediatric Nutrition in Developmental Disorders.* Springfield, Ill.: Charles C Thomas, 1978.
46. Nyhan, W.L., Fawcett, N., Ando, T., et al. Response to dietary therapy in B_{12} unresponsive methylmalonic acidemia. *Pediatrics* 51:539, 1973.
47. Childs, B., Nyhan, W.L., Borden, M., et al. Idiopathic hyperglycinemia and hyperglycinuria. A new disorder of amino acid metabolism. *Pediatrics* 27:522, 1961.
48. Ando, T., Rasmussen, K., Nyhan, W.L., et al. Propionic acidemia in patients with ketotic hyperglycinemia. *J. Pediatr.* 78:827, 1971.
49. Hsia, Y.E., Scully, K.J., and Rosenberg, L.E. Inherited propionyl-CoA carboxylase deficiency in 'ketotic hyperglycinemia.' *J. Clin. Invest.* 50:127, 1971.
50. Brandt, I.K., Hsia, Y.E., Clement, D.H., et al. Propionicacidemia (ketotic hyperglycinemia): Dietary treatment resulting in normal growth and development. *Pediatrics* 53:391, 1974.
51. Barnes, N.D., Hull, D., Balbogin, L., et al. Biotin-responsive propionicacidaemia. *Lancet* 2:244, 1970.
52. Auerbach, V.H., DiGeorge, A.M., Baldridge, R.C., et al. Histidinemia: A deficiency in histidase resulting in the urinary excretion of histidine and of imidazolepyruvic acid. *J. Pediatr.* 60:487, 1962.
53. Gatfield, P.D., Knights, R.M., Devereaux, M., et al. Histidinemia: Report of four new cases in one family and the effect of low histidine diets. *Can. Med. Assoc. J.* 101:465, 1969.
54. Stevens, F., and Ekvall, S. Histidinemia. Histidine alpha-deaminase deficiency. In S. Palmer and S. Ekvall, Eds., *Pediatric Nutrition in Developmental Disorders.* Springfield, Ill.: Charles C Thomas, 1978.
55. Scriver, C.R., Smith, R. J., and Phang, J.M. Disorders of proline and hydroxyproline metabolism. In J.B. Stanbury, J.B. Wyngaarden, D.S. Fredrickson, et al., Eds., *The Metabolic Basis of Inherited Disease,* 5th ed. New York: McGraw-Hill, 1983.
56. Harries, J.T., Piesowics, A.T., Seakins, J.W.T., et al. Low proline diet in type-I hyperprolinaemia. *Arch. Dis. Child.* 46:72, 1971.
57. Simila, S. Dietary treatment in hyperprolinemia type II. *Acta Paediatr. Scand.* 63:249, 1974.
58. Efron, M.L., Bixby, E.M., Palattao, L.G., et al. Hydroxyprolinemia associated with mental deficiency. *N. Engl. J. Med.* 267:1193, 1962.
59. Efron, M.L. Treatment of hydroxyprolinemia and hyperprolinemia. *Am. J. Dis. Child.* 113:166, 1967.
60. Knapp, A. Über eine neue, hereditäre, von Vitamin-B_6 abhängige Störung im Tryptophan-Stoffwechsel. *Clin. Chim. Acta* 5:6, 1960.
61. Tada, K., Yokoyama, Y., Nakagawa, H., et

al. Vitamin B_6-dependent xanthurenic aciduria. (The second report.) *Tohoku J. Exp. Med.* 95:107, 1968.
62. Barshaw, M., Brusilow, S., and Walser, M. Treatment of carbamyl phosphate synthetase deficiency with ketoanalogues of essential amino acids. *N. Engl. J. Med.* 292:1085, 1975.
63. Russell, A., Levin, B., Oberholzer, V.G., et al. Hyperammonaemia. A new instance of inborn enzymatic defect of the biosynthesis of urea. *Lancet* 2:699, 1962.
64. Mitchell, M., and Ekvall, S. Ornithine transcarbamylase deficiency. In S. Palmer and S. Ekvall, Eds., *Pediatric Nutrition in Developmental Disorders.* Springfield, Ill.: Charles C Thomas, 1978.
65. McMurray, W.G., Mohyruddin, F., Rossiter, R.J., et al. Citrullinuria: A new aminoaciduria associated with mental retardation. *Lancet* 1:138, 1962.
66. Allan, J.D., Cusworth, D.C., Dent, C.E., et al. A disease, probably hereditary, characterized by severe mental deficiency and a constant gross abnormality of amino acid metabolism. *Lancet* 1:182, 1958.
67. Smith, M.A. Argininosuccinic aciduria. In S. Palmer and S. Ekvall, Eds., *Pediatric Nutrition in Developmental Disorders.* Springfield, Ill.: Charles C Thomas, 1978.
68. Shih, V.E., Efron, M.L., and Moser, H.W. Hyperornithinemia and homocitrullinuria with ammonia intoxication, myoclonic seizures and mental retardation. *Am. J. Dis. Child.* 117:83, 1969.
69. Baron, D.N., Dent, C.E., Harris, H., et al. Hereditary pellagra-like skin rash with temporary cerebellar ataxia, constant renal aminoaciduria, and other bizarre biochemical features. *Lancet* 2:421, 1956.
70. Llenado, M., and Ekvall, S. Hartnup disease. In S. Palmer and S. Ekvall, Eds., *Pediatric Nutrition in Developmental Disorders.* Springfield, Ill.: Charles C Thomas, 1978.
71. Wollaston, W.H. On cystic oxide, a new species of urinary calculus. *Philos. Trans. R. Soc. Lond.* [*Biol.*] 100:223, 1910.
72. Milne, M.D., Asatoor, A.M., Edwards, K.D.G., et al. The intestinal absorption defect in cystinuria. *Gut* 2:323, 1961.
73. Dent, C.E., Friedmann, W., Green, H., et al. Treatment of cystinuria. *Br. Med. J.* 1:403, 1965.
74. Kolb, R.O., Earll, J.M., and Harper, H.A. 'Disappearance' of cystinuria in a patient treated with prolonged low methionine diet. *Metabolism* 16:378, 1967.
75. Mason, H.H., and Turner, M.E. Chronic galactosemia. *Am. J. Dis. Child.* 50:359, 1935.
76. Gabbay, K.H. The sorbitol pathway and the complication of diabetes. *N. Engl. J. Med.* 288:831, 1973.
77. Quan-Ma, R., Wells, H.J., Wells, W.W., et al. Galactitol in the tissues of a galactosemic child. *Am. J. Dis. Child.* 112:477, 1966.
78. Segal, S., and Cuatrecasas, P. The oxidation of C^{14} galactose by patients with congenital galactosemia. Evidence for a direct oxidative pathway. *Am. J. Med.* 44:340, 1968.
79. Guthrie, R.G. Screening for "inborn errors of metabolism" in the newborn infant—a multiple test program. *Birth Defects* 4(6):92, 1968.
80. Misuma, H., Wada, H., Kawakami, M., et al. Galactose and galactose-1-phosphate spot test for galactosemia screening. *Clin. Chim. Acta* 111:27, 1981.
81. Kromrower, G.M., and Lee, D.H. Long-term follow-up of galactosaemia. *Arch. Dis. Child.* 45:367, 1970.
82. Schapira, F., Gregori, C., Boue, J., et al. Prenatal diagnosis of galactosemia. *Biomedicine Express* 29(4):136, 1978.
83. Wenz, E., and Michel, M. Galactosemia. In S. Palmer and S. Ekvall, Eds., *Pediatric Nutrition in Developmental Disorders.* Springfield, Ill.: Charles C Thomas, 1978.
84. Donnell, G.N., and Bergren, W.R. The galactosemias. In D.N. Raine, Ed., *The Treatment of Inherited Metabolic Disease.* New York: Elsevier, 1974.
85. Segal, S.D. Disorders of Galactose Metabolism. In J.B. Stanbury, J.B. Wyngaarden, D.S. Fredrickson, Eds. *The Metabolic Basis of Inherited Disease,* 4th ed. New York: McGraw-Hill, 1978.
86. Gitzelman, R., Steinmann, B., van den Berghe, G. Essential fructosuria, hereditary fructose intolerance, and fructose-1,6-diphosphatase deficiency. In J.B. Stanbury, J.B. Wyngaarden, D.S. Fredrickson, et al., Eds., *The Metabolic Basis of Inherited Disease,* 5th ed. New York: McGraw-Hill, 1983.
87. Froesch, E.R., Wolf, H.P., Baitsch, H., et al. Hereditary fructose intolerance: An inborn error of fructose metabolism. *Am. J. Med.* 34:151, 1963.
88. Havel, R.J., Goldstein, J.L., and Brown, M.S. Lipoproteins and Lipid Transport. In P.K. Bondy and L.E. Rosenberg, Eds., *Metabolic Control and Disease,* 8th ed. Philadelphia: W.B. Saunders, 1980.
89. Glomset, J., Norum, K., and Gjone, E. Fa-

milial lecithin:cholesterol acyltransferase deficiency. In J.B. Stanbury, J.B. Wyngaarden, D.S. Fredrickson, et al., Eds., *The Metabolic Basis of Inherited Disease,* 5th ed. New York: McGraw-Hill, 1983.

90. Gjone, E., Blomhoff, J.P., and Skarbovik, A.J. Possible association between an abnormal low density lipoprotein and nephropathy in lecithin:cholesterol acyltransferase deficiency. *Clin. Chim. Acta* 54:11, 1974.
91. Steinberg, D. Phytanic acid storage disease (Refsum's disease). In J.B. Stanbury, J.B. Wyngaarden, D.S. Fredrickson, et al., Eds., *The Metabolic Basis of Inherited Disease,* 5th ed. New York: McGraw-Hill, 1983.
92. Refsum, S. Heredopathia atactica polyneuritiformis. *Acta Psychiatr. Scand.* [*Suppl.*] 38:9, 1946.
93. Refsum, S. Heredopathía atáctica polyneuritiformis reconsideración. *World Neurol.* 1:334, 1960.
94. Ackman, R.G., and Hooper, S.N. Isoprenoid fatty acids in the human diet: Distinctive geographical features in butterfats and importance in margarines based on marine oils. *Can. Inst. Food Sci. Technol. J.* 6:159, 1973.
95. Sen Gupta, A.K., and Peters, H. Isolation and structure determination of polybranched-chain fatty acids from fish oil. *Fette Seifen, Anstrichmittel* 68:349, 1966.
96. Steinberg, D., Mize, C.E., Herndon, J.H.K., Jr., et al. Phytanic acid in patients with Refsum's syndrome and response to dietary treatment. *Arch. Intern. Med.* 125:75, 1970.
97. Lundberg, A., Lilja, L.G., Lundberg, P.O., et al. Heredopathia atactica polyneuritiformis (Refsum's disease): Experiences of dietary treatment and plasmapheresis. *Eur. Neurol.* 8:309, 1972.
98. Stokke, O., and Eldjarn, L. Biochemical and dietary aspects of Refsum's disease. In P.J. Dyck, P.K. Thomas, and E.H. Lambert, Eds., *Peripheral Neuropathy,* vol. 2. Philadelphia: W.B. Saunders, 1975.
99. Seegmiller, J.E. Diseases of purine and pyrimidine metabolism. In P.K. Bondy and L.E. Rosenberg, Eds., *Metabolic Control and Disease,* 8th ed. Philadelphia: W.B. Saunders, 1980.
100. Seegmiller, J.E., Laster, L., and Howell, R.R. Biochemistry of uric acid and its relations to gout. *N. Engl. J. Med.* 168:712, 764, 821, 1963.
101. Hine, J. Hyperuricemia (Lesch-Nyhan syndrome). In S. Palmer and S. Ekvall, Eds., *Pediatric Nutrition in Developmental Disorders.* Springfield, Ill.: Charles C Thomas, 1978.
102. Ogryzlo, M.A. Hyperuricemia induced by high fat diets and starvation. *Arthritis Rheum.* 8:799, 1965.
103. Maclachlan, M.J., and Rodnan, G.P. Effects of food, fast and alcohol on serum uric acid and acute attacks of gout. *Am. J. Med.* 42:38, 1967.
104. Maloney, M.J., and Rosenberg, L.E. Inherited defects of B_{12} metabolism. *Am. J. Med.* 48:584, 1970.
105. Felix, J.S., and Demars, R. Purine requirement of cells cultured from humans affected with Lesch-Nyhan syndrome (hypoxanthine-guanine phosphoribosyltransferase deficiency). *Proc. Natl. Acad. Sci. U.S.A.* 62:536, 1969.
106. Baer, M.T. Folic acid deficiency. In S. Palmer and S. Ekvall, Eds., *Pediatric Nutrition in Developmental Disorders.* Springfield, Ill.: Charles C Thomas, 1978.
107. Hunt, A.D., Jr., Stokes, J., Jr., McCrory, W.W., et al. Pyridoxine dependency: Report of a case of intractable convulsions in an infant controlled by pyridoxine. *Pediatrics* 13:140, 1954.
108. Scriver, C.R., and Whelan, D.T. Glutamic acid decarboxylase in mammalian tissue outside the central nervous system and the possible relevance to vitamin B_6 dependency with seizures. *Ann. N.Y. Acad. Sci.* 166:83, 1969.
109. Kappas, A., Sassa, S., and Anderson, K.E. The porphyrias. In Stanbury, J.B., Wyngaarden, J.B., Fredrickson, D.S., et al., Eds., *The Metabolic Basis of Inherited Disease,* 5th ed. New York: McGraw-Hill, 1983.
110. Loo, Y.H., and Ritman, P. Phenylketonuria and vitamin B_6 function. *Nature* 213:914, 1967.
111. Berry, H.K. Inborn errors of metabolism. *J. Am. Diet. Assoc.* 49:44, 1966.
112. Rasmussen, H., and Anast, C. Familial hypophosphatemic rickets and vitamin D–dependent rickets. In J.B. Stanbury, J.B. Wyngaarden, D.S. Fredrickson, et al., Eds., *The Metabolic Basis of Inherited Disease,* 5th ed. New York: McGraw-Hill, 1983.
113. Palmer, S. Familial vitamin D–resistant rickets. In S. Palmer and S. Ekvall, Eds., *Pediatric Nutrition in Developmental Disorders.* Springfield, Ill.: Charles C Thomas, 1978.
114. Williams, T.F., and Winters, R.W. Familial (hereditary) vitamin D–resistant rickets

with hypophosphatemia. In J.B. Stanbury, J.B. Wyngaarden, and D.S. Fredrickson, Eds., *The Metabolic Basis of Inherited Disease,* 2nd ed. New York: McGraw-Hill, 1972.

115. Albright, F., Butler, A.M., and Bloomberg, E. Rickets resistant to vitamin D therapy. *Am. J. Dis. Child.* 54:529, 1937.
116. Albright, F., and Sulkowitch, H.W. The effect of vitamin D on calcium and phosphorus metabolism: Studies on four patients. *J. Clin. Invest.* 17:305, 1938.
117. Danks, D.M. Hereditary disorders of copper metabolism in Wilson's disease and Menkes' disease. In J.B. Stanbury, J.B. Wyngaarden, D.S. Fredrickson, et al., Eds., *The Metabolic Basis of Inherited Disease,* 5th ed. New York: McGraw-Hill, 1983.
118. National Academy of Sciences. *Zinc.* Subcommittee on Zinc, Committee on Medical and Biologic Effects of Environmental Pollutants. Division of Medical Sciences, Assembly of Life Sciences, National Research Council. Baltimore: University Park Press, 1978.
119. Nelder, K.H., Hagler, L., Wise, W. R., et al. Acrodermatitis enteropathica: A clinical and biochemical survey. *Arch. Dermatol.* 110: 711, 1974.
120. Moynahan, E.J. Acrodermatitis enteropathica: A lethal inherited human zinc-deficiency disorder. *Lancet* 2:399, 1974.
121. Nelder, K.H., and Hambidge, K.M. Zinc therapy of acrodermatitis enteropathica. *N. Engl. J. Med.* 292:879, 1975.
122. Michaelson, G. Zinc therapy in acrodermatitis enteropathica. *Acta Derm. Venereol.* (Stockh.) 54:377, 1974.
123. Palmer, S. Human zinc deficiency. In S. Palmer and S. Ekvall, Eds., *Pediatric Nutrition in Developmental Disorders.* Springfield, Ill.: Charles C Thomas, 1978.

Bibliography

Bondy, P.K., and Rosenberg, L.E., Eds. *Metabolic Control and Disease,* 8th ed. Philadelphia: W.B. Saunders, 1980.

Nyhan, W.L., Ed. *Heritable Disorders of Amino Acid Metabolism.* New York: John Wiley and Sons, 1974.

Palmer, S., and Ekvall, S., Eds. *Pediatric Nutrition in Developmental Disorders.* Springfield, Ill.: Charles C Thomas, 1978.

Raine, D.N., Ed. *The Treatment of Inherited Metabolic Disease.* New York: Elsevier, 1974.

Scriver, C.R., and Rosenberg, L.E. *Amino Acid Metabolism and Its Disorders.* Philadelphia: W.B. Saunders, 1973.

Stanbury, J.B., Wyngaarden, J.B., Fredrickson, D.S., et al., Eds. *The Metabolic Basis of Inherited Disease,* 5th ed. New York: McGraw-Hill, 1983.

Sources of Current Information

American Journal of Diseases of Children
Archives of Disease in Childhood
Journal of Inherited Metabolic Disease
Journal of Mental Deficiency Research
Journal of Pediatrics
New England Journal of Medicine
Pediatric Research
Pediatrics

11. Liver Disease and Alcoholism

The liver has a central function in nutrition and metabolism, and its malfunction has far-reaching effects. Malnutrition can be both a cause and a consequence of liver diseases, and nutritional care is important in their overall management.

NORMAL ANATOMY AND PHYSIOLOGY OF THE LIVER

The liver is the largest gland in the body, weighing 1 to 1.5 kg in an adult. It lies in the right upper quadrant of the abdominal cavity immediately below the diaphragm and against the right kidney and adrenal gland, lower esophagus, stomach, and intestine (see Fig. 5-1, p. 117). Its relationship to the vasculature of these organs is particularly important in the complications of some liver diseases.

Normal Liver Structure

The liver has two lobes, each with a separate blood supply. Their surfaces are closely apposed and they are enclosed in a common connective tissue capsule so that the two lobes are not visible externally.

Blood Supply

The blood vessels carrying blood to the liver enter from below at the *porta hepatis* or *hilus hepatis.* There are two blood supplies to the liver. The largest portion of blood (75 percent) enters the liver via the *portal vein,* which is formed from the mesenteric vein. This drains blood from the intestine, and the splenic vein drains blood from the spleen and stomach. The *hepatic artery* carries the remaining 25 percent of the blood but 50 percent or more of the liver's oxygen supply. It usually is a branch of the celiac trunk which arises from the aorta.

At the hilus, the connective tissue of the liver capsule extends up into the parenchyma of the liver and branches very much like the branches of a tree. The portal vein and hepatic artery follow the path of this connective tissue, also branching. At the ends of the branches, the blood from both sources flows into and merges in the *sinusoids,* capillarylike structures that are larger and more porous, thereby allowing protein to cross their walls. They are lined by endothelial cells but have no basement membrane. The sinusoids also have *Kupffer cells* attached to their interior walls. These are phagocytic cells of the reticuloendothelial system (see Chapter 4).

After the blood flows through the sinusoids, it is collected into the *central veins* of the liver. These drain into progressively larger veins and thence into the hepatic veins which leave the back of the liver to connect with the inferior vena cava.

The average rate of blood flow through the liver is 1,400 ml/min. There normally is very little resistance to blood flow through the liver; hepatic vein pressure is 0 mm Hg and portal pressure is approximately 8 mm Hg. Alterations in these pressures are significant in some liver conditions.

Hepatocytes

The parenchyma of the liver consists primarily of cells called *hepatocytes.* They exist in sheetlike *plates* which are two cells thick. When cut in cross section, they appear under the microscope as rows of cells called *hepatic cords.* The sinusoids exist on either side of the two-cell-thick structure. Thus, the blood is in intimate contact with the hepatocyte (Fig. 11-1). The Kupffer cells also are considered parenchymal but are present in much smaller numbers.

Drainage of Bile

Since bile is secreted by the liver, provision must be made for its drainage. For this purpose, very small ducts (*bile canaliculi*) exist between the two cells that represent the thickness of the hepatic plate. The bile is secreted into the canaliculi which drain successively into *canals of Hering, bile ductules,* and *bile ducts* in the portal tract. These structures compose the *biliary tree,* which follows the same course as the branching of the hepatic artery and portal vein. The flow, however, is in the opposite direction (see Fig. 11-1). Thus, the connective tissue, hepatic artery, portal vein, and bile ducts follow the same path. These are known as *portal tracts,* and they also contain lymphatics and nerves.

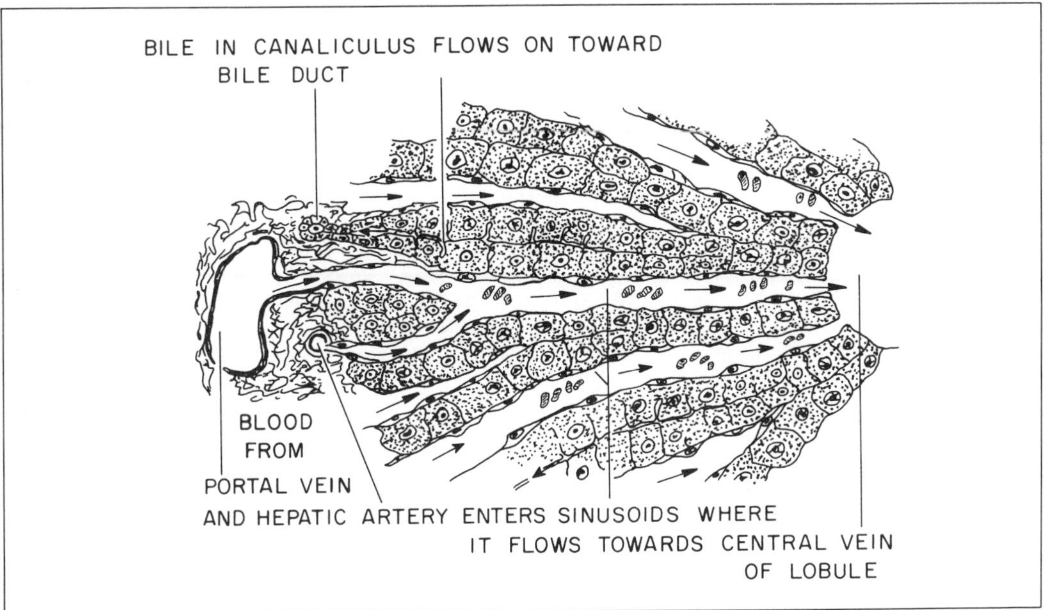

Figure 11-1. The flow of blood (indicated by arrows) from the portal vein and the hepatic artery (left) into sinusoids, lined by reticuloendothelium, that lie between hepatic cords; blood empties into the central vein (right). Also shown is the way that bile travels in the opposite direction in canaliculi to empty into bile ducts in portal areas. (Reprinted with permission from Ham, A.W., and Cormack, D.H., Histology, *8th ed. Philadelphia: J.B. Lippincott, 1979, p. 704.)*

Units of Structure

The basic unit of liver structure, which is easily seen with a microscope, is a *liver lobule.* It is roughly hexagonal and consists of a central vein surrounded by the hepatic plates, with three to six portal tracts visible at its edges (Fig. 11-2). An alternative structural unit is the *portal lobule,* which is visualized as a triangle with the portal tract in the center and a central vein at each angle (Fig. 11-2).

From a functional point of view, the liver can better be divided conceptually into *acini,* although an acinus is more difficult to see with a microscope. In concept, the central structure is the blood supply, rather than the central vein which accommodates drainage. The parenchyma consists of those cells supplied by one portal tract (see Fig. 11-2); a central vein thus may receive blood from more than one acinus. The acinus is a useful concept, since there are differences in the adequacy of the blood supply at various sites. Those cells closest to the central vein are exposed to blood with the least oxygen and the most carbon dioxide, whereas those closest to the smallest vessels of the blood supply prior to its entrance into the sinusoids are exposed to the freshest blood. The hepatocytes are unequal in other ways. They contain varying amounts of enzymes and so, presumably, they vary in their function. Hepatocytes nearest to the portal tract have high concentrations of glycolytic enzymes, whereas those near the central vein contain more enzymes involved in lipid metabolism. When hepatocytes are damaged, the damage can vary with the location of the cells.

Functions of the Liver

The liver has a variety of important functions. It controls the concentrations of many

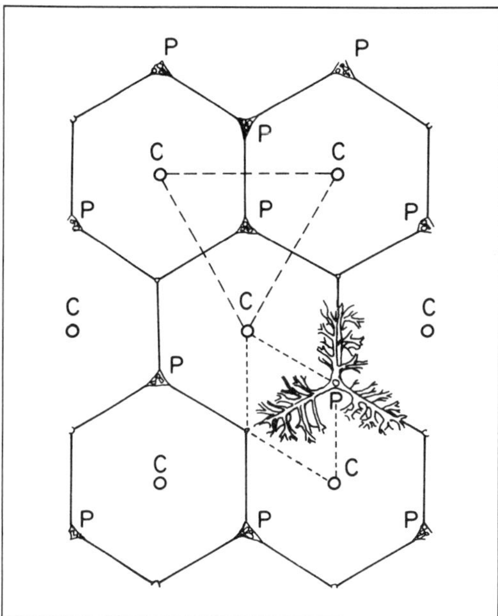

Figure 11-2. The hepatic lobules. The classic liver lobule is outlined with solid lines, the portal lobule with interrupted lines, and the liver acinus or functional unit with a dotted line. The branches of a portal vein and a hepatic artery from one portal area are shown at lower right. P = portal areas; C = central veins. (Reprinted with permission from Leeson, T.S., and Leeson, C.R., Histology, *4th ed. Philadelphia: W.B. Saunders, 1981, p. 391.)*

nutrients and disposes of many waste products in the bile. It also prepares materials for disposal in the urine. The liver synthesizes many substances and, through them, has extensive effects on digestion, colloid osmotic pressure, transport of metabolites, and blood coagulation. It also is an important storage depot.

Metabolic Functions

The liver receives directly from the intestine most of the absorbed nutrients that are products of digestion except for those absorbed into the lymphatic system (see Chapter 5). Thus, it is important in the metabolism of most nutrients. These metabolic processes are only summarized here. Further details may be obtained from elementary biochemistry textbooks.

Carbohydrate. The liver is the main, and sometimes the only, site of several aspects of carbohydrate metabolism. It receives almost all absorbed carbohydrate in the portal circulation. It stores glucose as glycogen (*glycogenesis*) and also breaks down glycogen to form glucose (*glycogenolysis*). It can form glucose from some amino acids (*gluconeogenesis*) and metabolizes hexoses other than glucose. These processes serve to provide a constant glucose supply to extrahepatic tissues, even though the exogenous supply of glucose is intermittent. The control of blood glucose concentration is described in more detail in Chapter 9. By taking up glucose the liver also prevents sudden changes in osmolality of body fluids following meals. In addition, it uses carbohydrates in the synthesis of mucopolysaccharides and synthesizes important metabolites via the hexose monophosphate shunt.

Protein. From the intestine, the liver receives amino acids, the sources of which are the diet, desquamated cells, and intestinal and pancreatic enzymes. The liver also receives endogenous amino acids in the blood. It extracts amino acids from the blood to varying degrees. Alanine uptake is very effective, and the glucogenic amino acids, in general, are taken up efficiently. The branched-chain amino acids—leucine, isoleucine, and valine—are not extracted by the liver but are allowed to enter the systemic circulation. The enzyme necessary for the metabolism of branched-chain amino acids are in the skeletal muscle, kidney, adipose tissue, brain, and other peripheral tissue, but not in the liver.[1]

The liver forms new nonessential amino acids by *transamination* and synthesizes a number of compounds containing nitrogen. Some of these are purines, pyrimidines, creatine, choline, coenzyme A, glutathione, porphyrins, glutamine, taurine, and carnosine. It degrades amino acids by *oxidative deamination,* producing alpha-keto acids and ammonia. *Urea synthesis,* which removes and detoxifies ammonia, occurs only in the liver.

The liver synthesizes structural and enzyme protein for liver function and is the source of much of the plasma protein. It is the only source of albumin and, as such, functions in the control of the colloid osmotic pressure. It is the principal site of synthesis of transferrin for iron binding and is the source of at least some ferritin. It also is the source of many factors necessary for blood coagulation, including prothrombin, fibrinogen, and factors V, VII, IX, and X.

Lipids. Lipids (fatty acids, triglycerides, phospholipids, cholesterol, and cholesteryl esters) normally make up approximately 5 percent of the weight of the liver. The liver is capable of synthesizing fatty acids, but most fatty acids are obtained from the diet or by release from adipose tissue. Regardless of the source, the liver is capable of using them to form triglycerides or phospholipids or to esterify cholesterol which it can synthesize from acetate.

The liver exports triglyceride to other tissue, a process that requires synthesis of apolipoproteins (see Chapter 8). This fact explains why liver protein metabolism is important in lipid release from the liver. The liver also oxidizes fatty acids to produce energy. In this process, it may produce large amounts of ketone bodies (see Chapter 9).

Vitamins. The liver has important functions related to many of the vitamins. Vitamin A is stored in the liver, and when it is released, it is bound to retinol-binding protein, which is synthesized in the liver. The liver is also the site of conversion of carotene to vitamin A. One of the steps in the activation of vitamin D_3 occurs in the liver. Vitamin D then is released attached to a binding globulin and is circulated to the kidney (see Chapter 7) where it is metabolized further. Through its action on vitamin D, the liver is important in the metabolism of calcium and phosphorus. It stores vitamin D and also functions in its disposal. Vitamin E and a small amount of vitamin K also are stored, as are some of the water-soluble vitamins for a short period.

Minerals. The liver stores iron and copper and recovers iron from discarded red blood cells (see Chapter 14). In addition, the liver is known to influence the metabolism of sodium, potassium, calcium, and chloride. Its influence on sodium metabolism will be discussed in greater detail later in connection with water balance (see pp. 448–449).

Alcohol. The liver is of major importance in the metabolism of alcohol. Because of the relationship between alcoholism and liver disease, alcohol metabolism will be described in detail under Alcoholism and Alcoholic Liver Disease (p. 445).

Protective and Detoxification Functions

The liver is associated with a number of processes by which it protects the body from deleterious substances. The phagocytic action of Kupffer cells has already been mentioned. The liver has a key role in the detoxification of exogenous and endogenous substances such as drugs, endogenous hormones, and toxins. The processes by which this is accomplished are described in Chapter 3. The removal of ammonia and the formation of urea may also be included among the liver's detoxification functions; its importance is described in more detail on page 445.

Digestion and Excretion

Since it synthesizes bile, the liver can be considered to have a role in digestion. The function of bile in digestion and absorption is described in Chapter 6. The bile is the vehicle for excretion of cholesterol and fat-soluble foreign materials. Bilirubin, the product of the breakdown of heme when red blood cells are discarded, also is excreted in the bile.

Circulatory and Other Functions

The liver has the capacity to serve as a reservoir for blood. It usually contains approximately 650 ml of blood but can expand or compress to alter its blood volume. The controlling mechanisms are not clear. The liver is a major source of lymph, producing lymph with a high protein content. It also serves as a hematopoietic organ in the fetus, but this function is confined to the bone marrow in the normal adult.

DIAGNOSIS OF LIVER DISEASE

There are numerous liver function tests based on the many metabolic functions of the liver. However, they are not specific for liver disease, and the results of many of these tests are influenced by extrahepatic factors. The tests may require analysis of blood, feces, or urine. They differ in their usefulness, some simply indicating the presence of disease or liver damage, others defining the extent of the diseases, and still others differentiating between specific hepatic diseases. Normal values are given in Appendixes D and E. Biochemical tests of liver function include tests for carbohydrate, lipid, and protein metabolism, detoxification, and excretion. Table 11-1 summarizes many of these tests but does not exhaust the possibilities.

A few tests are commonly associated specifically with liver functions. The sulfobromophthalein (*Bromsulphalein;* BSP) *retention test* measures the ability of the liver to concentrate and secrete the BSP dye. It is used as an overall assessment of liver function. Sulfobromophthalein is injected parenterally and then is bound to albumin, taken up by the liver, conjugated, and excreted in the bile. Abnormal retention indicates disease of the liver or biliary tract but does not differentiate between them. Normal retention is less than 5 percent of the dose in 45 minutes but may be higher in obesity, old age, pregnancy, and fever.

Another frequently used test is that for *serum bilirubin concentration.* Approximately 200 mg of bilirubin is formed daily from heme breakdown, and a small additional amount is obtained from myoglobin and cytochromes. The bilirubin is attached to albumin and carried to the liver from its site of origin. After uptake by the liver, it is conjugated with glucuronic acid, a reaction catalyzed by glucuronyltransferase, and excreted in the intestine in the bile. The serum concentration of bilirubin is measured by *van den Bergh's test,* which measures conjugated (*direct*) bilirubin and total bilirubin. Unconjugated (*indirect*) bilirubin then is obtained indirectly by subtraction. It is helpful in diagnosis to have both values to differentiate between biliary obstruction and hepatocyte disease. For example, increased unconjugated bilirubin indicates that the hepatocytes are decreased in number or incapable of normal conjugation. If the serum bilirubin is increased with proportionately more of the conjugated form, the hepatocytes must be capable of conjugation but the biliary tract may be obstructed, interfering with normal excretion.

When the liver cells are damaged, *changes in enzyme concentrations* appear in the blood. These changes may be the consequence of (1) an alteration in liver cell activity, (2) leakage from the cell, or (3) alterations in the rate of disappearance from the cell. No tests for serum enzymes are specific for detection of liver disease, but there are several that are reasonably useful. Table 11-1 lists a number of enzyme assays with some notes on the significance of the results.

Other useful diagnostic procedures include visualization of the liver following administration of a radioisotope that would concentrate in the liver (*scintiscan*) or visualization by *ultrasound* or *computerized tomography.*[2] *Angiography* visualizes the circulation. The procedure for visualizing the bile

Table 11-1. Tests of Liver Function

Function	Test	Comments
Carbohydrate metabolism	Glucose tolerance; glycogen reserves	Usually normal until disease is advanced; not helpful in differentiating between malfunction in carbohydrate metabolism in liver and other diseases
	Galactose tolerance	Sometimes useful; measures ability to clear galactose from circulation
Lipid metabolism	Serum cholesterol and cholesteryl esters	Total falls in severe injury; proportion of esters decreases; increases are seen in bile tract obstruction
	Serum lipoprotein X	Present in biliary obstruction
Protein metabolism	Blood urea nitrogen	Level changes in liver or kidney disease or malnutrition
	Blood ammonia	Increase occurs late in liver disease
	Blood amino acids	Increase occurs late in liver disease
	Serum protein concentrations	Decreased in liver or renal disease, protein-calorie malnutrition, protein loss from gastrointestinal tract
	Serum protein electrophoresis pattern	Changes may be useful in differential diagnosis of liver disease
	Prothrombin time	Depends on concentration of various clotting factors; decreases if liver cannot synthesize
Digestion	Serum bile acids	Measure of combined abilities to synthesize bile acids and clear them from blood
Detoxification and excretion	Bromsulphalein (BSP) retention	Used as overall assessment of liver function; measures ability to concentrate and secrete injected BSP; increased retention occurs in liver or biliary disease
	Indocyanin green	Alternative to BSP retention test
	Serum bilirubin (van den Bergh's test)	Measures ability to conjugate and excrete bilirubin
	Antipyrine, phenylbutazone, or labeled carbon dioxide for aminophenazone metabolism	Measures ability to produce enzymes for metabolism of these drugs
	Gamma-glutamyl transpeptidase	Elevated in severe liver or biliary tree disease; induced by drugs or alcohol (?); useful to monitor abstinence
Enzyme synthesis	Serum transaminases (SGOT and SGPT)	Increased in hepatocyte damage
	Serum glutamic acid dehydrogenase	Increased in alcoholic hepatitis and obstructive jaundice
	Serum alkaline phosphatase	Normally high in bile duct epithelium; serum levels increase in bile duct obstruction
	Serum 5′-nucleotidase	Elevated in obstructive biliary disease

Compiled from Price, C.P., and Alberti, K.G.M.M., Biochemical assessment of liver function. In R. Wright, K.G.M.M. Alberti, S. Karran, and G.H. Millward-Sadler, Eds., *Liver and Biliary Disease.* London: W.B. Saunders, 1979; Mezey, E., Diagnosis of liver disease by laboratory methods. In J.A. Halsted and C.H. Halsted, Eds., *The Laboratory in Clinical Medicine,* 2nd ed. Philadelphia: W.B. Saunders, 1981; and Byrne, C.J., Saxton, D.F., Pelikan, P.K., and Nugent, P.M., *Laboratory Tests. Implications for Nurses and Allied Health Professionals.* Menlo Park, Calif.: Addison-Wesley, 1981. SGOT = serum glutamic oxaloacetic transaminase; SGPT = serum glutamic pyruvic transaminase.

ducts and gallbladder is a *cholangiogram.* The physician may see some structures, particularly of the bile duct, by *endoscopy,* using a cannula.

METABOLIC AND MORPHOLOGICAL ALTERATIONS IN THE DISEASED LIVER

Many metabolic and morphological alterations are common to more than one liver disorder; some of these alterations will be described here, with a discussion of their relationship to symptoms of disease. A discussion of specific liver disorders will follow.

Morphological and Anatomic Disorders and Their Consequences

In the course of some liver diseases, particularly those of nutritional interest, there may be a loss of hepatocytes. This sometimes occurs within a short time and sometimes is the result of long-term degeneration. The fatty liver may be the first stage of the degenerative process. It is thought to be reversible at first. As the process continues, the normal architecture of the liver collapses, fibrosis develops (see Chapter 1), and the vascular bed is distorted.

Fibrotic and Nodular Liver

The hepatocyte is a stable cell—that is, it retains the ability to multiply—and the liver has remarkable powers of regeneration. Resections of 80 to 90 percent of the liver are replaced by enlarged and new cells in a very short time, although the factors that control this process are not understood very well. In the fibrotic liver, nonnecrotic hepatocytes attempt to regenerate the liver but cannot reinstate the normal architecture because the fibrotic bands get in the way. Instead, they multiply and form *nodules* of hepatocytes, but these do not have a normal relationship to the vascular system and cannot perform normally. Thus, there is *disorderly regeneration,* as described in Chapter 1.

Portal Hypertension, Ascites, and Varices

The fibrosis and nodules of regenerating hepatocytes together form a resistance to blood flow through the liver. The pressure in the portal vein rises as a consequence. When it exceeds 10 mm Hg, a collateral circulation develops between it and nearby veins so that blood can be diverted into the systemic veins. The veins with which the portal vein forms the collateral circulation are in the submucosa of the esophagus, stomach, and rectum, in the anterior abdominal wall, and the left renal vein, all of which drain into the vena cava. The collateral circulation develops by enlargement and proliferation of existing small blood vessels connecting these organs.

Portal hypertension can cause *ascites* (accumulation of fluid in the peritoneal cavity). Increased hydrostatic pressure in the portal vein in excess of the colloid osmotic pressure results in a transudation of fluid. Also, a block in the venous outflow from the liver causes an increased intrahepatic pressure with increased formation of hepatic lymph. When the capacity for lymph drainage is exceeded, the excess lymph exudes from the surface of the liver. Thus, the abdominal cavity becomes distended with high-protein fluid. The loss of protein from the blood lowers the colloid osmotic pressure, aggravating the problem. The pressure of this fluid accumulation can become so severe that it causes hernias and intestinal obstruction. Sometimes the hernia ruptures.

For the ascitic fluid to accumulate, renal excretion must be decreased. There are two mechanisms by which this may happen. In one, because of the loss of ascitic fluid from the circulation, the blood volume is decreased and renal perfusion declines. The renin-angiotensin-aldosterone system is activated (see Chapter 8), and the kidneys retain sodium. Thus, sodium retention would be secondary to ascites formation.[3] It has been suggested that the alternative mechanism involves renal retention of sodium as the primary abnormality.[4] Overflow of fluid then occurs when other conditions, such as portal hypertension, make it possible. The mechanism for increased sodium retention is not clear but probably is multifactorial, involving both aldosterone and renin.[3] It is possible, that the abnormal liver cannot inactivate aldosterone.[5]

The development of the collateral circulation is the cause of a number of added clinical manifestations. The high portal pressure is transferred to the systemic veins. In the esophagus, stomach, and intestine, the increased pressure causes *varices* (enlarged and tortuous veins such as those seen on the legs of some persons). Varices in the rectum result in hemorrhoids. Those in the esophagus or stomach may hemorrhage, contributing protein to the intestinal tract and exacerbating the tendency to neuropsychiatric disorders described later. Hemorrhage of varices is the immediate cause of death of a large number of patients with this condition, occurring in approximately one-third of patients with varices within 5 years. Only 20 to 40 percent survive.

Jaundice

Jaundice or *icterus* occurs when bilirubin is deposited in the tissues. The skin and sclera of the eyes become yellow owing to the presence of bilirubin. Jaundice can be caused by many conditions other than liver diseases. In the diseased liver, it often is the consequence of obstruction of the biliary tree. Also, bilirubin is transported on an albumin carrier, and reduced serum albumin causes bilirubin to be deposited in the tissue. Normal serum bilirubin is less than 1.0 mg/dl. In jaundice, it exceeds 2 mg/dl but may reach much higher levels. When the concentration reaches 18 to 20 mg/dl, deposition in the brain can cause brain damage.

Metabolic Disorders

Carbohydrate Metabolism

Liver damage can cause hypoglycemia, but this generally occurs only in fulminant disease or far-advanced chronic disease. It is assumed to result from a failure of gluconeogenesis but may be a consequence of reduced glycogenolysis. Patients with some liver diseases have decreased glycogen stores. In the alcoholic patient, reduced carbohydrate intake may contribute. In some patients, there is *insulin resistance* and *hyperglycemia*, but the mechanism is not clear.

Lipid Metabolism

Very-low-density lipoproteins, high-density lipoproteins, and lecithin-cholesterol-acyltransferase are synthesized in the liver. An alteration in any step in the process of lipid metabolism provides a potential mechanism for fat accumulation in the liver.[6] Possible alterations are listed here, and examples are given in parentheses:

1. Increased influx of fatty acids (diabetic ketosis; lipid mobilization from alcohol or corticosteroid intake)
2. Increased fatty acid synthesis (alcoholism; obesity)
3. Decreased fatty acid oxidation (alcoholism; obesity)
4. Increased availability of alpha-glycerophosphate for triglyceride esterification (alcoholism; obesity)
5. Decreased apolipoprotein synthesis necessary for lipoprotein formation (effects of selected toxic chemicals)
6. Impaired lipoprotein synthesis from available lipid and apolipoprotein (alcoholism)
7. Impaired lipoprotein release from the liver (alcoholism)

Liver injury may lead to decreased serum cholesterol as a consequence of decreased cholesterol or apolipoprotein synthesis or both. In biliary tract obstruction, serum cholesterol levels often increase. The effects of reduction of bile salts in the intestine as a consequence of obstruction are described in Chapter 6.

Protein and Nitrogen Metabolism

Changes in protein metabolism have important consequences in the patient with liver disease. These involve protein synthesis, amino acid metabolism, and the metabolism of urea and ammonia.

Protein Synthesis. In hepatic failure, depressed synthesis of plasma protein leads to *hypoproteinemia.* This condition can be exacerbated by increased plasma protein catabolism, internal bleeding, and increased urinary excretion of amino acids.

Urea and Ammonia Metabolism. Urea synthesis may be depressed as much as 90 percent in liver disease, since the activities of the necessary enzymes that occur in the liver are decreased. At the same time, the blood ammonia level rises. There are five principal mechanisms by which this can occur (Fig. 11-3):[6]

1. Amino acids in the intestine, from dietary protein or internal bleeding, are deaminated by intestinal bacteria.
2. Urine output falls in some liver disease (*hepatorenal syndrome*) and retained blood urea nitrogen diffuses into the intestine. Urease from bacteria then converts it to ammonia.
3. Removal of ammonia for urea synthesis is reduced as a result of decreased hepatic function.
4. Metabolic alkalosis and hypokalemia with decreased hydrogen ions accompany some liver disease. Ammonia produced from glutamine by the action of renal glutaminase is shunted into the circulation.

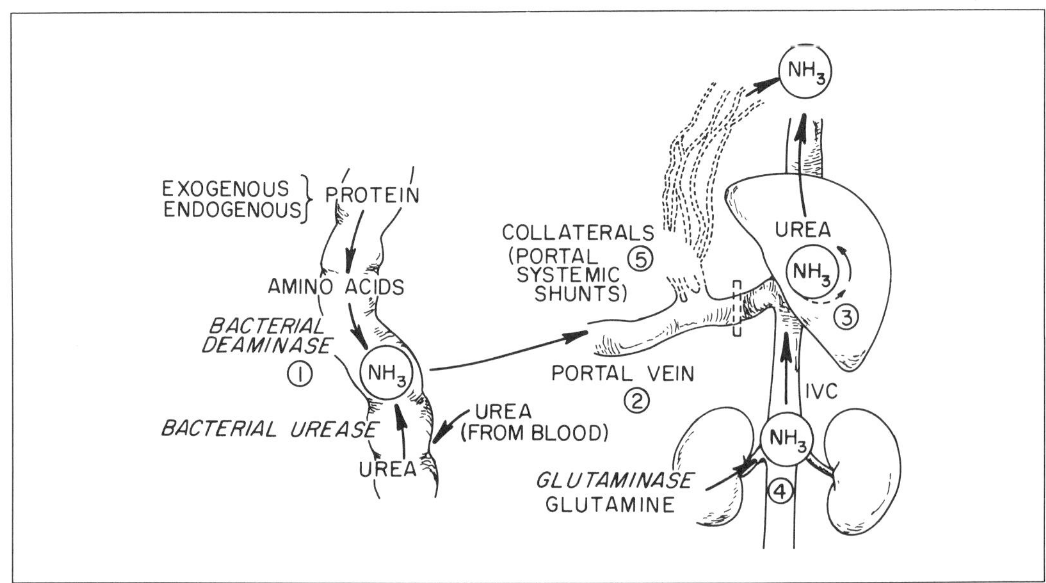

Figure 11-3. Major factors (steps 1 through 4) influencing the level of blood ammonia. In cirrhosis with portal hypertension, venous collaterals allow ammonia to bypass the liver (5), allowing for the entry of ammonia into the systemic circulation (portasystemic shunting). (Reprinted with permission from Alpers, D.H., and Isselbacher, K.J., Derangements of Hepatic Metabolism. In G.W. Thorn, R.D. Adams, E. Braunwald, et al., Eds., Harrison's Principles of Internal Medicine, *8th ed. New York: McGraw-Hill, 1977, p. 1578.)*

5. In the patient with portal hypertension, the blood in the venous anastomoses, which develop between the portal vein and systemic veins (portasystemic shunts), bypasses the liver. Sometimes, to reduce the danger of variceal hemorrhage, a portacaval shunt is created surgically, connecting the portal vein and the inferior vena cava. In either case, ammonia is not removed by the liver for detoxification.

Amino Acid Metabolism. The liver also affects the concentration and metabolism of amino acids from the blood. As amino acids come to it in the portal and hepatic blood, the liver takes them up to a varying extent. The branched-chain amino acids (BCAAs) are not absorbed by the liver but pass through to the systemic circulation. In sudden severe liver failure, the liver is unable to remove many of the amino acids from the plasma, and all amino acids except the BCAAs are increased in concentration. In chronic liver failure, there usually is an increase in the plasma concentrations of phenylalanine and tyrosine and also free (not total) tryptophan, and methionine, whereas BCAA concentrations are decreased. The normal ratio of BCAAs to aromatic amino acids (AAAs) in plasma is 3 or 4; in hepatic disease, it may be 1.0 or less.[7–9] It is not clear why this decrease occurs. Hyperinsulinemia may suppress muscle output of BCAAs, or there may be an increase in their oxidation outside the liver.[10] It also is possible that they are used by the kidney to form glucose in an attempt to compensate for loss of hepatic gluconeogenesis and thus maintain the blood glucose levels.

Protein Metabolism and Hepatic Encephalopathy. In patients with hepatic failure (*hepatic decompensation*), neuropsychiatric disturbances (*hepatic encephalopathy*) can occur. The clinical manifestations indicate that there are alterations in the transmission of impulses in the central nervous system (CNS). Hepatic encephalopathy is characterized by acute and temporary or chronic and sustained disturbances in consciousness and electroencephalographic (EEG) changes. These disturbances progress from mild personality changes, forgetfulness, day-night reversal of sleep, and deterioration in personal care to intellectual deterioration and confusion, stupor, and eventually to deep coma. Many patients have *asterixis,* a flapping tremor in the precoma stage, but it is not invariable and is seen in other diseases as well. *Fetor hepaticus* is a musty odor of the breath and urine in coma patients and in patients with extensive collateral shunting. The odor is believed to be caused by *mercaptans,* metabolites of methionine.

Acute and chronic hepatic encephalopathies. There are several circumstances in which hepatic encephalopathy occurs. They differ somewhat in their manifestations, so it is possible that there are differences in their etiology. If liver failure is sudden, such as in *acute fulminant hepatitis,* the patient develops *acute encephalopathy* and progresses through the symptoms within a very short period, sometimes in a few hours. The clinical manifestations are severe and often resemble psychiatric disorders. The causes generally are reversible and, if he or she survives, the patient may again become neurologically normal.

Chronic encephalopathy occurs in some patients with chronic liver disease. The patient has intermittent attacks without apparent cause, or an attack can be precipitated by identifiable factors. These include gastrointestinal bleeding, increased dietary protein, and azotemia, delivering more nitrogenous compounds to the liver. Hypokalemic alkalosis also precipitates encephalopathy by converting ammonium ion (NH_4) to ammonia (NH_3), thereby facilitating its diffusion across the blood-brain barrier. In some patients, the cause is excessive use of diuretics. Infection increases the sensitivity of the brain to ammonia and other nitrogenous compounds.

Pathogenesis of hepatic coma. The specific metabolic processes in the brain by which the neurologic symptoms are produced are not understood entirely, but the pathogeneses of hepatic coma in various conditions usually have some features in common. First, portal blood may be shunted around the liver either through spontaneously occurring shunts (*portasystemic*) or shunts that are created surgically (*portacaval*). Second, diminishing hepatic function usually contributes, but there are exceptions. Third, the etiologic agent responsible for producing the clinical manifestations originate in the gut; gut bacteria have some role in the syndrome, and the etiologic agent or agents may be nitrogenous. Finally, blood ammonia levels generally, but not invariably, correlate with the presence of encephalopathy but not with its severity.

Neurotransmitters. The identity of the etiologic agent is not known with certainty and is the subject of some very intriguing current research. To understand the theories of the specific causes of hepatic encephalopathy, some understanding of neurotransmitters is necessary.

Nerve impulses are transmitted from one neuron to another at *synapses* or from nerve to muscle at the *neuromuscular junction* (*motor end-plate*) (see Chapter 1). The end of the nerve fiber contains vesicles enclosing minute amounts of a *neurotransmitter.* When the nerve impulse (*depolarization wave*) reaches the end of the fiber at the synapse, the vesicles fuse with the cell membrane and release their contents into the gap or synaptic cleft between it and the next nerve fiber or muscle fiber. The transmitter combines with the membrane of the affected neuron or muscle and makes it more permeable to particular ions. If permeability to sodium ion is increased, a wave of depolarization is triggered in the affected cell. At some synapses, the flow of potassium or chlorine ion, which have an inhibitory effect, is increased.

There are a number of neurotransmitters, most of which are either monamines or peptides and therefore usually are products of amino acid metabolism. *Tyrosine* is oxidized in the adrenal medulla or nervous tissue to *3,4-dihydroxyphenylalanine* (*DOPA*). DOPA then is decarboxylated to *dopamine* (*dihydroxyphenylethylamine*) which is used as a transmitter in some neurons of the brain. Dopamine can be oxidized to produce *norepinephrine,* the transmitter in most sympathetic nerves. Norepinephrine is important in the CNS. Dopamine may also be methylated in the adrenal medulla to form *epinephrine,* using *methionine* as the methyl donor. Dopamine, epinephrine, and norepinephrine together are called *catecholamines.*

Adrenergic nerve fibers (those activated by epinephrine) have two different types of receptors, designated *alpha* and *beta.* Stimulation of these receptors may have opposite, and sometimes synergistic, effects. Norepinephrine has marked alpha-adrenergic receptor action and weaker beta-adrenergic receptor response. Epinephrine acts on both alpha-adrenergic and beta-adrenergic receptors. Adrenergic chemicals were studied first in the peripheral nervous system but also have demonstrated central effects in the brain.

Serotonin (5-hydroxytryptamine), formed from *tryptophan,* occurs primarily outside the nervous system (see Chapter 6) but acts as a neurotransmitter in some neurons in the CNS. It cannot cross the blood-brain barrier and therefore must be synthesized within the brain. *Acetylcholine,* a common transmitter between neurons that synapse outside the CNS, is formed from choline and acetyl-coenzyme A (acetyl-CoA). Another transmitter is *4-aminobutyrate* or *gamma-aminobutyric acid* (*GABA*), which is formed from L-glutamate by transamination and increases chloride ion passage when released, producing an inhibitory effect. *Glycine* is an inhibitory transmitter. *Glutamate* and *aspartate* are excitatory.

With this knowledge of neurotransmitters we now can explore the relationship of protein metabolism and hepatic encephalopathy. In hepatic encephalopathy, there is an abnormality in central neurotransmission. For many years, it was believed to be the result of toxic effects of ammonia on the brain even though the blood ammonia concentration and depth of coma are poorly correlated. Because of this poor correlation, it was suggested by some investigators that ammonia was not important in the etiology or was not the primary cause.[11] However, it now is agreed that ammonia is a toxic substance. In addition, in hepatic disease there apparently are changes in the blood-brain barrier or the brain itself that make the brain more sensitive to ammonia. Other researchers have suggested that coma results from the effect on the brain of mercaptans, short-chain fatty acids,[12,13] or of a synergism between the fatty acids and ammonia.[14]

It has been suggested that amino acids themselves, as well as amino acid metabolites, are the toxic materials. Normally these substances would be taken up by the liver, but in patients with portasystemic shunts, they bypass the liver and reach the brain, increasing the production of false neurotransmitters and possibly resulting in encephalopathy.[15]

Phenylalanine and tyrosine, it should be remembered, are precursors of catecholamines, and tryptophan is a precursor of serotonin. Products of microbial metabolism of tyrosine and tryptophan in the intestine include amines, indoles, and other substances that are weak or *false neurotransmitters.* Among these are *tyramine* and *octopamine.* Octopamine, produced from phenylalanine, tyrosine, or tyramine, has been studied in some depth and shown to be increased in the blood at levels that correlate well with the severity of the coma. *Phenylethanolamine,* another false neurotransmitter from phenylalanine, also increases. It is proposed that these substances are taken up by the nervous system, compete with true neurotransmitters, and create a widespread disturbance in neurotransmission.

The specific mechanisms by which alterations in amino acid concentrations alter neurotransmission is not entirely clear. Obviously, the need is for a theory that accounts for all the facts, including provision for a role for ammonia and the derangements in plasma amino acid concentrations. Current proposals are summarized here, but it is important to remember that these are subject to change with continuing research.

Using information largely from the research by Fischer,[16] we begin with the supposition that ammonia in the blood is increased and there is an apparent change in the blood-brain barrier by which its penetrability is altered, leading to an increase in ammonia levels in the brain. This ammonia is detoxified by astrocytes (the stroma cells in the brain) by forming glutamine from glutamic acid:

$$\underset{\text{Glutamic Acid}}{\begin{array}{l} COOH \\ | \\ CHNH_2 \\ | \\ CH_2 \\ | \\ CH_2 \\ | \\ COOH \end{array}} + NH_3 = \underset{\text{Glutamine}}{\begin{array}{l} COOH \\ | \\ CHNH_2 \\ | \\ CH_2 \\ | \\ CH_2 \\ | \\ CONH_2 \end{array}} \longrightarrow + H_2O$$

When glutamine leaves the cells and returns to the circulation (the theory continues), it exchanges with tyrosine, tryptophan, and methionine at the cell membrane so that they increase in concentration in the brain. Thus, ammonia contributes indirectly to the accumulation of these amino acids in the brain, which in turn alters the neurotransmitter balance in the brain. Tyrosine is the main precursor of norepinephrine, but in hepatic failure, excess tyrosine or phenylalanine appear to cause an accumulation of octopamine rather than increased synthesis of norepinephrine.[11,15] There is a depletion of norepinephrine during hepatic coma. In hepatic failure, there also is a disturbance in serotonin metabolism. Glutamate, an excitatory transmitter, is decreased, presumably having been used to detoxify the ammonia.

Tryptophan, present in the brain in increased quantities, is metabolized to serotonin. The increased serotonin, which is inhibitory, may be taken up in place of norepinephrine or dopamine. Gamma-aminobutyric acid, also inhibitory, has been shown to be increased in the blood plasma in patients in hepatic coma but has not yet been studied in the brain.

Branched-chain amino acids are neutral amino acids that are capable of competing with the AAAs at the blood-brain barrier. Presumably, they could reduce the entrance of the AAAs and thus cause disturbances in neurotransmission.

If these proposals are correct, they would, as pointed out by their authors,[17] account for the role of ammonia and the altered amino acid ratios, since both would affect neurotransmission. They would also explain why reduction of serum ammonia and restoration of normal amino acid ratios are effective in treating hepatic coma.

The effects of administering ornithine salts of the keto acid analogues of the BCAAs were compared with the effects of the BCAAs themselves in patients with portasystemic encephalopathy. Patients receiving the ornithine salts had the more significant improvement.[18] The reason for this is not known, and further investigation of the metabolic processes in the CNS obviously is needed.

There are those who disagree with the theory that the changes in amino acid pattern cause encephalopathy; they argue that the changes in plasma amino acid concentrations can occur along with encephalopathy but are not necessarily its cause.[19] Nevertheless, changes in amino acid concentrations are the basis for some of the newer nutritional care procedures discussed later in this chapter (see pp. 464–465).

Vitamin Metabolism

Low levels of folate,[20] thiamine, riboflavin, niacin, pyridoxine, vitamin B_{12}, and biotin[21] are commonly seen in patients with chronic hepatic failure. Folate is the most frequently deficient vitamin. Deficiencies of fat-soluble vitamins also are found frequently.[22] Poor diet, malabsorption, and metabolic aberrations are contributing causes.[20–23]

The expected clinical consequences of vitamin deficiency are seen in these patients. These include bleeding tendencies (vitamin K), night blindness (vitamin A), bone disorders (vitamin D), peripheral neuropathy (thiamine), glossitis and cheilosis (riboflavin), pellagra and Wernicke's encephalopathy (thiamine and niacin), and megaloblastic anemia (folate and vitamin B_{12}).[20–23]

Malabsorption in Liver Disease

Malabsorption is a common finding in patients with liver disease. Suggested causes include abnormal intestinal flora, increased pressure in the portal vein and lymphatics, and pancreatic insufficiency, but the specific mechanisms have not been determined.

VIRAL HEPATITIS

Viral hepatitis is a transmissible disease that is considered a serious public health problem. As such, it is the subject of much cur rent research.

Epidemiology

Viral hepatitis can be caused by three or more viruses. The most common disease is called *hepatitis A* or *infectious hepatitis,* occurring in approximately 60 percent of cases. *Hepatitis B,* formerly called serum hepatitis, occurs in 25 percent. Other forms of hepatitis currently are called *non-A, non-B hepatitis.* The liver can also be affected by other viruses.

Hepatitis A has a short incubation period. It often is transmitted via fecal contamination of milk, water, or raw shellfish and is seen primarily in children and young adults.

Hepatitis B has a long incubation period. It is transmitted parenterally, often by contaminated needles, and thus is a particular problem in drug addicts. It also is contracted during tattooing. Hepatitis B is of great concern in hemodialysis. The non-A, non-B viral disease is tentatively designated as *hepatitis C*, but probably there are multiple viruses and diseases. It is transmitted in blood transfusions.

Clinical Manifestations

Clinical manifestations of the various forms of viral hepatitis are similar but vary in severity. Hepatitis A usually begins acutely but is mild, whereas hepatitis B is more insidious in onset but prolonged and more severe. At first, there is a *prodromal period* (indicating the approach of the disease) in which the patient is easily fatigued and experiences anorexia and nausea. Some cases go unrecognized throughout, but others progress to clinical jaundice. This probably occurs in less than 5 percent of patients with hepatitis A virus, and liver function tests usually return to normal in 2 months. Hepatitis B is not only more prolonged but is more likely to progress to acute fulminant hepatitis with a 75 to 80 percent death rate. Chronic hepatitis develops in 5 to 10 percent of cases. Patients who advance to the recovery period may have fatigue, malaise, lassitude, and depression for weeks or months.

Nutritional Care

There are no specific antiviral agents for hepatitis. Treatment consists of bed rest, diet, and corticosteroid drugs. There is not complete agreement on the best diet, but the usual recommendations are as follows:

1. Provide calories generously, usually 3,000 to 4,000 kcal for an adult. This requires careful attention, since patients often are anorexic and nauseated. If the patient is vomiting, intravenous dextrose solutions are used. Sometimes amino acids are included.
2. Include 300 to 400 g of carbohydrate and 1.5 to 2.0 g of protein/kg of body weight to spare the liver and provide for repair.
3. Restrict fat only if it causes nausea or anorexia. Otherwise, a moderate amount of fat to make the diet acceptable is permitted. The generous intake of energy and protein is more important than fat restriction.
4. Cater to the patient's preferences in order to increase intake.
5. Take precautions against the spread of infection to others via the patient's tray.
6. Advise the patient to avoid alcohol for 4 to 6 months, although there is only marginal evidence that this influences the outcome.[24]

ALCOHOLISM AND ALCOHOLIC LIVER DISEASE

Alcoholism affects 9 million to 11 million people in the United States and has a number of social, economic, and physiologic consequences. Serious liver disease is among its effects; therefore, it will be discussed in some detail.

Alcohol Intake

Ethyl alcohol or *ethanol* (CH_3CH_2OH) is widely used as a social beverage, but its abuse is a major problem. *Alcoholism* is the excessive consumption of alcohol accompanied by alcohol dependence. Its effects may be divided into *acute effects*—that is, those resulting shortly after intake—and *effects of chronic abuse.*

The same dose-response relationship exists for alcohol as for other drugs (see Chapter 3). There is a minimum dose below which there are no observable effects, whereas at higher doses, effects are dose-related. Effects depend on the amount of the drug at the receptor site which, in turn, is a function of the magnitude and frequency of the dose. When speaking of alcohol intake, the effect depends on the alcohol content of the beverage a person drinks, how much, and how often.

Alcoholic beverages may be divided, for purposes of this discussion, into three categories—beer, wine, and distilled liquor. From a practical point of view, their consumption can be considered in terms of "drinks." In addition to their differences in taste and kilocalorie content, they also differ in alcohol and water content.

Some average figures can be used for illustrative purposes. The alcohol content of beer may be given in a percentage of weight to volume. Let us assume that a person is drinking a typical 12-oz. can of beer. Beer is, on the average, 3.8% alcohol. For ease of calculation, we also assume 30 ml/oz. Thus, one can of beer will contain 360 ml × 0.038 or 13.4 g of alcohol. If alcohol is considered as a percentage of volume to volume, the percentage of alcohol usually is approximately 4.5 to 5 percent.

The alcohol content of unfortified wine is 12 to 14 percent. This percentage also indicates weight per volume. A typical drink of wine might be 5 oz. or 150 ml. Thus, 150 ml × 0.12 = 16.0 g of alcohol. Fortified wines—that is, sherry or port—are prepared by the addition of brandy, so that their alcohol content may be 20 percent or more. Among so-called skid row alcoholics, a variation of fortified wines is popular. When these sweet wines are prepared, fermentation of the sugar is halted by the addition of concentrated alcohol. The wine thus has both a high sugar and a high alcohol content that often is substituted for food almost completely. However, it has no protein and essentially no vitamin or mineral content.

The alcohol content of distilled beverages, such as whisky, rum, gin, or brandy, is more variable. It is measured in *proof degrees,* the definition of which varies from one country to another. In the United States, 1 proof equals 0.5% alcohol. Therefore, 80-proof whisky contains 40% alcohol. Other distilled beverages vary from 35 to 50% alcohol or 70 to 100 proof. The customary measure is a jigger, the content of which is 1½ oz. or 45 ml. Thus, a jigger of 80-proof whisky taken as is or in a mixed drink would contain 45 ml × 0.40 or 18 g of alcohol.

Absorption and Distribution

Alcohol is a small, un-ionized molecule that is completely miscible with water and also somewhat fat-soluble. Its absorption and distribution follow the usual principles that apply to drugs with similar properties (see Chapter 3). It crosses membranes by diffusion, dependent on the concentration gradient. It is absorbed largely from the stomach and more rapidly from the upper small intestine. The rate of absorption from the stomach can be influenced by the presence of food or water in the stomach and by the stomach emptying time.

Most alcohol is carried in the body water. As a consequence, blood alcohol content is used as a basis for calculation of the content in tissue, in which it exists in proportion to the water content of the tissue.

Metabolism and Excretion

Approximately 5 percent of ingested alcohol can be excreted from the body in urine, expired air, feces, sweat, and milk. The remaining 95 percent is first oxidized to acetaldehyde by one of at least three pathways.[25]

1. The enzyme *alcohol dehydrogenase* (ADH) is used in the *ADH system* in the reaction:

$$\underset{\text{(ethanol)}}{CH_3CH_2OH} + NAD \xrightarrow{\text{Alcohol dehydrogenase}} \underset{\text{(acetaldehyde)}}{CH_3CHO} + NADH + H^+ \quad \textbf{(1)}$$

This reaction occurs almost entirely in the liver and is the rate-limiting step in the metabolism of alcohol. Approximately 15 mg of ethanol can be metabolized per hour, a rate reached when blood alcohol is approximately 10 mg/dl.

2. The *microsomal ethanol oxidizing system* (*MEOS*) also converts a portion of the ethanol to acetaldehyde using a cytochrome protein.[26] The overall reaction is:[25]

$$CH_3CH_2OH + NADPH + H^+ + O_2 \xrightarrow{\text{MEOS}} CH_3CHO + NADP^+ + 2H_2O \quad \textbf{(2)}$$

Like other microsomal oxidizing systems, this system seems to be inducible—that is, it increases in activity in the presence of large amounts of alcohol.[27] It may become of greater significance in chronic alcoholism.

3. The third system uses *catalase* as an enzyme in the presence of hydrogen peroxide by the following reactions:[28]

$$CH_3CH_2OH + H_2O_2 \xrightarrow{\text{Catalase}} CH_3CHO + 2H_2O \quad \textbf{(3)}$$

The hydrogen peroxide may be generated from either hypoxanthine or NADPH as follows:

$$\text{Hypoxanthine} + H_2O + O_2 \xrightarrow{\text{Xanthine oxidase}} \text{xanthine} + H_2O_2 \quad \textbf{(4)}$$

or

$$NADPH + H^+ + O_2 \xrightarrow{\text{NADPH oxidase}} NADP^+ + H_2O_2 \quad \textbf{(5)}$$

Following the oxidation of alcohol by one of these routes, the acetaldehyde is oxidized to acetate by *aldehyde dehydrogenase* in the following reaction:

$$CH_3CHO + NAD^+ + H_2O \xrightarrow{\text{Aldehyde dehydrogenase}} CH_3COOH + NADH + H^+ \quad \textbf{(6)}$$

Acetaldehyde oxidation occurs in the liver and in other tissues containing aldehyde dehydrogenase. Alcohol thus contributes to the body pool of acetyl-CoA. In the process of converting 1 g of ethanol to carbon dioxide and water, the body obtains 7.1 kcal. It also is important to note that there is an increase in the NADH/NAD ratio. The overall reaction is:

$$C_2H_5OH + 3O_2 \rightarrow 2CO_2 + 3H_2O + 18\ ATP \quad \textbf{(7)}$$

The relative importance of these three pathways is the subject of some debate. The weight of opinion is that alcohol dehydrogenase is responsible for the oxidation of most alcohol. The importance of the involvement of the MEOS is controversial. Overall, the evidence suggests that ADH is the only active enzyme at low ethanol concentration but, at higher concentrations (those above 10 mmol/L) ADH accounts for 60 percent and MEOS for 40 percent.[25] This seems to leave no role for catalase. However, it has been suggested that catalase may be involved in pathologic conditions, when there is increased purine breakdown and formation of H_2O_2.[29] The role of catalase in alcohol metabolism in pathologic conditions requires further investigation.

The major pathway for alcohol oxidation, then, provides us with acetaldehyde and hydrogen to consider when we examine the next steps in the metabolism of alcohol. First, we will consider the hydrogen (Fig. 11-4).

The main pathway for the hydrogen metabolism requires transfer of hydrogen into the mitochondria where it is oxidized for energy production, supplanting fat. Ethanol oxidation in the liver is obligatory—that is, it takes precedence. The lipids, which would otherwise be oxidized, accumulate, producing a fatty liver. The excess hydrogen can also be used for the synthesis of fatty acids and alpha-glycerophosphate with subsequent formation of triglyceride, also contributing to the fatty liver. Pyruvate obtained in the process of gluconeogenesis is reduced to

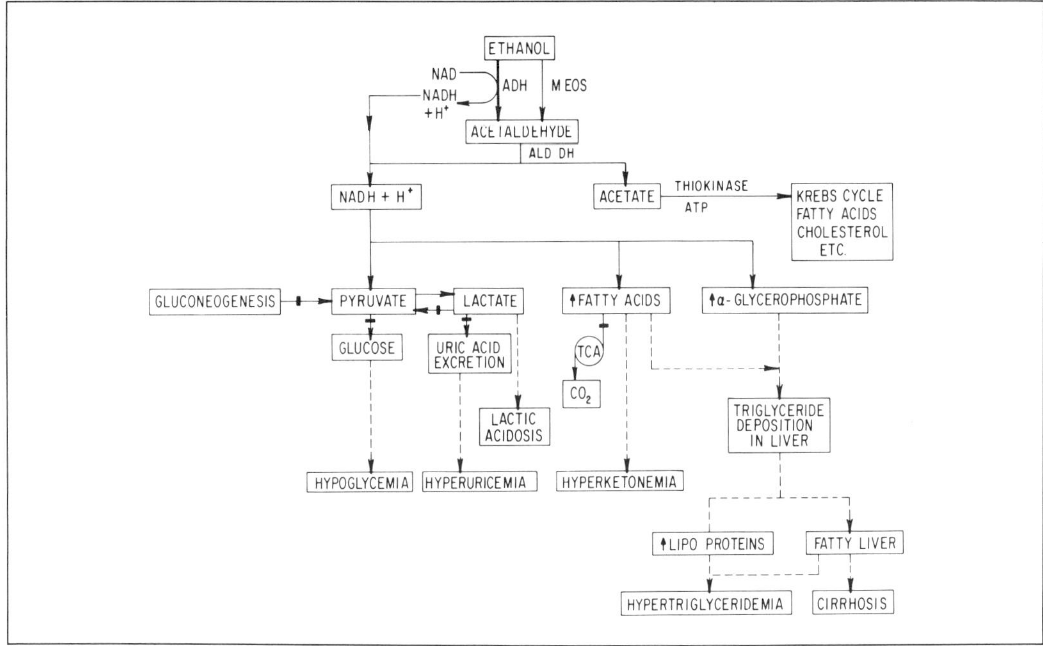

Figure 11-4. Effects of ethanol on metabolism. ADH = alcohol dehydrogenase; MEOS = microsomal ethanol oxidizing system; ALD DH = aldehyde dehydrogenase.

lactate instead of being used for glucose synthesis. In the alcoholic who has not been eating, liver glycogen reserves, which are important for maintaining normal blood glucose concentrations, will also be depleted and hypoglycemia then can develop (see Chapter 9). The increased lactic acid can interfere with uric acid excretion, precipitating an attack of gout in susceptible individuals.

The liver must now dispose of the lipid, if possible. To do this, it must assemble the lipid into lipoproteins (see Chapter 8). This is facilitated by proliferation of the smooth endoplasmic reticulum and increased activity of the necessary enzymes. As a result, there is a tendency for increased production of lipoprotein even when alcohol is not immediately involved. This reaction is the basis for the recommendation for abstinence in hyperlipoproteinemia.

The liver can also dispose of excess fat by converting it to ketone bodies, as described in Chapter 9. In some patients, this can result in a condition similar to diabetic ketoacidosis.

Acetaldehyde, the other product of alcohol dehydrogenase activity, is converted into acetate and then to acetyl-CoA. This occurs primarily in the liver mitochondria, although a small amount of acetaldehyde escapes into the blood and is metabolized in other tissues. Acetaldehyde may be central in the process of liver damage by decreasing mitochondrial functions.[30] It is reported to interfere with protein synthesis in the heart and has effects on the brain. It has been suggested that acetaldehyde may be the substance primarily involved in the predisposition to alcoholism and in the development of alcohol dependence.[30] Some individuals develop a limited tolerance to alcohol — that is, it requires a slightly larger dose to achieve a given pharmacologic effect on the CNS. The basis for this may be the induction of the MEOS so that ingested alcohol is metabolized faster and more must be drunk to achieve a given blood alcohol level.

Nutritional Status of the Alcoholic

Alcoholism is a major cause of malnutrition. The reasons for this are threefold. First, alcohol interferes with central mechanisms that regulate food intake, and food intake decreases. Second, toxic effects and adaptive responses to ethanol interfere with the absorption, metabolism, or storage of nutrients. Various organs, primarily the liver and brain, can be damaged in this process; the cardiovascular, endocrine, immune, and hematopoietic systems also can be damaged. Third, the nutrient content of the diet often is depressed, even if total energy intake is adequate. The nonalcohol calories in the diet of the chronic alcoholic equal 70 percent or less of their caloric need. In addition, their energy intake often is in the form of pure carbohydrate and few other nutrients are provided. Excessive alcohol intake may provide less energy than an equicaloric amount of carbohydrate. As the MEOS is induced, it produces heat rather than ATP.

Food Intake and Alcoholism

Hunger and appetite are somewhat dependent on the amount of alcohol ingested. Light alcohol intake stimulates appetite, whereas excessive alcohol intake tends to cause anorexia, leading eventually to malnutrition. Other influences on food intake include socioeconomic factors and the user's psychological state. Funds to buy alcoholic beverages can be a major consideration, since alcoholics with limited incomes are known to buy alcohol in place of food.

Effects of Alcohol on Digestion and Absorption

Heavy alcohol intake has a detrimental effect on the gastrointestinal tract, liver, and pancreas, and malabsorption can occur even in the absence of liver disease. Large amounts of ethanol have a dose-dependent and direct toxic effect on the gastrointestinal mucosa, with resultant disaccharidase deficiency and disordered mucosal transport, as well as malabsorption of folate, thiamin, vitamin B_{12}, fat-soluble vitamins, calcium, magnesium, long-chain fatty acids, and amino acids.[31-38]

Effects of Chronic Alcoholism on Nutrient Metabolism

Dietary deficiencies are seen frequently in alcoholics. In addition, alcohol may affect nutrient metabolism via its injurious effects on the liver and its influence on other organs and pathways. For example, it decreases protein synthesis, especially in the pancreas,[39] and glucose uptake and glycogen formation in muscle.

Some changes in mineral metabolism are seen. Magnesium has been of particular interest, since the symptoms of magnesium deficiency and acute alcohol withdrawal (*delirium tremens*) are similar. A precise role for magnesium deficiency in delirium tremens has not been established, but the existence of a relationship is generally accepted.[40]

Various metabolic alterations, including abnormal pancreatic function, lead to changes in vitamin absorption and utilization. Thiamine deficiency is common. Supplementation is ineffective because alcohol interferes with thiamine metabolism. The most severe form of thiamine deficiency is *Wernicke's encephalopathy,* characterized by visual disorders, ataxia, confusion, and coma. This condition is thought to be a thiamine dependency syndrome in which vigorous treatment with thiamine and general nutritional support is required in conjunction with alcohol withdrawal. Despite treatment, some patients progress to a chronic degenerative condition known as *Korsakoff's psychosis* characterized by poor memory for recent events. The sequence sometimes is called *Wernicke-Korsakoff syndrome.* Other neurologic deficits associated with nutritional deficiency in alcoholics include *peripheral neuropathy* (thiamine and vitamin B_6 deficiency) and *pellagrous psychosis* (niacin deficiency).

Folate deficiency also occurs frequently in chronic alcoholics and presents important hematologic problems. Alcohol interferes with folate absorption, storage, and conversion to its active form.[41] Ethanol interferes with vitamin B_6 metabolism, too, and decreases intestinal absorption of fat-soluble vitamins. Vitamin A absorption and metabolism are altered.

Acute Adverse Effects of Alcohol Intoxication

The acute neurologic effects of alcohol intoxication are dose-related, progressing from euphoria, relief from anxiety, and removal of inhibitions to ataxia, impaired vision, lack of muscle coordination, impaired reaction time, faulty judgment, and uninhibited behavior. If alcohol intake continues, it can progress from an anesthetic dose to lethal levels very quickly, but the anesthetic effect usually prevents intake of a lethal dose. It is important to remember that ethanol is a depressant, not a stimulant. The specific mechanisms by which ethanol produces these effects is unknown.

The causes of hangover also are incompletely understood. Effects usually are worse following the intake of alcoholic beverages containing many *congeners* (pharmacologically active molecules other than ethanol, including higher alcohols and benzene). Bourbon, whisky, rum, and brandy are high in congeners, whereas vodka is low. Hangover severity has also been related to the amount of metabolic acidosis and the degree of dehydration. These effects will occur in the novice drinker as well as in the chronic alcoholic.

Alcoholic Liver Disease

Alcoholic liver disease occurs in three forms—steatosis (fatty liver), alcoholic hepatitis, and cirrhosis.

Steatosis

Steatosis is seen in more than 80 percent of chronic alcoholics. This process of fatty metamorphosis was described in Chapter 1. Symptoms include malaise, anorexia, vomiting, weakness, and tenderness of an enlarged liver. More severely affected patients may show evidence of portal hypertension, fluid retention, and bleeding varices. Usual laboratory results include increased BSP retention and elevated serum globulin and transaminases. Serum albumin is depressed.

Fatty liver can often be treated by bed rest, abstinence from alcohol, and an adequate diet. With such treatment, fatty infiltration and abnormal serum bilirubin and enzyme levels disappear in 4 to 6 weeks. Abnormal BSP retention and serum albumin concentrations that persist may indicate residual liver impairment, but this condition is not known to lead to cirrhosis.

Alcoholic Hepatitis

Alcoholic hepatitis is less common than steatosis, occurring in approximately 30 percent of chronic alcoholics, but it is not necessarily a sequal to the fatty liver. It frequently is precipitated after a bout of heavy drinking. Symptoms include fatigue, weakness, anorexia, fever, and hepatomegaly. Laboratory results show elevated transaminases and glutamate dehydrogenase and decreased prothrombin time. The hepatocytes are necrotic, with an inflammatory reaction and hyaline degeneration (see Chapter 1). Some patients proceed to liver failure and encephalopathy. Alcoholic hepatitis can be fatal or can lead to chronic liver disease and cirrhosis.

Nutritional care may be similar to that provided for fatty liver. Some patients, especially those with vomiting and fever, require fluid and electrolyte therapy (see Chapter 12).

Alcoholic Cirrhosis

Alcoholic cirrhosis (*Laennec's cirrhosis*) develops in approximately 10 percent of chronic alcoholics who have a daily intake of 160 g of ethanol for 10 years. It is described in detail in the section titled Cirrhosis. *Hepatoma* (primary liver cancer) develops in 5 percent or more of the patients with Laennec's cirrhosis.

Nutritional Care of Alcoholics

Over the long term, alcoholics, whether they are abstinent or not, should have a diet adequate in all nutrients. Meals often are more acceptable if they are small and more frequent. Energy content of the diet should be individualized to maintain normal weight. Protein, fat, carbohydrate, and sodium are given as tolerated by the condition of the liver. Vitamin and mineral supplements are necessary if laboratory values indicate a deficiency, but there is no need for excessive nutrient medication.

During withdrawal, a chronic alcoholic may need parenteral support to correct fluid and electroylyte imbalance and hypoglycemia. Oral feeding should begin as soon as possible. Milk may be avoided if intestinal damage has resulted in lactose intolerance.

Several nutrition-related problems may arise in newly abstinent alcoholics. Hypoglycemic episodes, for example, may recur for several years. Some patients find it helpful to eat large breakfasts. Some patients are reported to develop a craving for sweets. It has been suggested that this may be a substitute for alcohol. When alcohol intake stops, secretion of antidiuretic hormone increases, leading to overhydration; therefore, fluid restriction may be necessary.

Some patients are treated with disulfiram to decrease their dependency on alcohol. Disulfiram interferes with the metabolism of acetaldehyde to acetate, and alcohol intake then causes unpleasant symptoms (see Chapter 3). In addition to avoiding alcoholic beverages, it is important for the patient to avoid inadvertent alcohol intake in food. Some foods to be avoided are wine vinegar, apple cider, foods cooked in wine, and flamed desserts.

The chronic alcoholic who continues to drink must understand that good nutrition will not prevent tissue damage from the alcohol, although it may moderate the severity of the damage if part of it was caused by malnutrition. Food-alcohol incompatibilities are summarized in Table 3-14.

Fetal Alcohol Syndrome

Serious effects on the infant are observed following alcohol intake by the pregnant woman. This syndrome is described in Chapter 16.

CIRRHOSIS

Cirrhosis is a generic term rather than a single specific disease. A recent concise definition states that it is a *diffuse process characterized by fibrosis and a conversion of normal architecture into structurally abnormal nodules.*[42,43] It is an irreversible *stage* in the evolution of many chronic liver diseases, although its process can sometimes be arrested if the etiologic agent is known and can be removed.

Etiology

There are many possible causes of cirrhosis. Chronic alcoholism is the most common in North America. Other causative drugs and toxins include isoniazid, methotrexate, and exposure to an assortment of industrial chemicals. Infections, particularly hepatitis B and C, and autoimmune diseases are other causes. Various metabolic disorders lead to cirrhosis and are discussed in other chapters. These include hemochromatosis, Wilson's disease, galactosemia, type 4 glycogen storage disease, tyrosinosis, urea cycle disorders, and abetalipoproteinemia (see Chapters 10 and 14). Biliary obstruction from biliary atresia, cystic fibrosis (see Chapter 6), or gallstones, and vascular factors interfering with the outflow of hepatic blood (*Budd-Chiari syndrome*) are additional causes, as is intestinal bypass (see Chapter 15). In some cases, the etiology is unknown.

The specific type of cirrhosis sometimes varies with the cause. Chronic alcoholism leads to Laennec's cirrhosis. On a worldwide basis, the most frequently seen form of the disease is *postnecrotic cirrhosis.* Its cause is not always known but its incidence is high in underdeveloped countries, and patients often have a history of hepatitis.

Classification

There is no ideal classification of cirrhotic diseases. They often are grouped by etiology. An alternative classification is by morphological appearance. In the latter system, the liver may be *micronodular* with nodules less than 3 mm in diameter, separated by fine fibrous bands, or *macronodular* with larger nodules, or it may have *mixed nodules* of varying size.

Pathogenesis

Cirrhosis evolves slowly, often over many years, but occasionally its progress is rapid or intermittent. It usually is the consequence of some etiologic agent that is applied for a long period, causing cell damage and cell death. These, in turn, evoke the mechanisms of disorderly regeneration and repair, including fibrosis, as described in Chapter 1.

Clinical Manifestations

Fibrosis and the presence of nodules throughout the liver are required for diagnosis of cirrhosis.[44] The liver has a large reserve capacity, and there is often a long period in the progress of the disease when the patient is asymptomatic. Common presenting symptoms are malaise and lethargy, dyspepsia, bloating, nausea, vomiting, and anorexia. The clinical manifestations vary somewhat with the etiology but merge as the disease progresses. Advanced cirrhosis is dominated by liver failure, portal hypertension, ascites, edema, variceal bleeding, hemorrhages, secondary infections, and hepatic encephalopathy.[44] Additional complications of cirrhosis are hepatocellular carcinoma and renal failure.

In some patients, a progressive renal failure known as *hepatorenal syndrome* may follow gastrointestinal bleeding, infections, or excessive diuresis. The cause of this complication is unknown, but mortality is very high. Death occurs in uremia, hepatic coma, or from gastrointestinal hemorrhage.

Nutritional Care

Specific treatment of cirrhosis is aimed at removing the etiologic agent. Abstinence from alcohol is necessary in alcoholic cirrhosis. If the cause of cirrhosis is drug toxicity, use of the drug must be discontinued immediately. Hemochromatosis and Wilson's disease require the elimination of iron and copper, respectively. Some other etiologic agents respond to drug therapy.

General Nutritional Support

Nutritional care in cirrhosis is important since the use of drugs is limited by the reduced ability of the liver to metabolize them. Nutritional care is planned to support healing and regeneration of the damaged liver and to prevent or manage life-threatening complications. General nutritional support of the patient *without* impending encephalopathy consists of a high-calorie diet, 45 to 50 kcal/kg of body weight per day to minimize endogenous protein catabolism, with 1 g or less of protein per kilogram of body weight. The protein is included to maintain nitrogen balance and provide for liver repair, but the amount is not increased so that encephalopathy is not precipitated. If the patient has ascites, the calorie and protein content must be based on an estimate of body weight from which the weight of the ascites fluid has been subtracted.

The form in which the protein is given may be important. There is some evidence that cirrhotic patients tolerate the protein from dairy products and vegetable proteins better than that from other sources.[45] The basis for this difference may lie in the respective amino acid patterns of the various proteins.[46] Vegetable proteins contain less methionine and fewer AAAs than do other proteins. They also may change the bacterial flora of the gut.[47] Given the proposed role of ammonia in the pathogenesis of hepatic encephalopathy, foods that contain preformed ammonia are omitted. Among these are various cheeses, salami, bacon, ham, ground beef, and gelatin. Analysis of ammonia in a number of foods has been provided by Rudman et al.[46]

The diet should contain 300 to 400 g of carbohydrate to spare protein. Fat can be offered in moderation in order to make the diet more palatable but should be restricted if there is evidence of jaundice. A patient weighing 60 kg might, for example, be given a diet containing 400 g of carbohydrate, 60 g of protein, 90 g of fat, and 2,650 kcal. Because the patient often is anorexic or nauseated, the foods might be offered in four to six smaller meals or the patient might be given liquid supplements. To encourage food intake, the patient's preferences should be considered, and the patient should be consulted and encouraged frequently by the nutritional care specialist.

In addition to these general procedures, other modifications may be indicated by complications of the particular disease.

Esophageal and Gastric Varices

In a patient with esophageal and gastric varices, a diet reduced in roughage may be used to avoid damage to the mucosa and resultant gastrointestinal bleeding. At the same time, the patient must avoid constipation, since straining at the stool may cause hemorrhage. For this purpose, fluid intake should be maintained and potassium intake should be generous, with ample intake of fruit or fruit juice. A soft, low-fiber diet is used. Lactulose, employed in the prevention of encephalopathy, is helpful. Meals should be small and frequent, and patients are advised to eat slowly and to chew their food well.

If the patient has an esophageal hemorrhage, the bleeding can sometimes be stopped on an emergency basis by inserting into the esophagus an appliance called a *Sengstaken-Blakemore tube.* It is a balloonlike device that can be inflated to stop the bleeding by pressure. Supportive treatment includes parenteral fluids and electrolytes, blood transfusions, and cleansing enemas to remove blood from the intestinal tract, thus preventing ammonia intoxication.[48]

Resumption of oral feeding, when it is possible, should be approached cautiously. Clear liquids, tea, water, and broth may first be given hourly or every 2 hours. All liquid should be at room temperature or cooler. The diet may be progressed from a full liquid diet to a nonroughage soft diet to a general nonroughage diet as tolerated. Small frequent meals may be helpful. Other modifications mandated by damage to the liver must be continued.

Ascites and Edema

Minimal fluid retention may disappear with bed rest alone; ascites disappears if the causes are removed. Therefore, the primary objective in the treatment of patients with ascites and edema is to improve liver function. The diet is sodium-restricted, often to

250 to 500 mg/day. The sodium restriction is more severe than that used in renal and cardiovascular disease because diuretic drugs can be used only with caution in the cirrhotic patient. A potassium-sparing diuretic is used, if any. There is controversy concerning fluid restriction. It may be restricted to a volume equivalent to urine output the previous day. The objective is a weight loss of 0.5 to 1.0 kg/day. Others suggest unrestricted fluid intake as long as sodium intake is restricted and there is no evidence of further fluid retention.

Hepatic Encephalopathy

Nutritional care of patients with hepatic encephalopathy currently is divided into categories of *established* or *experimental* treatments.

Established Treatments. As the number of functioning hepatocytes declines, the established treatment is to restrict protein intake to 40 g/day or less, if necessary, to avoid encephalopathy. The protein must be distributed throughout the day. Maintenance of nitrogen balance is difficult if not impossible. The patient's anorexia is a complicating problem.

Precipitating factors must be removed or corrected. Standard therapy has centered on the gut, to reduce its protein content, alter the intestinal flora, or affect the rate of absorption of amino acids or their metabolites. *Neomycin* or another nonabsorbable antibiotic to reduce intestinal bacteria may be administered so that more protein, needed for liver regeneration, can be included in the diet. However, neomycin contributes to malabsorption. *Lactulose* is a nonabsorbable disaccharide which produces an acidic diarrhea, reducing bacterial action. It also may depress absorption of aromatic amino acids.[11] If there is gastrointestinal bleeding, it must be stopped.

In impending encephalopathy, the protein in the diet is reduced as necessary, to 20 g or even none. If the patient is in a coma, no protein is given. In cases of prolonged coma, the patient is fed intravenously.

Fat emulsions apparently may be used safely in parenteral fluids. They are hydrolyzed by lipoprotein lipase in capillaries, and fatty acids are oxidized by the liver.[49] Excess carbohydrate, however, must be converted to fat and exported as lipoprotein by the liver. Thus, large amounts of carbohydrates may cause a fatty liver, and partial substitution of fat for some of the carbohydrate will reduce the amount of fat that actually remains in the liver. A high carbohydrate content also presents a problem to patients with carbohydrate intolerance.

As the patient's metabolism is corrected and the neurologic symptoms subside, his or her protein intake can be increased cautiously, by 10 to 15 g/wk up to a maximum of 1 g/kg or 85 g.

Fat tolerance during oral feeding may be determined by trial and error by the patient and nutritional care specialist. Some patients, particularly those with biliary cirrhosis, have a greater tolerance for medium-chain triglycerides. Other patients tolerate the fat in dairy products well.

Experimental Treatments. Experimental treatments are of three types. The administration of levodopa as a medication to provide a source for dopamine and norepinephrine has been reported to be helpful in some patients. Its use is controversial.

The manipulation of amino acid concentrations currently is considered experimental. The use of a special formulation, a hypertonic dextrose solution high in BCAAs (37 to 50 percent) and low in AAAs, has been proposed for intravenous use. In theory, this formulation, known as *F080,* would have the following effects:

1. Reduce muscle catabolism, promote muscle protein synthesis, and thus reduce plasma AAAs
2. Reduce AAA uptake at the blood-brain

barrier by providing BCAAs to compete for uptake
3. Improve hepatic protein synthesis and regeneration, thus reducing plasma AAAs
4. Help satisfy peripheral energy needs, reduce protein catabolism, and therefore reduce ammonia production, which in turn would reduce brain glutamine and the exchange of glutamine for AAAs in the brain

As much as 120 g of protein per day has been given in this manner.

An alternative experimental approach is to feed the patients alpha-keto analogues of the BCAAs. These analogues are presumed to be transaminated, with glutamine as the nitrogen donor. The transamination is not dependent on the liver.

For patients with impending encephalopathy or following recovery, other products are available. It must be recognized that 40 g of protein may not be sufficient to maintain nitrogen balance, but more severe reductions are likely to cause protein catabolism and the release of AAAs. For these patients, liquid supplements containing increased amounts of branched-chain amino acids and reduced AAAs are helpful. Two such products, *Hepatic-Aid* and *Travasorb Hepatic* are now available (see Appendix L). Hepatic-Aid comes in a pudding form, also. Nothing is known yet of the effects of these products on long-term survival.

Feeding Techniques

Decisions about feeding methods to be used require consideration of the degree of organ failure, gastrointestinal function, and electrolyte and fluid tolerance, nutritional status, and the ability of the patient to eat conventional foods. The consumption of conventional foods can be limited by anorexia and encephalopathy.[21,50] In addition, the restriction of protein, sodium, fluid, and food consistency may make the diet unpalatable.[51] Nonetheless, a great amount of food is necessary to provide adequate energy.

The careful attention of and imaginative meal planning by the nutritional care specialist are needed to encourage a patient's adequate nutrient intake. Small frequent meals usually are necessary, as are supplements of high-calorie formulas. A number of supplements containing carbohydrate polymers are useful for this purpose (see Appendix J).

If the patient's intake remains insufficient, complete formula feeding by tube or as a supplement to meals may be instituted. Particular care is necessary, especially if the patient has esophageal varices. Available prepared formulas listed in Appendix L for general use contain too much sodium and water and sometimes too much protein for many patients with hepatic disease. Instead, *modular formulas,* those tailor-made to the tolerance of the individual patient, may be used.[52] Products useful in preparation of such formulas include Casec as a source of protein, Polycose, Moducal, or Sumacal as a source of carbohydrate, and MCT oil or Microlipid to supply fat.[52] Information on these and other products useful for this purpose is listed in Appendix K.

The formulas high in BCAAs, Hepatic-Aid and Travasorb Hepatic, are usable for tube feeding, also. These two products differ in some important ways. Travasorb Hepatic contains 10.6% protein, the nitrogen of which is approximately 50% BCAA. It also contains vitamins and minerals to provide 100 percent of the Recommended Dietary Allowances if 2,300 kcal are given. It contains 1.1 kcal/ml at the recommended dilution, and its osmolarity is 650 mOsm/L. The caloric density may be inadequate for patients whose fluid must be restricted. The inclusion of minerals reduces the potential for modifying the formula. Hepatic-Aid, on the other hand, provides 10.3% protein with 36 percent of the nitrogen as BCAA. It is essentially free of vitamins and minerals, so these must be added if the formula is used for a long period. Its osmolarity is 950 mOsm/L at the recommended dilution, requiring slow administration. The caloric density, 1.6 kcal/ml, may be an advantage for use with patients who require fluid restriction.

Abnormal hepatic function may reduce the ability to synthesize tyrosine from phenylalanine and cystine from methionine.[53] Travasorb Hepatic and Hepatic-Aid are free of both cystine and tyrosine, so these amino acids may have to be supplemented for some patients.[51]

When patients have regained the ability to tolerate 40 g of protein per day with stable fluid and electrolyte status, they might be given a casein-based formula at less cost.[51] Products that have been found useful are Magnacal, Isocal, and Ensure.[51]

Patients who are comatose for long periods may be fed intravenously. This procedure is discussed in Chapter 12.

Specific Forms of Cirrhosis

Laennec's Cirrhosis

Laennec's cirrhosis is also known as *alcoholic, fatty,* or *portal cirrhosis,* although the disease does not always resemble these descriptive terms exactly. It is the type most frequently seen in the United States and Canada and usually is associated with chronic alcoholism.

Etiology. Many studies have linked chronic alcoholism with Laennec's cirrhosis, but the amount of alcohol intake, in terms of quantity or duration, that will cause this disease is unknown. A pint of whisky or several quarts of wine daily for 5 to 10 years is typical in these patients.

At one time, it was thought that the condition was caused by the malnutrition common to alcoholics. However, the investigations of Salaspuro and Lieber[54] have shown that Laennec's cirrhosis can develop in the presence of adequate nutrition. Nevertheless, since many alcoholics are malnourished, the currently held view is that *malnutrition* is a contributory factor to the liver cell damage.

Only 10 to 20 percent of chronic alcoholics develop cirrhosis. As a consequence, it has been suggested that some patients have a *genetic predisposition* to its development.

Clinical Manifestations. Laennec's cirrhosis is a progressive disease, but if the patient strictly avoids alcohol and is treated properly, it can often be arrested and some repair may take place. Then, the 5-year survival rate is approximately 60 percent. If alcohol intake continues, the survival rate is 40 percent in 5 years.

At first, the liver is enlarged with much fatty infiltration. The fat disappears with therapy unless the patient continues alcohol intake. As the disease progresses, hepatocytes are destroyed and septa of connective tissue appear in the lobules. Some regeneration occurs, forming the nodules. A decrease in fatty infiltration and reduction in the liver cell mass causes the liver to become shrunken and hard as the disease progresses. If the disease is not arrested, the number of liver cells dwindles until the disease progresses to irreversible *end-stage cirrhosis.*

The liver has a large reserve capacity, and often liver damage proceeds for many years before symptoms occur. Presenting symptoms are insidious in onset and may consist of fatigue, weakness, anorexia, jaundice, edema, and ascites. If alcohol intake continues, the disease progresses with fever, nausea, and vomiting. Jaundice deepens, ascites becomes more severe, and neurologic symptoms occur, progressing to weakness, portal hypertension, and a general worsening of other symptoms. Many patients die in hepatic coma, often precipitated by hemorrhage of esophageal varices or by infection.

Laboratory findings include increased BSP retention and elevated transaminases and alkaline phosphatase in serum. Serum albumin is depressed, as are clotting factors. White and red blood cells are decreased in number, possibly from a direct effect of alcohol on the bone marrow. Serum ammonia is elevated, and serum electrolytes are deranged in patients with ascites.

Nutritional Care. General nutritional care of patients with Laennec's cirrhosis is as described previously for cirrhotic patients. In addition, since the patient is likely to be an alcoholic and therefore may be malnourished, nutritional care must include abstinence from alcohol, if possible, and correction or prevention of malnutrition. The direct toxic effects of alcohol on digestion, absorption, and metabolism of nutrients must be considered. Nutritional care in malabsorption disorders is described in Chapter 6.

Postnecrotic Cirrhosis

The cause of postnecrotic cirrhosis is unknown, but it is preceded by hepatitis in many individuals. In some cases, it follows infections or exposure to industrial chemicals or other toxic materials. In other cases, evidence indicates that nutritional factors are involved in the cirrhotic process.[55]

Clinical manifestations are variable but can include symptoms similar to hepatitis or can consist of abdominal pain, ascites, jaundice, portal hypertension, and variceal hemorrhage. Laboratory tests show hyperbilirubinemia, BSP retention, elevated transaminases and alkaline phosphatase in serum, and elevated gamma globulin, but depressed albumin. Deficiencies of clotting factors are common, as is anemia.

Nutritional care requires avoidance of excess protein and control of ascites. Other aspects of care are rest and avoidance of drugs, except in some cases that respond to corticosteroids. Infections must be treated promptly, and portal hypertension may be treated surgically if there is variceal hemorrhage.

Biliary Cirrhosis

Biliary cirrhosis is a disorder in which there is impaired bile excretion, progressive destruction of the small bile ducts, and parenchymal destruction centered around the bile ducts. The disease is classified as primary or secondary. The cause of *primary biliary cirrhosis* is unknown but may be an autoimmune or endocrine disorder. It occurs almost exclusively in middle-aged women. *Secondary biliary cirrhosis* occurs as a consequence of the obstruction of the bile duct.

Clinical manifestations of biliary cirrhosis include severe pruritis (itching), prolonged progressive jaundice, and hepatomegaly. Because bile flow is compromised, patients have steatorrhea and diarrhea by the mechanism described in Chapter 6. The patients also develop xanthomas and xanthelasma (see Chapter 8). Laboratory tests show elevated serum levels of cholesterol, other lipids, and alkaline phosphatase. Lipoprotein X also is found. There is a chronic inflammation of hepatocytes around the portal ducts and the interlobular ducts. The disease progresses for months or years, and cirrhosis is a late phase.

In the secondary disease, treatment consists of correction of the obstruction. The primary disease is incurable and progressive. Patients succumb, on the average, 6 to 7 years following the onset of symptoms.

In addition to those items previously described in relation to cirrhotic disease in general, nutritional care includes the following features:

1. A high-calorie diet
2. Reduction of dietary fat to 30 to 40 g/day, especially if the patient has steatorrhea
3. Fat-soluble vitamins, given parenterally

Patients may have edema, ascites, and esophageal varices. If so, their diets should be modified accordingly.

Case Study: Alcoholic Cirrhosis

Mr. K, a 39-year-old man, was brought to the hospital emergency room when he began vomiting blood in a nearby bar. The immediate need was, of course, to stop the bleeding. The patient was admitted to the hospital as a bed patient.

The admission examination found the patient to be approximately 8 kg under desirable weight, slightly dehydrated, and jaundiced. The abdomen was distended, and the liver was firm and enlarged. There was a moderate pedal edema. The following values were obtained in laboratory tests:

Serum alkaline phosphatase	12 Bodansky units
SGOT	208 units/ml
SGPT	172 units/ml
Serum albumin	2.8 g/dl
Serum bilirubin, total	8.7 mg/dl
Serum sodium	145 mEq/L
Serum magnesium	1.3 mEq/L
Serum potassium	3.2 mEq/L

The patient admitted to heavy alcohol use for the last 10 years. He said he had experienced abdominal pain, loss of appetite, and chronic fatigue for the last month. Mr. K was given a soft diet containing 70 g of protein, 1,000 mg of sodium, 3,000 kcal, and 1,000 ml of fluid per day in six equal feedings. Multivitamin supplements and a potassium-sparing diuretic were prescribed.

Three days later, the patient became lethargic and mentally confused. He had EEG changes and a flapping tremor. Treatment included neomycin and magnesium citrate. The diuretic was discontinued, and all protein in his diet was eliminated. At this time, laboratory results were as follows:

Serum potassium	3.2 mEq/L
Serum sodium	154 mEq/L
Blood urea nitrogen	6 mg/dl

In another 3 days, Mr. K was mentally alert, and his diet prescription was changed to 10 g of protein, 500 mg of sodium, 500 ml of fluid, and 2,000 kcal. Protein was increased at a rate of 5 g every other day up to 50 g; with increases above this level, blood ammonia began to rise, and so the diet was maintained at 50 g of protein.

On discharge from the hospital, the patient was referred to the mental health counselor and the alcoholic abuse clinic.

Exercises

1. Compare each of the laboratory values with normal values.
2. What abnormalities of liver function are indicated by each of the following: serum albumin, transaminases, alkaline phosphatase, serum bilirubin, serum sodium.
3. If the patient drank 750 ml of 80-proof whisky daily, how much alcohol would he get? How many kilocalories would he get from this source?
4. Why were vitamin supplements given to this patient?
5. Explain the pathogenesis of the patient's encephalopathy, jaundice, and fluid retention.
6. Give the rationale for each diet modification.
7. What diet do you think was recommended to this patient when he was discharged from the hospital?

References

1. Khatra, B.S., Chawla, R.K., and Sewell, L.W., Rudman, D. Distribution of branched-chain and keto acid dehydrogenase in primate tissue. *J. Clin. Invest.* 59:558, 1977.
2. Wright, R., Alberti, K.G.M.M., Karran, S., and Millward-Sadler, G.H., Eds. *Liver and Biliary Disease.* London: W.B. Saunders, 1979.
3. Wilkinson, S.P., and Williams, R. Ascites, electrolyte disorders and renal failure. In R. Wright, K.G.M.M. Alberti, S. Karran, and G.H. Millward-Sadler, Eds., *Liver and Biliary Disease.* London: W.B. Saunders, 1979.
4. Leiberman, F.L., Denison, E.K., and Reynolds, T.B. The relationship of plasma volume, portal hypertension, ascites, and renal sodium retention in cirrhosis. The overflow theory of ascites formation. *Ann. N.Y. Acad. Sci.* 170:202, 1970.
5. Frankes, J.T. Physiologic considerations in the medical management of ascites. *Arch. Intern. Med.* 140:620, 1980.
6. Alpers, D.H., and Isselbacher, K.V. Derangements of hepatic metabolism. In G.W. Thorn, R.D. Adams, E. Braunwald, et al., Eds., *Harrison's Principles of Internal Medicine,* 8th ed. New York: McGraw-Hill, 1977.
7. Wu, C.V., Gollman, G., and Butt, H.R. Changes in free amino acids in the plasma

during hepatic coma. *J. Clin. Invest.* 34:845, 1955.

8. Fischer, J.E., Yoshimura, N., James, J.H., et al. Plasma amino acids in patients with hepatic encephalopathy: Effects of amino acid infusions. *Am. J. Surg.* 127:40, 1974.
9. Rosen, H.M., Yoshimura, N., Hodgman, J.M., and Fischer, J.E. Plasma amino acid patterns in hepatic encephalopathy of differing etiology. *Gastroenterology* 72:483, 1977.
10. Soeters, P.B., and Fischer, J.E. Insulin, glucagon and amino acid imbalance and hepatic encephalopathy. *Lancet* 2:880, 1976.
11. Fischer, J.E. Portasystemic encephalopathy. In R. Wright, K.G.M.M. Alberti, S. Karran, and G.H. Millward-Sadler, Eds., *Liver and Biliary Disease.* London: W.B. Saunders, 1979.
12. Takahashi, Y. Serum lipids in liver disease. Liver disease and the relationship of serum lipids and hepatic coma. *Jpn. J. Gastroenterol.* 60:571, 1963.
13. Chen, S., Mahadevan, V., and Zieve, L. Volatile fatty acids in the breath of patients with cirrhosis of the liver. *J. Lab. Clin. Med.* 75:622, 1970.
14. Zieve, F.J., Zieve, L., Doizaki, W.M., and Gilsdorf, R.B. Synergism between ammonia and fatty acids in the production of coma. *J. Pharmacol. Exp. Ther.* 191:10, 1974.
15. Fischer, J.E., Rosen, H.M., and Ebeid, A.M. The effect of normalization of plasma amino acids on hepatic encephalopathy in man. *Surgery* 80:77, 1976.
16. Fischer, J.E., and Bower, R.H. Nutritional support in liver disease. *Surg. Clin. North Am.* 61:653, 1981.
17. Bernardini, P., and Fischer, J.E. Amino acid imbalance and hepatic encephalopathy. *Annu. Rev. Nutr.* 2:419, 1982.
18. Herlong, H.F., Maddrey, W.C., and Walser, M. The use of ornithine salts of branched chain keto acids in portal systemic encephalopathy. *Ann. Intern. Med.* 93:945, 1980.
19. Morgan, M., and Sherlock, S. Presented in discussion at the Conference on Fulminant Hepatic Failure, Washington, D.C., Feb. 7–8, 1977.
20. Halsted, C.H., Robles, E.A., and Mezey, E. Intestinal malabsorption in folate-deficient alcoholics. *Gastroenterology* 64:526, 1973.
21. Leevy, C.M., Baker, H., and Tenhorne, W. B-complex vitamins in liver disease of the alcoholic. *Am. J. Clin. Nutr.* 16:339, 1965.
22. Morgan, A.G., Kellcher, V., Walker, B.E., and Losowsky, M.S. Nutrition in cryptogenic cirrhosis and chronic aggressive hepatitis. *Gut* 17:113, 1976.
23. Mezey, E. Liver disease and nutrition. *Gastroenterology* 74:770, 1978.
24. Wright, R., and Millward-Sadler, G.H. Acute viral hepatitis. In R. Wright, K.G.M.M. Alberti, S. Karran, and G.H. Millward-Sadler, Eds., *Liver and Biliary Disease.* London: W.B. Saunders, 1979.
25. Badawy, A.A.-B. The metabolism of alcohol. *Clin. Endocrinol. Metab.* 7:247, 1978.
26. Orme-Johnson, W.H., and Ziegler, D.M. Alcohol mixed function oxidase activity of mammalian liver microsomes. *Biochem. Biophys. Res. Commun.* 21:78, 1965.
27. Loomis, T. The pharmacology of alcohol. In N.J. Estes and M.E. Heinemann, Eds., *Alcoholism,* 2nd ed. St. Louis: C.V. Mosby, 1982.
28. Keilin, D., and Hartree, E.F. Properties of catalase. Catalysis of coupled oxidation of alcohols. *Biochem. J.* 39:293, 1945.
29. Lundquist, F. Enzymatic pathways of ethanol metabolism. In J. Trémolières, Ed., *International Encyclopedia of Pharmacology and Therapeutics.* Sec. 20, *Alcohol and Alcoholism,* vol. 1. Oxford: Pergamon Press, 1970.
30. Lieber, C.S. The metabolism of alcohol. *Scientific American* 234:25 (1976).
31. Roe, D.A. *Alcohol and the Diet.* Westport, Conn.: AVI, 1979.
32. Shanbour, L.L. Effects of ethanol on the determinants of intestinal transport. *Alcohol. Clin. Exp. Res.* 3:142, 1979.
33. Kuo, Y.-J., and Shambour, L.L. Effects of ethanol on sodium, 3-O-methyl glucose and L-alanine transport in the jejunum. *Am. J. Dig. Dis.* 23:51, 1978.
34. Perlow, W., Baraona, E., and Lieber, C.S. Symptomatic intestinal disaccharidase deficiency in alcoholics. *Gastroenterology* 72:680 (1977).
35. Halsted, C.H., Robles, E.A., and Mezey, E. Decreased jejunal uptake of labeled folic acid (^{3}H-PGA) in alcoholic patients: Roles of alcohol and nutrition. *N. Engl. J. Med.* 285:701, 1971.
36. Thomson, A.L., Baker, H., and Leevey, C.M. Patterns of ^{35}S-thiamine hydrochloride absorption in the malnourished alcoholic patient. *J. Lab. Clin. Med.* 76:34, 1970.
37. Worthington-Roberts, B. Alcoholism and Malnutrition. In N.J. Estes and M.E. Heinemann, Eds., *Alcoholism,* 2nd ed. St. Louis: C.V. Mosby, 1982.
38. Israel, Y., Valenzuela, J.E., Salazar, I., and Ugarte, G. Alcohol and amino acid transport in the human small intestine. *J. Nutr.* 98:222, 1969.

39. Sinclair, H.M. Nutritional aspects of alcoholism. *Proc. Nutr. Soc.* 31:117, 1972.
40. Flink, E.B., Shane, S.R., Jacob, W.H., and Jovans, J.E. Some aspects of magnesium deficiency and chronic alcoholism. In V.M. Sardesai, Ed., *Biochemical and Clinical Aspects of Alcohol Metabolism.* Springfield, Ill.: Charles C Thomas, 1969.
41. Hellman, R.S., and Steinberg, S.E. The effects of alcohol on folate metabolism. *Annu. Rev. Med.* 33:345, 1982.
42. Anthony, P.P., Ishak, K.G., Nayak, N.C., et al. The morphology of cirrhosis. *J. Clin. Pathol.* 31:395, 1978.
43. Anthony, P.P., Ishak, K.G., Nayak, N.C., et al. The morphology of cirrhosis: Definition, nomenclature and classification. *Bull. WHO* 55:521, 1977.
44. Millward-Sadler, G.H., and Wright, R. Cirrhosis: An appraisal. In R. Wright, K.G.M.M. Alberti, S. Karran, and G.H. Millward-Sadler, Eds., *Liver and Biliary Disease.* London: W.B. Saunders, 1979.
45. Greenberger, N.J., Carley, J., Schenker, S., et al. Effect of vegetable and animal protein diets in chronic hepatic encephalopathy. *Am. J. Dig. Dis.* 22:845, 1977.
46. Rudman, D., Smith, R.B., Salam, A., et al. Ammonia content of food. *Am. J. Clin. Nutr.* 26:487, 1970.
47. Misra, P. Hepatic encephalopathy. *Med. Clin. North Am.* 65:209, 1981.
48. Conn, H.O. Cirrhosis. In L. Schiff and E.R. Schiff, Eds., *Diseases of the Liver,* 5th ed. Philadelphia: J.B. Lippincott, 1982.
49. Wretlind, A. Current states of Intralipid and other fat emulsions. In H.C. Meng and D.W. Wilmore, Eds., *Fat Emulsion in Parenteral Nutrition.* Chicago: American Medical Association, 1976.
50. Hurlow, A. Diet in the treatment of liver disease. *J. Hum. Nutr.* 31:105, 1977.
51. Wade, J.E., Echenique, M., and Blackburn, G.L. Enteral feeding in liver failure. In I.D. Johnston, Ed., *Second Bermuda Symposium on Clinical Nutrition.* Lancaster, England: MTP Press, 1983.
52. Smith, J., Horowitz, J., Henderson, J.M., and Heymsfield, S. Enteral hyperalimentation in undernourished patients with cirrhosis and ascites. *Am. J. Clin. Nutr.* 35:56, 1982.
53. Rudman, D., Kutner, M., Ansley, J., et al. Hypotyrosinemia, hypocystinemia, and failure to retain nitrogen during total parenteral nutrition of cirrhotic patients. *Gastroenterology* 81:1025, 1981.
54. Salaspuro, M.P., and Lieber, C.S. Alcoholic liver disease. In R. Wright, K.G.M.M. Alberti, S. Karran, and G.H. Millward-Sadler, Eds., *Liver and Biliary Disease.* London: W.B. Saunders, 1979.
55. Cossa, J.P., and Teti, S.P. Nutritional support of the patient in hepatic failure. *Nutr. Supp. Serv.* 1:39, 1981.

Bibliography

Davidson, C.S., Ed. *Problems in Liver Diseases.* New York: Stratton Intercontinental Medical Book Co., 1979.

Estes, N.J., and Heinemann, M.E. *Alcoholism,* 2nd ed. St. Louis: C.V. Mosby, 1982.

Leiber, C.S., Ed. *Metabolic Aspects of Alcoholism.* Lancaster, England: MTP Press, 1977.

Roe, D.A. *Alcohol and the Diet.* Westport, Conn.: Avi, 1979.

Schiff, L., and Schiff, E.R., Eds. *Diseases of the Liver,* 5th ed. Philadelphia: J.B. Lippincott, 1982.

Wright, R., Alberti, K.G.M.M., Karran, S., and Millward-Sadler, G.H., Eds. *Liver and Biliary Disease.* London: W.B. Saunders, 1979.

Sources of Current Information

Alcoholism: Clinical and Experimental Research
Hepato-Gastroenterology
Hepatology

VI. Disorders Causing Increased Nutrient Needs

12. Nutrition in Hypermetabolic Conditions

Bruce M. Wolfe, M.D., and Wayne I. Yamahata, M.D.

Malnutrition or, more precisely, undernutrition not only follows reduced food intake but also may occur if the patient has increased need even in the presence of an amount of food intake that is adequate under normal circumstances. Many of the earlier chapters in this text described conditions in which the patient becomes malnourished as a result of anorexia or inability to ingest, digest, or absorb nutrients. In this chapter, we will consider conditions in which malnutrition may be caused by increased, unmet needs for nutrients. Particular emphasis will be placed on conditions classified as *hypermetabolic* or *hypercatabolic,* such as major surgery, major traumatic injuries, or *sepsis* (the presence of pathogenic organisms or their toxic metabolites). These conditions have a common effect in that they impose stress on the body. The consequences and factors unique to each of these stresses will be described. Cancer is another hypermetabolic illness, but because a number of unique aspects of nutritional care are associated with it, cancer is considered separately in the next chapter.

Fluid and electrolyte balance is another concern in hypermetabolic patients. This type of problem also occurs in many other conditions, including diabetes mellitus and gastrointestinal, renal, cardiovascular, and hepatic diseases. Fluid and electrolytes are integral parts of nutrition, and disturbances in their balances are a common denominator in many conditions that require nutritional management. Therefore, it is important that the nutritional care specialist understand the general principles of fluid and electrolyte balance.

THE HYPERMETABOLIC RESPONSE

Metabolic Effects of Starvation

The metabolic response to deficient nutrient intake is described here, since studies of metabolism in starvation are helpful in understanding metabolism in hypermetabolic conditions as well as in conditions in which the food intake of patients is decreased. Energy expenditure continues in starvation despite the lack of energy intake. It measures approximately 1,800 kcal/day in a normal human and the energy must be mobilized from body stores. As shown in Fig. 12-1, certain tissues—most notably the nervous system, red blood cells, bone marrow, phagocytes, fibroblasts, and the renal medulla—require glucose as their source of energy. Approximately 180 g of glucose must be supplied to these tissues. Under normal circumstances, the brain metabolizes 100 to 150 g of glucose to carbon dioxide and water each day,[1] and the other tissues metabolize 30 to 40 g of glucose to lactate and pyruvate.[2,3] The lactate is recycled to glucose using energy, and the pyruvate can be a substrate for gluconeogenesis or for formation of ATP. During normal nutrition, the skeletal muscle, heart, and renal cortex primarily use glucose. The liver derives much energy from the oxidation of free fatty acids to ketones.

Figure 12-1. Approximate daily flow of fuels in a fasting human, emphasizing amino acid release from muscle as a source of glucogenic substrate for liver. ~P = energy; RBC = red blood cells; WBC = white blood cells. (From Cahill, G.F., Jr., Physiology of insulin in man. Diabetes *20:787, 1971. Reproduced with permission from the American Diabetes Association, Inc.)*

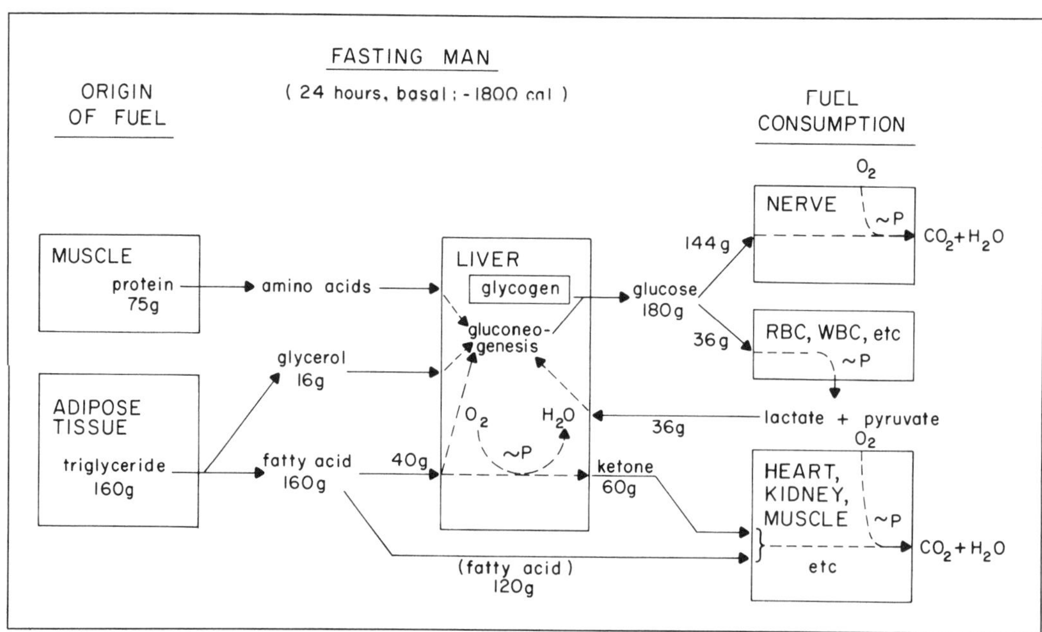

Early Starvation

In early starvation, the glycogen reserves are depleted quickly. Body fat, though, contains large energy stores in most patients. It would be ideal if all of the energy needs in starvation could be met from stored carbohydrate and fat, but studies have shown that in starvation this is not the case. Once the liver glycogen reserves are exhausted, the body adjusts by hydrolyzing skeletal muscle protein and using the amino acids as sources of glucose (see Fig. 12-1).

Gluconeogenesis occurs mainly in the liver and kidney.[4] In the liver, the main substrate is alanine, which comes to the liver from the muscle via the glucose-alanine cycle.[5] In the muscle, the branched-chain amino acids, leucine, isoleucine, and valine, are transaminated to provide most of the nitrogen for synthesis of alanine from pyruvate.[6] The alanine circulates to the liver,[7] where it is used for gluconeogenesis;[6] urea is the main by-product. In the kidney, the main substrate for gluconeogenesis is glutamine,[8] but other amino acids can be converted to glutamine by transamination, with ammonia as the main by-product. Approximately half of the total glucose is derived from the kidney as starvation continues.[4] The primary source of glucose in early starvation is the increased rate of gluconeogenesis.

In early starvation, and persisting for 5 to 7 days, the urinary nitrogen excretion is approximately 12 g/day, of which 80 to 90 percent is urea. This loss represents a deficit of approximately 75 g of protein or 360 g of lean wet tissue per day. During 7 days of starvation, as much as 500 g of protein or 5 percent of the total body intracellular protein may be lost. Important metabolic proteins are lost, such as those in the plasma and liver and the digestive enzymes.[9,10] Extracellular protein in bone matrix, tendons, and other supporting structures turns over slowly and so generally is preserved.

For each 1,800 kcal, 160 g of adipose tissue are metabolized.[2] Lipolysis releases free fatty acids and glycerol. The glycerol may provide approximately 18 g of glucose per day.[2] The free fatty acids serve as an energy source for the Cori cycle and as a source of acetyl CoA, increasing the conversion of pyruvate to oxaloacetate.[11,12] Some fatty acids are metabolized via ketone bodies.

Prolonged Starvation

In prolonged starvation (Fig. 12-2), adaptive mechanisms conserve protein by enabling a greater portion of the energy needs to be met by fat metabolism, with a decreased requirement for glucose. The production of ketone bodies from fatty acids is accelerated, and the brain gets a significant proportion of its energy from these ketones. Muscle protein continues to be catabolized but at a decreased rate, thus prolonging survival. During prolonged starvation, protein catabolism falls to 20 g/day and the efficiency of amino acid reuse increases so that urea nitrogen excretion decreases. The principal energy substrate is adipose tissue, with 60 percent of calories derived from the metabolism of fat to carbon dioxide, 10 percent from the metabolism of free fatty acids to ketone bodies, and 25 percent from the metabolism of ketone bodies.

Metabolic rate and total energy expenditure decrease and are manifested by decreased activity, increased sleep, and decreased body temperature. If starvation continues, the body loses most of the intercostal muscles necessary for respiration. It becomes impossible to clear pulmonary secretions, and the patient may die of pneumonia and respiratory failure.[13]

Metabolic Effects of Injury or Sepsis

The metabolic response to injury or sepsis resembles the response to starvation in some respects but differs in others (Fig. 12-3). The metabolic rate is increased and tissue *catabolism* (breakdown into simpler compounds) predominates over *anabolism* (synthesis), resulting in a net destruction of tissue called the *catabolic response.*

Continued catabolism, particularly of protein, impairs the capacity to recover from

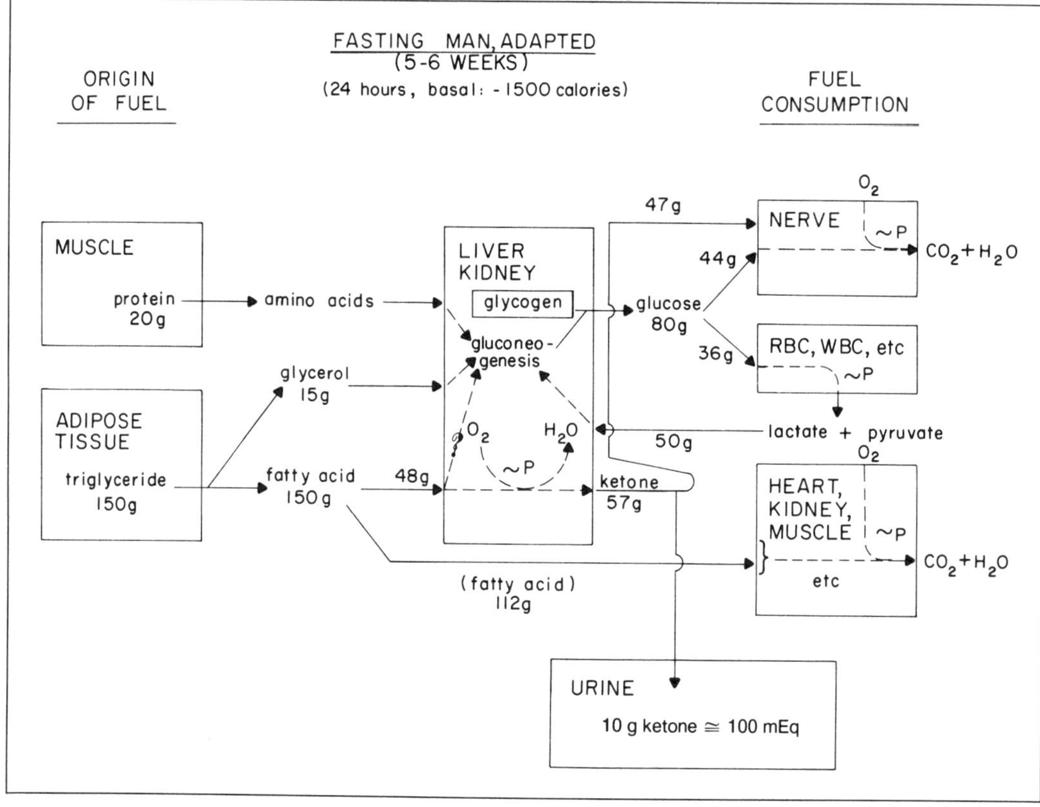

Figure 12-2. Substrate metabolism in a human after a prolonged period of fasting (5 to 6 weeks). ~ P = energy; RBC = red blood cells; WBC = white blood cells. (From Cahill, G.F., Jr., Starvation in man. Reprinted with permission of the New England Journal of Medicine *282:669, 1970.)*

injury or illness, since many aspects of recovery are dependent on active protein synthesis. For example, healing of traumatic or surgical wounds, tissue repair, replacement of red blood cells and lost plasma protein (as in hemorrhage), and immune response to infection are all processes of synthesis of new protein.

In the presence of a hypermetabolic condition with inadequate nutritional support, protein-calorie malnutrition may occur as marasmus, kwashiorkor, or marasmic kwashiorkor. Methods of identifying these conditions during nutritional assessment have been described in Chapter 2.

The mechanisms by which stressful stimuli cause an increase in the metabolic rate are not understood completely but have been studied in burned subjects. It is suggested that a stimulatory mediator may arise from the burn wounds and act on the hypothalamus. Since the metabolic rate has been decreased in burned experimental animals when prostaglandin synthesis was inhibited, the data strongly suggest that prostaglandins are the mediators affecting the hypothalamus.[14] In addition, prostaglandins have been found to be elevated in burn wound exudate and lymph.[15] In the stimulated hypothalamus, the ventral medial nucleus is the origin of sympathetic impulses that stimulate the liver, pancreas, and adrenal glands. The resulting hormonal changes help restore circulation, if it is depressed, and provide energy to the cells to prolong survival.

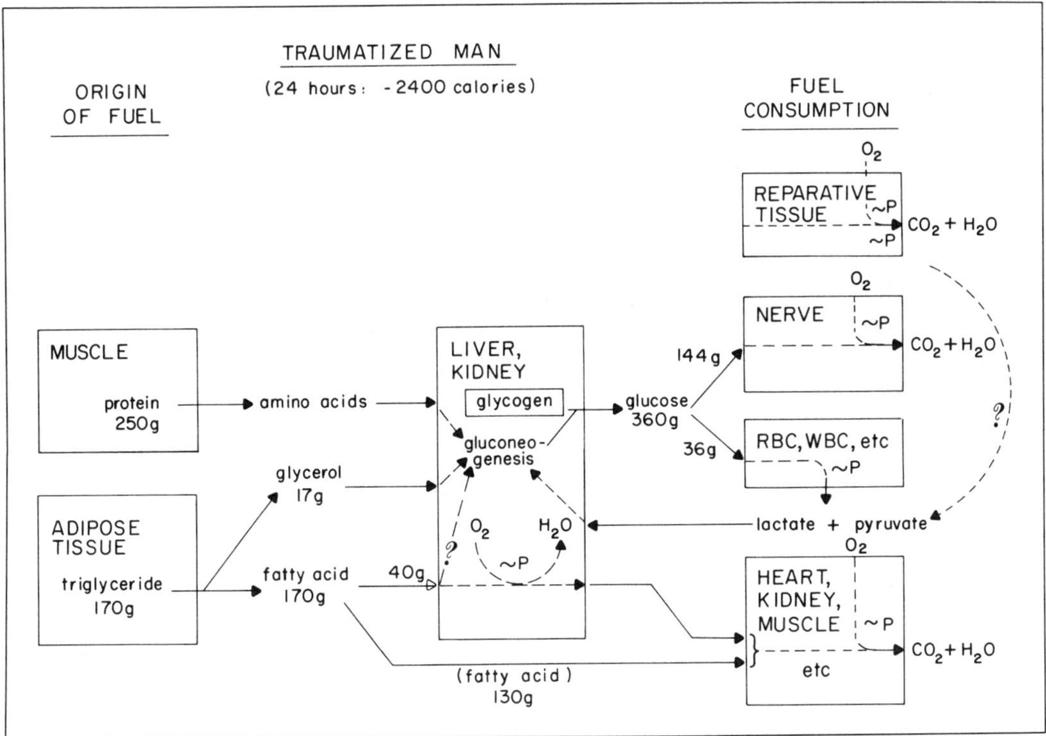

Figure 12-3. Estimation of daily fuel flux in a severely traumatized human. ~ P = energy; RBC = red blood cells; WBC = white blood cells. (Reprinted with permission from Cahill, G. Carbohydrates. In Symposium on Total Parenteral Nutrition. Nashville, Tenn., 1/17–19, 1972. *Chicago: American Medical Association, 1972. Pp. 50–51.)*

The metabolic consequence of this response to trauma and sepsis are reasonably well defined, although not all of the mechanisms have been established. The response was characterized by Cuthbertson[16] using nitrogen balance studies in subjects with fractures. Excretion of as much as 40 g of nitrogen in the urine per day, equivalent to approximately 1 kg of muscle, is not unusual in traumatized adults,[17] and depletion of lean body mass occurs rapidly. As much as 20 percent of body protein may be lost in 2 weeks following a major injury. This is an amount much in excess of the amount of tissue injured. Other pathways of loss are transudates, exudates, wound drainage, intestinal losses, and hemorrhage in which 30.4 g of nitrogen are lost per liter of blood.

At the same time that these losses are occurring, most hypercatabolic conditions are characterized by increases in the synthesis of *acute-phase proteins.* These include fibrinogen, complement, and various globulins. The function of many of these proteins in the body's defense mechanisms is not understood completely, but some possibilities include amplification of the immune response, aid in tissue repair, removal of hemoglobin from lysed red cells, and the minimizing of further tissue damage from phagocytosis.[18,19] Protein also is required for tissue repair. Both of these categories of anabolic processes are superimposed on the normal needs for homeostasis.

The rate of anabolism is, however, slower than the rate of catabolism, resulting in a net protein loss. Skeletal muscle makes the major contribution to both anabolic activity and gluconeogenesis, with lesser contributions from the skin and lower intestine.

In the body's response to trauma, hypermetabolism is associated with negative nitrogen balance and increased oxygen consumption, whereas in chronic starvation, the metabolic rate decreases in response to diminished nutrient intake. This constitutes a major difference between the response to trauma and the response to starvation. With an increased metabolic rate, there may be impairment of the usual metabolic pathways for use of energy sources.

Alterations in endocrine function play a major role in mediating the response to trauma. Several hormones are involved. *Catecholamine* secretion is particularly increased by stress and persists as long as the stress continues.[20] The consequences of the action of the increased catecholamines include an elevation in the metabolic rate and the production of hyperglycemia. Catecholamines also stimulate *glucagon* release. Increased circulating levels of glucagon are found consistently in stressed patients, whereas serum insulin may be depressed.[21] These changes, too, contribute to the production of hyperglycemia.

The catecholamine and glucagon responses are immediate. An acutely injured patient may have *hypovolemia* (diminished blood volume), and so blood flow to the central nervous system may be decreased. Consequently, a higher concentration of nutrients in the blood is necessary so that the brain can extract sufficient nutrients from the limited flow. The development of hyperglycemia, then, appears to be protective in cases of acute injury.

Catecholamines also stimulate adrenocorticotropic hormone (ACTH) release, resulting in increased glucocorticoid levels,[20] which may be two to five times normal and may last 7 to 10 days in minimal injury or for months in prolonged stress.[22-24] These corticoids increase lipolysis, amino acid mobilization, and glucagon release and inhibit protein synthesis and insulin secretion.[3,25-27] *Growth hormone* levels also are increased. The effects of glucocorticoid and growth hormone are not felt as quickly as the catecholamine and glucagon responses, but both contribute to the hyperglycemia.

When blood glucose levels are high, the normal physiologic response is an increase in insulin release and inhibition of glucagon. In the traumatized patient, however, hyperglucagonemia persists despite the presence of hyperglycemia. The glucagon stimulates gluconeogenesis in the liver. Cortisol is synergistic with glucagon in the stimulation of gluconeogenesis, so that their combined actions significantly increase urea formation and nitrogen loss.

The traumatized patient has an increased rate of glucose uptake by peripheral tissue and an increased release of lactate which is circulated to the liver and resynthesized into glucose via the Cori cycle. Thus, glucose metabolism may be limited to anaerobic glycolysis, an inefficient means of metabolizing glucose for energy. The mechanisms of this altered metabolism are currently being investigated and may involve a failure of entry of carbon fragments into the tricarboxylic acid cycle.

The metabolism of fatty acids and the resulting acetyl-CoA is even less well understood than the altered glucose metabolism. Based on the observation that glucose supports nitrogen balance as well as, if not better than, fat emulsion during acute stress, it is believed that defects in fatty acid metabolism do occur in cases of injury or sepsis.

All of these metabolic events combine in accelerating the rate of development of malnutrition. If the patient has insufficient nutrient intake, these metabolic effects of stress are added to the metabolic effects of starvation. The simultaneous occurrence of diminished intake and hypermetabolic conditions is common in hospitalized patients.

Fluid and Electrolyte Balance

The preservation of normal fluid and electrolyte balance is hormone-mediated. Impulses from the hypothalamus to the posterior pituitary gland stimulate production of *antidiuretic hormone* (ADH). The increased ACTH and the renin-angiotensin system, which is stimulated in hypovolemia, affect the secretion of *aldosterone.* An increase in aldosterone and ADH secretion then results in sodium reabsorption and osmotic reabsorption of fluid, thereby increasing fluid volume.

NUTRITIONAL REQUIREMENTS IN HYPERMETABOLIC ILLNESS

The formulation of a nutritional support plan for patients with a hypermetabolic illness requires the assessment of the patient's nutritional status and the severity of the stress, an estimate of the likely duration of the stress, and consideration of the patient's age. The techniques for nutritional assessment were described in Chapter 2. These same methods are applicable to hypermetabolic patients; however, the need for nutritional support is obvious in patients whose critical illness is coupled with a lack of food intake. Detailed assessment procedures rarely are necessary in these circumstances to establish the nutritional status. However, nutritional assessment is useful in such patients to monitor the efficacy of nutritional therapy.

To formulate a nutritional care plan, an estimate must be made of the patient's nutrient requirements. These requirements must take into consideration normal maintenance needs, the increased needs related to the hypermetabolic conditions, and the needs for repair and repletion.

Energy

Formulas and procedures that are useful in estimating the basal metabolic rate (BMR) in a normal healthy subject have limitations when applied to hospitalized patients. Patients are affected by a number of variables that increase or decrease the metabolic rate. The most influential factors in determining energy expenditures are the injuries or disease processes themselves and the activity of the patient. Recent food intake may raise the BMR by 5 to 15 percent. Conversely, fasting or nutritional depletion may decrease the BMR by as much as 30 percent. This presumably is the result of diminished thyroid stimulation and decreased sympathetic activity that occur during fasting. Loss of active metabolic tissue also may play a role. Fever can be most influential, with a 10 to 13 percent increase in heat production for each degree centigrade that the body temperature rises. Finally, pain, fear, and anxiety may contribute to additional energy expenditure.

In practice, the basal energy expenditure (BEE) of a normally nourished hospitalized patient is estimated to be at least 10 percent greater than the estimated BMR of the patient when he or she is not ill. The minimally elevated expenditure can be attributed to eating and to some limited physical activity and usually is referred to as *resting metabolic expenditure* (RME) or BEE (see Chapter 2). The BEE can be elevated, sometimes spectacularly, by the effects of illness or injury.

A number of tables and charts predicting the effects of injury or illness on energy expenditure have been published. One of these is provided as Table 12-1. As might be expected, the values given in different tables are variable and should be used as general guidelines only.

These tables and charts theoretically include only minimal physical activity. If physical activity is above minimal, an additional factor must be included. These *activity energy expenditures* increase the BEE by approximately 20 percent in patients who are largely confined to bed and 30 percent for the more ambulatory patients.[28] Thus, the equations for BEE given in Chapter 2 must be adapted to include corrections for activity and for injury or illness:

$$\text{BEE for men} = (66 + 13.7W + 5H - 6.8A) \times \text{activity factor} \times \text{injury factor} \quad \textbf{(1)}$$

Table 12-1. Increase in Energy Expenditure and Nitrogen Excretion Following Injury or Illness

Type of Injury or Illness	% Increase above BEE	Urinary Nitrogen (g/kg/day)[a]
Elective surgery	24	0.214
Skeletal trauma	32	0.317
Blunt trauma	37	0.332
Head trauma and steroids	61	0.338
Sepsis	79	0.368
Burns	132	0.360

Reprinted with permission from Long, C.L., Schaffel, N., Geiger, J.W., et al., Metabolic response to injury and illness: Estimation of energy and protein needs from indirect calorimetry and nitrogen balance. *J.P.E.N.* 3:453, 1979.

BEE = basal energy expenditure.

[a] Normal urinary nitrogen measures 0.085 g/kg/day.

BEE for women

$$(655 = 9.6W + 1.7H - 4.7A) \times \text{activity factor} \times \text{injury factor} \quad \mathbf{(2)}$$

where W = weight in kilograms; H = height in centimeters; A = age in years.

The activity factor is 1.2 if a patient is confined to bed or 1.3 if the patient is allowed to be out of bed. The injury factors are as follows: minor operation, 1.2; skeletal trauma, 1.35; major sepsis, 1.6; or severe thermal burn, 2.1.

These formulas may be made more precise by substituting specific values from other tables for the injury factor, but it is more important to remember that these equations are, at best, only broad guidelines. The nutritional care specialist must be alert for signs of caloric excess or deficiency in patients and must adjust the regimens accordingly.

In addition to the ongoing increased expenditure in hypermetabolic patients, the dimensions of any existing deficits must also be considered. Both protein and energy must be supplied in amounts in excess of expenditure if lost tissue is to be restored. There are no firm criteria established to determine the amount in excess of current expenditure that should be provided to depleted patients. In general, patients who are not energy deficient are given 20 percent more than the expenditure for current needs, whereas patients exhibiting substantial energy deficits are provided with up to 40 percent more energy than the current level of expenditure. Occasionally, 60 percent excess is recommended,[29] but this amount rarely is given.

Protein

The requirement for protein is poorly defined in patients with hypermetabolic conditions. Protein intake usually is increased above the minimum requirements for healthy adults, provided the patient has normal cardiac, renal, and hepatic function. Intakes of from 1 to 2 g of protein per kilogram of body weight per day are commonly used. For the great majority of patients, 1.2 to 1.5 g/kg/day is sufficient. Higher intakes are used for children.

Protein-Energy Ratio

Since energy is needed to support anabolism, the nitrogen-calorie ratio must be considered. Healthy people with a relatively high energy expenditure due to activity require increased energy intake, although their protein requirement is not known to be increased. An adequate diet in such subjects may have a nitrogen-energy ratio of 1:300 (1 g of nitrogen per 300 kcal) or more.

In contrast, hospitalized patients are thought to have higher protein requirements despite their relative inactivity. The nitrogen-energy ratio that supports optimal use of amino acids for protein synthesis in these patients has been estimated to be from 1:100 to 1:180.[30] The ratio of nitrogen to energy supplied must be raised in patients with disorders of nitrogen metabolism or disposal, as in hepatic or renal disease. A daily weight increase of 0.5 to 1 lb. is the maximum possible increase in lean tissue. Weight gain in excess of this amount represents water or fat.

Micronutrients

Little is known about the requirements for vitamins in hypermetabolic diseases. As a consequence, large increases to therapeutic doses of many vitamins have been recommended. There is, however, little evidence of a need for significantly increasing a patient's intake of ascorbic acid or the B vitamins.

Vitamin A is transported from the liver bound to retinol-binding protein (RBP). Protein deficiency decreases RBP and, thus, serum retinol levels. If large amounts of vitamin A are given to a patient deficient in RBP, there is a rise in plasma levels of vitamin A ester associated with lipoprotein. This is the form that apparently causes the symptoms of toxicity, even in the case of moderate elevation of intake.[31] The nutritional care specialist should be alert for signs of toxicity when large doses of vitamin A are prescribed. Appropriate dosage of vitamin A in the hypermetabolic patient is unknown and requires investigation.

Cellular destruction from trauma or the subsequent catabolic response is accompanied by losses of potassium, phosphate, magnesium, sulfur, zinc, creatine, creatinine, and uric acid.[32] After surgery or trauma, patients will often be dehydrated and have decreased blood volume. Immobilization of a large part of the body affects calcium and phosphorus turnover as well as nitrogen metabolism. Following fractures, there is a great calcium loss, but the negative calcium balance is not corrected by administration of calcium.

It is clear that fluid and electrolyte disorders occur frequently in hypermetabolic illness. In view of their common occurrence and their importance, they will be considered in greater detail in the next section.

FLUID AND ELECTROLYTE BALANCE

Water accounts for 50 to 70 percent of total body weight in the adult of normal weight. Usually the percentage is somewhat lower in women than in men, who generally have a lower fat content and greater muscle mass. In extremely obese individuals, the proportion of water may be much lower. The amount of water, as a percentage of body weight, decreases with age. The newborn infant may consist of 75 to 80 percent water, which decreases to 65 percent in 1 year.

The water in the body is divided into three compartments. Water within the cells, or *intracellular fluid* (ICF), makes up approximately two-thirds of the total body water or 40 percent or so of total body weight. The other third of total body water, or approximately 20 percent of total body weight, is the *extracellular fluid* (ECF), which is divided into the water that exists between the cells (*interstitial fluid*) and that which is in the *plasma.* A simple distribution in a typical 70-kg man is shown in Table 12-2.

The largest proportion of ICF is in the skeletal muscle mass. Its chemical composition is known only approximately, but the major cations are potassium and magnesium. The major anions are phosphate and protein.

The interstitial fluid is divided into two subcategories. One portion is considered to be nonfunctional or slowly equilibrating. It consists of the water in connective tissue and transcellular water—that is, the amount in cerebrospinal fluid and in the joints. The second subcategory equilibrates more rapidly with other body fluids. The normal composition, then, is similar in interstitial fluid and plasma; sodium, chloride, and bicarbonate are major ions. Plasma also contains protein, found only in small amounts in interstitial fluid. The normal composition of body fluid compartments is given in Table 12-3.

Table 12-2. Typical Fluid Distribution in a Healthy 70-Kg Man

Compartment	Fluid Volume (ml)	% Body Weight
Intracellular	28,000	40
Extracellular, total	14,000	20
Plasma	(3,500)	(5)
Interstitial	(10,500)	(15)
Total	42,000	60

Normal Fluid and Electrolyte Exchanges

Under normal conditions, an individual consumes 2,000 to 2,500 ml of water daily, of which approximately 75 percent is taken as liquid by mouth. Some of the remaining 25 percent or so is contained in solid food. Meats, for example, are 50 to 75 percent water, and fruits and vegetables may be as much as 95 percent water. Water also is obtained as a result of metabolic processes; this is known as *metabolic water.* Metabolism produces 0.6 ml of water per gram of carbohydrate, 0.41 ml/g of protein, and 1.07 ml/g of fat.

Daily water losses normally average 250 ml in feces, 800 to 1,500 ml in urine, and 600 to 900 ml as insensible loss (water vapor from the skin [75 percent] and lungs [25 percent]). Insensible water loss may be greatly increased by exercise. A typical fluid balance is shown in Table 12-4.

Maintenance Therapy

Some patients are temporarily unable to take food or fluids by mouth but do not have abnormal fluid or electrolyte losses, abnormal renal function, or preexisting imbalances. The need of these patients is for provision of normal requirements.

The daily *water* needs of these patients are equal to the total loss of water each day. All sources of water and all routes of loss must be considered. At least 500 ml of urine must be produced each day to excrete a usual solute load of 600 mOsm. Adding the insensible losses of 600 to 900 ml, the patient must then be given 1.25 to 1.50 liters of water per day. Since insensible losses may be higher in the hospital environment, a common practice is to provide 35 ml/kg of body weight per day. Thus, a 70-kg man would need 2,450 ml.

An alternative method is to calculate need on the basis of body weight: 100 ml/kg for the first 10 kg of body weight, 50 ml/kg for the next 10 kg, and 25 ml/kg for the remaining weight. Using this method, the 70-kg man would receive 2,750 ml of fluid. These estimates may be used for older children as well, but are not appropriate for infants and young children.

A greater volume of urine production will be needed if the patient is hypercatabolic and is producing a greater solute load or is incapable of maximum urine concentration. Intestinal losses of approximately 250 ml and insensible losses of 500 to 800 ml are added to the total need.

If the patient has abnormal losses, the volume of that fluid must also be included in the calculation of fluid need, to prevent de-

Table 12-3. Typical Normal Composition of Body Fluid Compartments

Ions	Intracellular Fluid (mEq/L)	Interstitial Fluid (mEq/L)	Plasma (mEq/L)
Cations			
Sodium	10	144	142
Potassium	150	4	4
Calcium		3	5
Magnesium	40	2	3
Total	200	153	154
Anions			
Chloride		114	103
Bicarbonate	10	30	27
Sulfate, phosphate	150	3	3
Organic acids		5	5
Protein	40	1	16
Total	200	153	154
Osmotic pressure (mOsm/L)	305.00	300.75	296.50

Table 12-4. Representative Fluid Balance

Water Intake	(ml)	Water Loss	(ml)
Sensible		*Sensible*	
Oral fluids	1,500	Urine	1,500
Solid foods	700	Intestinal	250
Insensible		*Insensible*	
Metabolic water	250	Lungs and skin	700
Total	2,450		2,450

velopment of a deficit. Some of these losses include the following:

1. There may be increased evaporation from the skin as a result of fever, high room temperature with low humidity, or hyperventilation. These and sweat losses are difficult to estimate. Approximately 500 ml/day may be lost if the body temperature is elevated to 38°C., and losses may be approximately 500 ml/day if the room temperature is higher than 32°C. Evaporative losses may be replaced with 5% glucose in water, and losses in sweat, by hypotonic saline.

2. Gastrointestinal losses are incurred if the patient is vomiting or has diarrhea, a draining fistula, or similar losses of gastrointestinal fluids. The composition of gastrointestinal secretion is given in Table 12-5, which also indicates electrolyte replacement needs.

3. Internal shifts may cause fluid to be sequestered in some compartments, creating a deficit in others, even if the amount of total body water is not altered. Replacement needs may be greatly increased in patients with infectious diseases such as peritonitis, in those with pancreatitis, extensive burns, nephrotic syndrome, enteritis, ileus, or portal vein thrombosis, and in surgical patients in the postoperative period.

4. Urinary losses of fluid, sodium, or potassium may be excessive in a variety of renal diseases, in patients receiving corticosteroid medication, and in hyperaldosteronism.

In hypermetabolic conditions, *sodium* normally is well preserved by the kidney, but losses continue in the feces and sweat. Approximately 70 mEq of sodium ion or 4 g of sodium chloride per day usually will provide replacement and prevent a deficit.

Potassium excretion in the urine, normally 20 to 60 mEq/L, continues at the rate of 30 to 40 mEq/day even if the patient has been on a potassium-free diet for as long as a week. In addition, approximately 10 mEq are excreted in stools and sweat. These amounts can be replaced by at least 40 mEq of potassium. Commonly, 60 mEq or more are given if renal function is normal.

Table 12-5. Electrolyte Composition of Gastrointestinal Secretions and Other Body Fluids

	Electrolytes (mEq/L)			
Fluid	Sodium	Potassium	Chloride	Bicarbonate
Saliva	20–46	16–23	24–44	12–18
Gastric juice	31–90	3.6–5.5	100–105	24.6–28.8
Bile	134–156	3.9–6.3	83–110	38
Pancreatic juice	113–153	2.6–7.4	54–95	110
Small intestine (by suction)	72–120	3.5–6.8	69–127	30
Ileal fluid	90–140	6–30	82–125	25–30
Feces	<10	<10	<15	<15
Sweat	18–97	1–15	18–97	0
Cerebrospinal fluid	135–147	2.5–3.4	116–132	21–25

Modified from Lockwood, J.S., and Randall, H.T., The place of electrolyte studies in surgical patients. *Bull. N.Y. Acad. Med.* 25:228, 1949; Randall, H.T., Water and electrolyte balance in surgery. *Surg. Clin. North Am.* 32(3):445, 1952; and Maxwell, M.H., and Kleeman, C.R., Eds., *Clinical Disorders of Fluid and Electrolyte Metabolism*, 2nd ed. New York: McGraw-Hill, 1972.

Therapy for Fluid and Electrolyte Imbalances

In some circumstances, abnormalities of body fluid balance do occur. They generally are classified as disturbances in volume, concentration, or composition. Although they do not ususally occur separately, each will be described in turn for greater clarity.

Volume Disturbances

Extracellular fluid volume deficit or *hypovolemia* can develop in patients in the circumstances previously described and may be accompanied by increased, decreased, or normal electrolyte levels. Signs of volume depletion are given in Table 12-6. Laboratory values show increased blood urea nitrogen (BUN), serum creatinine, and hematocrit. Urine chloride is less than 10 mEq/L and urine specific gravity is high.

Let us assume a patient (Patient 1, described in Table 12-7) as an example in estimating replacement need. A common procedure to calculate fluid deficit is to assume that Mrs. M.G. is approximately 50 percent water, since she is a young adult woman. She has lost 6 kg. The deficit of total body water can be determined by the following calculations:

Normal body weight × 50% = 55 kg × 0.5 = 27.5 liters total body water

Present body weight × 50% = 49 kg × 0.5 = 24.5 liters total body water

Fluid deficit = 27.5 − 24.5 = 3.0 liters

Table 12-6. Clinical Manifestations of Fluid and Electrolyte Imbalances

Fluid or Electrolyte	Clinical Manifestations of Deficit	Clinical Manifestations of Excess
Extracellular fluid volume	Increased pulse rate; decreased body temperature; increased respiration rate; anorexia; nausea and vomiting; weight loss (500 ml of fluid = 1 lb.); urine flow <20–40 ml/hr; systolic blood pressure 10 mm Hg less when standing than when supine; dry skin; dry mucous membrane; fatigue, apathy; longitudinal wrinkles in skin; depressed fontanel in infant; shock and coma if very severe deficit	Puffy eyelids; peripheral edema; ascites; pleural effusion; pulmonary edema; acute weight gain; increased central venous pressure; dyspnea; tachycardia (symptoms vary with cause)
Sodium	Abdominal cramps; anorexia; diarrhea; lethargy; apprehension; confusion; convulsions; coma	Firm rubbery tissue turgor; dry sticky mucous membranes; oliguria; agitation, convulsions
Potassium	Muscle weakness (skeletal, intestinal, heart, respiratory); cardiac arrhythmias; electrocardiographic abnormalities; apnea and respiratory arrest; nephropathy; nausea; paralytic ileus	May be none. Symptoms similar to hypokalemia. Muscle weakness; intestinal colic; diarrhea; Oliguria, anuria; electrocardiographic changes
Calcium	Muscle cramps; tingling of fingers; tetany; convulsions	Nausea and vomiting; relaxed muscles; kidney stones; pathologic fractures; bone pain; cardiac arrest; stupor, coma
Magnesium	Hyperactivity; neuromuscular irritability; tremor; disorientation; convulsions	Anorexia, weight loss; loss of muscle tone; depression
Bicarbonate	Metabolic acidosis: weakness; deep, rapid breathing; shortness of breath; disorientation, coma	Metabolic alkalosis: depressed respiration; hypertonic muscles; tetany
Carbonic acid	Respiratory alkalosis: deep, rapid breathing; tetany; unconsciousness	Respiratory acidosis: decreased respiration; disorientation

Table 12-7. Case Report: Mrs. M.G., Prolonged Vomiting

Sex	Female			
Age	29 years			
Normal weight	121 lb (55 kg)			
Present weight	105 lb (49 kg)			
Blood pressure	95/65			
Arterial blood gases				
	Current	Normal		
pH	7.5	7.34–7.45		
Pao_2	85 mm Hg	80–100 mm Hg		
$Paco_2$	45 mm Hg	35–45 mm Hg		
Bicarbonate ions	33 mEq/L	24–31 mEq/L		
	Serum		Urine	
	Current	Normal	Current	Normal
Sodium	115 mEq/L	136–145 mEq/L	26 mEq/L	40–90 mEq/L
Potassium	1.9 mEq/L	3.5–5.0 mEq/L	65 mEq/L	20–60 mEq/L
Chloride	75 mEq/L	100–106 mEq/L	8 mEq/L	40–120 mEq/L
Urea nitrogen	43 mg/dl	8–25 mg/dl		
Creatinine	1.7 mg/dl	0.7–1.5 mg/dl		
Specific gravity			1.03	1.003–1.030

Pao_2 = arterial oxygen tension; $Paco_2$ = arterial carbon dioxide tension.

In the ensuing 24 hours, the patient will also need replacement of daily sensible and insensible losses. If we calculate maintenance need on the basis of normal body weight, Mrs. M.G.'s total need is 3 liters plus 2,375 ml or slightly more than 5 liters. Generally, at least half of this should be replaced within 24 hours. More severe deficits are replaced intravenously.

The opposite condition, *volume excess* or *hypervolemia,* occurs in cardiac or renal insufficiency. It can occur when water and electrolytes shift from interstitial space to the plasma. It usually is treated with fluid and sodium restrictions and diuretics. It may be iatrogenic. The exact procedure for treatment depends on the cause (see Chapters 7 and 8).

Concentration Disturbances

Because sodium is the dominant ion in the ECF, sodium concentration dominates the osmotic pressure. It is important to recall that sodium moves water, so that a sodium deficit in the ECF (actually in the plasma, since that is the only place it can be measured) will cause fluid to move into the ICF to stabilize the osmotic pressure. Sodium excess in the plasma will draw water from the ICF. Thus, concentration disturbances are disorders of sodium concentration. The normal amount of sodium ion in the plasma is 142 mEq/L (see Table 12-3).

Hyponatremia (*sodium deficit, low-sodium syndrome,* or *hypotonic dehydration*) is seen in patients who have lost water and electrolytes or who have received an excessive amount of dextrose in water or other sources of sodium-free water. The condition is defined by a serum sodium level of less than 130 mEq/L. Identifiable signs of hyponatremia (see Table 12-6) can occur only when the condition is severe and include oliguria progressing to anuria and increased intracranial pressure.

In Mrs. M.G. (see Table 12-7), the total sodium deficit can be calculated first by determining her deficit in sodium concentration (normal sodium concentration [142] [obtained from Table 12-3] minus measured serum sodium [115]), and then multiplying the result by her present fluid volume of 24.5 liters:

$$(142 - 115 \text{ mEq/L}) \times 24.5 \text{ liters} = 661.5 \text{ mEq}$$

In addition to this 661.5 mEq, the sodium in her fluid loss of 3 kg must be provided as well as the 90 mEq which will be lost in the next 24 hours: 3 liters × 142 mEq = 426 mEq for a total of 661.5 + 426 + 90 mEq or 1,177.5 mEq. Other losses associated with her illness must be added to this amount.

Hypernatremia (*pure water deficit* or *hypertonic dehydration*) is seen in patients who are unable to obtain water or ask for it. It occurs in diabetes insipidus or in patients given tube feedings without adequate water. Signs of hypernatremia are listed in Table 12-6. If serum sodium is less than 160 mEq/L, water may be given orally, but in more marked hypernatremia, sodiumfree intravenous fluid, such as 5% dextrose in water, may be used.

The volume of water necessary to correct hypernatremia may be calculated:

$$\frac{\text{Normal serum sodium} \times \text{normal TBW}}{\text{Measured serum sodium}} = \text{Current TBW}$$

where TBW = total body water. **(3)**

In a patient weighing 70 kg, assuming that person is 60 percent water, total body water equals 42 liters. If the patient's serum sodium is 162 mEq/L, current TBW is calculated using this equation:

$$\frac{142 \text{ mEq} \times 42 \text{ liters}}{162 \text{ mEq}} = 36.8 \text{ liters}$$

The deficit thus is 42 − 36.8 or 5.2 liters.

Composition Disturbances

Changes in concentration of ions other than sodium can occur without significantly altering the osmotic pressure; therefore, they are classified as changes in composition rather than concentration. A number of disorders are included in this category. Their clinical manifestations are given in Table 12-6.

Hypokalemia. Hypokalemia can occur as a consequence of severe vomiting, malabsorption, chronic renal disease, metabolic disorders, or poor nutrition. Clinical manifestations rarely develop until serum potassium levels have fallen below 3.0 mEq/L. Potassium depletion cannot be estimated on the basis of serum potassium alone, since that value varies with the acid-base balance. Serum potassium increases in acidosis and decreases in alkalosis. Moderate deficits may be replaced orally, usually with 10% potassium chloride mixed with fruit juice and given after meals to reduce gastric irritation. When the deficit is severe or if oral intake is not possible, intravenous therapy may be necessary.

In either case, since ECF levels of potassium are less than 2 percent of the total body potassium, the deficit is estimated on the basis of total body weight. A woman's total body potassium is approximately 35 mEq/kg of body weight. Therefore, Mrs. M.G.'s total potassium (see Table 12-7) may be calculated:

$$35 \text{ mEq} \times 55 \text{ kg} = 1{,}925 \text{ mEq}$$

Since she has a weight deficit of 6 kg or 11 percent of her normal body weight ($6/55 \cong .11$). Thus, an additional amount of potassium must be added, as follows:

$$1{,}925 \text{ mEq} \times .11 \cong 212 \text{ mEq}$$

The amount of potassium lost daily as a further consequence of her illness must be added, also. If her losses were 50 mEq, for example, her replacement need would be 1,925 + 212 + 50 or 2,187 mEq. Because of the effect of potassium on the heart and other muscles, the deficit must be made up slowly, over a period of 2 to 3 days or as much as a week. During this time, the daily losses of 40 to 60 mEq must be added to the amount being replaced.

Hyperkalemia. Hyperkalemia accompanies renal failure, burns, infections, and other catabolic conditions and also occurs in acidosis. It can be iatrogenic from sources such as penicillin and blood transfusions. In hyperkalemic patients, the underlying cause is treated, and potassium administration, including dietary sources, are stopped. To avoid the effects of hyperkalemia (see Table 12-6), insulin often is given to increase cellular uptake of glucose and potassium. An intravenous solution of sodium lactate, calcium gluconate, and dextrose in water is used less often. Calcium gluconate antagonizes the effects on the heart. Lactate is metabolized into bicarbonate, thereby raising the blood pH. This shift, combined with the glucose, helps to move potassium back into the cells.

Treatment may involve removing potassium from the body, forcing potassium into the cells, or antagonizing potassium's effects. The use of *cation exchange resins* removes potassium ion slowly. In extreme circumstances, hemodialysis may be used. Sodium bicarbonate, sometimes provided as sodium lactate, causes movement of potassium ion into the cells very rapidly, as do glucose infusions. Calcium, which antagonizes the cardiac and neuromuscular effects of hyperkalemia, may be injected as 10% calcium gluconate. This is a temporary measure, however, and should be followed by the other forms of therapy.

Hypocalcemia. Hypocalcemia is defined as a serum calcium level of less than 8 mg/dl. It is seen in malabsorption syndromes, acute pancreatitis, infections, intestinal fistulas, and hypoparathyroidism. Intravenous 10% calcium gluconate or 10% calcium chloride is used in treatment. Losses from gastrointestinal drainage may be particularly high; these patients may require 400 to 500 mg/day. Coexisting hypomagnesemia must be corrected simultaneously to reverse hypocalcemia.

Hypercalcemia. Hypercalcemia is seen most often in hyperparathyroidism and cancer of the bone. Calcium levels are lowered by dilution when other ECF deficits are treated.

Hypomagnesemia. Hypomagnesemia occurs in malabsorption syndromes, gastrointestinal losses, and deficient magnesium intake. Replacement of magnesium is provided with 10 to 40 mEq of the sulfate salt per 24 hr.

Hypermagnesemia. Hypermagnesemia can accompany renal insufficiency or excessive use of magnesium-containing drugs such as some laxatives and antacids. The condition may be treated with a slow calcium infusion to counteract the neuromuscular effects plus isotonic saline to stimulate urine flow and magnesium excretion.

Hypochloremia. Hypochloremia can be produced in severe vomiting with loss of hydrogen and chloride ions. Needs can be replaced when intravenous sodium chloride is administered. Bicarbonate serves as the replacement anion in metabolism when chloride is deficient.

Hydrogen and Bicarbonate Ion Imbalances. Hydrogen and bicarbonate ion (acid-base) imbalances are classified as metabolic acidosis or alkalosis and respiratory acidosis or alkalosis. Only the metabolic disorders are ordinarily treated intravenously.

Usually, carbon dioxide, which can form carbonic acid, is excreted by the lungs and has no net effect on the pH of the blood, but the body also produces approximately 70 mEq of *nonvolatile* or *fixed acid* daily from sulfur-containing amino acids or incompletely oxidized carbohydrate and fat. This material must be excreted in the urine.

Metabolic acidosis. In metabolic acidosis, serum bicarbonate is less than 24 mEq/L, plasma pH is less than 7.35, and the patient retains fixed acid or loses base. Hyperventilation, which is a compensatory mechanism, causes a fall in Pco_2.

In calculating the bicarbonate deficit, the ECF space is used. The normal serum bicarbonate level is 26 mEq/L. If a 65-kg man has a plasma bicarbonate level of 16 mEq/L, we can calculate his deficit as 26 − 16 or 10 mEq/L. The ECF constitutes approximately 20 percent of his total body weight or 13 liters. Theoretically, then, his bicarbonate deficit equals 10 mEq/L × 13 liters or 130 mEq. One liter of 1/6 molar sodium lactate provides 166 mEq. Sometimes, the physician elects to use bicarbonate directly. It can be added to dextrose and water from ampules containing 45 mEq/50 ml.

Metabolic alkalosis. Metabolic alkalosis occurs in the loss of hydrogen ion, most commonly from prolonged vomiting or gastric suction, in postoperative patients, or from excessive intake of antacids. Metabolic alkalosis usually is defined as a plasma bicarbonate level in excess of 29 mEq/L, plasma pH higher than 7.45, and a potassium level of less than 4 mEq/L. Comparison of these values with those of Mrs. M.G. (see Table 12-7) indicates that she has metabolic alkalosis. The body attempts to compensate for this condition by retaining CO_2 via shallow breathing, and Pco_2 rises to 44 to 48 mm Hg.

Treatment is influenced by the cause and accompanying imbalances. When the patient has prolonged vomiting, saline and potassium chloride infusions are used. The sodium reduces hydrogen ion excretion in the kidneys, and the chloride frees bicarbonate for renal excretion. The vomiting patient will also have lost potassium, which is replaced along with the chloride.

Other Nutritional Concerns in Fluid and Electrolyte Imbalances

The nutritional care specialist should be aware that these fluid and electrolyte alterations affect the desire for food and water. Anorexia is seen in potassium or protein deficit and in hypercalcemia. Thirst is seen in sodium excess, hypercalcemia, and in blood volume deficit whether it is due to hemorrhage or heart failure. Absence of thirst occurs in sodium deficit.

METHODS OF NUTRITIONAL SUPPORT

Once estimations of nutrient expenditures and intake requirements are made, the patient's capacity for achieving that intake by standard dietary means must be evaluated. If it appears feasible for the patient to take a sufficient amount of food and fluid from the hospital menu, he or she may, for example, be given a diet with increased protein and energy content plus any other modifications required by his or her specific conditions. High-protein, high-calorie supplements (see Chapter 2 and Appendix K) between meals often are useful. The patient's intake should be monitored carefully to be certain that intake is commensurate with need.

If, over a period of days, the patient's intake is insufficient to meet his or her needs, more active nutritional support by means of enteral tube feeding may be undertaken. A combination of tube feeding and standard meals may be used. These methods have been described in Chapter 2. If they are inadequate, parenteral feeding becomes necessary. It, too, may be used as a supplement to other methods or as the sole method of feeding, depending on the circumstances.

Specific guidelines to determine when patients require alternative nutritional support have not been developed. In general, if the interval of relative or total starvation has been or is expected to be 2 weeks or longer, or if protein-energy malnutrition is identified at the time of assessment, active nutritional support is indicated. Well-nourished patients with brief intervals of starvation do not require special nutritional support. Up to 7 days of relative starvation is well tolerated and is not thought to impair recovery in the initially well-nourished patient.

In the strict meaning of the term, *parenteral nutrition* refers to the provision of nutrients by any route that does not involve the intestinal tract. It includes, for example, intramuscular injections of vitamins. In common usage, however, parenteral nutrition generally refers to the intravenous route. It may be used for partial or total nutritional support for a brief period, for an extended time, or for life. There are three fundamental types of intravenous feeding: (1) supplemental nutrition into a peripheral vein, (2) total nutrition into a central vein, or (3) total nutrition into a peripheral vein. The amount of energy that must be provided intravenously is crucial in determining the method to be used.

Supplemental Peripheral Venous Alimentation

Isotonic solutions of low concentration for short-term supplementation or substitution for oral intake may be given into a peripheral vein. These solutions are used to maintain fluid and electrolyte balance but provide only a limited supply of energy substrates. Sometimes, low concentrations of amino acids are included.

Categories of Intravenous Fluids

For maintenance or correction of fluid and electrolyte balance, there are four categories of intravenous fluids that are most often used in supplemental peripheral venous alimentation. Each of these is described briefly, so that the nutritional care specialist becomes familiar with the purpose for which the physician orders their use and the nutrients provided.

Dextrose in water solutions (Table 12-8) provide calories and water. The dextrose is hydrated (glucose monohydrate) and yields only 3.4 kcal/g. As a consequence, each liter of 5% dextrose in water (D5W) provides only 170 kcal (1,000 × 0.05 × 3.4). To supply more energy, a higher concentration of dextrose would be needed but would cause irritation in the vein. When D5W is infused, the dextrose is metabolized rapidly, leaving water to reduce plasma osmotic pressure. Water then moves from the plasma into the cells. The use of D5W, then, is primarily for replacement of volume deficits, not as an energy source.

Saline solutions (see Table 12-8) are available in several concentrations. A concentration of 0.9% sodium chloride often is referred to as *isotonic saline, normal saline,* or *physiologic saline.* It has the tonicity of plasma (308 mOsm/L) but its sodium ion and chloride ion contents are higher in concentration than in plasma. This is necessary because other plasma ions are lacking. Isotonic saline is used to replace ECF deficits, to treat sodium depletion, and to treat metabolic alkalosis. *Hypotonic saline* (0.45% sodium chloride) supplies normal salt and water requirements, whereas *hypertonic saline* (3% or 5% sodium chloride) is used in small amounts to treat water overload and severe sodium depletion.

Dextrose in saline solutions (see Table 12-8) contain both dextrose and sodium chloride in the same solution. A mixture of 5% dextrose in 0.45% saline is used to replace fluid losses and to assess the adequacy of renal function. Mixtures of 5% or 10% dextrose in normal saline provide replacement of sodium ion and chloride ion and some kilocalories to reduce catabolism.

Multiple electrolyte solutions (see Table 12-8) are used for maintenance or replacement. Maintenance solutions contain approximately normal needs, whereas replacement solutions contain some electrolytes in excess of normal needs. Almost all contain potassium and either lactate, citrate, or acetate, which are metabolized to bicarbonate. These solutions are used in cases of gastrointestinal losses, burns, acidosis, dehydration, or sodium depletion.

Table 12-8. Characteristics of Intravenous Fluids

	Cations			Anions					
Type of Fluid	Sodium (mEq/L)	Potassium (mEq/L)	Calcium (mEq/L)	Chloride (mEq/L)	Bicarbonate (mEq/L)[a]	Kilocalories per Liter	pH (approximate)	Osmolarity (mOsm/L)	Notes
Dextrose in water solutions									
5% dextrose in water						170	4.8	252	5%: No replacement of electrolytes or correction of fluid deficits
10% dextrose in water						340	4.7	505	10%, 20%, 50%: Hypertonic solutions act as osmotic diuretics, increasing body fluid loss
20% dextrose in water						680	4.8	1,010	
50% dextrose in water						1,700	4.6	2,525	All: Dextrose provides calories
Dextrose in saline solutions									
5% dextrose and 0.2% sodium chloride	34			34		170	4.6	320	All: Provides calories, water, sodium, and chloride. Dextrose provides calories.
5% dextrose and 0.45% sodium chloride	77			77		170	4.6	406	5%, 0.45%: Used to treat hypovolemia and to promote diuresis in dehydrated patients
5% dextrose and 0.9% sodium chloride	154			154		170	4.4	559	
10% dextrose	154			154		340	4.8	812	

chloride									
0.9% sodium chloride	154			154		0	6.0	154	0.9%: Widely used as a routine electrolyte replacement solution or to correct mild metabolic acidosis
3% sodium chloride	513			513		0	4.5–7.0	1,026	3%, 5%: Used for correction of severe salt depletion only
5% sodium chloride	855			855		0	4.5–7.0		
Multiple electrolyte solutions									
Ringer's solution	147	4	5	155		0	4.0–7.5	309	Replaces potassium, calcium, sodium, and chloride; chloride is in excess of normal plasma level
Lactated Ringer's solution (Hartmann's)	130	4	3	109	28	9	6.5	273	Closely resembles ECF
5% dextrose in lactated Ringer's	130	4	3	109	28	179	5.1	524	Replaces ECF deficits; replaces losses from vomiting or gastric suction
10% dextrose in lactated Ringer's solution	130	4	3	109	28	349	4.9	776	Dextrose provides calories
1.9% Darrow's solution	122	35		104	53				Useful in treatment of acidosis and potassium deficiency; useful in diarrhea and diabetic coma

ECF = extracellular fluid.

[a] Or its equivalent in lactate, acetate, or citrate.

Other available solutions sometimes used contain alcohol, artificial plasma extenders, ammonium chloride, and calcium gluconate.

All intravenous solutions can be classified as hypertonic, isotonic, or hypotonic in the same manner as described for the saline solutions. Hypertonic solutions contain electrolytes in excess of the concentrations in plasma and are used to provide replacement. Hypertonic solutions are 5% dextrose in normal saline, 5% dextrose in Ringer's lactated injection, and 10% or 20% dextrose in water. Isotonic solutions are used to expand ECF volume. Normal saline, D5W, and Ringer's lactated solution are isotonic. Hypotonic solutions are useful to shift fluid from plasma to the interstitial fluid. The primary example is half-normal (0.45%) saline.

Energy Supply

The energy supply available from the solutions used for supplemental peripheral venous feeding is limited for two reasons. First, the total amount of solution that can be administered per day is limited by the danger of fluid overload. Second, the osmolality of the solution must be low, since highly concentrated solutions cause inflammation and sclerosis in the vein at the site of the administration. Consequently, 5% to 10% glucose solutions are used for administration into peripheral veins. Since each liter of intravenous solution of 5% glucose provides 170 kcal, 9 liters of solution would be required to meet a minimal maintenance requirement of 1,500 kcal/day. This amount of solution is unlikely to be tolerated. Hence, as a source of energy, supplemental peripheral venous feeding is useful only for patients who need limited support for a short period.

As an alternative, Blackburn et al.[33] have suggested the use of a glucose-free amino acid solution to reduce the stimulation for insulin release. The procedure is known as *protein-sparing therapy.* Assuming that the patient has adequate fat reserves, the reduced insulin levels would result in increased fat mobilization for energy, reduce the mobilization of amino acids for energy, and make the administered amino acids available for protein synthesis. The method has not been generally accepted as standard procedure. In the opinion of many clinicians, the high cost of amino acids compared to glucose is not justified by the limited advantage gained.

Total Parenteral Nutrition

Some patients need more nutritional support than can be provided by supplemental peripheral venous alimentation. For these patients, more aggressive nutritional support has become available in recent years. The procedure is commonly referred to as *total parenteral nutrition* (*TPN*). As is implied by its name, TPN may be used as the sole means of feeding the patient, or it may supplement enteral feeding.

A major difference between intravenous and enteral feeding is that the intravenous feeding enters the systemic circulation directly, rather than entering the portal circulation and the lymphatic system. However, because the intestinal tract, with its digestive function, is bypassed in intravenous alimentation, the nutrients must be provided in a predigested state. The significance of this altered route of entry of nutrients has not been determined. It apparently does not affect nutritional requirements, but immune function and a number of functions of the gastrointestinal tract, including exocrine pancreatic function, intestinal mucosal enzyme content, and gallbladder contraction, may be depressed. These changes are believed to be reversible when enteral feeding is resumed, but resumption of enteral feeding should be done cautiously if the duration of TPN has been prolonged.

Total parenteral nutrition is a complex and expensive procedure with potential risks and complications. Therefore, it is undertaken only if adequate nutrient intake via the gastrointestinal tract is impossible or inadvisable. Examples of conditions in which TPN may be appropriate are listed in Table 12-9. Gastrointestinal conditions in which TPN might be useful were described in Chapters 5 and 6.

Most institutions establish a nutritional support service to provide the necessary meticulous attention for TPN patients. The professionals involved in the service vary, but a nutritional support service usually consist of at least a physician, nurse, nutritional care specialist, and pharmacist. Sometimes, a social worker, physical therapist, administrator, and secretary also are included. The nutritional care specialist on the nutritional support service must have a thorough knowledge of nutrition and an appreciation of the methods, problems, and risks involved in TPN. He or she has a particularly important role in monitoring the patient's nutritional status during the course of the TPN feeding and in providing appropriate nutritional support during the weaning process. These subjects will now be described briefly, with emphasis on central venous feeding.

Table 12-9. Indications for Use of Total Parenteral Nutrition

Unavailability of the gastrointestinal tract
Short bowel syndrome
Obstruction
Ileus
Malabsorption
Chronic vomiting
To minimize gastrointestinal function
Inflammatory bowel disease
Fistulas
Intractable diarrhea and failure to thrive
Acute pancreatitis
Preoperative repletion of patients who have lost more than 10–15% body weight
Patients who cannot meet energy needs by oral intake
Hypermetabolism: major surgery or trauma, major burns, or sepsis
Protein-losing gastroenteropathy
Extreme weakness
Anorexia and unwillingness to eat: cancer, chemotherapy, radiotherapy, psychological depression, or anorexia nervosa
Disturbances of nitrogen metabolism
Reversible liver failure
Acute and chronic renal failure
Nonterminal coma

Central Venous Alimentation

Placement of the Catheter. Insertion of the catheter is a surgical procedure. The catheter commonly is placed into the right or left subclavian vein and then threaded into the superior vena cava. Sometimes the internal jugular vein is used as the starting point for catheter insertion. For relatively short-term TPN, a typical line consists of a 16-gauge percutaneous intravenous catheter (Intracath). Percutaneous stiffer catheters are not suitable for patients requiring TPN for many months or for life because of the danger of thrombosis, erosion of the wall of the vein, and infection. Instead, a silicone rubber *catheter* is inserted for long-term use. These catheters are less reactive and are soft and flexible. They are approximately 90 cm long. Part of the catheter lies in a subcutaneous tunnel and emerges just lateral to the sternum at approximately the fourth or fifth rib. In this position, the patient can see and care for it, and it does not interfere with clothing.

Preparation and Administration of the Solution. All TPN solutions must be sterile and are prepared in the pharmacy using aseptic techniques. Standard procedure for their administration to the hospitalized patient infuses the solutions steadily over a 24-hour period, beginning with 50 ml/hr the first day, 75 ml/hr the second day, and progressing to 125 ml/hr the third day and thereafter. An infusion pump usually is considered preferable to regulate the flow, although gravity drip administration may be used.

Composition of Solutions. To provide a large quantity of nutrients within a volume of fluid that the patient can tolerate, it is necessary to use a hyperosmolar solution that has a higher concentration of the nutrients in a smaller total volume. All required nutrients must be provided in the infusate.

Amino acids. The sources of amino acids used most commonly in TPN are mixtures of crystalline amino acids. Representative commercially available amino acid mixtures are listed in Table 12-10. The amino acid content of each mixture is available from the manufacturer. Those containing all the essential amino acids along with ten or twelve nonessential amino acids similar to egg protein promote best utilization for protein synthesis.[34] The body has a limited capacity to synthesize arginine, so arginine is included in the infusate.[35] Infants require histidine, and premature infants are deficient in cystathionase, the enzyme that converts methionine to cystine; therefore, cystine is essential.[36] A product especially formulated to meet the needs of patients with renal disease contains only the essential amino acids.

Recent work has suggested that the branched-chain amino acids (BCAAs), leucine, isoleucine, and valine, may have special properties that are significant in nutritional support. In the glucose-intolerant, hypermetabolic patient, muscles can use BCAAs to meet their energy requirements.[37] A small amount of BCAAs can be metabolized directly by the muscle for energy, but most must be metabolized in the liver. The use of BCAA supplementation currently is under investigation. A high concentration of BCAAs with a low concentration of aromatic amino acids may be useful in reversing coma in hepatic encephalopathy (see Chapter 11). Amino acid mixtures altered to meet these needs may be useful in TPN of patients with hepatic disease. Other special formulations for treatment of specific diseases may be forthcoming as our knowledge improves.

Carbohydrate. Carbohydrate to provide sufficient energy substrate is provided in the form of dextrose solutions. They are available in concentrations of up to 70 percent. Carbohydrates other than glucose, including fructose, have been used as energy sources, but no advantage of their use has been established. Amino acids are not considered sources of energy in the patients being replenished, since the objective is to have these patients retain rather than deaminate amino acids for energy.

Lipids. Lipids may be included at either of two levels, a low level sufficient to prevent essential fatty acid (EFA) deficiency or a larger amount which will contribute significantly to the kilocalorie content of the infusate. If lipids are given only to prevent EFA deficiency, two to four 500-ml bottles (2 to 4 units) of 10% fat emulsion per week are sufficient. If these are not provided, EFA deficiency is seen in the form of circular skin lesions, hair loss, delays in wound healing,

Table 12-10. Commercially Available Sources of Amino Acids for Total Parenteral Nutrition

Product	Manufacturer	Amino Acid Concentration (%)	Osmolarity (mOsm/L)
Aminosyn	Abbott Laboratories	3.5, 5.0, 7.0, 8.5, 10.0	406 500 700 850 1,000
Freamine II	American-McGaw	3.0, 8.5	405 810
Nephramine[a]	American-McGaw	5.4	440
Travasol	Travenol Laboratories	3.5, 5.5 8.5, 10.0	
Vamin	Pharmacia, Canada	7	
Veinamine	Cutter Laboratories	8	950

[a] Contains only essential amino acids plus histidine.

and abnormalities in liver function. Changes in the unsaturated fatty acid ratios (triene-tetraene ratio) indicative of deficiency can be seen as early as 4 days following the use of an EFA-deficient formula.

Lipid can provide up to 60 percent of the total caloric need. The recommended daily dose is 1 to 2 g/kg/day. It is given in combination with glucose, since lipid alone might maintain body fat while allowing protein loss via gluconeogenesis. The use of lipids as an energy source is somewhat controversial; nonprotein calories are provided primarily as glucose in most large centers. The rationale for the routine infusion of greater amounts of fat in TPN is as follows:

1. Provision of nonprotein calories as glucose and fat most closely resembles a normal diet.
2. The impairment of glucose metabolism induced by catabolic states suggests that a portion of the intake should be substituted with fat.
3. Provision of glucose as an energy source results in greater production of carbon dioxide per unit of energy than does fat.

On the other hand, there are arguments favoring continuation of the predominant use of glucose as the nonprotein energy source in TPN, with limitation of fat intake to amounts sufficient to avoid EFA deficiency. These arguments include the following:

1. There are questions regarding the efficacy of fat as an energy source to support protein metabolism in catabolic patients. Although defects in the complete oxidation of glucose in catabolic states have been identified, studies of the efficacy of glucose and fat in the support of nitrogen balance in catabolic patients have suggested that glucose is more effective. Patients who are not severely catabolic appear to achieve similar nitrogen balance with glucose or with a portion of the intake as fat.
2. Complications specific to the infusion of fat emulsions may include impairment of the diffusion of gas across the alveolocapillary membrane in the lung, impairment of immune function, and impairment of blood coagulation. However, widespread use of currently available fat emulsions is remarkably free of complications.
3. Glucose is an inexpensive energy source. The cost to a hospital pharmacy to prepare an intravenous solution as either 10%, 20%, or 30% glucose varies only slightly. In contrast, the production of infusates containing fat emulsions is an expensive process. The substitution of fat calories for a portion of glucose calories in TPN has a major impact on the cost of delivery of the feeding.

Lipid products for parenteral use are described in Table 12-11. When administered, the lipid is not mixed with the glucose–amino acid solution but is run into a catheter from a separate bottle. The separate lines are connected just before they enter the vein. Starting infusion rates may be 1 ml/min. for ½ hour and then increased to 125 ml/hr.

Transient side effects of lipid infusion do occur. They include chills, shivering, fever, vomiting, and chest and back pain. Alternative methods of administration may avoid these side effects. It has been claimed that application of corn oil or safflower oil to the skin will supply some of the requirement. For those patients in whom some intake by mouth is possible, 2 to 5 tsp. of an appropriate vegetable oil taken orally will prevent EFA deficiency.

The *energy-nitrogen ratio* in the final formula is an important consideration. A sufficient amount of energy from nonprotein sources must be provided so that amino acids are used for anabolic processes rather than as a source of energy. There remains some controversy on the best amount to use. A common current practice is to provide a ratio of at least 120 : 1, that is 120 nonprotein

Table 12-11. Lipid Emulsions for Total Parenteral Nutrition

Product	Lipid Concentration (%)	Osmolarity (mOsm/L)	Kcal/ml	pH[a]	Composition	Fatty Acid Content (%)
Intralipid (Cutter Laboratories)	10 20	280 330	1.1 2.0	7.5 7.5	Soy oil in water; 1.2% phosphatide; 2.5% glycerol	Linoleic, 55; linolenic, 8; other, 37
Liposyn (Abbott Laboratories)	10 20	300 340	1.1 2.0	8.0 8.3	Safflower oil in water; 1.2% phosphatide; 2.5% glycerol	Linoleic, 78; linolenic, 0.5
Travamulsion (Travenol Laboratories)	10	270	1.1	5.5–9.0	Soy oil in water; 1.2% phosphatide; 2.5 glycerin	Linoleic, 56; linolenic, 6; other, 38

[a] Adjusted with sodium hydroxide.

kilocalories per gram of nitrogen. For example, let us assume that a patient is receiving 1 liter of 8.5% Freamine. This would contain 85 g of amino acids which are 16% nitrogen. The nitrogen content thus is 85 × 0.16 or 13.6 g. In order to receive at least 120 kcal/g of nitrogen, the patient needs 1,632 kcal (13.6 × 120). One liter of 20% dextrose in water (D20W) contains 200 g of dextrose, yielding 3.4 kcal/g or 680 kcal/L. One 500-ml unit of 10% Intralipid contains 450 kcal. Thus, the patient might be given 500 ml of 10% Intralipid, which contain 450 kcal, and 2 liters of D20W, which contain 1,360 kcal, to total 1,810 kcal or 133 kcal/g of nitrogen.

Vitamins and minerals. All requirements for *vitamins* must be met, but complete agreement on the amounts to be given has not been reached. Although it is unclear whether vitamin requirements are increased in stressed patients, patients with surgical or traumatic wounds are assumed to need increased amounts of vitamin C for wound healing. Overdosage with vitamins A and D have led to documented cases of toxicity.

A number of multivitamin products are commercially available for parenteral use, but none provides all the necessary vitamins. In a typical procedure, 10 ml/day of a commonly used product such as MVI-12 or M.V.C. 9+3 is added. Vitamin K is given as a separate injection, 5 mg intramuscularly once weekly. It is needed particularly by patients receiving oral antibiotic therapy and by those with malabsorption syndromes. Serum levels of vitamins should be monitored at intervals, and doses should be adjusted accordingly.

Requirements for *minerals* are not known specifically. Since losses must also be replaced, requirements of individual patients may vary widely. Deficits must be replaced as described in the section on Therapy for Fluid and Electrolyte Imbalances (p. 484). Approximately 80 percent of hospitalized patients, however, may be managed with standardized formulations. Some electrolytes are included in the commercial amino acid preparations. Patients receiving antibiotics may receive significant amounts of sodium from that source.[38]

Potassium is the principal intracellular cation that tends to be lost when muscle is catabolized during elevated gluconeogenesis. Potassium deficiency prevents growth,[39] and repletion of 1 kg of lean muscle mass requires 145 to 155 mEq of potassium or 75 mEq/day. Daily urinary potassium excretion of 40 to 60 mEq/day must also be provided for. Therefore, daily needs are 120 to 160 mEq/day or approximately 50 mEq/L of infusate. Patients with compromised renal function will not tolerate this amount and so a smaller dose is administered carefully. Potassium is added to the infusate as the chloride, phosphate, or acetate.

Magnesium acts as a cofactor and is taken up intracellularly. At maximum rates of anabolism, 15 to 30 mEq/day have been recommended to meet the requirement.[38–40] It is given as the sulfate.

Phosphate is needed for protoplasm formation. A commonly administered amount is 30 mEq/day. It is used for synthesis of membrane phospholipids and high-energy phosphate bonds. It also is important in bone formation. The amount recommended varies widely, with a greater amount required if the patient is very depleted,[40,41] and a lesser amount if renal function is impaired. Phosphate is given as sodium or potassium salt.

Sodium must be provided to replace *obligatory* (unavoidable) urinary losses and to maintain sodium concentration in the ECF. For maintenance, 50 mEq of sodium per liter of TPN infusate usually is sufficient.[38] Since formation of 1 g of protoplasm is accompanied by expansion of 0.8 ml of ECF volume, an additional 70 mEq of sodium is provided during anabolism. Less sodium is given to patients with cardiovascular or renal insufficiency. Sodium usually is administered as the chloride or acetate.

Chloride balance is maintained if sodium chloride is used. Acidotic patients are given *acetate*,[38] which serves as a bicarbonate precursor, rather than bicarbonate itself, which is not compatible with other ions in TPN solutions. A commonly used protocol specifies a 4 : 1 chloride-acetate ratio. If requirements for chloride are increased in the patient with large losses from a gastrostomy or nasogastric tube, chloride may be given as both sodium and potassium chloride.

Calcium is required to maintain calcium balance, normal parathyroid function, and bone mineralization, but the requirement in TPN is not known. It is provided as calcium gluceptate, chloride, and gluconate in amounts of 200 to 400 mg/day (10 to 20 mEq/day).[40] Immobilization increases urinary excretion of calcium.

Iron may be included at levels of 1 to 2 mg/day[42] but is not always added to a TPN solution. If a deficiency of iron exists, it may be given to the TPN patient intramuscularly as Imferon. The requirement for parenteral iron may be calculated using the following formula:[43]

$$\text{Milligrams of iron} = 0.3W \times \frac{(100 - \text{Hb})}{0.148} \quad \textbf{(4)}$$

where W = body weight in pounds; Hb = hemoglobin in grams per deciliter of blood.

Of the trace elements, *zinc* has been studied most extensively. It is necessary as a cofactor for many enzymes. It quickly migrates to rapidly dividing cells, but the mechanism of its action in repair is not known. Nevertheless, low serum zinc levels have been associated with poor repair and chronic skin ulceration (*decubitus ulcers* or so-called bed sores).

Copper deficiency has been reported in patients on long-term TPN,[44] but exact requirements are not known. Chromium[41] and selenium[45] deficiencies have also been reported.

Addition of 4 mg of zinc and 1 mg of copper or more per day often is recommended. It is recommended also that zinc levels be increased up to 300 μg/kg for premature infants. Small bowel zinc losses of 12 mg/L of fluid and diarrheal zinc losses of 17 mg/L of fluid must be replaced.[46] Requirements for other trace elements, including selenium, vanadium, molybdenum, nickel, tin, arsenic, silicon, and cadmium, are not known yet, but deficiencies of these elements in TPN patients have not been reported. Solutions containing trace elements for intravenous use are commercially available.

Most institutions have a standard protocol for inclusion of vitamins and minerals in TPN feedings which is used unless there are orders to the contrary. Assuming this type of standard procedure, a TPN order might read, "1 liter of 10% Intralipid and 2 liters of supplemental solution composed of 1 liter of D20W and 1 liter of 8.5% Freamine amino acid solution per day. IV rate: 83 ml/hr supplemental solution and 42 ml/hr Intralipid."

Complications. There are a number of possible complications of central venous alimentation. A major complication is infection, which can progress from the catheter site and cause general sepsis. Fungal infections, such as *Candida*, and bacterial contamination with *Staphylococcus aureus* or *Staphylococcus epidermidis* occur. Technical complications include *pneumothorax* (air in the thoracic cavity), *hemothorax* (blood in the thoracic cavity), hematoma, embolism, perforation of the vein, and injuries to the phrenic nerve or thoracic duct.

Most metabolic complications are avoidable. Hyperglycemia may ensue if the glucose infusion rate is too rapid. It also precedes the onset of sepsis and is seen in patients receiving steroid drugs. Unchecked hyperglycemia may lead to hyperosmolar nonketotic coma (see Chapter 9). This complication is avoidable by diminishing the rate of infusion of glucose or by adding insulin to the infusion if blood glucose measures 250 mg/dl.

Hypoglycemia can occur if the infusion rate is decreased too rapidly when the feeding is being discontinued. The infusion should be tapered off slowly over a period of 1 to 2 hours, allowing insulin secretion rate to subside. Hypoglycemia can occur also when the infusion stops because of mechanical problems.

Excess energy intake may be detrimental. The development of acute fatty infiltration of the liver associated with mild to moderate hepatic dysfunction has been attributed to excess energy supply. Excess provision of energy as glucose may result in respiratory failure. Infused glucose must be cleared from the circulation. Glucose that cannot be oxidized must be converted to fat once glycogen stores are saturated. The conversion of glucose to fat yields carbon dioxide as a metabolic by-product, but the reaction does not produce energy. Thus, as increasing loads of glucose are infused, carbon dioxide production divided by oxygen consumption (the *respiratory quotient*) may rise rapidly to values greater than 1. Respiratory failure requiring ventilatory assistance or difficulty in weaning patients from respirators may occur if excess glucose is provided. This complication can be avoided by limiting the kilocalorie content of the infusate to that which covers only the need.

Insufficient or excessive administration of electrolytes also may cause complications. Deficiencies of trace elements, vitamins, and essential fatty acids have been reported, as have overdoses of fat-soluble vitamins and trace elements. These become less common as our knowledge of requirements improves.

Peripheral Venous Alimentation

Indications for TPN by peripheral vein are the same as those for TPN by central vein, but the technique for peripheral venous alimentation avoids the risks of the central route. It also avoids some of the problems of the hyperosmolar solutions, since solutions used in peripheral venous alimentation have lower osmolarity. This lower osmolarity, however, reduces the energy supply per given volume. Thus, peripheral venous feeding is usable for patients whose needs are likely to be short-term (7 to 10 days) and whose requirements are more modest than those that can be met via a central line. The patient must also be able to tolerate a larger fluid load than would be required with central venous alimentation.

It often is recommended that the final concentration of dextrose not exceed 5%. To achieve this, 10 to 20% dextrose solutions are mixed with a 5% crystalline amino acid solution. The osmolarity of this solution is approximately twice that of plasma and will cause phlebitis in 24 to 36 hours.

Two procedures are available to avoid this problem while still providing sufficient energy. One is the use of a fat emulsion, and the other is the use of hydrocortisone plus heparin. A 10% fat emulsion (see Table 12-11) infused along with the dextrose–amino acid solution is reasonably well tolerated. Infusion of 1,500 ml each of dextrose–amino acid solution and 10% fat emulsion in 24 hours will provide 1,950 kcal, 10 g of nitrogen, and 3 liters of water with a nonprotein calorie–nitrogen ratio of 90:1. This will maintain a stable patient. For malnourished or hypermetabolic patients, a 20% fat emulsion and a large amount of amino acids may meet the need. If this is not the case, a central venous catheter will be required.

An alternative to the use of fat emulsion gives a solution of 2.5% amino acid in 6.5% dextrose with an osmolarity of 900 mOsm, three times normal. To protect the vein, 5 mg of hydrocortisone and 500 units of heparin are added to each liter. In 3 liters of solution, the patient will receive 12.4 g of nitrogen and 780 kcal. This is supportive for the stable patient but is clearly inadequate for the patient with increased needs.

There are several limitations to the use of peripheral venous alimentation for total support. The amount of fat that can be administered is limited to approximately 2 g/kg/day. If this amount is exceeded, the incidence of thrombocytopenia and fat embolism is increased. The total kilocalorie supply thus is restricted.

The administration of 10% glucose plus 5% amino acids provides approximately 500 kcal/L or approximately 3,000 kcal in 6 liters. With the lipid, a total of 4,500 kcal may be achieved, but the patient must be able to tolerate a large fluid load. This is not the case in patients with renal disease, for example. Patients with respiratory disorders in which pulmonary edema must be avoided also are usually fluid-restricted.

Nevertheless, peripheral venous alimentation is useful in several circumstances:

1. For short-term support in patients whose energy needs are moderate
2. When risks of central venous TPN are great
3. When supplemental, rather than total, nutrition is needed
4. Occasionally, as an intermediate method when weaning a patient from central venous TPN

Parenteral Nutrition in Specific Conditions

Diabetes. Patients with diabetes who normally require insulin will require insulin in conjunction with TPN. The goal in diabetic patients who are unable to eat is to continue to make glucose available as a fuel that can be metabolized for cellular energy. If glucose is not available, then acceleration of proteolysis and use of endogenous amino acids for energy requirements will lead to profound negative nitrogen balance. Diabetics should receive at least their daily maintenance dose of insulin and frequently require greater doses during stress.

Renal Failure. Patients with renal failure and a hypermetabolic condition require special consideration. Patients with chronic renal failure commonly have varying degrees of protein deficiency; chronic losses of amino acids occur during hemodialysis, and limitation of protein intake is a common dietary recommendation in chronic renal failure (see Chapter 7). Acute renal failure associated with catabolic illness necessitates careful consideration of the requirements for protein synthesis and repair as supported by amino acids versus the need to minimize protein turnover and urea formation. The rate of urea formation and thus the rate of rise of urea nitrogen concentration in the plasma during acute renal failure may be reduced to a minimum by provision of minimal amounts of amino acids and enough glucose to meet energy requirements. The use of essential amino acids alone to minimize urea formation is controversial. Such mixtures may be effective in avoiding the need for dialysis.

Hepatic Failure. Patients with hepatic failure may become difficult to manage nutritionally if hepatic encephalopathy or coma occur. Patients with hepatic impairment may be managed by instituting parenteral nutrition at a cautious protein intake, such as 0.5 g/kg per day or less, with careful monitoring of cerebral function. If the given level of protein can be infused without impairing the level of cerebral function, it may then be considered appropriate and may be raised slowly as long as there is no mental deterioration.

The accumulation of toxic amounts of ammonia resulting from an inability to convert ammonia to urea contributes to the cerebral effects of hepatic failure (see Chapter 11). More recently, it has been shown that patients in hepatic coma have an abnormal blood amino acid pattern (Chapter 11). Infusion of a TPN solution with decreased aromatic amino acids and increased BCAAs results in dramatic improvement in cerebral function.[47]

Respiratory Failure. Respiratory failure can occur in many circumstances. For example, some patients have *impairment in the movement of the thorax or lungs* as a result of respiratory center depression, diseases of the neuromuscular junction, or respiratory muscles or from conditions that restrict the movement of the chest wall or lungs. Other patients have *diseases of the lungs* themselves, resulting in loss of compliance. In others, *airway obstruction* occurs in such conditions as chronic bronchitis, emphysema, or bronchial asthma.

These patients are acutely ill, and recent studies have demonstrated that many are malnourished.[48] In some of these patients, the work of breathing against a resistance is increased, contributing to the energy deficit. In any case, the severely malnourished patient who is not adequately fed may catabolize his or her respiratory muscles, thereby exacerbating the condition and increasing the difficulty of weaning the patient from the ventilator.

Other nutrition-related factors include depression of immune function in the malnourished patient, which may place the ventilator-assisted patient at high risk of respiratory infection. Some ventilator-assisted patients receive corticosteroids to reduce bronchospasm or sometimes for other purposes. These medications further reduce immune function and also depress protein synthesis. There is a high incidence of ileus and gastrointestinal hemorrhage in these patients.

The nutritional needs of ventilator-assisted patients are not known specifically, but studies suggest that oxygen consumption (energy requirement) is increased. Driver et al.[49] report that the patient needs 2,500 to 3,000 kcal/day to maintain good nutrition and improve the rate of weaning from the ventilator. A further increase is needed in the presence of sepsis, fever, and trauma. However, overfeeding should be avoided. When excess carbohydrate is converted to fat, producing a respiratory quotient greater than 1.0, the increase in carbon dioxide production places an additional demand on the respiratory system and makes weaning from the ventilator more difficult, for the reasons previously explained.

Enteral feeding is recommended for these patients provided the tube from the ventilator is so placed that the patient does not aspirate the feeding. Parenteral feeding is required if aspiration cannot be prevented and in cases of prolonged ileus.

Monitoring the TPN Patient

The TPN patient is monitored closely. The nutritional care specialist should observe carefully those items that are relevant to nutrition. Baseline data, obtained before TPN is begun, usually include a complete blood count, blood glucose, serum creatinine, blood urea nitrogen, and serum electrolytes, albumin, transaminases (serum glutamic oxaloacetic transaminase [SGOT] and serum glutamic pyruvic transaminase [SGPT]), calcium, phosphorus, and magnesium. During TPN, blood glucose, electrolytes and urea nitrogen are obtained three times per week. Other tests are obtained weekly or at less frequent intervals to detect metabolic complications.

Weaning the Patient from TPN

The nutritional care specialist plays a particularly important role when the patient is being weaned from TPN. The patient normally is weaned gradually as enteral intake (by tube or by mouth) slowly increases. Reductions in the rate of TPN infusions are made in appropriate proportion to enteral intake. Total parenteral nutrition has the potential to diminish appetite, but oral intake of food is more often depressed by incomplete recovery from the condition necessitating the TPN.

Patients who need TPN permanently may manage their condition at home if they are emotionally stable. Patients who are candidates for home TPN are taught catheter care, how to mix and administer the solution, and how to monitor fluid and electrolyte balance.

SEPSIS

Sepsis (the presence of pathogenic microorganisms or their toxins in blood or tissue) from catheter contamination and many other infections is accompanied by fever and an increase in metabolic rate. *Fever* is defined as an increase in central body temperature. It occurs in response to infection, inflammation, or both. Heat stroke and increased intracranial pressure which cause *hyperthermia* (increased body temperature) are not classified as fevers. In these two conditions, body temperature rises because the "thermostat" that controls body temperature fails and so temperature control is lost. In a fever, the normal setting of the thermostat is at a higher point as a result of the toxins released by an infectious or inflammatory process. Other factors that can alter body temperature are drugs, some hormones, and ionic changes in the posterior hypothalamus.

The *preoptic area* of the hypothalamus in the brain contains sites that detect changes in body temperature, integrating responses from the thermal receptors of the body. The preoptic area stimulates the anterior or posterior hypothalamus to increase and prevent heat loss. The hypothalamus, then, serves as the thermostat. It normally is set at approximately 37°C. (98.6°F.). Under normal conditions, when the body temperature rises, the body's heat-losing mechanisms are activated. These include vasodilation and sweating. Conversely, when the body temperature drops, heat-producing responses such as shivering and vasoconstriction are initiated.

In a fever, the thermostat in the hypothalamus is set at a higher temperature. Mechanisms for heat production and heat conservation are activated and body temperature rises until the new setting is reached. At that time, the balance is maintained at the new higher setting.

Agents that Produce Infection or Inflammation

Any agent that produces an infection or inflammation or both is a *pyrogen.* Pyrogens may be endogenous or exogenous. *Exogenous pyrogens,* which produce a fever when introduced into the body, include bacteria, viruses, fungi, and other microorganisms. *Endogenous pyrogens* are produced within the body and may include damaged tissue, necrotic cells, and antigen-antibody reactions, including graft rejection.

The agent believed to be primarily responsible for fever in humans is an endogenous pyrogen (EP) found in various phagocytic cells. These include leukocytes, macrophages in the lungs and peritoneum, and Kupffer cells of the liver.[50] When EP is released, it circulates via the bloodstream. According to one theory, EP stimulates prostaglandin E_1 from the hypothalamus.[51] Prostaglandin E_1 then stimulates the release of norepinephrine which stimulates adenyl cyclase production. Adenyl cyclase catalyzes conversion of ATP to cAMP, which, in turn, alters the calcium-to-sodium ratio in the hypothalamus, thus altering its firing rate. This resets the thermostat to a higher level and produces a fever.

Body heat is produced by an increase in the metabolic rate. This is accomplished by stimulation of the sympathetic nervous system, thyroid hormone secretion, and shivering.[52] The accelerated metabolic activity increases the demand for oxygen and nutrients. Metabolic waste products build up. Excess carbon dioxide stimulates respiration, removing carbon dioxide and water. Fluid loss may eventually cause dehydration, with dry skin, dry mucous membranes, sunken eyeballs, and a concentrated urine of small volume. Intracellular potassium is lost, and sodium and chloride move into the cell.

If the fever is prolonged, body proteins are catabolized, with decreased activity, malaise, weakness, muscle aching, and albuminuria. Anorexia, fat catabolism, ketosis, and acidosis also may occur, although sepsis may slow the development of ketosis; it is not known whether fever has any beneficial effects. It can be very debilitating but does not appear to destroy microorganisms.[50,53] During the febrile period, the patient's nutritional status should be assessed at intervals. Fluids, electrolytes, proteins, and energy supplies must be adequate.

Specific Infectious Diseases

Some infectious diseases have unique characteristics that require consideration in nutritional care.

Typhoid fever is rare in the United States and Canada but does occur occasionally. It is caused by bacteria *Salmonella typhosa,* which enter the patient via the gastrointestinal tract. Common sources are water or food contaminated by feces from a carrier. The organism penetrates the intestinal wall and produces inflammation of the lymph nodes and spleen. It also may localize in the lungs, gallbladder, central nervous system, or kidney. The principal locale is in the Peyer's patches of the small intestine, sometimes causing intestinal hemorrhage or perforation. The accompanying fever is very high.

Primary treatment is with antibiotics. The patient may need parenteral glucose solution to maintain fluid balance. A high-calorie, low-residue diet is recommended when oral intake is possible.

Poliomyelitis became rare once an effective vaccine was made available; however, it, too, does occur sometimes. It may be nonparalytic or paralytic. Paralytic poliomyelitis may present special nutritional problems. One form is bulbar poliomyelitis in which cranial nerves are affected. Symptoms include dysphagia, difficulty in chewing, inability to swallow, loss of gag reflex, and loss of movement of palatal and pharyngeal muscles. Respiratory paralysis is the most life-threatening aspect, and patients may require a mechanical respirator. Complications of this disease include urinary tract infections and renal stones.

Nasogastric tube feeding may be necessary. To reduce renal stone formation, it often is recommended that the diet be low in calcium (0.5 mg/day or less) with no milk. Fluid intake should be generous.

Tuberculosis is a chronic disease caused by *Mycobacterium tuberculosis.* It usually occurs in the lungs but may also be found in bones, kidneys, or lymph nodes. Malnutrition, diabetes, measles, chronic cortiocosteroid therapy, and general debility are predisposing factors to progression of the disease.

The principal drug used in treatment of tuberculosis is isoniazid (INH) which interferes with DNA synthesis and intermediary metabolism of the bacillus. Isoniazid increases the urinary excretion of pyridoxine and can cause a vitamin deficiency. Supplementary doses of 25 to 50 mg of pyridoxine per day are given.

The usual recommended diet for the patient with tuberculosis contains kilocalories for maintenance of normal body weight with generous allowances of protein, minerals, and vitamins to promote healing. If patients are hospitalized for long periods, attention to their personal preferences is important.

THE PATIENT UNDERGOING MAJOR SURGERY

Nutritional care of the surgical patient can be divided into the preoperative and postoperative periods.

Preoperative Nutrition

Nutritional deficiences should be corrected and reserves established if time permits prior to surgery. Obese patients should be reduced, if possible, while assuring adequate protein intake.

In the immediate preoperative period, nothing is given by mouth for at least 8 hours, since food in the stomach may interfere with the surgical procedure, lead to vomiting and aspiration, and increase gastric retention. If surgery is on the gastrointestinal tract itself, the patient may not be fed for several days preoperatively to remove all fecal matter. These patients may be given a chemically defined diet (see Appendix L) during this interval.

Postoperative Nutrition

A surgical patient commonly undergoes a brief postoperative period of starvation. This is well tolerated if the patient is well nourished before the surgery. In the immediate postoperative period, fluid, electrolytes, and some energy are provided intravenously. When the gastrointestinal tract begins to function, oral feeding can begin. In minor surgery, diet as tolerated is given as soon as the patient is fully reactive. In more extensive surgery, the patient may be given a clear liquid diet and then progress through full liquid and soft diets to the house diet, according to tolerance. The patient should be advanced to solid foods as rapidly as possible (see Chapter 2).

For patients who are malnourished prior to surgery or who have extensive periods of inadequate intake postoperatively, additional support can be provided with supplements and tube feeding (see Chapter 5) or with parenteral nutrition as previously described. Specific procedures for nutritional care are described elsewhere for patients undergoing surgery of the upper and lower digestive system (see Chapters 5 and 6) and for those with cancer (see Chapter 13).

THE BURN PATIENT

The nutritional care of burn patients requires special attention for a number of reasons. Nutritional requirements are higher among burn patients than in any other single group of hospitalized patients. At the same time, intake is decreased significantly. If these needs are not met, the time required for full recovery from extensive burns is so prolonged that the patient becomes seriously depleted. If vigorous nutritional support is not provided, healing is delayed and infection is more common. There also is considerable weight loss, decreased immunocompetence with increased susceptibility to infection, and inability to maintain the work of breathing, leading to multiple organ failure and increased mortality.

Estimation of the Extent of Injury

The severity of burns is determined by the depth of the burn wound and the percent of body surface area burned. A *first-degree burn* involves only the epidermis (the outermost, nonvascular layer of the skin). First-degree burns are characterized by erythema (redness), which may appear several hours after the injury. Sunburn is an example of a first-degree burn. Because the tissue damage is superficial, systemic manifestations are mild. Pain and some edema are the chief manifestations. These burns heal in 5 to 10 days.

Second-degree burns involve all of the epidermis and a portion of the *dermis* or *corium* (the fibrous inner layer of the skin, containing blood vessels, nerves, glands, and hair roots). The dermis extends between the epidermis and subcutaneous fat. Thus, these burns are *partial-thickness burns.* Preservation of epidermal appendages, including sweat glands and hair follicles, makes regeneration of epithelium possible unless infection supervenes. These wounds are characterized by blisters and accompanied by considerable subcutaneous edema. Superficial second-degree burns may heal uneventfully in 10 to 14 days, whereas deeper second-degree burns may require 25 to 35 days for healing. Thus, skin grafting may be used on these wounds.

Third-degree burns are *full-thickness burns,* wounds in which the entire dermis down to the subcutaneous fat is destroyed and thrombosis of small vessels in the underlying tissue occurs. Coagulation necrosis (see Chapter 1) produces the *eschar,* a dry, leathery, inelastic slough composed of the former elements of the skin. As all of the elements of the skin are destroyed, the functions of the skin are lost entirely. These functions include retention of heat and moisture and formation of a barrier against invasive infection. Untreated third-degree burns routinely become infected. Third-degree burns have no epithelial elements remaining and require skin grafting for wound closure.

The extent of burn injury commonly is expressed as the percent of body surface area burned. First-degree burn areas generally are not included in this percent determination. Diagrams that map the percent of specific areas of body surface are available to facilitate accurate estimation of percent of body burned. The "rule of nines" may be used for a rough estimation of body surface area in adults. In this system, each of the upper extremities is considered to have 9 percent of the body surface, the lower extremities, 18 percent each, the anterior and posterior trunk, 18 percent each, the head, 9 percent, and the perineum, 1 percent. This formula is not accurate in children.

At the time of initial evaluation, the distinction between second-degree and third-degree burns may be difficult. Preservation of the sensation of touch and pain in a burn wound suggests preservation of at least a portion of the dermal elements and indicates a second-degree burn. The burn wound that is anesthetic or numb suggests destruction of all elements of the skin and is presumed initially to represent a third-degree burn.

Minor burns include those partial-thickness burns of less than 10 percent of the body surface and full-thickness burns of less than 2 percent of the body surface. Hospitalization usually is not required, and nutritional intake is easily maintained. Small full-thickness burns about the face or hands, however, may require hospitalization for specialized treatment but generally do not cause sufficient systemic metabolic response to impair nutritional intake. Partial-thickness or full-thickness burns of 10 to 20 percent of the body surface area require hospitalization. Generally, sepsis can be avoided in these patients, and the nutritional consequences are not severe. Burns of greater than 20 percent of the body surface area severely alter the metabolic response and increase the challenge of accomplishing adequate nutritional care. Children, particularly infants, require hospitalization and aggressive nutritional therapy for smaller burn wounds than do adults. In general, the survival rate declines with increasing depth of burn, area of burn, and with advancing age.

Pathophysiology of Burn Injury

Effects on the Skin

The skin has important functions in preventing heat and water loss and preventing the invasion of pathogenic organisms. Both of these functions are lost when the body surface is burned. Great care must be taken to prevent infection in deep second-degree and third-degree burns.

Normal skin contains lipids which limit the loss of water by evaporation to 700 to 1,000 ml/day. This protection is lost in the burned area, and water losses through the area of a full-thickness burn may be as high as 200 ml/m^2/hr. Formerly, it was believed that each gram of water loss was accompanied by heat loss of 0.58 kcal and that, in major burns, total energy loss by this route could reach 7,000 kcal/day. For this reason, burn centers maintain a warmer and more humid environment. There is recent evidence, however, that evaporative water loss is not the primary mediator of increased caloric expenditure. When evaporative water loss was prevented in one investigation, metabolic rate did not decrease consistently.[54] Therefore, the evidence now suggests that hypermetabolism, rather than evaporative heat loss, is the primary mechanism for increased energy need, as it is in other forms of trauma.

The evaporated water is essentially free of electrolytes. If fluid is not replaced, the patient may develop hypertonic dehydration. The burn injury also causes a significant increase in capillary permeability, mostly in and around the site of the injury but also in other areas. Fluid and protein rapidly escape from the circulatory system. Blood volume decreases and interstitial fluid volume increases to create edema. In addition, some fluid and protein are lost from the burn surface. In extensive third-degree burns, the fluid loss can approach 10 percent of the body weight, primarily in the first 24 hours. In 48 hours, resorption of edema fluid occurs.

Effects on Blood Cells and the Vascular System

The effect of loss of blood volume in burn patients is the same as that which occurs in hemorrhagic shock. Ischemia of the kidneys may cause oliguria and acute tubular necrosis.

At the same time, red cell mass declines by approximately 10 percent in the first 24 hours following deep burns, as a result of damage or destruction of cells in the burn area and as a consequence of dehydration. Later, red cell production may be depressed. Total losses may reach 185 percent of normal over the course of the illness.

Hemodynamic and Metabolic Effects

Hemodynamic and metabolic changes in burn patients occur in three phases. For the first 48 hours, there is the *hypovolemic* or *shock phase.* This is followed by a *hypermetabolic phase* until the wound closes. An *anabolic phase* succeeds wound closure.

In the early shock phase, the patient has tachycardia, hypotension, and subnormal cardiac output. The changes in renal function are largely the effects of hypovolemia, renal vascular restriction, and adrenocortical hormone activity. Inadequate therapy may result in acute renal failure.

Endocrine effects are those already described for other forms of trauma (see p. 478) but are of greater magnitude and return to normal only when the wound is closed.[55] The summation of these effects and evaporative heat losses results in severe negative energy and nitrogen balances. Increases in caloric requirements of 4,000 kcal or more have been documented. Positive nitrogen balance is achieved only when the wound is closed.

Other factors that contribute to changes of nutritional status are:

- The occurrence of infection.
- Surgical procedures, such as skin grafting.
- Curling's ulcer (an acute gastric ulcer with bleeding), which possibly is the result of ischemia. Patients are given antacids to maintain gastric pH above 5. If hemorrhage occurs, vagotomy and partial gastrectomy may be necessary.
- Adynamic ileus, which prevents oral feeding for a variable period. The increased catacholamine levels cause vasoconstriction in the splanchnic bed, slowing peristalsis.

Management of the Burn Patient

Early treatment of a patient with a major burn includes establishment of an airway with a tracheostomy if necessary, insertion of a urinary catheter, administration of analgesic drugs, antibiotics, and tetanus immunization, care of the wound, and fluid replacement. The type of fluids given vary with the circumstances, but several formulas are available as guidelines in estimating therapy. One formula, for example, estimates fluid and electrolytes as follows:

Volume of fluid to be administered in the first 24 hours = 4 ml Ringer's lactated solution × W × %BSA burned **(5)**

where BSA = body surface area; W = body weight in kilograms.

According to this formula, a 70-kg man with a burn over 40 percent of his body would require 11.2 liters of fluid to replace his loss (4 × 70 × 40). The difficulties of treatment with this volume of fluid are obvious.

The goal in long-term therapy of burn patients is to accomplish healing of all the burn wounds. A variety of techniques are used, including prevention of infection and allowance for spontaneous healing of partial-thickness burns. Full-thickness burn management requires removal of the eschar and application of split-thickness skin grafts taken from an area of unburned skin elsewhere on the body. Excision of the eschar (*debridement*) and application of skin grafts may be done as early as a few hours following injury to as late as several weeks postinjury. Patients with burns of 50 percent of the body surface area can be expected to require many weeks for ultimate recovery, because skin graft donor sites may have to heal and serve a second time to provide sufficient skin for grafting and wound coverage.

Specific formulas for estimation of nutritional requirements in burn patients have been devised. These formulas consider the size of the burn wound, because the extent of burn wound correlates closely with the severity of the hypermetabolism. During the course of hospitalization, as burn wounds heal and the percent of body surface area unhealed decreases, the energy expenditures may be adjusted downward.

The Curreri formulas have been widely used to estimate daily nutritional requirements.[56,57] Energy requirement is determined as follows:

Kilocalories required for 24 hours = (25 kcal × W) + (40 kcal × %BSA burned) **(6)**

Protein losses also are increased significantly. In addition to the loss of protein via muscle catabolism in stress, the burn patient can lose large amounts of protein through the burn wound. This loss may average 1 to 3 g or more for each percent of burn.[58,59] The Curreri formula for estimation of desirable protein intake is:

$$\text{Grams of protein per 24 hours} = (1 \text{ g/kg of body weight} + (3 \text{ g} \times \%\text{BSA burned}) \quad \textbf{(7)}$$

Using these formulas, our 70-kg man with the 40 percent burn would need ([25 × 70] + [40 × 40]) 3,350 kcal and 190 g of protein ([1 × 70] + [3 × 40]).

These formulas are considered to overestimate need. An alternative method consists of calculating ideal caloric intake and then establishing protein intake based on a kilocalorie-to-nitrogen ratio of 150:1 or 200:1. One gram of nitrogen equals 6.25 g of protein. Assuming 150 kcal per gram of nitrogen, our 70-kg man then would receive the following:

$$3{,}350/150 \cong 22.3 \text{ g nitrogen per 24 hours}$$
$$22.3 \times 6.25 \cong 140 \text{ g protein per 24 hours}$$

Remember that these formulas provide an estimate only. Patient progress must be monitored carefully.

The burned patient represents a challenge to the nutritional care specialist. The patient's energy and protein needs are considerable, and great encouragement is needed to increase food intake owing to the patient's discomfort and depression. The patient is not fed until the postinjury ileus resolves, usually in 36 to 48 hours. In addition, the many surgical procedures require that the patient fast in preparation for anesthesia. The missed meals can represent a substantial loss. Despite these problems, most burn patients are able to eat considerable amounts of food in a high-protein, high-calorie diet with frequent feedings and between-meal supplements. Attention must be paid to the patient's preferences to make the food as appealing as possible.

A patient with burns over more than 40 percent of his or her body seldom eats enough to met the increased needs. Tube feeding may be used to supplement oral intake. The location of the tube depends on the location of the burn. A nasogastric tube cannot be used for a patient with burns about the head and neck. Patients who are eating reasonably well may receive tube feedings during sleep, whereas those who are eating poorly or not at all may be fed continuously.

Supplementation of nutrient intake by intravenous infusion may be employed in burn patients, but in some burn centers it is avoided if possible. The primary reasons for this policy are the danger of infection and the limitation of access sites in patients burned over a large area. Nutritional intake is a higher priority, however, so that if enteral feeding is unsuccessful, parenteral feeding is used.

References

1. Ferrendelli, J.A. Cerebral utilization of nonglucose substrates and their effect in hypoglycemia. In F. Plum, Ed., *Brain Dysfunction in Metabolic Disorders.* New York: Raven Press, 1974.
2. Cahill, G.F., Jr., Herrera, M.G., Morgan, A.P., et al. Hormone-fuel interrelationships during fasting. *J. Clin. Invest.* 45:1751, 1966.
3. Levine, R., and Haft, D.E. Carbohydrate homeostasis. *N. Engl. J. Med.* 282:175, 1970.
4. Owen, O.E., Felig, P., Morgan, A.P., et al. Liver and kidney metabolism in prolonged starvation. *J. Clin. Invest.* 48:574, 1969.
5. Saudek, C.D., and Felig, P. The metabolic events of starvation. *Am. J. Med.* 60:117, 1976.
6. Felig, P., Owen, O.E., Wahren, J., and Cahill, G.F., Jr. Amino acid metabolism during prolonged starvation. *J. Clin. Invest.* 48:548, 1969.
7. Mallette, L.E., Exton, J.H., and Park, C.R. Effects of glucagon on amino acid transport and utilization in the perfused rat liver. *J. Biol. Chem.* 244:5724, 1969.
8. Pitts, R.F. Renal production and excretion of ammonia. *Am. J. Med.* 36:720, 1964.

9. Whipple, G.H. *The Dynamic Equilibrium of Body Proteins.* Springfield, Ill.: Charles C Thomas, 1956.
10. Filkins, J.P. Lysosomes and hepatic regression during fasting. *Am. J. Physiol.* 219:923, 1970.
11. Exton, J.H. Gluconeogenesis. *Metabolism* 21:945, 1972.
12. Elman, R. *Parenteral Alimentation in Surgery.* New York: Hoeber Medical Division, Harper and Row, 1947.
13. Shils, M.E., and Randall, H.T. Diet and nutrition in the care of the surgical patient. In R. S. Goodhart and M.E. Shils, Eds., *Modern Nutrition in Health and Disease,* 6th ed. Philadelphia: Lea and Febiger, 1980.
14. Herndon, D.N., Wilmore, D.W., Mason, A.D., Jr., and Pruit, B.A., Jr. Humoral mediators of nontemperature-dependent hypermetabolism in 50% burned adult rats. *Surg. Forum* 28:37, 1977.
15. Arturson, G. Prostaglandins in human burn-wound secretion. *Burns* 3:112, 1977.
16. Cuthbertson, D.P. The disturbance of metabolism produced by bony and non-bony injury, with notes on certain abnormal conditions of bone. *Biochem. J.* 24:1244, 1930.
17. Cahill, G.F., Jr., Felig, P., and Marliss, E.B. Some physiological principles of parenteral nutrition. In C.L. Fox, Jr., and G.G. Nahas, Eds., *Body Fluid Replacement in the Surgical Patient,* part IV. New York: Grune and Stratton, 1970.
18. Wannemacher, R.W., Jr. Protein metabolism (applied biochemistry). In H. Ghadimi, Ed., *Total Parenteral Nutrition.* New York: John Wiley and Sons, 1975.
19. Powanda, M.C. Changes in body balance of nitrogen and other key nutrients: Description and underlying mechanisms. *Am. J. Clin. Nutr.* 30: 1254, 1977.
20. Egdahl, R.J. Pituitary-adrenal response following trauma to the isolated leg. *Surgery* 46:9, 1959.
21. Iverson, J. Adrenergic receptors and the secretion of glucagon and insulin from the isolated perfused canine pancreas. *J. Clin. Invest.* 52: 1202, 1973.
22. Hume, D.M. The neuro-endocrine response to injury: Present status of the problem. *Ann. Surg.* 138:548, 1953.
23. Moore, F.D., Steenburg, R.W., Ball, M.R., et al. Studies in surgical endocrinology: I. The urinary excretion of 17-hydroxycorticoids and associated metabolic changes, in cases of soft tissue trauma of varying severity and in bone trauma. *Ann. Surg.* 141: 145, 1955.
24. Ross, H., Johnston, I.D.A., Welborn, T.A., and Wright, A.D. Effect of abdominal operation on glucose tolerance and serum levels of insulin, growth hormone and hydrocortisone. *Lancet* 2:563, 1966.
25. Clark, E. Effect of cortisone upon protein synthesis. *J. Biol. Chem.* 200:69, 1953.
26. Perley, M., and Kipnis, D.M. Effects of glucocorticoids on plasma insulin. *N. Engl. J. Med.* 274:1237, 1966.
27. Marco, J., Calle, C., Roman, D., et al. Hyperglucagonemia induced by glucocorticoid treatment in man. *N. Engl. J. Med.* 288:128, 1973.
28. Killey, J.M. Energy requirements of the surgical patient. In W.F. Ballinger, J.A. Collins, J.A. Drucker, et al., Eds., *Manual of Surgical Nutrition.* Philadelphia: W.B. Saunders, 1973.
29. Dudrick, S.J., Jensen, T.G., and Rowlands, B.J. Nutritional support: Assessment and indications. In M. Dietel, Ed., *Nutrition in Clinical Surgery.* Baltimore: Williams and Wilkins, 1980.
30. Kinney, J.M. Energy requirements for parenteral nutrition. In J.E. Fischer, Ed., *Total Parenteral Nutrition.* Boston: Little, Brown, 1976.
31. Smith, F.R., and Goodman, D.S. Vitamin A transport in human vitamin A toxicity. *N. Engl. J. Med.* 294:805, 1976.
32. Moore, F.D. Homeostasis: Bodily changes in trauma and surgery. In D.C. Sabiston, Ed., *Davis-Christopher Textbook of Surgery,* 11th ed. Philadelphia: W.B. Saunders, 1977.
33. Blackburn, G.L., Flatt, J.P., Clowes, G.H.A., and O'Donnell, T.E. Peripheral intravenous feeding with isotonic amino acid solutions. *Am. J. Surg.* 125:447, 1973.
34. Bergstrom, K., Blomstrand, R., and Jacobson, S. Long term complete intravenous nutrition in man. *Nutr. Metab.* 14(Suppl.):118, 1972.
35. Shenkin, A., and Wretlind, A. Parenteral nutrition. *World Rev. Nutr. Diet.* 28:1, 1978.
36. Deitel, M., Sauve, Sr. F., Alexander, M.A., et al. A crystalline amino acid solution for total parenteral nutrition. *Can. J. Hosp. Pharm.* 30:175, 1977.
37. Freund, H., Yoshimura, N., Lunetta, L., and Fischer, J.E. Role of branched chain amino acids in decreasing muscle metabolism in vivo. *J.P.E.N.* 2:48A, 1978.
38. Sheldon, G.F., and Kudsk, D.A. Electrolyte requirements in total parenteral nutrition. In M. Deitel, Ed., *Nutrition in Clinical Surgery.* Baltimore: Williams and Wilkins, 1980.
39. Cannon, P.R., Frazier, L.E., and Hughes, R.H.

Influence of potassium on tissue protein synthesis. *Metabolism* 1:49, 1952.
40. Fischer, J.E. Nutritional management. In J.L. Berk, J.E. Sampliner, J.S. Artz, and B. Vinocur, Eds., *Handbook of Critical Care.* Boston: Little, Brown, 1976.
41. Meng, H.C. Parenteral nutrition: principles, nutrient requirements, techniques and clinical applications. In H.A. Schneider, C.E. Anderson, and D.B. Coursin, Eds., *Nutritional Support of Medical Practice.* Hagerstown, Md.: Harper and Row, 1977.
42. Deitel, M., and Macdonald, L.D. Current concepts of intravenous Hyperalimentation. In H.H. Draper, Ed., *Advances in Nutritional Research,* Vol. 3. New York: Plenum, 1980.
43. Weinsier, R.L., and Butterworth, C.E., Jr. *Handbook of Clinical Nutrition.* St. Louis: C.V. Mosby, 1981.
44. Karpel, J.T., and Peden, V.H. Copper deficiency in long-term parenteral nutrition. *J. Pediatr.* 80:32, 1972.
45. McClain, C.J. Trace metal abnormalities in adults during hyperalimentation. *J.P.E.N.* 5:424, 1981.
46. Shils, M.E. Guidelines for total parenteral nutrition. *J.A.M.A.* 220:1721, 1972.
47. Fischer, J.E., Funovics, J.M., Aguirre, A., et al. The role of plasma amino acids in hepatic encephalopathy. *Surgery* 78:276, 1975.
48. Driver, A.G., and Le Brun, M. Iatrogenic malnutrition in patients receiving ventilatory support. *J.A.M.A.* 244:2195, 1980.
49. Driver, A.G., McAlevy, M.T., and Burgher, L.W. Nutritional support of patients with respiratory failure. *Nutritional Support Services* 1:26, 1981.
50. Atkins, E., and Bodel, P. Fever. *N. Engl. J. Med.* 286:27, 1972.
51. Rosendorff, C. Neurochemistry of fever. *S. Afr. J. Med. Sci.* 41:23, 1976.
52. Guyton, A.C. *Textbook of Medical Physiology,* 5th ed. Philadelphia: W.B. Saunders, 1976.
53. Bickley, H.C. *Practical Concepts in Human Disease.* Baltimore: Williams and Wilkins, 1974.
54. Zawicky, B.E., Spitzer, K.W., Mason, A.D., Jr., and Johns, L.A. Does increased evaporative water loss cause hypermetabolism in burned patients? *Ann. Surg.* 171:236, 1970.
55. Wilmore, D.W. Nutrition and metabolism following thermal injury. *Clin. Plast. Surg.* 1:603, 1974.
56. Curreri, P.W., Richmond, D., Marvin, J., and Baxter, C.R. Dietary requirements of patients with major burns. *J. Am. Diet. Assoc.* 65:415, 1974.
57. Batchelor, A.D.R., Sutherland, A.B., and Colver, C.G. Sodium balance studies following thermal injury. *Br. J. Plast. Surg.* 18:130, 1965.
58. Nylen, B., and Wallenius, G. The protein loss via exudation from burns and granulating wound surfaces. *Acta Chir. Scand.* 122:97, 1961.
59. Soroff, H.S., Pearson, E., and Artz, C.P. An estimation of the nitrogen requirements for equilibrium in burned patients. *Surg. Gynecol. Obstet.* 112:159, 1961.

Bibliography

Berk, J.L., Sampliner, J.E., Artz, J.S., and Vinocur, B., Eds. *Handbook of Critical Care.* Boston: Little, Brown, 1976.

Deitel, M., Ed. *Nutrition in Clinical Surgery.* Baltimore: Williams and Wilkins, 1980.

Fischer, J.E., Ed. *Total Parenteral Nutrition.* Boston: Little, Brown, 1976.

Grant, J.P. *Handbook of Total Parenteral Nutrition.* Philadelphia: W.B. Saunders, 1980.

Wilson, J.L., Ed. *Handbook of Surgery,* 5th ed. Los Altos, Calif.: Lange Medical, 1973.

Sources of Current Information

Annals of Surgery
JPEN. Journal of Parenteral and Enteral Nutrition
Nutrition Support Services
Surgery

13. Nutrition and Cancer

Cancer is the second most common cause of death in adults and children in the United States, preceded only by cardiovascular disease in adults and accidents in children. The medical specialty that is concerned with cancer is *oncology.*

A *neoplasm* or *tumor* is a relatively autonomous growth of tissue. It occurs only in multicellular organisms where its growth is uncontrolled by the mechanisms that govern normal growth. The growth may be by cell division or by synthesis of macromolecules and apparently is unrelated to the demands of the host.

REPRODUCTION OF THE NORMAL CELL

To understand the nature of neoplastic growth, we need to review normal cell division. The reproductive cycle in the cell is represented in Fig. 13-1.

Mitosis (the M phase), or cell division, is divided into four steps known as *prophase, metaphase, anaphase,* and *telophase. Interphase* (the period between cell divisions) is divided into (1) the *first growth period* (G_1), in which the cell size increases following the previous division; (2) *synthesis* (S), in which chromosomes reproduce; and (3) the *second growth period* (G_2), in which cells rearrange for division.

This cycle applies only to continuously dividing (*labile*) cells such as those in the crypts of Lieberkühn in the intestines (see Chapter 1). A second group of cells are the *permanent* cells, which lose their ability to divide once they reach a certain stage in their development. Erythrocytes and neutrophils are among these. There is also a third group, the *stable* cells, that enter a quiescent stage, the *G_0 phase* (see Fig. 13-1), in which they do not divide but remain capable of doing so if stimulated. In the liver, for example, cells

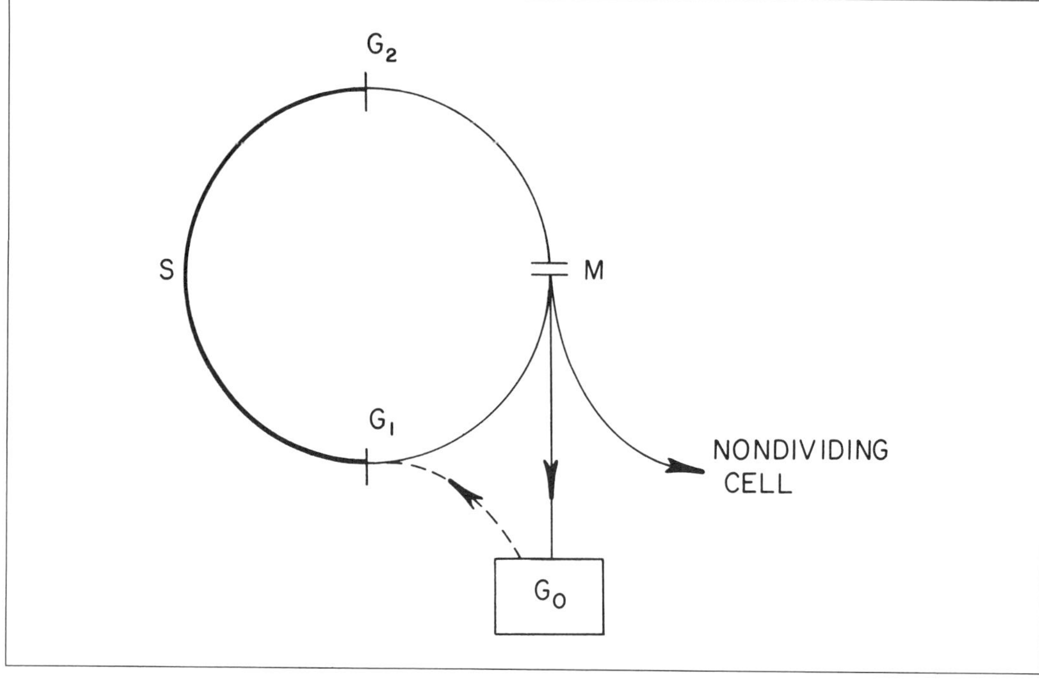

Figure 13-1. The cell cycle. M = mitosis, from prophase through telophase; G_1 = interval between completion of mitosis and onset of DNA synthesis; S = period of DNA replication; G_2 = interval between completion of DNA synthesis and mitosis; G_0 = quiescent cells that can be stimulated to synthesize DNA and divide. (From Baserga, R., Ed., Biochemistry of Cell Division, *1969, p. 4. Courtesy of Charles C Thomas, Publisher, Springfield, Ill.)*

will divide following partial hepatectomy. Some of the reasons which have been given for prolonged resting phases include cell crowding, contact inhibition, undernutrition, hypoxia, and effects of accumulation of metabolites or other substances.

Neoplasms can arise only in cells that have the ability to proliferate—that is, labile and stable cells. Cancer cells apparently have the same components of the cell cycle but do not respond similarly to the control mechanisms. Undernutrition, for example, interferes with growth in a child, but a cancer continues to grow in an undernourished host.

CLASSIFICATION OF NEOPLASMS

Neoplastic diseases are believed to be a group of disorders rather than one disease and have been classified according to their behavior. *Benign tumors* are circumscribed, encapsulated growths of cells that usually are well differentiated. They tend to grow slowly but may cause obstruction or atrophy of adjacent tissue as a result of pressure. They may be fatal when they occur at some sites, such as in the brain. They also sometimes become malignant. *Malignant tumors* (or *cancers*) often contain less-well-differentiated cells. They usually grow more rapidly and tend to invade surrounding tissue. In addition, malignant tumor cells may be released and be carried by the blood or lymph to distant sites where secondary tumors, known as *metastases*, appear.

Neoplasms also are named for the tissue from which they arise (Table 13-1). Some examples of benign tumors classified according to the tissue from which they arise are *fibroma* (from fibrous tissue), *chondroma* (from cartilage), and *adenoma* (from glandu-

Table 13-1. Examples of Neoplasms According to the Histogenetic Classification

Tissues of Origin	Benign	Malignant
Epithelial neoplasms		
Epidermis	Epidermal papilloma	Epidermal carcinoma
Stomach	Gastric polyp	Gastric carcinoma
Biliary tree	Cholangioma	Cholangiocarcinoma
Adrenal cortex	Adrenocortical adenoma	Adrenocortical carcinoma
Connective tissue neoplasms		
Fibrous tissue	Fibroma	Fibrosarcoma
Cartilage	Chondroma	Chondrosarcoma
Bone	Osteoma	Osteogenic sarcoma
Fat	Lipoma	Liposarcoma
Smooth muscle	Leiomyoma	Leiomyosarcoma
Skeletal muscle	Rhabdomyoma	Rhabdomyosarcoma
Neoplasms of the hemopoietic and immune systems		
Lymphoid tissue	Brill-Symmers disease	Lymphosarcoma (lymphoma) Lymphatic leukemia Reticulum cell sarcoma Hodgkin's disease
Thymus	Thymoma	Thymoma
Granulocytes		Myelocytic leukemia
Erythrocytes	Polycythemia vera	Erythroleukemia
Plasma cells		Multiple myeloma
Neoplasms of the nervous system		
Glia	Astrocytoma Oligodendroglioma	Glioblastoma multiforme
Meninges	Meningioma	Meningeal sarcoma
Neurons	Ganglioneuroma	Neuroblastoma
Adrenal medulla	Pheochromocytoma	Pheochromocytoma
Neoplasms of multiple histogenetic cellular origin		
Breast	Fibroadenoma	Cystosarcoma phylloides
Kidney		Wilms' tumor
Ovary, testis, etc.	Dermoid cyst (benign teratoma)	Malignant teratoma
Miscellaneous neoplasms		
Melanocytes	Nevus	Melanoma
Placenta	Hydatidiform mole	Choriocarcinoma
Ovary	Granulosa cell tumor Cystadenoma	Granulosa cell tumor Cystadenocarcinoma
Testis		Seminoma

Reprinted with permission from Pitot, H.C., *Fundamentals of Oncology,* 2nd ed. New York: Marcel Dekker, 1981, p. 25.

lar tissue). Tumors may be classified according to the histologic type (for example, *cystic,* or *follicular*). They sometimes are named after their discoverer. Two of the best known of these are *Hodgkin's disease* in the lymph tissue and *Wilms' tumor* in the kidney, both malignant processes.

Another classification system refers to the embryonic origin. Malignant tissues from ectoderm and endoderm are called *carcinomas,* and those from mesoderm are *sarcomas.* If malignant cells appear very primitive and resemble embryonic tissue, the tumor is called a *blastoma,* as in *neuroblas-*

toma. Those tumors derived from two cell layers are *carcinosarcomas,* and those from all three cell layers are *teratomas.* Sometimes terms are combined to be more specific about a tumor's source: examples are *adenocarcinoma, chondrosarcoma,* and *liposarcoma.* Obviously, the suffix *-oma* indicates a tumor. An exception to this is the *granuloma,* a non-neoplastic growth that occurs in response to inflammation. *Leukemia* refers to malignant growth of blood cells.

Cancers also are graded or "staged," using one of several available systems. One of the most commonly used is the *TNM system.* It provides a description of the cancer according to the size of the primary *t*umor, the involvement of adjacent lymph *n*odes, and the number of *m*etastases. The system varies somewhat with the identity of the primary tumor, but in general T_1 is a small, relatively circumscribed tumor, whereas T_4 indicates invasion of neighboring structures. N_0 designates no regional lymph node involvement. The other extreme of the scale, N_4, indicates involvement of multiple regional lymph nodes. M_0 indicates that no distant metastases are known, and M_1 designates their presence. Thus, $T_1N_0M_0$ indicates a small primary tumor with no regional lymph node involvement or known metastases, whereas $T_4N_4M_1$ indicates a large primary tumor, extensive lymph node involvement, and evidence of metastases.

NATURAL HISTORY OF NEOPLASTIC GROWTH

A sequence of change in the morphology of some cells has been observed in the genesis of cancer:

1. *Metaplasia* is replacement of one cell type with another. For example, in cases of irritation or inflammation of a mucosal surface, the underlying cells may differentiate into squamous cells instead of columnar cells. Frequently, this is a precancerous change. It may precede the development of a tumor by years.

2. *Dysplasia* or *anaplasia,* an alteration in adult cells with changes in their size, shape, or arrangement also is precancerous. It, too, can precede tumor development by months or years.

3. *Hyperplasia* is an increase in the number of cells. It occurs normally in fetal growth, wound healing, callus formation, and in the bone marrow, crypt cells of the intestine, and the basal layer of the skin. Abnormal hyperplasia usually occurs in neoplastic disease but is not required. Instead, the tissue may synthesize excess quantities of macromolecules.

4. *Neoplasia*—uncontrolled, progressive multiplication of cells—constitutes the fully developed disease.

Each primary tumor progresses independently, even in the same animal. In addition, characteristics of a particular tumor, such as growth rate, invasiveness, metastatic tendency, responsiveness to hormones, morphology, and *karyotype* (the arrangement of chromosomes) change independently.

When a tumor changes from benign to malignant or becomes more malignant, there is a change in morphology and activity. It is believed that, rather than a change in all cells, a few cells grow and metabolize faster and thus become predominant.

The mechanisms by which a tumor invades surrounding tissue is unknown. Factors involved may include proteolysis, decreased pH, differences in osmotic pressure, and others. Metastases tend to follow the routes of blood and lymph. Those carried in the blood usually are found first in the small capillaries at new sites.

PATHOGENESIS OF CANCER

Cancer cells are derived from normal cells. A current theory proposes that *carcinogenesis* (the process of cancer production) occurs in two stages, *initiation* and *promotion.* The initiation phase consists of a *mutation* (a transmissible alteration in a gene) in the cell, which then becomes neoplastic. Presumably, the mutation occurs in genes that regulate cell production. Such a mutation could account for the irreversible nature of the neoplastic change, the tendency for the tumor cells to reproduce, and the great variety of tumors. However, a neoplastic cell can remain dormant for years. The dormant cell may later be activated in the promotion phase. Promoters are agents that alter gene expression, but the exact nature of promotion is not understood clearly.

Both initiators and promotors are believed to be environmental factors in almost all cases. If this is so, then the majority of cancers are preventable. The initiation phase of carcinogenesis is theorized to be irreversible, but the action of promoters is time-dependent and dose-dependent. The theory further states that if an environmental promoter is present in very low dose or is applied for only a short period, its effects may subside. An initiator or promotor that is widespread in the environment, present in larger quantities, and difficult to avoid would be a particular hazard. Some agents are thought to be both initiators and promoters and are called *complete carcinogens.*

ETIOLOGY OF CANCER

A wide variety of agents are thought to be initiators or promoters in carcinogenesis, including chemicals, microorganisms, and radiation. Although a large number of chemicals are known to be carcinogenic, they have no common structure or mode of action. Most carcinogenic agents contained in food are chemical agents.

Nutrition and Diet

Dietary and nutritional factors are thought to influence the incidence of cancer via three general mechanisms in animals, but their effects in humans are understood less clearly. First, food items may provide a source of carcinogens or potentially carcinogenic substances. In foods, there are two categories of mutagens that may be carcinogenic, those that are naturally occurring and those that occur as the result of processing. Mutagens that are the result of processing include products of bacterial, fungal, or chemical action, products of cooking, additives, and contaminants such as pesticide residues, agricultural contaminants, and products of fuel combustion. Carcinogenic contaminants and additives which may be used in processing are assumed to be avoidable if they can be identified and eliminated from use. There are four categories of naturally occurring mutagens. One group consists of *alkaloids* or *flavonoids,* which occur in edible plants. A second category is *aflatoxin* B_1, which is produced by *Aspergillus flavus,* a contaminant mold that may grow in grains and peanuts stored in warm, humid environments. It is a *hepatocarcinogen* (causes liver cancer) but is not a common problem in the United States. *Polycyclic hydrocarbons,* produced in cooking methods that result in charred or browned protein foods, also can be carcinogenic. Lastly, *nitrosamines* are *gastrocarcinogenic* (causing stomach cancer). These are formed from amines present in some foods plus nitrites added to some fish or meat as a preservative. Nitrites can also be produced by reduction of nitrates in vegetables.

Another general mechanism by which foods may affect the occurrence of cancer is by influencing the formation of carcinogens. Some nutritive factors are reported to be carcinogenic and others, anticarcinogenic. Vitamin C inhibits the conversion of nitrates to nitrosamines, and thus is anticarcinogenic in nitrite-containing foods.[1] Derivatives of vitamin A, antioxidant food additives such as butylated hydroxytoluene (BHT), ethoxyquin, or coumarin, and some materials in the cabbage family (*Brassica*) are thought to be anticarcinogenic. However, the modes of action of these dietary factors are unknown. It has been suggested that they may alter the intestinal flora (fiber, meat), the mixed function oxidase system, and other enzyme systems (meat, fat, indoles in vegetables, trace elements, and antioxidants), the endocrine or immune systems (fats, total energy), the availability of substrates for neoplastic growth, or the rate of activation of the carcinogen.

Caloric restriction in animals has been associated with a low incidence of most neoplasms,[2] although the incidence of hepatic tumors is increased. Mitosis during caloric restriction may be inhibited by energy deficit or hormonal changes. The effects of diminished energy intake in humans is unknown, but it has been reported that, in individuals who are 25 percent or more overweight, there is a 33 percent increase in the incidence of tumors.

A third mechanism by which some foods modify the effects of carcinogens is by affecting concentration in the bowel (fiber), exerting an effect on transport (fiber, alcohol), or inhibiting promotion (vitamin A, carotene). Increased intake of animal fat or protein have been associated with increased incidence of malignancies of the colon.[2-4] Increases in colon cancer have also been associated with low dietary fiber.[5-6] It is hypothesized that high-fiber foods pass through the gut quickly, allowing less time for the intestinal flora to produce carcinogens or for carcinogens to act on intestinal cells. Alternatively, colon cancer may arise following potentiation of carcinogens by increased amounts of bile acids, production of which is stimulated by dietary fat. Fiber may be anticarcinogenic by binding fecal bile acids.

Other relationships between diet and cancer have been reported. Pickled vegetables, potatoes, salted fish, and abrasive food grains have been associated with an increase in gastric cancers.[7] Alcohol appears to act as a promoter, associated with cancer of the liver, mouth, larynx, and esophagus, particularly in smokers.[8,9]

Risk factors in humans cannot be extrapolated from effects in animals. In general, dietary factors are believed to be promoters, not initiators. The observed relationships between diet and cancer do not identify the specific carcinogen involved, and mechanisms are unknown; therefore, there are no generally accepted diet recommendations for the prevention of cancer. However, Wynder[10] has suggested that the "prudent diet" recommended for prevention of cardiovascular disease may also be useful for prevention of cancer. In any case, knowledge of carcinogens in food may be important in answering a client's questions in nutritional counseling.

Hormone-Nutrient Interactions

There is some evidence that hormones are involved in carcinogenesis and that nutrition may influence their action. Among the most common cancers are those of tissues whose growth is hormone-regulated—the breast, uterus, and prostate. It is not believed, however, that hormones are primary carcinogens. Instead, they might have an effect on the cells that render them susceptible to the primary agent.[11] The relationship of nutritional factors to hormone action are unclear, but it is known that obesity alters the metabolism of estrogen, a hormone associated with cancers of the vagina, uterus, breast, and liver.[12] Fat intake has also been associated with endometrial cancer.[13] Obese postmenopausal women convert a larger portion of androstenedione from the adrenal cortex to estrone than do thin women, and higher estrone levels indicate increased risk of endometrial cancer.[14] Increased dietary fat and increased kilocalorie intake have been associated with breast cancer,[15-17] and dietary fat, with prostate cancer.[18]

Stress

There may be a relationship between the incidence of cancer and stress. Possible mechanisms are stress damage to the thymus or other parts of the immune system or a hormonal effect involving the hypothalamus, pituitary gland, and adrenal cortex.

Radiation

Radiation may be carcinogenic under appropriate circumstances. It can cause chromosomal damage with abnormal repair. Sources of ionizing radiation in the environment include x-rays, radioactive materials used in diagnostic tests or in the work place, and exposure to atomic wastes. Ultraviolet light from sunlight is a nonionizing radiation which has been reported to be associated with an increased incidence of skin cancer. It is not known whether microwaves are carcinogenic. The predominant current opinion states that radiation is an initiator.

Inflammation and Infections

Chronic inflammation, some infectious agents (such as parasitic worms), and a number of *oncogenic* (tumor-causing) *viruses* also are carcinogenic. An oncogenic virus is a mass of chromosomes with six genes or less plus a protein coat. It adds to a cell new genetic material which may express itself as a malignancy. Oncogenic viruses have been identified in animals, but their importance in human cancer is unknown. One controversial theory states that chemical carcinogens act by activating an oncogenic virus.

HOST EFFECTS ON CARCINOGENESIS

In children, the cause of cancer may involve a genetic predisposition plus environmental influences in utero or during the neonatal period. The incidence of cancer increases with age, with a particular increase in later middle age and in old age. It is not known whether this occurs as a consequence of longer exposure to factors in the environment or is inherent in the aging process. Sex, too, is known to have an influence, since the type of cancer varies in men and women, even when genital system cancers are not included.

METABOLIC AND NUTRITIONAL ALTERATIONS IN MALIGNANCY

A malignancy can affect the patient's nutritional status in three ways. First, it may have a general systemic effect. Second, depending on its location, it may have local effects on specific organs. Finally, cancer therapy often affects nutritional status.

Systemic Effects

As malignancy progresses, cancer cells tend to become less differentiated. This does not mean, however, that the "dedifferentiated" cell is equivalent to the cells in the developing embryo. One of the important differences is that embryonic development is controlled very precisely, whereas malignancies do not respond to these controls. Cancer cells do tend to become less like their tissue of origin. As growth proceeds, different types of neoplasms become more alike, with many similarities in their metabolism. Thus, we can describe some metabolic alterations that are seen commonly in patients with neoplastic disease, regardless of the specific tissue involved.

The major symptom complex common to neoplastic disease is *cachexia,*[19,20] characterized by anorexia, tissue wasting, weakness, impaired organ function, apathy, water and electrolyte imbalance, and decreased resistance to infection.[19] The patient becomes so emaciated that he or she appears to die of starvation. The severity of cachexia is not related entirely to the size, site, or type of neoplasm. The etiology of the tissue catabolism in most patients is not entirely clear.

Possibilities for consideration are, of course, decreased energy intake, increased energy expenditure, or both. It is thought that, in most patients, decreased intake probably is predominant, since many of the characteristics of cachexia can be overcome by increasing food intake.

Decreased Food Intake

In some patients there are mechanical barriers to food intake, such as those that can occur in cancers of the head and neck, esophagus, gastrointestinal tract, or adjacent organs. Even when mechanical barriers are not present, the nutrient intake in most cancer patients tends to decrease, primarily as a result of anorexia.[21,22] In fact, anorexia sometimes appears so early that it is the warning symptom that leads to the original diagnosis.

The mechanisms for the production of anorexia are not understood entirely. Abnormalities of taste and smell occur in proportion to the tumor burden and probably contribute to decreased food intake.[23–26] The abnormalities frequently encountered include an increased threshold for sweet taste and a lower threshold for bitter taste. Thus, patients must have sweeter food to taste the sweetness. The increased bitter taste causes early difficulty in eating protein foods, especially beef and pork. Fish and poultry are tolerated for a longer period, but patients also may find these unacceptable as the disease progresses.

The mechanisms producing these abnormalities still are under investigation. DeWys[21] has suggested that cell renewal in the taste buds is decreased in the patient with cancer, causing the elevated sweet threshold. Zinc deficiency may cause an increase in some thresholds, whereas altered plasma amino acids may lower the threshold for bitter taste.[24]

Patients also complain of a feeling of fullness, sometimes after only a few bites of food. Decreased gastrointestinal secretion, slowing digestion, and atrophy of the epithelium or muscle wall of the intestinal tract may be the mechanisms altering the sense of fullness.

Certain metabolites also are thought to affect food intake. Serotonin, synthesized from tryptophan, is known to stimulate the satiety center in the brain of rats and reduce their food intake. Krause et al.[27] postulate a mechanism which begins with a meal containing carbohydrate to induce plasma insulin release. As a result of this release, peripheral amino acid use is increased, and tryptophan in the blood is transferred across the blood-brain barrier, thereby competing with the branched-chain amino acids (BCAAs). When plasma BCAAs are reduced, tryptophan can be transported into the brain faster; this increases the brain serotonin level, presumably causing a reduction in food intake by stimulating the satiety center. This theory raises the possibility that food intake may be stimulated by administering BCAAs, but whether this is effective in humans is not yet known.

Other metabolites that possibly affect food intake are lactate, fatty acids, peptides, oligonucleotides, and imbalances of amino acids. These may act via an effect on neuroendocrine cells or on the hypothalamus and other central nervous system cells.[28] Hormonal changes, particularly insulin resistance, and psychological factors stimulating catecholamine release also may reduce appetite (see Chapter 15).

Altered Metabolism and Competition for Nutrients

Decreased food intake does not account entirely for the weight changes seen in cancer patients. Weight loss often is disproportionate to the decrease in nutrient intake and may occur even in the presence of seemingly normal intake. It may occur at a rate in excess of that seen in starvation,[29] suggesting either alterations in host metabolism, decreasing efficiency of nutrient use, or competition for nutrients between host and tumor in which the tumor prevails.

It is obvious that neoplastic tissue competes successfully for nutrients, since tumor growth commonly is seen even though the host is wasting.[30] The tumor has a high energy requirement to maintain sodium and potassium gradients,[31] to support protein synthesis, and to supply substrates for growth. This increased fuel consumption results in an increased resting metabolism in the tumor-host complex.[32–34] Increases of 35 to 74 percent have been reported,[35] but in many patients, the total tumor burden is not thought to be large enough to produce the observed amount of wasting unless the metabolism of the tumor is very inefficient, which may be the case.

In addition, it is speculated that the patient's metabolism is altered to meet the energy demands of the tumor. There is a systemic insulin resistance,[36,37] with decreased peripheral glucose uptake and decreased formation of glycogen.[38] At the same time, gluconeogenesis is increased.[39,40]

Many tumors have a particularly accelerated rate of glycolysis and lactic acid production.[41] The glycolysis of each mole of glucose provides 2 moles of ATP, but this ATP is used by the tumor. The lactic acid produced is returned to the liver and kidney, resynthesized to glucose via the Cori cycle, and recycled back to the tumor. This process requires the expenditure of 6 moles of ATP. There is increased or poorly regulated gluconeogenesis from the lactate in the liver, which may be the consequence of insulin resistance. The resulting increase in Cori cycle activity in cancer patients causes a total loss of 8 moles of ATP to the host.[39,40] Although it has been argued that this is not a significant loss,[42] it may also be argued that the oxidative metabolism of 1 mole of lactate could have yielded 30 moles of ATP which now are lost.

The patient's lipid metabolism may be abnormal as well. Serum free fatty acids are elevated, but clearance of lipid is increased.[43] At the same time, fat stores are depleted. The mechanism involved in the apparent increased mobilization of lipids is unknown, but some evidence suggests that tumors produce lipolytic substances.[44] The severe fat wasting may also be the result of the high energy expenditure. A shift from carbohydrate to lipid metabolism may be the result of alterations in insulin, glucagon, and catecholamine balance.[45]

Cancer patients have altered protein metabolism. There is decreased protein synthesis in the host, with a decrease in serum albumin[46] and many enzymes.[37] It is not known to what extent these are the consequence of substrate deficiency and decreased synthesis or of increased catabolism. The mechanisms for nitrogen conservation in starvation (see Chapter 12) appear to remain intact. Nevertheless, nitrogen loss in the host persists, even when amino acid and energy intakes are adequate.

Tumors have a great capacity to concentrate amino acids and have been called a "nitrogen trap."[33,47] The nitrogen turnover in a tumor is very low—that is, the amino acids are not recycled. Protein synthesis is increased, whereas amino acid breakdown, gluconeogenesis and urea cycle enzymes are depressed. Purine, pyrimidine, and DNA synthesis are increased, but degradation of purines and pyrimidine is diminished. As a consequence of these factors, patients with rapidly growing cancers may be in a positive nitrogen balance although they are losing weight.

Tumors not only retain exogenous proteins efficiently, but animal experiments have shown that they grow at the expense of the host. They draw some protein from host body tissue, largely from skeletal muscle.[48] The tumor thus contains even more nitrogen than was retained for positive nitrogen balance. Some tumors appear to have a special capacity to degrade selected essential amino acids, thereby producing an amino acid imbalance. Another possibility is that rapidly growing tumors have a heightened ability to concentrate amino acids or take up circulating proteins, such as albumin. Some protein is lost as the result of increased gluconeogenesis in the host.[49] The extent to which a tumor is a metabolic drain contributing to tissue wasting in the human host is unclear.

Additional effects on protein metabolism are indicated by the finding of novel proteins and peptides in the urine of patients with advanced cancer.[50,51] The activities of a number of enzymes of host tissue also are affected by the presence of neoplasms, even at distant sites. The mechanism by which this occurs is unknown.[51]

Fluid often is retained as neoplastic disease advances, masking tissue loss, although clinical edema may not be evident. In these circumstances, body weight is not useful as an indicator of nutritional status.

Overall, the metabolism of the cancer patient differs from that seen in starvation. Whereas healthy subjects show a decrease in basal metabolic rate (BMR) and decreased oxidative metabolism in starvation, BMR in cancer patients often increases and oxygen consumption persists in the postabsorptive period. The patient thus is hypermetabolic, and in many respects, metabolism resembles that described in Chapter 12.

Interrelationships of Nutritional Status and Systemic Effects of Cancer

It has been shown that improved nutrition accelerates tumor growth, but these experiments were done in animals with large transplanted tumors. In human patients with spontaneous tumors, no acceleration of tumor growth was observed following improved nutrition.[52] It has been suggested that inducing a deficiency of essential amino acids might impede tumor growth; however, this approach has not been successful since it also deprives normal tissue. Although the host and tumor are interdependent in some ways, they also are independent of each other to a great extent. A neoplasm, once it reaches a certain size, continues to grow regardless of the nutritional needs of the host. Therefore, nutritional deprivation harms the host more than it harms the tumor.

Effects on Specific Organ Systems

In addition to their systemic effects, cancers may have other effects which depend on their specific location, particularly in the digestive system.[53,54] Gastric carcinomas can cause losses of blood and other protein-rich fluids. Nausea and vomiting develop as a result of obstruction in the gastrointestinal tract and can lead to fluid, electrolyte, and protein losses. Intestinal damage can result in malabsorption with steatorrhea, diarrhea, lactase deficiency, and protein-losing enteropathy. Reduced intake may produce alterations in the intestinal mucosa known as *cancer enteropathy.* Pancreatic insufficiency caused by neoplastic growth can lead to impairment of nutritional status. (See Chapter 6 for nutritional care in these conditions.) Cancer of the liver may cause decreased albumin production with consequent hypoalbuminemia. Prothrombin deficiency also occurs in carcinoma of the liver, if the liver is unable to synthesize prothrombin or if decreased bile production interferes with vitamin K absorption.

Some malignancies affect nutrition by secreting one or more hormones in pharmacologic quantities. Some of these conditions, described in Chapters 5 and 6, include Zollinger-Ellison syndrome, pancreatic cholera, carcinoid syndrome, and villous adenoma. Medullary carcinoma of the thyroid secretes excess thyrocalcitonin which causes diarrhea by stimulating jejunal mucosal secretion of fluids and electrolytes. Bronchogenic and oat cell carcinomas cause fluid and electrolyte imbalances, as do carcinoma of the adrenal cortex or corticotropin-secreting tumors in the lung.

Neoplasms of the central nervous system have less specific effects. The mental symptoms may interfere with food intake in a variety of ways.

Nutritional Consequences of Cancer Therapy

The nutritional deprivation seen in the cancer patient is aggravated by therapy. There are three major approaches to anticancer therapy, all of which have nutritional significance: *surgery, radiation,* and *chemotherapy. Immunotherapy* is a promising approach that will probably be used more frequently in the future with further development of techniques. *Hyperthermia* is an experimental method which could result in significant energy loss.

Surgery

The systemic effects and nutritional implications of surgery in cancer patients is the same as that seen in other surgical patients (see Chapter 12). Patients sometimes develop complications among which are fistulas, obstruction, and sepsis. Other complications can arise, depending on the specific site of the resections. For example, patients with resections of the oropharynx or esophagus may become dependent on tube feedings. Dumping syndrome, malabsorption, fluid and electrolyte losses, and ostomies may follow resections of the stomach or various parts of the intestinal tract. Nutritional care in these conditions is described in Chapters 5 and 6.

Radiation Therapy

Radiation disrupts the chemical bonds required in DNA reproduction and synthesis,[55] thus interfering with reproduction of dividing cells. It may be used in the form of x-rays or radioactive isotopes to produce *gamma rays* or atomic particles such as *electrons* (from *beta emitters*), *neutrons,* or *protons.* Radiation is used to treat tumors that respond to doses which are tolerable to normal tissues or those that can be targeted so that overlying tissue is not damaged. A typical protocol for treatment provides for radiation therapy 5 days/wk for 4 to 6 weeks. The treatment has its greatest effect on cells in the G_2 or M phase of the cell cycle.

Radiation is used for approximately half of all cancer patients, often in combination with chemotherapy. It can cause severe anorexia, nausea, and sometimes vomiting. Tumors of the central nervous system can produce changes in mental function leading to decreased food intake. Increased intracranial pressure can cause nausea and vomiting. Cerebral edema may follow radiation therapy and exacerbate the symptoms.

When radiation is applied to the head or neck, an altered and unpleasant or decreased sense of taste and alterations in the sense of smell may be caused by damage to the taste buds and olfactory receptors.[56,57] In rats, radiation has been shown to cause the release of histamine, producing very strong learned taste aversions. These taste aversions can be blocked by administering an antihistamine to the animal prior to exposure to radiation. Levy et al.[58] proposed that the histamine production after radiation exposure represented the physiologic basis of radiation-induced taste aversions and noted that *humans treated with antihistamines immediately after radiation exposure showed a marked decline in incidence of nausea, vomiting, irritability, anorexia, and similar symptoms of radiation sickness.* Normal taste acuity returns 1 to 2 months following treatment.

Mucositis (inflammation of the mucosal lining of the mouth and pharynx) can cause severe pain and reduce food intake. Xerostomia can result from damage to the salivary glands, and that saliva which is produced may be particularly thick and viscous. The development of rampant caries, periodontal disease, and *osteoradionecrosis* (necrosis of the bone due to excessive radiation) often occurs.

Radiation to the organs of the thorax, the esophagus, lungs, or mediastinum may cause esophagitis, dysphagia, nausea, stenosis, or fistulas. Low-dose radiation to the stomach is tolerated reasonably well and usually creates few problems, but high-dose radiation may cause ulceration with bleeding, vomiting, and weight loss.[59] The usual ulcer regimens are not effective, and partial gastrectomy may be necessary.[60] Radiation damage to the pancreas is rare.

Irradiation of the abdomen or pelvic region for gastrointestinal or genitourinary tract cancer tends to denude the mucosal lining and cause a loss of intestinal villi. There are changes in the vascular bed with intimal thickening, interfering with blood circulation. In addition to nausea, vomiting, and anorexia, steatorrhea and diarrhea are common. These conditions develop as early as 2 weeks after treatment begins. Other effects include strictures and obstructions, inflammation, ulcers, fistulas, thromboses, and acute or chronic enteritis or colitis. Whereas some of these effects are temporary, long-term injury also can result from radiation therapy. Ulceration, for example, can develop a month to a year after radiation is terminated.

Chemotherapy

Chemotherapy involves the use of antineoplastic drugs which disrupt the reproductive cycle of cells. These drugs affect cancer cells and normal cells in the same way. The mechanisms by which they do this include:

- Interference with the synthesis of purines and pyrimidines for incorporation into the nucleic acids necessary for DNA synthesis
- Disruption of normal DNA structure or replication of RNA
- Prevention of normal cell division by causing spindle damage
- Creation of a hormone imbalance
- Making essential amino acids unavailable

There are six general categories of antineoplastic agents, and each group functions a different way to interfere with cell reproduction. *Alkaloids,* obtained from plants, disorganize the chromosome spindles during mitosis. Examples of alkaloids are vincristine and vinblastine. *Alkylating agents,* such as nitrogen mustard and cyclophosphamide, bind with DNA, RNA, or some enzymes to interfere with cell division. *Antimetabolites* block reactions necessary to produce precursors to DNA synthesis. This category includes methotrexate, which reduces available folic acid, and 6-mercaptopurine, 5-fluorouracil, and cytosine arabinoside. Some *antibiotics,* such as mithramycin, bleomycin, and doxorubicin, interfere with the structure or function of DNA or other cell structures. The *antineoplastic enzyme* asparaginase interferes with the reactions necessary to produce a required amino acid. *Hormones* may affect the cell or otherwise interfere with cell metabolism by altering the hormone balance. These include estrogens, androgens, progestins, and prednisone. The sites of action of the major classes of chemotherapeutic drugs are shown in Fig. 13-2.

The *log kill hypothesis* is used as a basis for chemotherapy. It assumes that a single dose kills a constant proportion, up to 99.9 percent, of the tumor cells. Repeated doses further reduce the number of neoplastic cells. A single surviving malignant cell, however, can multiply and eventually kill the host. Therefore, the maximum tolerable dose is used in a series that is repeated. In addition, it is common to use several antineoplastic agents for their synergistic effects. Since the treatment consists of repeated doses over a period of time, nutritional effects must be expected to occur for weeks or months.

The effectiveness of chemotherapeutic agents depends on their greater toxicity to cancer cells than to normal cells. Unfortunately, all existing agents are toxic to normal cells to some extent, and their use is limited by this toxicity. Since most antineoplastic drugs interfere with cell reproduction, it follows that they affect cells that are reproducing, including reproducing normal cells. A major toxic effect is on the bone marrow, manifested by *leukopenia* (deficiency of leukocytes), *thrombocytopenia* (insufficient platelets), and *anemia.* These conditions limit the dose that may be used. When the red

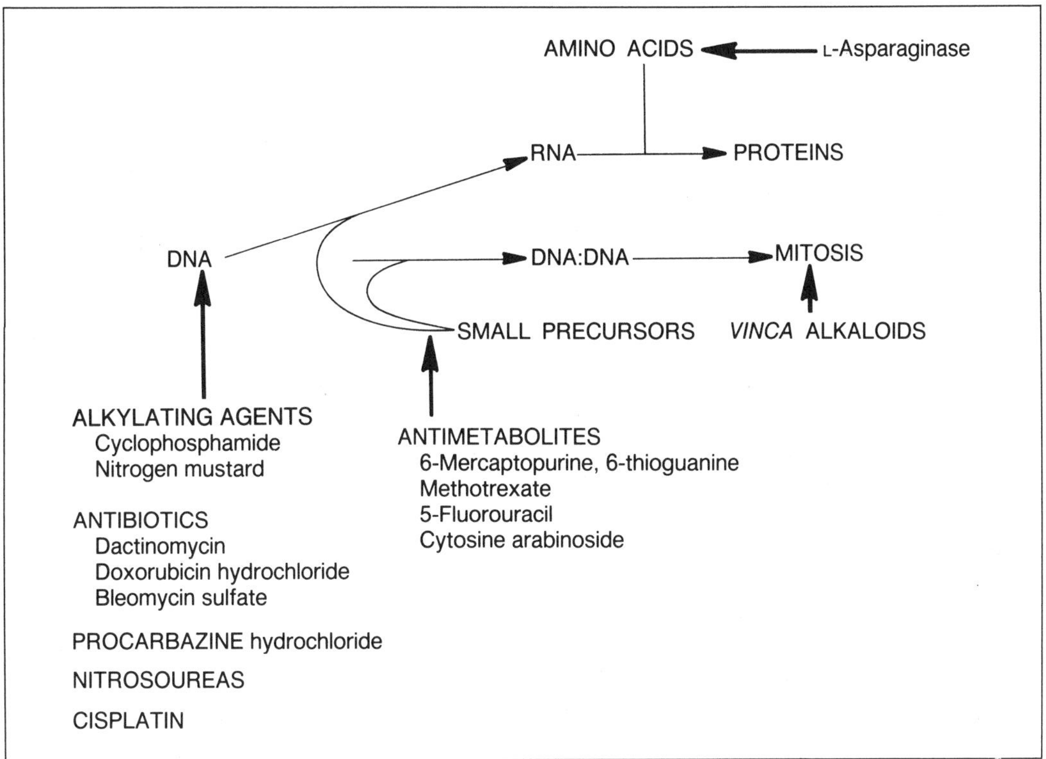

Figure 13-2. Site of action of chemotherapeutic agents. (Reprinted with permission from Cline, M.J., and Haskell, C.M., Cancer Chemotherapy, *3rd ed. Philadelphia: W.B. Saunders, 1980, p. 3.)*

blood cell and platelet count is reduced severely, the therapy must be stopped until the cells multiply sufficiently. This is one of the major reasons that antineoplastic drugs are used in repeated series with intermittent recovery periods.

Antineoplastic drugs extensively affect the nutritional status of the patient. They have many effects on the gastrointestinal tract, since the lining is constantly renewed (Table 13-2). Toxic effects include oral ulcerations, glossitis, stomatitis, and mucositis, all of which cause severe pain during food intake. Nausea, vomiting, and diarrhea are seen commonly with all classes of antineoplastic drugs. They are believed to be the result of drug effects on a *chemoreceptor trigger zone* in the brain.[61,62] Anorexia with decreased food intake also usually occurs. Aversions to specific foods eaten before a treatment that caused gastrointestinal discomfort have been shown to develop. Some drugs cause altered taste sensations. Diarrhea occurs as a side effect of some drugs, and constipation is a side effect of others. Other nutrition-related side effects of chemotherapy include hepatotoxicity, electrolyte imbalances, and nephrotoxicity. Products of destroyed cancer cells and some of the drugs, especially alkylating agents, may be nephrotoxic.

In studies of the effects of nutritional status on a patient's response to antineoplastic drugs, it has been shown that cachectic patients respond poorly to chemotherapy, largely because they are unable to tolerate the usual doses. Hence, nutritional status both influences and is influenced by these agents.

Table 13-2. Nutrition-Related Side Effects of Chemotherapy

Chemotherapeutic Agent	Nausea	Vomiting	Anorexia	Diarrhea	Inflammation or Ulceration of Oral Cavity	Other
Amethopterin (methotrexate, MTX)	X	X–	X	X	X	Gastrointestinal ulcerations; abdominal pain; hepatotoxicity; cirrhosis
L-Asparaginase (Elspar, L-ASP, crasnitin, amidohytrolate, colaspase)	X	X	X			Hepatic dysfunction; pancreatitis; allergy
5-Azacytidine (Aza-CR, 5-AZE, ladakamycin [investigational])	XX	XX		X		
Bleomycin sulfate (Blenoxane, Bleo, BLM-2)	X	X–			X	
Busulfan (Myleran, BUS, BSF, BAN)	X	X			X	
Carmustine (BCNU, BiCNU)	XX	XX	X	X		
Chlorambucil (Leukeran, CHL, CB-1348)	X	X–		X		
Cisplatin (*cis*-platinum, Platinol, DDP, CPDD, PDD, CPD, CACP)	XX	XX	X			
Cyclophosphamide (Cytoxan, Endoxan, CYT, CTX, CYC, CPM)	XX	XX	X	X	X	Abdominal or epigastric pain
Cytosine arabinoside (cytarabine, ARA-C, Cytosar-U, CA)	X	X		X	X	Gastrointestinal ulcerations
Dacarbazine (DTIC-Dome, DIC, imidazole carboxamide)	XX	X				
Dactinomycin (ACT-D, ACT, DSCT, ACD, Cosmegen)	XX	XX	X	X	XX	Abdominal pain
Daunomycin hydrochloride (daunorubicin, DNR, rubidomycin, Cerubidine)	XX	X	X		X	Abdominal or epigastric pain
3-Diazauridine	X	X	X			Gastrointestinal atrophy and necrosis
Doxorubicin hydrochloride (Adriamycin)	XX	X	X	X	XX	
Etoposide (VP 16–213, Ethylidene-Lignan P, EPEG [investigational])		X				
5-Fluorouracil (5-FU, fluorouracil, Adrucil, Efudex, Fluoroplex)	X	X	X	XX	XX	
Hexamethylmelamine (HMM, HXM)	XX	XX	X			
Hydroxyurea (Hydrea, HYD, HU, HUR)	X	X–		X	X	Constipation
Lomustine (CCNU, CeeNU)	XX	XX	X	X		
Mechlorethamine hydrochloride (nitrogen mustard, Mustargen, HN_2HN2)	XX	XX	X	X–		

tional])						
Methylglyoxalbisguanyl hydrazone (methyl GAG, methyl GBG, MGBG, MGGH, mitoguazone)				X		
Mithramycin (Mithracin)	XX	X	X	X		Hepatotoxicity
Mitomycin (Mutamycin, Mitomycin C, MTC, Ametysin)	X	X				
Neocarzinostatin	X	X				
Piperazinedione (Merck compound 593A [investigational])	X	X				
Procarbazine hydrochloride (methyl hydrazine, Matulane, Ibenzmethyzin, MIH)	X	X				Gastrointestinal ulceration
Razoxane	X	X				
Rubidizone	X	X				
Semustine (methyl CCNU, meCCNU)	XX	X	X		X	
Streptozocin (Streptozotocin)	XX	XX	X	X		
Teniposide (VM-26, Thenylidine-Liganan-P, PTG)	X	X				
6-Thioguanine (6-TG, Tabloid)	X	X−		X	X	
Triethylenethiophosphoramide (Thiotepa, THIO, TESPA, TSPA)	X	X				
Vinblastine sulfate (Velban, VBL, Velbe, Vinkaleukoblastine sulfate)	X	X			X	Ileus
Vincristine sulfate (VCR, Oncovin, LCR, leucocristine sulfate)	X	X			X	Ileus; abdominal pain
Hormones						
Adrenocorticoids (prednisone, Medrol)						Weight gain; increased appetite; fluid retention; gastrointestinal ulcers
Androgens (Halotestin, Teslac, Depo-Testosterone, Deca-Durabolin, Methosarb)	X	X				Fluid retention; liver damage
Antiestrogens (tamoxifen citrate)	X	X				(Transient)
Estrogens (diethylstilbestrol [DES], TACE, Stilphostrol)	X	X				Fluid retention

Information compiled from: Visconti, J.A., *Drug-Food Interactions.* Columbus: Ross Laboratories, 1979; Wollard, J.J., Ed., *Nutritional Management of the Cancer Patient.* New York: Raven Press, 1979; Carter, S.K., Nutritional problems associated with cancer chemotherapy. In G.R. Newell and N.M. Ellison, Eds., *Nutrition and Cancer: Etiology and Treatment.* New York: Raven Press, 1981; See Lasley, K., and Ingnoffo, R.J., *Manual of Oncology Therapeutics.* St. Louis: C.V. Mosby, 1981; Donaldson, S.S., and Lenon, R.A., Alterations of nutritional status. Impact of chemotherapy and radiation therapy. *Cancer* 43:2036, 1979; U.S. Public Health Service, National Cancer Institute, *Chemotherapy and You.* NIH Publication No. 81-1136. Washington, D.C.: U.S. Department of Health and Human Services, 1980.

X = present; X− = minimal; XX = extreme.

CAUSE OF DEATH FROM CANCER

Although the effects of cancer are poorly understood, certain factors are recognized as being among the immediate causes of death in cancer victims. Cachexia is the primary cause of death in many, or perhaps most, cancer patients. Other causes are (1) organ failure, especially renal; (2) obstruction of a vital organ, airway, or blood vessel; (3) increased intracranial pressure; (4) circulatory system effects such as hemorrhage, stroke, or embolus; and (5) infection.[63]

NUTRITIONAL MANAGEMENT OF THE CANCER PATIENT

In considering nutritional management in cancer, the question must be asked whether nutritional support to prevent or treat malnutrition makes any difference in the final analysis. Weight loss has been shown to be a good predictor of complications and death,[64,65] but it is unclear whether nutritional intervention increases the survival time or rate of cure. It *is* clear that nutritional support is well tolerated by the cancer patient and that it is possible to improve nutritional status in these patients.

Nutritional intervention can cause nitrogen retention and weight gain, although complete reversal of the tendency toward cachexia is rare. It decreases susceptibility to infection by supporting defense mechanisms, including delayed hypersensitivity, cough, mucous protection of membranes, and ciliary function.[66,67] It also helps to minimize the symptoms of high-dose radiation and chemotherapy, making it possible to complete the course of treatment.[68–71] The advantages of nutritional intervention allow patients to be more active and have an increased feeling of well-being. As a consequence, nutritional support now is commonly used as an adjunct to other forms of therapy to at least improve the quality of life.

The role of the nutritional care specialist in the oncology unit is less firmly established than is the need for nutritional support. A recent survey indicated that, although physicians regarded the nutritional care specialist as the primary source of nutrition information, they believed that they, not the nutrition specialist, should relay the information to the patient.[72] Nutritional care specialists must be more assertive in demonstrating their value in direct care of the cancer patient.

Nutritional Assessment

All cancer patients should be considered to be at risk of malnutrition. Nutritional assessment should be done early and repeated at intervals, but the procedures used may have to be altered from the general guidelines given in Chapter 2. An initial screening of all oncology patients, without anthropometric measurements, has been recommended by some oncologists,[71,73] whereas others recommend the extensive use of anthropometric measurements.[74] Risk factors to be considered during assessment include alcoholism, poor dentition, decreased appetite, nausea, vomiting, and diarrhea. In determining risk, plans for treatment must be taken into account even if the patient is not currently malnourished. Patients who will be treated by surgery, radiation, or chemotherapy should receive preventive support. Oncology patients receiving the house diet should also be a concern of the nutritional care specialist. Although there may be no indication for restriction of specific foods, increased need and reduced intake may place them at risk.

Patients who are found to be at risk in the initial screening should be assessed in depth, including a detailed diet history. Plans for nutritional support should be integrated with dental and mouth care. The financial resources of and facilities to provide an adequate diet for ambulatory patients must also be considered.

Nutritional Care

The procedures for nutritional care of each patient must be individualized, since needs vary from one patient to another, with the progress of the disease, and with the treatments used. It is not possible to establish a protocol that can be applied to all patients. Nevertheless, some guidelines can be provided:

Nutritional support is necessary to correct poor nutritional status, but in the cancer patient, it may also be used in anticipation of future problems. The nutritional care specialist should make every effort to prevent the weight loss typical of many cancer patients. In patients who are already depleted, repletion, although more difficult, should be attempted. For maintenance, 2,000 kcal/day often are sufficient, whereas repletion may require 3,000 to 4,000 kcal/day. Protein for maintenance may be 90 to 100 g/day, whereas repletion may require 100 to 200 g/day.

Oral feeding is recommended if the gastrointestinal tract is functional and oral intake is tolerated. Particular approaches to anorexia include the use of small frequent meals with foods of high nutrient density and individualization of the diet for the patient's needs and preferences. The patient needs personal attention and encouragement to eat.

Bloating sometimes occurs and may be related to the type of food eaten. The elimination of fried, greasy, and fatty foods,

Table 13-3. Oral Nutritional Guidelines During Cancer Therapy

Criteria	Diet Suggestions	Supplements	Poorly Tolerated Foods
Stomatitis	Liquid to soft: low-fat milk, melons, peeled cucumber, grapes, fruit ades, blenderized canned soda pops; 1% Dyclone solution to deaden mouth	Polycose, Precision, Isocal, Ensure	Juices, milk and milk products, meats, bread products, nuts, crisp and raw fruits and vegetables
Salivary changes			
Viscous, mucous saliva production	Liquids: hot tea with lemon, Kool-Aid popsicles, canned soda pops, lemon pudding. Swab mouth 10 minutes before meals with cotton swab coated with meat tenderizer	Polycose if well diluted	Milk and milk products, milk shakes, ice cream, liquid Jello, viscous liquids such as Precision
Decreased salivation	Regular with high moisture content: beverages served with food, sauces, gravies, casseroles, chicken, and fish; saliva stimulants such as sugarless lemon drops and gum	Polycose, Ensure, Isocal, Precision, Sustacal, Instant Breakfast	Dry foods, bread products, meats such as beef, pork, and lamb
Taste sensation changes	Regular with strongly flavored food emphasized: highly spiced foods such as pizza, spaghetti, pickles, olives, and barbecued meats; foods with texture; emphasis on odor and eye appeal	Fruit-flavored and chocolate-flavored supplements	Bland foods, milkshakes, ice cream, plain meats, and foods without texture
Gastrointestinal alterations	Liquid to soft; high-protein, high-calorie: alterations in lactose, fat, and fiber content	Nonmilk supplements, Polycose, MCT Oil	Raw fruits and vegetables, milk and milk products, and highly spiced foods

Adapted with permission from Aker, S., Oral feedings in the cancer patient. *Cancer* 43:2105, 1979.

gas-producing foods, milk, carbonated beverages, and chewing gum may help.

The patient's diet may be modified to reduce pain, avoiding very hot or cold foods, decreasing spices and acidic foods, and providing foods with a smooth texture. A rinse containing an analgesic sometimes is given before meals to reduce pain. Patients with a dry mouth may be given more liquid foods and provided with an artificial saliva. Other suggestions are given in Table 13-3. A decrease in sucrose in the diet is helpful in caries prevention.

If intake of usual foods cannot be maintained at a level sufficient to maintain normal weight, supplemental feedings often are used. Tube feedings may be used to replace or supplement oral intakes if these are inadequate. Nasogastric tubes, however, may be refused by the patient with oral inflammations. Some patients have gastrostomies or jejunostomies for feeding. If they cannot be fed in this way, intravenous hyperalimentation is used.

Low-fiber, high-fiber, or soft diets and other modifications may be indicated by a patient's specific symptoms. In patients receiving antineoplastic drugs, an increase in fluid intake is indicated to improve renal excretion of drugs and the products of cell breakdown, reduce the incidence of urinary infection, and replace losses from gastrointestinal disturbances, fevers, and infections. This may present particular problems in the patients with chewing and swallowing difficulties. Care of renal disease may also be needed. Patients receiving cyclophosphamide should receive 2 to 3 liters of fluid per day. Nutritional management of the patient who has radiation injury to the liver is the same as for hepatitis (see Chapter 11). The terminal cancer patient should be provided with any food requested and any food that makes the patient comfortable.

Because nutritional care of the cancer patient must be individualized to meet the needs of the specific patient, the nutritional care specialist must have extensive skill and knowledge. Many of the techniques used in the management of gastrointestinal symptoms were described in Chapters 5 and 6, and so they are not repeated here. Procedures for nutritional support with supplements, tube feedings, and total parenteral nutrition are included in Chapters 5 and 12.

SPECIAL CONSIDERATIONS IN LEUKEMIA

Leukemia is a general term referring to a neoplastic disease of the blood-forming tissues. It is characterized by a significant increase in the numbers of leukocytes or their precursors. The lymphocytes do not function normally. In addition, the lymphoid tissue of the spleen, liver, lymph nodes, and bone marrow enlarge and proliferate. Clinical manifestations include anemia, thrombocytopenia, tendency to bleed from the nose, gums, joints, and other internal organs, increased incidence of skin infections and pneumonia, heat intolerance, and exhaustion.

Leukemias are broadly classified as *acute* or *chronic* according to the duration and rate of progression of the disease and also according to the type of cell involved. *Lymphocytic leukemia* involves lymphocytes and lymphoblasts, whereas *myelocytic leukemia* involves the granulocytes. The features of these main types of leukemia are described in Table 13-4.

The cause of leukemia is unknown, but contributing factors are largely those seen in other forms of cancer: ionizing radiation, exposure to carcinogenic chemicals, or viruses. Heredity is thought to be a factor, since there is an increased incidence in the siblings of leukemia patients. An increased incidence accompanying Down's syndrome (see Chapter 16) also indicates genetic involvement.

Cure of leukemia rarely is achieved, and the aim of treatment usually is remission. *Remission* is defined as relief of symptoms,

Table 13-4. Characteristics of the Main Types of Leukemia

Type	Age and Sex Incidence	Onset of Symptoms	Treatment	Prognosis
Acute lymphocytic leukemia	Most commonly 3–4 years old; rare after age 15. Slightly increased among men	Sudden onset; symptoms rarely present more than 6 weeks prior to diagnosis	Very responsive to chemotherapy	5-year survival: 50%. Some indefinite disease-free survivors; slightly poorer prognosis in adults
Chronic lymphocytic leukemia	Most commonly 50 to 70 years old; rare before age 35; increased incidence with age. Greatly increased among men	Symptoms may not interfere with life of patient for years	Not very responsive to chemotherapy; main treatment is to fight infections	Variable; median survival is 7 years
Acute myelogenous leukemia	Most commonly young adults, but nearly equal frequency among all age groups. Slightly increased among men	Onset of symptoms may be abrupt, but usually a prodromal period of 1 to 6 months	Similar to acute lymphocytic leukemia, but needs increased chemotherapy (more resistant to treatment)	Untreated, median survival: 2 months. Treated, median survival: 13 months
Chronic myelogenous leukemia	Most commonly 30 to 50 years old; uncommon before age 20. Slightly increased among men	Usually gradual	Chemotherapy, splenectomy (for splenic enlargement)	Median survival: 3 to 5 years, but eventually all reach blastic crisis

Reprinted with permission from Saunders, B., Nutritional management of the leukemia patient. In J.J. Wollard, Ed., *Nutritional Management of the Cancer Patient.* New York: Raven Press, 1979, p. 121.

normal red blood cell and platelet counts, and the maintenance of competent white blood cells with as low a count of leukemic cells as possible.

Since the leukemic cells are spread throughout the body, surgical excision is not possible. The most frequently used form of treatment is chemotherapy. The drugs used have the various side effects previously described (see Table 13-2), and nutritional care must be that indicated by the side effects. In addition, since many leukemia patients are children, the diet must be adjusted for age.

A newer treatment begins with *whole body irradiation* or higher-dose chemotherapy. This procedure is intended to kill all leukemic cells, but it also kills normal white blood cells, leaving the patient vulnerable to infection. It is followed by a bone marrow transplant. Within a few hours after whole body irradiation, nausea, vomiting, diarrhea, and fever occur. These subside in 1 to 3 days. *Parotitis* (inflammation of the parotid gland) and pancreatitis occur and subside within 1 to 3 days. They may be followed by mucositis, which can endure for several weeks. The patient usually is fed parenterally to avoid infection and to maintain good nutritional status until his or her immunity is reestablished and oral intake increases sufficiently.

A serious complication of bone marrow transplant occurs if the grafted cells, which are immunocompetent, recognize the *host*—that is, the patient—as "foreign." The condition is known as *graft-versus-host disease*

Table 13-5. Sample Diet Progression in Graft-Versus-Host Disease

Approximate Days Following Onset	Intravenous Feeding	Oral Feeding
0–16[a]	Kcal/day: 1.8 × BEE Protein, as crystalline amino acids: 2 g/kg IBW for adults; 2.5–3.0 g/kg IBW for children. Fat emulsion: 500 ml/day for adults; 250 ml/day or a maximum of 4 g/kg IBW for children.	None
17–25[a]	Continue as above	60 ml every 2 to 3 hours of iso-osmotic low-residue beverages.
26–34[a]	Continue as above	Add one solid food every 3 to 4 hours. Foods must be low in fiber, low in acid, low in fat, free of gastric irritants, and contain minimal amounts of lactose. Fat should not exceed 20 to 40 g/day. Include pectin-containing foods.
35–80[a]	As necessary to meet nutritional needs.	Low fiber, low acid, no gastric irritants, minimal amounts of lactose; less than 40 g of fat per day if fat is malabsorbed.
81 or later[a]	Discontinue when nutritional needs are met by oral intake	Add foods containing fiber, lactose,[b] or acids one at a time. Add only one food per day, in order of patient's preference. If patient has no steatorrhea, liberalize fat content.

BEE = basal energy expenditure; IBW = ideal body weight.

[a] Or as tolerated.

[b] Add lactase (LactAid [SugarLo Co.]) to reduce lactose concentration in dairy products.

(*GVHD*). The grafted cells create a severe immune response which affects the skin, liver, lymphoid cells, and gut. Symptoms include nausea, vomiting, anorexia, abdominal pain, and secretory diarrhea. The intestinal lesions resemble celiac disease, Crohn's disease, or chronic ulcerative colitis. Abnormal liver function also may occur, with reduced bile salt production resulting in steatorrhea.

A diet regimen based on experience with a large number of patients has been suggested.[75] These recommendations are summarized in Table 13-5. Patients receive total parenteral nutrition through a central line, sometimes for an extended period (see Table 13-5). This support is continued while oral intake increases from liquid formulas to a low-fat, low-lactose, low-fiber, low-acid diet. The diet is liberalized as tolerated.

Most patients are receiving steroid medications which can induce osteoporosis. They should ingest 1,200 to 1,500 mg of calcium and 400 IU of vitamin D daily. High-potassium foods may be needed to provide 3,000 mg/day to patients with diarrhea. Supplements may be needed in addition.

Immunotherapy is a new form of treatment which is used as an adjunct to other treatments. It attempts to stimulate the body's immune system to attack the cancer cell as a foreign cell. Side effects include chills, fever, malaise, and nausea. Small frequent feedings with a large amount of fluid are helpful.

Case Study: Leukemia and Chemotherapy*

Mrs. R. is a 32-year-old woman who was admitted with a recent diagnosis of acute myelogenous leukemia and fever. She is to be started on chemotherapy. The patient complains of vomiting, loss of appetite, mucositis, and oral lesions, and denies feeling nauseous. Her chart includes the following information:

Procedures: Multiple bone marrow aspirates
Medications

Serax
ARA-C
Daunorubicin
Trilafon
Nembutal
Lomotil
Neutra-Phos
K-Lor
Tobramycin sulfate
Ticarcillin disodium
Amphotericin B
Mycostatin
Xylocaine 2% Viscous Solution
Mylanta

Laboratory values

Admission:

Red blood cell count	$3.12 \times 10^6/mm^3$
Hemoglobin	9.0 g/dl
Hematocrit	27.3 percent
White blood cell count	$2.3 \times 10^3/mm^3$
Blood urea nitrogen	2 mg/dl
Serum cholesterol	103 mg/dl
Others	Within normal limits

Three weeks later:

Serum albumin	2.8 g/dl
Serum calcium	8.2 mg/dl
Serum phosphate	1.8 units/dl
Serum creatinine	0.4 mg/dl
Others	Unchanged

Height: 5 ft 3 in.
Weight

Usual	47.7–50 kg
At admission	46.4 kg
At 3 weeks	44.3 kg

Without dentures: Secondary lesions
Social history: Married; lives with husband and 15-year-old son. Works as a hairdresser.
Food dislikes: "Thick foods," gravies, mayonnaise, fish, spicy foods.

Exercises

1. How does each laboratory value compare to normal values?
2. Give the purpose of each medication.
3. What nutrition problems would you anticipate as a result of chemotherapy?
4. Using the information given, how would you assess the patient's nutritional status?
5. What diet would you recommend?
6. What are the advantages of preventing weight loss?

* Adapted from a case study provided by Mary Ellen Collins, R.D., of Brigham and Women's Hospital, Boston, Mass.

References

1. Rawson, R.W. The role of nutrition in the etiology and prevention of cancer. *Nutr. Cancer* 2:17, 1980.
2. Colman, K.C. Nutrition and cancer. In J.R. Richards and J.M. Kinney, Eds., *Nutritional Aspects of Care of the Critically Ill.* Edinburgh: Churchill Livingstone, 1977.
3. Carroll, K.K., and Khor, H.T. Dietary fat in relation to tumorigenesis. *Prog. Biochem. Pharmacol.* 10:308, 1970.
4. Wynder, E.L., and Reddy, B.S. Metabolic epidemiology of colorectal cancer. *Cancer* 34:801, 1974.
5. Burkitt, D.P. Epidemiology of cancer of the colon and rectum. *Cancer* 28:3, 1971.
6. Burkitt, D.P. Benign and malignant tumors of the large bowel. In D.P. Burkitt and H.C. Trowell, Eds., *Refined Carbohydrate Foods and Disease.* London: Academic, 1975.
7. Weisburger, J.H., Reddy, B., Hill, P., et al. Nutrition and cancer—on the bearing on causes of cancer of the colon, breast, prostate,

and stomach. *Bull. N.Y. Acad. Med.* 56:673, 1980.

8. Wynder, E.L., Covey, L.S., Mabucki, K., and Mushinski, M. Environmental factors in cancer of the larynx. *Cancer* 38:1591, 1976.
9. Chronic effects of alcohol. *Br. Med. J.* 2:381, 1978.
10. Wynder, E.L. The dietary environment and cancer. *J. Am. Diet. Assoc.* 71:385, 1977.
11. Berenblum, I. Established principles and unresolved problems in carcinogenesis. *J. Natl. Cancer Inst.* 60:723, 1978.
12. Lipsett, M.B. Interaction of drugs, hormones and nutrition in the causes of cancer. *Cancer* 43:1967, 1979.
13. Armstrong, B., and Doll, R. Environmental factors and cancer incidence and mortality incidence in different countries with special reference to dietary practices. *Int. J. Cancer* 15:617, 1975.
14. MacDonald, P.C., Edman, C.D., Hemsell, D.L., et al. Effect of obesity on conversion of plasma androstenedione to estrone in postmenopausal women with and without endometrial cancer. *Am. J. Obstet. Gynecol.* 130:448, 1978.
15. Carroll, K.K., Gammel, E.B., and Plunkett, E.R. Dietary fat and mammary cancer. *Can. Med. Assoc. J.* 98:590, 1968.
16. Drasar, B.S., and Irving, D. Environmental factors and cancer of the colon and breast. *Br. J. Cancer* 27:167, 1973.
17. Hems, G. Epidemiological characteristics of breast cancer in middle and late age. *Br. J. Cancer* 24:226, 1970.
18. Jackson, M.A., Ahluwalia, B.S., Herson, J., et al. Characterization of prostatic carcinoma among blacks: A continuation report. *Cancer Treat. Rep.* 61:167, 1977.
19. Theologides, A. Nutritional management of the patient with advanced cancer. *Postgrad. Med.* 61:97, 1977.
20. Costa, G., and Donaldson, S.S. Effects of cancer and cancer treatment on the nutrition of the host. *N. Engl. J. Med.* 300:1471, 1979.
21. DeWys, W.D. Anorexia in cancer patients. *Cancer Res.* 37:2354, 1977.
22. DeWys, W.D. Anorexia as a general effect of cancer. *Cancer* 43:2013, 1979.
23. DeWys, W.D. Taste and feeding behavior in patients with cancer. In M. Winick, Ed., *Nutrition in Cancer.* Current Concepts in Nutrition, vol. 5. New York: John Wiley and Sons, 1977.
24. DeWys, W.D., and Walters, K. Abnormalities of taste sensation in cancer patients. *Cancer* 36:1888, 1975.
25. DeWys, W.D. Changes in taste sensation and feeding behavior in cancer patients: A review. *J. Hum. Nutr.* 32:447, 1978.
26. Nielsen, S.S., Theologides, A., and Vickers, A.M. Influence of food odors on food aversions and preferences in patients with cancer. *Am. J. Clin. Nutr.* 33:2253, 1980.
27. Krause, R., James, H., Humphrey, C., et al. Cancer anorexia: A plasma amino acid–mediated phenomenon. Presented at the First European Congress on Parenteral and Enteral Nutrition, Stockholm, September 1979.
28. Theologides, A. Anorexia-producing intermediary metabolites. *Am. J. Clin. Nutr.* 29:552, 1976.
29. Douglas, H.O. Hyperalimentation in gastrointestinal cancer. *Contemp. Surg.* 13:35, 1978.
30. Munro, H.N. Tumor-host competition for nutrients in the cancer patient. *J. Am. Diet. Assoc.* 71:380, 1977.
31. Levinson, C., and Hemping, H.G. The role of ion transport in the regulation of respiration in Ehrlich mouse ascites—tumor cells. *Biochim. Biophys. Acta* 135:306.
32. Warnold, I., Lundholm, K., and Schersten, T. Energy balance and body composition in cancer patients. *Cancer Res.* 38:1801, 1978.
33. Waterhouse, C. How tumors affect host metabolism. *Ann. N.Y. Acad. Sci.* 230:86, 1974.
34. Waterhouse, C.L., Fenninger, L.D., and Keutmann, E.H. Nitrogen exchange and caloric expenditure in patients with malignant neoplasm. *Cancer* 4:500, 1951.
35. Kisner, D.L., and DeWys, W.D. Anorexia and cachexia in malignant disease. In G.R. Newell and N.M. Ellison, Eds., *Nutrition and Cancer: Etiology and Treatment.* Progress in Cancer Research and Therapy, vol. 17. New York: Raven Press, 1981.
36. Marks, P., and Bishop, J. The glucose metabolism of patients with malignant disease and of normal subjects as studied by means of an intravenous glucose tolerance test. *J. Clin. Invest.* 36:254, 1957.
37. Kisner, D., Hamosh, M., Blecker, M., et al. Malignant cachexia: Insulin resistance and insulin receptors. *Proc. Am. Assoc. Cancer Res.* 19:199, 1978.
38. Lundholm, K., Holm, G., and Schersten, T. Insulin resistance in patients with cancer. *Cancer Res.* 33:4665, 1978.
39. Holroyde, C.P., Gabuzda, T.G., Putnam, R.C., et al. Altered glucose metabolism in metastatic carcinoma. *Cancer Res.* 35:3710, 1975.
40. Waterhouse, C. Lactate metabolism in patients with cancer. *Cancer* 33:66, 1974.

41. Fenninger, L.D., and Mider, G.B. Energy and nitrogen metabolism in cancer. *Adv. Cancer Res.* 2:229, 1954.
42. Young, V.R. Energy metabolism and requirements in the cancer patient. *Cancer Res.* 37:2336, 1977.
43. Wright, C.J., Duff, J.H., McLean, A.P.H., and MacLean, L.D. Regional capillary blood flow and oxygen uptake in severe sepsis. *Surg. Gynecol. Obstet.* 132:637, 1971.
44. Liebelt, R.A., Liebelt, A.G., and Johnstone, H.M. Lipid mobilization and food intake in experimentally obese mice bearing transplanted tumors. *Proc. Soc. Exp. Biol. Med.* 138:482, 1971.
45. Stein, T.P. Cachexia, gluconeogenesis and progressive weight loss in cancer patients. *J. Theor. Biol.* 73:51, 1978.
46. Steinfield, J.L. I^{131}-albumin degradation in patients with neoplastic disease. *Cancer* 13:974, 1960.
47. Mider, G.B., Tesluk, J., and Morton, J.J. Effects of Walker Carcinoma 256 on food intake, body weight and nitrogen metabolism of growing rats. *Acta Unio Int. Contra Cancrum* 6:409, 1948.
48. Buzby, G.P., Mullen, J.L., Stein, T.P., et al. Host-tumor interaction and nutrient supply. *Cancer* 45:2940, 1980.
49. Gold, J. Cancer cachexia and gluconeogenesis. *Ann. N.Y. Acad. Sci.* 230:103, 1974.
50. Rodman, D., Del Rio, A., Akgun, S., and Frumin, F. Novel proteins and peptides in the urine of patients with advanced cancer disease. *Am. J. Med.* 46:174, 1969.
51. Theologides, A. Cancer cachexia. *Cancer* 43:2004, 1979.
52. Mullen, J.L., Buzby, G.P., Gertner, M.H., et al. Protein synthesis dynamics in human gastrointestinal malignancies. *Surgery* 87:331, 1980.
53. Lawrence, W. Effects of cancer on nutrition: Impaired organ system effects. *Cancer* 43:2020, 1979.
54. Leffall, L.D. Summary of the informal discussion of impaired organ system effects of cancer on nutrition. *Cancer Res.* 37:2379, 1977.
55. Welch, D. Nutritional consequences of carcinogenesis and radiation therapy. *J. Am. Diet. Assoc.* 78:467, 1981.
56. Conger, A.D. Loss and recovery of taste acuity in patients irradiated to the oral cavity. *Radiat. Res.* 53:338, 1973.
57. Cooper, G.P. Receptor origin of the olfactory bulb response to ionizing radiation. *Am. J. Physiol.* 215:803, 1968.
58. Levy, C.J., Carroll, M.E., Smith, J.C., and Hofer, K.G. Antihistamines block radiation-induced taste aversions. *Science* 186:1044, 1974.
59. Roswit, B. Complications of radiation therapy: The alimentary tract. *Semin. Roentgenol.* 9:51, 1974.
60. Bowers, R.F., and Brick, I.B. Surgery in radiation injury of the stomach. *Surgery* 22:20, 1947.
61. Borison, H.L. Area postrema: Chemoreceptor trigger zone for vomiting—is that all? *Life Sci.* 14:1807, 1974.
62. Cockel, P. Anti-emetics. *Practitioner* 206:56, 1971.
63. Warren, S. The immediate cause of death in cancer. *Am. J. Med. Sci.* 184:610, 1932.
64. Costa, G., and Donaldson, S. The nutritional effects of cancer and its therapy. *Nutr. Cancer* 2:22, 1980.
65. Buzby, G.P., Mullen, J.L., Matthews, D.C., et al. Prognostic nutritional index in gastrointestinal surgery. *Am. J. Surg.* 139:160, 1979.
66. Copeland, E.M., MacFadyen, B.V., and Dudrick, S.J. Effect of intravenous hyperalimentation on established delayed hypersensitivity in the cancer patient. *Ann. Surg.* 184:60, 1976.
67. Newhouse, M., Sanchis, J., and Bienenstock, J. Lung defense mechanisms. *N. Engl. J. Med.* 295:990, 1976.
68. Copeland, E.M., MacFadyen, B.V., MacComb, W.S., et al. Intravenous hyperalimentation in patients with head and neck cancer. *Cancer* 35:606, 1975.
69. Copeland, E.M., Suchon, E.A., MacFadyen, B.V., et al. Intravenous hyperalimentation as an adjunct to radiation therapy. *Cancer* 39:609, 1977.
70. Filler, R.M., Jaffe, N., Cassady, J.R., et al. Parenteral nutritional support in children with cancer. *Cancer* 39:2665, 1977.
71. Copeland, E.M., Daly, J.M., and Dudrick, S.J. Nutrition as an adjunct to cancer treatment in the adult. *Cancer Res.* 37:2451, 1977.
72. Cooper-Stephenson, C., and Theologides, A. Nutrition in cancer: Physicians' knowledge, opinions and educational needs. *J. Am. Diet. Assoc.* 78:472, 1981.
73. Shils, M.E. Principles of nutritional therapy. *Cancer* 43:2093, 1979.
74. Harvey, K.B., Bothe, A., and Blackburn, G.L. Nutritional assessment and patient outcome during oncological therapy. *Cancer* 43:2065, 1979.
75. Gauvreau, J.M., Lenssen, P., Cheney, C.L., et al. Nutritional management of patients with

intestinal graft-versus-host disease. *J. Am. Diet. Assoc.* 79:673, 1981.

Bibliography

Buzby, G.P., Mullen, J.L., Stein, T.P., et al. Host-tumor interaction and nutrient supply. *Cancer* 45:2940, 1980.

Carson, J.A.S., and Gormican, A. Taste acuity and food attitudes of selected patients with cancer. *J. Am. Diet. Assoc.* 70:361, 1977.

Hegedus, S., and Pelham, M. Dietetics in a cancer hospital. *J. Am. Diet. Assoc.* 67:238, 1975.

Munro, H.N. Tumor-host competition for nutrients in the cancer patient. *J. Am. Diet. Assoc.* 71:380, 1977.

Newell, G.R., and Ellison, N.M., Eds., *Nutrition and Cancer: Etiology and Treatment.* Progress in Cancer Research and Therapy, vol. 17. New York: Raven Press, 1981.

Oram-Smith, J.C., Stein, T.P., Wallace, H.W., and Mullen, J.L. Intravenous nutrition and tumor-host protein metabolism. *J. Surg. Res.* 22:499, 1977.

Pitot, H.C. *Fundamentals of Oncology,* 2nd ed. New York: Marcel Dekker, 1981.

Suen, J.Y., and Myers, E.N., Eds. *Cancer of the Head and Neck.* New York: Churchill Livingstone, 1981.

Theologides, A. Pathogenesis of cachexia in cancer. *Cancer* 29:484, 1972.

Theologides, A. Anorexia-producing intermediary metabolites. *Am. J. Clin. Nutr.* 29:552, 1976.

vanEys, J., Seelig, M.S., and Nichols, B.L., Jr. *Nutrition and Cancer.* New York: SP Medical and Scientific Books, 1979.

Wollard, J.J., Ed. *Nutritional Management of the Cancer Patient.* New York: Raven Press, 1979.

Sources of Current Information

British Journal of Cancer
Cancer
Cancer Research
International Journal of Cancer
Journal of the National Cancer Institute
JPEN. Journal of Parenteral and Enteral Nutrition
Nutrition and Cancer
Radiation Research

14. Nutritional Anemias

Robert B. Rucker, Ph.D.

Anemia most often implies a reduction in the quantity of *hemoglobin* or in the number of *red cells* (*erythrocytes*) in blood. Its major pathophysiologic effect is a reduction in the oxygen-carrying capacity of blood which can lead to tissue *hypoxia* (low oxygen content). Signs of anemia are common to many diseases and disorders; therefore, anemia is a symptom of disease rather than a disease itself.

Almost all forms of anemia involve nutrition in their treatment. In this chapter, some of the major types of anemias will be described and the roles of various nutrients in *erythropoiesis* (production of red blood cells) and hemoglobin synthesis will be discussed. Normal values are given in Appendix F. Nutrients such as iron, folic acid, vitamin B_{12}, protein, and ascorbic acid are very important to normal red blood cell and hemoglobin formation; defective erythropoiesis may result from defects in the metabolism of copper, vitamin A, vitamin E, niacin, pyridoxine, riboflavin, and thiamine. Fortunately, the understanding of how this diverse array of nutrients may alter normal erythropoiesis or hemoglobin synthesis is facilitated by the knowledge that many nutrients act through related mechanisms. Steps involved in the development of erythrocytes and the synthesis of hemoglobin are described in the following sections. It is important to understand the key features of these steps to understand the mechanisms that underlie nutrition's role in the treatment of anemias.

ERYTHROPOIESIS AND HEMOGLOBIN SYNTHESIS

Developmental Features of Red Blood Cell Formation

The first signs of vascular system development occur during the third week of embryogenesis. As described in Chapter 4, the cells associated with the development of the vascular system are *mesenchymal* (mesodermal) in origin. The mesenchymal cells destined to become hemoglobin-synthesizing cells (*erythroblasts*) first form unique clusters of cells called *blood islands.* In the fetus, the blood islands are initially confined to the yolk sac, spleen, and liver. However, by the fourth month of development, erythropoiesis also occurs in bone. Throughout fetal development, erythropoiesis is both *medullary* (in the bone marrow) and *extramedullary* (in tissues other than bone). After birth, the bone marrow progressively takes over the function of erythropoiesis so that, in young children and adults, significant extramedullary erythropoiesis usually is observed only under abnormal circumstances.[1,2] Figure 14-1 illustrates the expansion and regression of hematopoietic or erythropoietic tissue during fetal and adult life. With time, hematopoietic function from medullary sources is progressively reduced, as only replacement of red blood cells is needed by the time that adolescent growth is completed. In bone marrow, the major types of blood cells are derived from progenitor or *stem cells,* as described in Chapter 4.

Major factors that influence red blood cell development and formation are (1) the concentration of hemoglobin within the cell, (2) *erythropoietic stimulating factor,* also referred to as *erythropoietin,*[3] and (3) the supply of essential nutrients (Fig. 14-2).

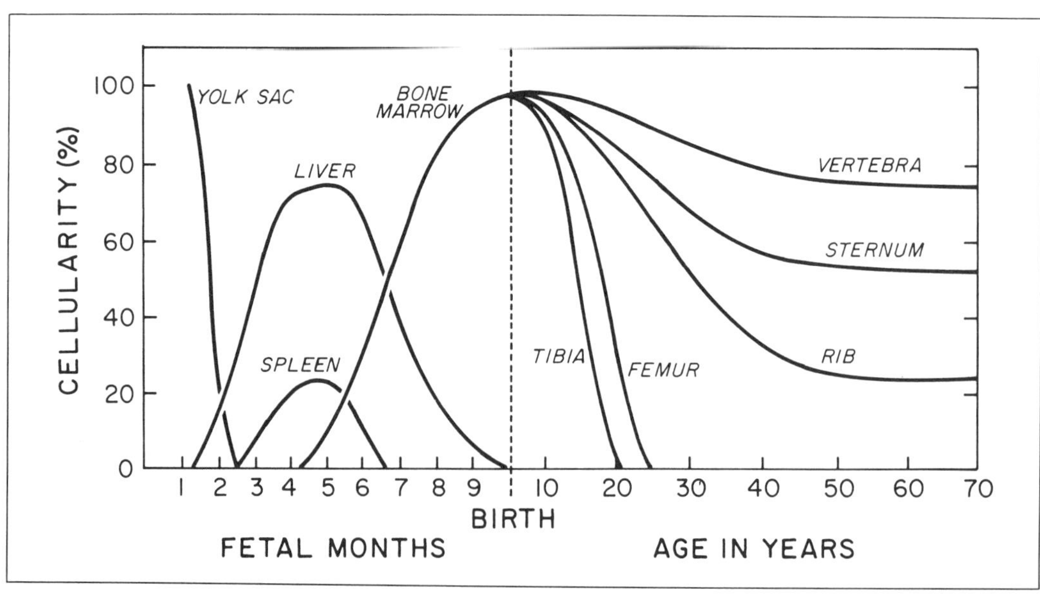

Figure 14-1. Relative contribution of different hematopoietic tissues to and time course of red blood cell production during fetal and adult life. (Adapted with permission from Ersley, A.J., and Gabuzda, T.G., Pathophysiology of Blood, *2nd ed. Philadelphia: W.B. Saunders, 1979, p. 3.)*

Red Blood Cell Maturation and Turnover

Role of Erythropoietin

Erythropoietin causes an acceleration in the maturation of erythroid-committed cells to form erythroblasts. When tissue oxygen tension is low, the kidney releases an enzyme that activates an inactive erythropoietin precursor found in plasma. Once activated, erythropoietin stimulates erythrocyte maturation. Erythropoietin also influences hemoglobin synthesis by stimulating the synthesis of messenger RNA (mRNA) for hemoglobin. Figure 14-3 depicts the role of erythropoietin in the erythroid cell cycle. It is based on observations that a loss of red blood cells and increased hypoxia cause an increase in net erythropoietin production.[3]

Role of Hemoglobin

The concentration of hemoglobin and byproducts of hemoglobin synthesis also are

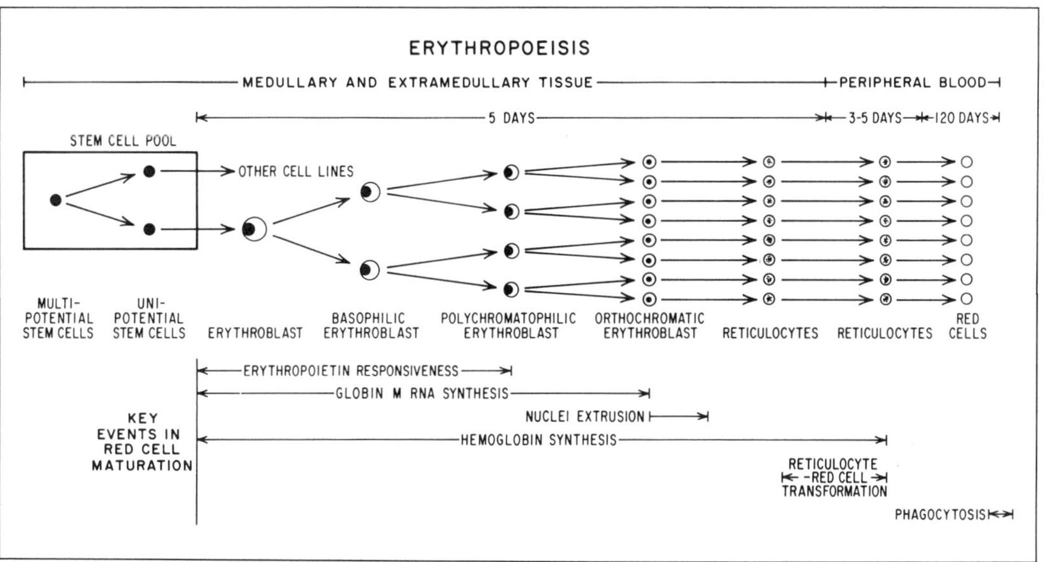

Figure 14-2. Stepwise maturation of erythroid cells. From the stem cell pool, multipotential stem cells differentiate into cells of a given cell line. In the erythroid series, the erythroblast is the first distinguishable cell which quickly divides to form a series of daughter cells (basophilic, polychromatophilic, and orthochromatic erythroblasts). Basophilic and polychromatophilic daughter cells are responsive to erythropoietin. At the orthochromatic stage, the nucleus of the cell is extruded and there is transformation to reticulocytes. Reticulocytes then are released into peripheral blood and transform into mature red blood cells. Approximate times for some of these transformations are given, as well as some key events in the various steps of red blood cell maturation.

important in the regulation of erythropoiesis.[1] High concentrations of hemoglobin cause relatively fewer cell divisions to take place before an erythroblast is transformed into a reticulocyte. Further, the concentration of hemoglobin acts as an internal negative feedback control on hemoglobin synthesis. Thus, both hemoglobin concentration and erythropoietin can influence considerably the steps in red blood cell maturation.

The first form of the erythroid cell, the *pronormoblast,* is a large cell containing a nucleus that occupies approximately 75 percent of the cell. The terms *basophilic, polychromatophilic,* and *orthochromatic* indicated in Fig. 14-2 are used to describe the changes in cellular characteristics that accompany the increased hemoglobin content and stepwise reduction in cellular and nuclear size during maturation. The cellular color change progresses from blue to red. At the orthochromatic stage the nucleus of the erythroblast is extruded, giving rise to cells called *reticulocytes.*[2] A *reticulum* is a network, and reticulocytes have netlike fibers in the cytoplasm.

Reticulocytes are young red blood cells still capable of synthesizing hemoglobin. They contain mRNA and the machinery for protein synthesis but no nucleus and little or no DNA. They are the most immature cells that normally appear in circulating blood and lose their potential for hemoglobin synthesis as they transform into mature red blood cells, erythrocytes. When stimulated by erythropoietin and when hemoglobin synthesis is optimal, the time required for these various processes is only a few days. The erythrocyte or red blood cell, however, normally persists in the circulation for several months.

At the point when hemoglobin synthesis is nearly completed, the reticulocyte penetrates the vascular linings of bone marrow

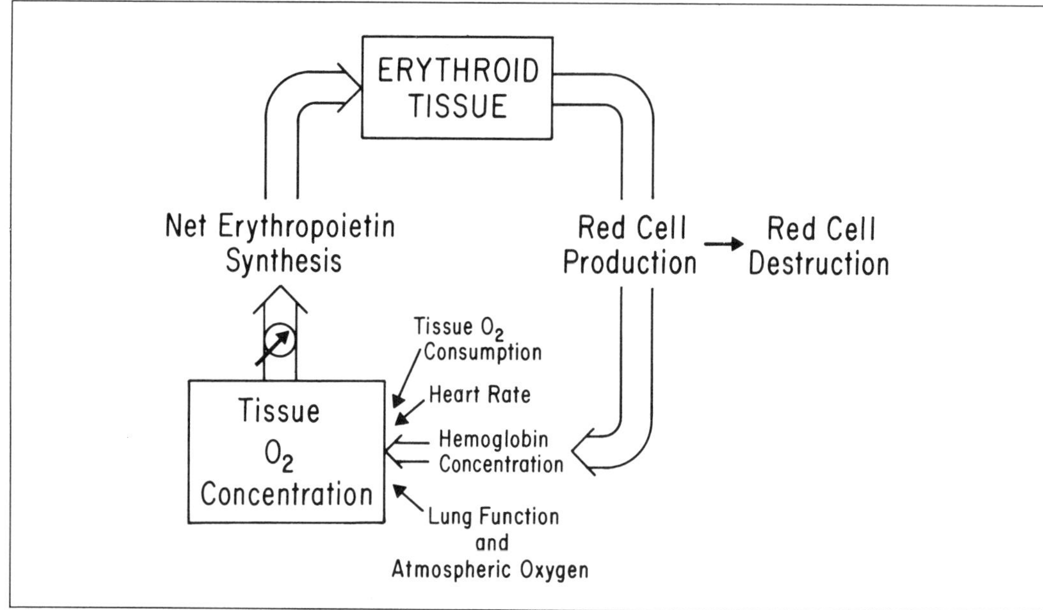

Figure 14-3. Regulation of erythroid cell maturation by erythropoietin. The body tissue concentration of oxygen (O_2) is influenced by numerous factors, such as O_2 consumption by the tissue, heart rate, hemoglobin concentration, and lung function. When the tissue concentration of O_2 is lowered, erythropoietin precursors in circulation are activated to stimulate formation of new red blood cells.

and enters into the circulation. It takes on the shape of a red blood cell, a biconcave disk, and loses its protein synthetic activity. Its metabolic activity now is governed largely by the initial content of nutrients which gradually are depleted as the cell ages.

Erythrocytes remain in the circulation for approximately 120 days before they are destroyed by phagocytic processes. With shape changes due to denaturation and the abnormal packing of hemoglobin, aged red blood cells become vulnerable to phagocytic action of macrophages in organs such as the spleen and liver (Fig. 14-4).[4]

Hemoglobin Synthesis and Degradation

Since erythroid cell maturation is controlled in part by hemoglobin concentration, it is important to appreciate some of the steps in hemoglobin biosynthesis.[5] Hemoglobin is composed of four protein subunits. The oxygen-binding capacity of hemoglobin depends on the appropriate association of two identical subunits and two other subunits that may or may not be identical. For example, in normal adults, 95 percent of the hemoglobin is composed of two identical subunits, designated as alpha chains, and two identical subunits, designated as beta chains. Other nonalpha chains predominate in hemoglobin during fetal development and in certain diseases, such as thalassemia (Fig. 14-5). The chemical characteristics of the protein or *globin* subunits are different enough so that it is possible to distinguish fetal blood from adult blood by a variety of clinical procedures.

Before these subunits are converted to active hemoglobin, there is need for the attachment of *heme.* Heme consists of a porphyrin ring structure that contains *iron.* The synthesis of heme occurs in the mitochondria of pronormoblasts. Nutritional deficiencies, such as iron or pyridoxine deficiency, often cause decreased heme biosynthesis. Details regarding these relationships

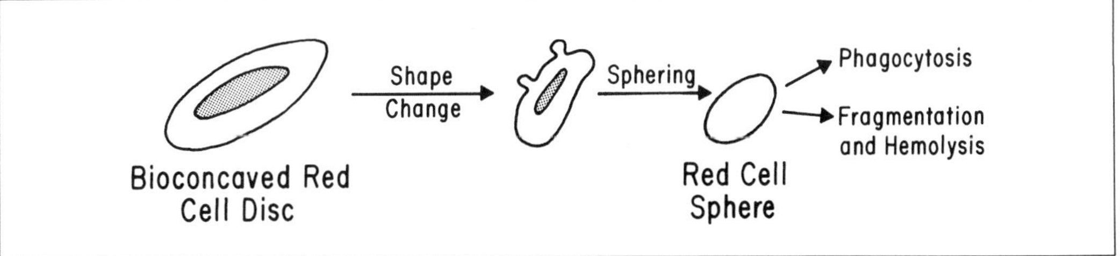

Figure 14-4. Steps in the destruction of the red blood cell. The aged red blood cell transforms from a biconcave disk into a sphere. The spheres are trapped in the fenestrated vasculature of organs such as the spleen. The trapping then is followed by phagocytosis. Some red blood cells also are fragmented as they penetrate small capillaries and are lost owing to hemolytic processes.

Figure 14-5. The change in globin chains during intrauterine development. (Reprinted with permission from Bunn, H.F., Forget, B.G., and Ranney, H.M., Human Hemoglobins. *Philadelphia: W.B. Saunders, 1977, p. 107. As adapted from Rucknagel, D.L., and Laros, R.K., Jr., Hemoglobinopathies. Genetics and implications for studies of human reproduction.* Clin. Obstet. Gynecol. *12:49, 1969; and Bunn, H.F., Hemoglobin I. Structure and function. In W.S. Beck, Ed.,* Hematology, *2nd ed. Cambridge, Mass.: MIT Press, 1977.)*

are discussed more completely in the following sections. The importance of heme lies in its ability to bind oxygen. Thus, factors that influence heme synthesis can ultimately influence systemic oxygen concentration.

When red blood cells are fragmented, the hemoglobin that is released from the red cell is degraded by lysosomal proteinases. The heme portion undergoes several modifications that give rise to products which are excreted via bile. As shown in Fig. 14-6, heme is first degraded to biliverdin and eventually to bilirubin. When heme is degraded in nonhepatic tissue, bilirubin is released into circulation and binds to albumin. Following its transport to the liver, it mixes with the liver pool of bilirubin and normally is excreted via the bile. Elevated blood

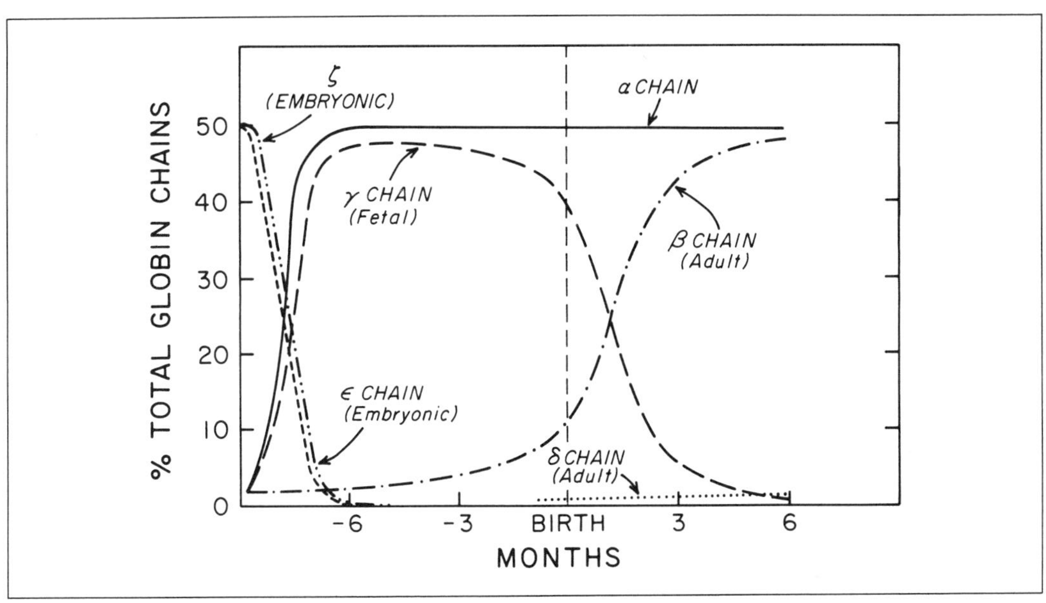

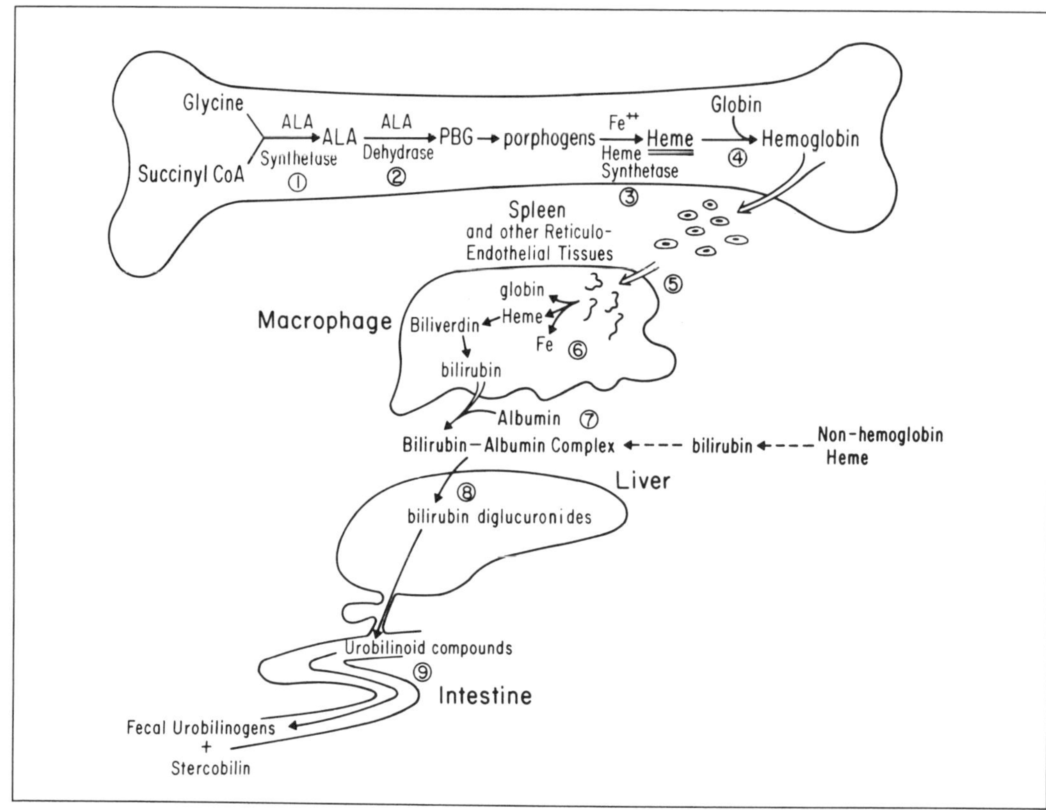

Figure 14-6. Summary of the major steps involved in heme synthesis and degradation. The initial steps (1 and 2) take place in the mitochondria of erythroid cells and require first the synthesis of alpha-aminolevulinic acid (ALA) and porphobilinogen (PBG). The third step comes at the end of the pathway and represents the site where iron is inserted into heme. Heme then combines with each of the four globin chains of hemoglobin in the red blood cell. After the red blood cell has served its function (step 4), it is degraded (step 5). Iron is released, globin is degraded, and heme first is converted to biliverdin (step 6) and then is transported to the liver (step 7) for eventual elimination (steps 8 and 9). CoA = coenzyme A.

plasma levels of bilirubin often serve as a clinical marker for liver damage and biliary obstruction (see Chapter 11).

Important Nutrients Involved in Erythropoiesis

Many nutrients influence the rate of red blood cell formation and hemoglobin synthesis. The body's need for iron,[6] folic acid, vitamin B_{12}, and other vitamins[7] is closely related to synthesis of new red blood cells and hemoglobin.

Iron

The iron required for synthesis of a normal concentration of hemoglobin to replace 1 percent of the red blood cell mass (the amount lost each day) is approximately 25 mg. Most of this iron comes from internal storage or is released from degraded hemoglobin. The released iron usually is stored in liver, spleen, and muscle, bound to the intracellular protein complexes *ferritin* or *hemosiderin*. The term *hemosiderin* is used for poorly defined iron-protein complexes in cells. The presence of hemosiderin in high amounts in liver or the release of ferritin into circulation often indicates excessive or optimal iron storage.

An important feature of iron regulation is the consistent reuse of internal stores of iron. Iron is not readily excreted from the body, and the major losses of iron occur only when red blood cells or epithelial cells are lost. Entry of iron from intestinal mucosal cells, however, is rapid when the body stores of iron are low. To a degree, intestinal cells appear to be able to sense when the body stores of iron are low or elevated, and they regulate iron absorption accordingly.

Iron is transported in circulation by the protein *transferrin.* The erythroblasts in bone marrow are known to have receptors for transferrin. Once associated with these receptors, iron is taken up by the erythroblast and transported to mitochondria for eventual use in heme synthesis. Intestinal absorption is controlled in part by the amount of iron that is bound to circulating transferrin.

With respect to the internal circulation of iron, plasma contains enough transferrin to bind approximately 300 to 400 μg of iron per deciliter of blood. In normal individuals, however, only 30 percent or so of this capacity is reached. Normally, this level of 30 percent saturation is maintained by the continual entry of iron from the intestine.

Approximately 70 percent of the body's iron ultimately is delivered for hemoglobin synthesis, and the other 30 percent is directed toward the synthesis of other iron-containing proteins such as myoglobin and various oxidases. When iron is needed for erythropoiesis or by other iron-requiring cells, the removal of iron from transferrin is very efficient. For example, erythroid marrow receives only 5 percent of the cardiac output but extracts 85 percent of the circulating iron. When a cell is saturated with enough iron, it no longer takes up iron efficiently or stores it as ferritin for future use. With a deficiency of dietary iron, there is first a reduction in the saturation of transferrin, which is followed by a reduction in the iron associated with cellular ferritin. These losses subsequently lead to reduced net heme synthesis and, in turn, reduced hemoglobin synthesis.

Another dimension of iron absorption and metabolism is the body's ability to use iron from differing food sources. The relative absorption or availability of iron is related in part to the solubility of iron complexes derived from digestion of food. Iron complexed from foods of animal origin often are more soluble and available than iron complexes from foods of plant origin (Table 14-1).

Folic Acid and Vitamin B_{12}

Folic acid and vitamin B_{12} are important factors in erythropoiesis.[7] These vitamins are involved in purine synthesis, thymidine synthesis, and ultimately, DNA and RNA synthesis (Fig. 14-7). With deficiencies of either folic acid or vitamin B_{12}, the pronormoblast cannot divide normally and its rate of maturation is decreased.

A variety of metabolic and nutritional conditions can promote deficiencies of either vitamin B_{12} or folic acid. Some of these conditions are listed in Table 14-2. They include the impaired synthesis of *intrinsic factor,* a protein derived from the gastric mucosa that is essential for B_{12} absorption, and impaired

Table 14-1. Absorption of Iron from Diets Containing Different Proportions of Foods of Animal Origin

Type of Diet	Assumed Upper Limit of Iron Absorption by Normal Individuals (%)
<10% of calories from foods of animal origin	10
10–25% of calories from foods of animal origin	15
>25% of calories from foods of animal origin	20

Reprinted with permission from FAO/WHO, *Requirements of Ascorbic Acid, Vitamin D, Vitamin B_{12}, Folate, and Iron.* World Health Organization Technical Report Series No. 452, 1970, p. 50.

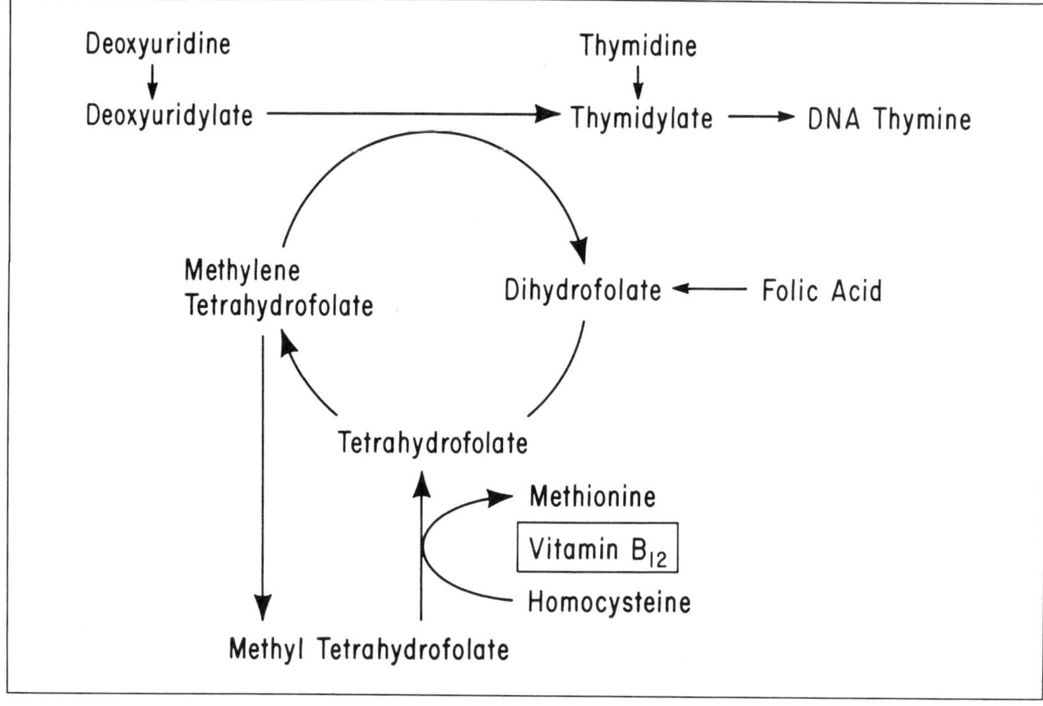

Figure 14-7. Interrelationship between folic acid and vitamin B_{12}. Elevated plasma methyl tetrahydrofolate levels are observed in patients with vitamin B_{12} deficiency due to the inability to convert methyl tetrahydrofolate to tetrahydrofolate or other active forms of folic acid. Because of this lack of active intracellular folates, there is reduced conversion of deoxyuridylate to thymidylate. Unused folate is "trapped" as methyl tetrahydrofolate. Note that the tetrahydrofolate form of the vitamin is the active form. The dihydrofolate form of the vitamin must first be reduced to tetrahydrofolate.

folic acid absorption. Folic acid is found in many foods as polyglutamyl folic acid or conjugated folate. Factors that inhibit activity of intestinal conjugase, an enzyme responsible for the cleavage of glutamyl residues from polyglutamyl folate, interfere with folic acid absorption. These points will be raised again in the section Megaloblastic Anemias (p. 545).

Other Nutrients

In addition to iron, folic acid, and vitamin B_{12}, many other nutrients are involved in erythropoiesis and hematopoiesis. *Pyridoxine* is a cofactor for the enzyme alpha-aminolevulinic acid synthetase (see Fig. 14-6). A deficiency of pyridoxine can result in decreased heme synthesis and, eventually, anemia. Impaired red blood cell formation may also be observed in severe vitamin C, niacin, and thiamine deficiencies.

The dietary intake of *vitamins E* and *A* may also influence erythropoiesis and red blood cell integrity. Vitamin A toxicity can cause changes in red blood cell membranes which, in some instances, result in anemia because of increased red cell destruction. On the other hand, vitamin A deficiency appears to cause an increased accumulation of iron in storage tissues so that iron is not readily released for hematopoiesis. Vitamin E protects red blood cell membranes from oxidative damage. Red blood cell membranes tend to rupture more easily in the presence of oxidants when the vitamin E concentration in the red cell membrane is reduced. There also are reports from experimental animal studies that suggest that de-

Table 14-2. Typical Reasons for Vitamin B_{12} and Folic Acid Deficiency

Category	Etiologic Mechanisms	Category	Etiologic Mechanisms
Vitamin B_{12} deficiency		*Folic acid deficiency (cont'd.)*	
Decreased absorption	Poor diet Intrinsic factor deficiency Pernicious anemia Gastrectomy (total and partial) Destruction of gastric mucosa by caustics Anti–intrinsic factor antibody in gastric juice Abnormal intrinsic factor molecules Intrinsic intestinal disease and selective malabsorption syndromes Ileal resection, ileitis (ileum is site for B_{12} absorption) Sprue, celiac disease Infiltrative intestinal disease (lymphoma, scleroderma, etc.) Drug-induced malabsorption Competitive parasites Fish tapeworm infestation Bacteria in diverticula of bowel, blind loops (bacteria compete for B_{12}) Chronic pancreatic disease	Decreased requirement	Intrinsic intestinal disease Anticonvulsants, oral contraceptives
Increased requirement	Pregnancy Neoplastic disease Hyperthyroidism	Increased requirement	Pregnancy Infancy Hyperactive hematopoiesis Neoplastic disease Skin disease
Folic acid deficiency		Blocked activation	Folic acid and B_{12} antagonists (various chemotherapy drugs) Metabolic inhibitors Purine synthesis: 6-mercaptopurine, 6-thioguanine Pyrimidine synthesis: 6-azauridine Thymidylate synthesis: 5-fluorouracil Deoxyribonucleotide synthesis: hydroxyurea, cytosine arabinoside Inborn errors Lesch-Nyhan syndrome Hereditary orotic aciduria Deficiency of formiminotransferase, methyltransferase, and the like Unexplained disorders Pyridoxine-responsive megaloblastic anemia Thiamine-responsive megaloblastic anemia Erythremic myelosis (Di Guglielmo syndrome)
Decreased absorption	Poor diet Alcoholism Infancy Hemodialysis Intestinal short circuits Steatorrhea Sprue, celiac disease		

creased activity of alpha-aminolevulinic acid synthetase is associated with vitamin E deficiency. This role, however, is secondary to the more important one of protection of the lipid-rich membranes of red blood cells from oxidative damage.

Decreased protein synthesis due to severe protein deficiency can also result in impaired red blood cell formation. This fact is one of the bases for the use of hemoglobin concentration in nutritional assessment, as described in Chapter 2. Finally, *essential fatty acid* deficiency has also been reported to cause alterations in red blood cell membrane composition and structural integrity. A list of some of the anemias and presumed mechanisms involving deficiency of selected nutrients are given in Tables 14-3 and 14-4.

Table 14-3. The Anemias

Anemias due to decreased red blood cell production
- Normocytic anemias
  - From primary bone marrow failure
    - Aplastic anemia
    - Myelopathic (e.g., leukemia-related) anemias
  - From secondary causes
    - Chronic inflammation
    - Uremia
    - Hepatic disease
    - Endocrine disorders
- Megaloblastic (macrocytic) anemias
  - From primary nutritional deficiencies
    - Vitamin B_{12}
    - Folic acid
    - Thiamine and pyridoxine (rare)
  - From secondary causes
    - Drugs acting as B_{12} and folate antagonist
    - Orotic aciduria
    - Erythroleukemias
    - Pernicious anemias
- Microcytic anemias
  - From primary nutritional deficiencies
    - Iron
    - Pyridoxine (sideroblastic anemia)
    - Ascorbic acid and vitamin A deficiency
  - From other causes
    - Hemorrhage
    - Forms of thalassemia
    - Drugs and heavy metal intoxication (e.g., lead, cadmium)

Anemias due to increased destruction of red blood cells
- Hemoglobinopathies
  - Sickle cell anemia
  - Thalassemia
- Hemolytic anemias
  - From primary nutritional deficiencies: vitamin E
  - From secondary causes
    - Favism
    - Glucose-6-phosphate dehydrogenase deficiency
    - Drugs
    - Mechanical damage
    - Infection (e.g., malaria)
    - Immunologic disorders

THE ANEMIAS

A classification of anemias is given in Table 14-3. It is emphasized that the general term *anemia* is defined relative to standards that are derived from studies on large populations; therefore, there is no definitive separation between anemic and nonanemic patients. Further, anemia most often is the secondary manifestation of a disease. Although the underlying cause of an anemia may not be nutritional in origin, usually some type of nutritional management is important in the treatment of the anemia.

Normocytic Anemias

The term *normocytic anemia* is used to decribe the condition in which cell size, cell hemoglobin concentration, and reticulocyte count are within normal limits, but the *hematocrit* (packed cell volume or proportion of cells in blood) is low.[8] Normocytic anemias usually are the result of a decreased proliferation of red blood cells from bone marrow. This is *bone marrow failure* in the sense that red blood cells are not released at a normal rate, so there are fewer cells, but the cells that are released have a normal appearance.

Normocytic anemias are the least well understood of all of the hematologic disorders. One form of normocytic anemia is *aplastic anemia.* It is an anemia in which the bone marrow appears to be morphologically and functionally hypoplastic—that is, the amount of functional marrow is decreased. Aplastic anemias often are unresponsive to medicinal iron. They may be caused by ionizing radiation or by drugs and chemical agents such as benzidine, chloramphenicol, selected antimicrobial drugs, and drugs used as anticonvulsants. In rare instances, the use of aspirin or even chemicals in hair dyes have been known to cause aplastic anemia. When aplasticlike anemias are seen in childhood, they usually are genetic in origin. When they are seen in adults, they sometimes are associated with renal failure and thymomas (a relatively rare form of thymic tissue cancer). In patients with chronic renal disease, the red blood cell life span often is shortened, and there may be decreased net erythropoietin production.

The treatment of anemias associated with diseases such as chronic renal failure usually is directed at treatment of the primary disease (see Chapter 7). Often, normocytic anemia associated with the diseases given in Table 14-3 are mild. If the anemia is severe, *blood transfusions* are used to correct the anemia. The transfusions generally are performed to "buy time" until remission occurs. Diets modified to provide additional nu-

Table 14-4. Mechanisms by Which Common Nutrition-Related Anemias Are Promoted

Anemia	Causative Nutrient or Food Component Deficiency	Mechanism
Macrocytic	Vitamin B_{12} and folic acid	Decreased DNA synthesis that retards or inhibits cell division
	Thiamine and pyridoxine	Presumed to be related to decreased DNA synthesis owing to impaired purine synthesis
Microcytic	Iron	Reduced heme synthesis and, subsequently, hemoglobin synthesis
	Ascorbic acid	Presumed to be related to decreased iron utilization
	Vitamin A	Presumed to be related to increased iron storage so that iron is not available for heme synthesis
	Vitamin E	Presumed to be related to decreased heme synthesis
	Pyridoxine	Reduced heme synthesis
	Lead	Reduced heme synthesis
	Copper	Reduced iron use and release for heme synthesis
	Cadmium	Reduced iron and copper use
Hemolytic	Vitamin E	Impaired integrity of red blood cell membrane, which leads to increased susceptibility to damage by oxidants

trients usually are not helpful. The blood transfusion itself can supply iron and other nutrients. Thus, the potential always exists for iron toxicity with repeated transfusions, since the body has no way to eliminate excess iron. One pint of blood contains approximately 250 mg of iron, so fifteen transfusions or more can double the total body iron content of 3.5 g. Obviously, medicinal iron therapy is not needed in these circumstances. Therefore, apart from supplementing the diet with B vitamins such as folic acid and vitamin B_{12}, any diet therapy for the patient with normocytic anemia is not directed at the anemia but at the primary disease or condition underlying the anemia. However, the patient may profit from a diet reduced in dietary iron.

Megaloblastic Anemias

Megaloblastic (large primitive cell, or macrocytic) *anemias* usually are the result of a deficiency of vitamin B_{12} or folic acid or are caused by drugs or conditions that interfere with folic acid and vitamin B_{12} metabolism.[9] For example, megaloblastic anemias may be secondary to enteropathies, such as tropical sprue or gluten sensitivity, or to drug-induced disorders of DNA synthesis, particularly drugs such as methotrexate that act as folic acid antagonists. As described earlier, there is retarded development of the pronormoblasts in megaloblastic anemia which causes a decrease in the rate of erythroblast maturation to reticulocytes and erythrocytes. Megaloblastic cells are easily detected because of their larger size and nuclear content. Abnormal megaloblasts also are often packed with hemoglobin but contain fragmented remnants of nuclear material. The term *megaloblast* denotes any myeloid cell in the leukocyte series that is in transition before mitosis.

The classic form of megaloblastic anemia is *pernicious anemia* which is caused most often by the inability to produce sufficient intrinsic factor. Pernicious anemia was first described in 1855 at Guy's Hospital in England by Thomas Addison. The term *addisonian pernicious anemia* sometimes is used to distinguish true pernicious anemia (decreased intrinsic factor production) from *non-addisonian pernicious anemia* (decreased production of intrinsic factor owing to gastrectomy or lesions of the gastric mucosa). There is a higher incidence of the disease in Scandinavians, a relatively inbred population. The current thought is that pernicious anemia is an autoimmune disorder (see Chapter 4) caused by the presence of the high amounts of anti–intrinsic factor antibodies in serum and gastric juice. There are also very rare forms of juvenile pernicious anemia in which there is failure of intrinsic factor secretion or the production of biologically inert intrinsic factor.

Vitamin B_{12} is efficiently stored, and several years may pass before clear signs of macrocytic anemia due specifically to vitamin B_{12} deficiency are observed. Only in very strict vegetarians, however, should a simple deficiency of vitamin B_{12} be observed, since foods of plant origin do not contain vitamin B_{12} unless contaminated by soil and bacteria. Most often, diet-related macrocytic anemias are due to folic acid deficiency. In contrast to vitamin B_{12}, folic acid may be depleted from the body in 2 to 4 months. Moreover, the absorption and metabolism of folic acid appears to be influenced by a broader spectrum of enteropathies and drug-related problems (particularly those associated with alcohol).

Before initiating nutritional therapy, it is important that the cause of the megaloblastic anemia be determined. For example, administration of only folic acid in the presence of a primary vitamin B_{12} deficiency may correct, in part, the megaloblastic anemia, but it will not correct other signs of vitamin B_{12} deficiency, such as progressive nervous tissue degeneration.

Symptoms of megaloblastic anemia common to both vitamin B_{12} and folic acid deficiency are weakness, dyspnea, and intestinal disorders characterized by either diarrhea or constipation. Other common signs of water-soluble vitamin deficiencies, as well as the clinical signs of macrocytic anemia, may be present. If vitamin B_{12} deficiency is the underlying cause of the anemia, the peripheral and central nerve degeneration may first appear as numbness and tingling in the extremities, diminution of vibratory or postural sense, poor muscle control, or poor memory.

When there is no underlying genetic or systemic cause of megaloblastic anemia, usually a normal diet with increased amounts of protein, iron, vitamin B_{12}, and folic acid is all that is required to correct the condition. With a simple deficiency of vitamin B_{12} or folic acid, recovery is rapid (Fig. 14-8).

Microcytic Anemia

Microcytic (small cell) *anemia* usually is the result of decreased hemoglobin biosynthesis.[5] Red blood cells that are not fully packed with hemoglobin are fairly small. Also, they sometimes do not have the dark red color of normal red blood cells, thus the term *hypochromic microcytic* is used to describe their appearance. *Hypochromic* connotes less color or pigmentation.

Iron deficiency is a major cause of microcytic anemia. For an adult consuming 2,500 calories/day, 10 to 20 mg of iron usually is adequate, assuming that at least 10 percent of the total ingested iron is absorbed. Excessive blood loss, pregnancy, and menstrual losses of iron increase demands for iron. For example, during pregnancy there is expansion of the mother's hemoglobin mass that requires approximately 0.5 to 1.5 mg of absorbed iron per day in addition to the normal requirement. The formation of the placenta, cord, and fetus requires another 400 mg of total iron over the course of pregnancy. The loss of blood at delivery (usually 500 to 600 ml) requires an additional 300 to 350 mg of total iron. Thus, the total iron costs of pregnancy in excess of the normal basal requirements of 1 to 2 mg of absorbed iron per day is equal to approximately 4 mg/day. The hypothetical needs for iron under differing conditions of pregnancy are summarized in Fig. 14-9.

In the early stages of iron deficiency, ferritin stores are depleted and iron absorption increases. Typical of all true anemic states, weakness and dyspnea may occur. A severe iron deficiency also may cause structural and functional changes in epithelial tissues. Another common sign is thin and flat fingernails that eventually take on a spoon-shaped appearance. Gastric ulcers and achlorhydria may occur.

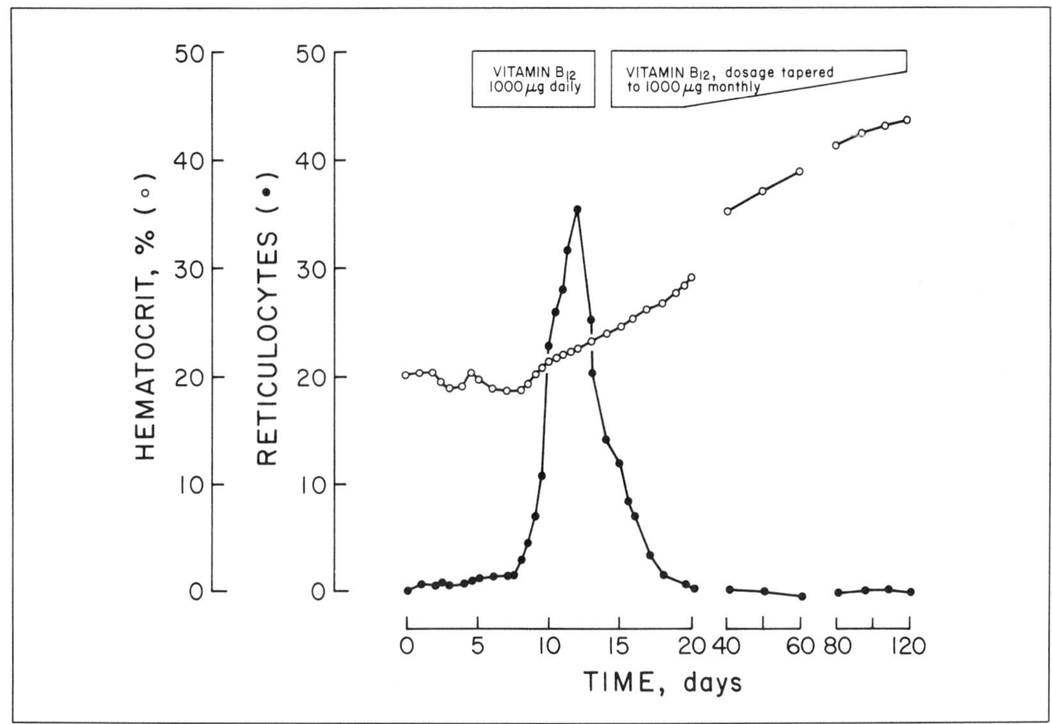

Figure 14-8. Time course for changes in reticulocyte count and hematocrit level during treatment of pernicious anemia with vitamin B_{12}. (Reprinted with permission from Beck, W.S., and Goulian, N., Drugs effective in nutritional anemia and other megaloblastic anemias. In J.R. DiPalma, Ed., Drill's Pharmacology in Medical Practice, *4th ed. New York: McGraw-Hill, 1971, p. 1073.)*

Although iron is best absorbed when little food is given, excessive amounts of elemental iron or iron salts without food can cause gastric irritation; therefore, it is best to administer iron supplements at or following a meal. The gastrointestinal side effects of iron supplements may also be minimized by increasing the supplement slowly over a few days until the required amount is reached. The amounts of iron that are given often amount to 1 to 2 mg/kg of body weight (100 to 200 mg/day). With a simple iron deficiency, this amount usually causes a rapid stimulation of heme synthesis and hemoglobin synthesis. Parenteral administration of iron may be necessary for patients who are unable to take iron orally.

It should be emphasized that in extremely high doses, iron can be very toxic, particularly in children. Doses of 3 to 10 g/day are known to be fatal. High amounts of iron can cause metabolic acidosis and *cirrhosis*—that is, damage to the parenchymal cells in a number of tissues because of the inability of these tissues to store excessive amounts of iron.

It has become increasingly clear that iron plays an important role in the general *host defense mechanisms* of the body against infection. With low levels of iron intake, it has been argued that certain cells involved in host defense, such as leukocytes, do not function optimally. On the other hand, it is documented that a number of bacterial organisms are highly responsive and proliferate in an environment rich in iron. For example, *Salmonella* and *Mycobacterium tuberculosis* undergo significant proliferation in the presence of iron. The concentration of iron in

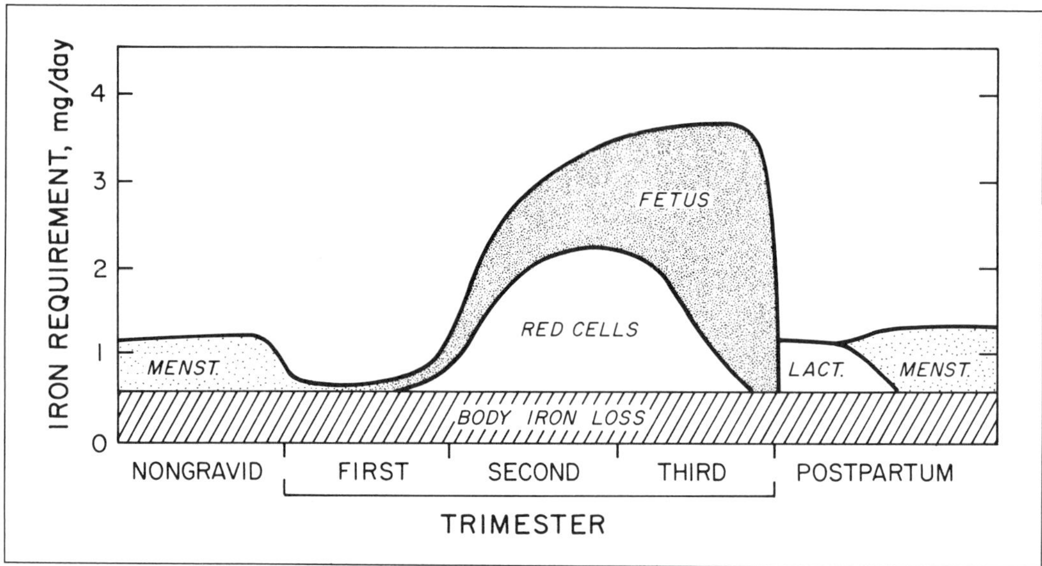

Figure 14-9. The change in iron requirement during pregnancy. Note that the values are for the absorbed iron requirement. Given common food sources, the actual dietary iron intake should be five to ten times the amounts indicated. Menst. = menstruation; Lact. = lactation. (Redrawn and reprinted with permission from Bothwell, T.H., and Finch, C.A., Iron Metabolism. *Boston: Little, Brown, 1962, p. 309.)*

liver, spleen, and other storage tissues often increases with infection, and the amounts of circulating iron decrease. This phenomenon is thought to be a host defense mechanism against infection. As a consequence of the decrease in circulating iron, however, anemia may result from chronic infection. Some clinicians now believe that excessive iron supplementation should be approached cautiously, particularly if the iron supplementation is recommended for only a mild anemia and there are signs of bacterial infection.[10]

Hypochromic microcytic anemia may arise from severe protein deficiency such as that seen in kwashiorkor, intoxication with heavy metals such as lead, and in deficiencies of vitamin A, vitamin E, copper, or pyridoxine. Copper deficiency causes iron to accumulate in storage tissues so that the delivery of iron to bone marrow is impaired. Likewise, pyridoxine deficiency can cause anemia even in the presence of a high level of iron in serum and tissue. Pyridoxine-dependent anemia is distinctive because of the accumulation of iron in erythroblasts. With a decrease in heme synthesis (see Fig. 14-6), iron remains in the mitochondria of erythroblasts and forms inorganic iron complexes. Erythroblasts that contain an excess of iron are called *sideroblasts.* These cells are identified in the laboratory by staining for iron. Sideroblastic anemia can also be a result of inherited defects in the formation of alpha-aminolevulinic acid or defects in other steps in the heme pathway. It should be appreciated, however, that neither copper nor pyridoxine deficiency occur frequently in humans.

The mechanisms by which many heavy metals or deficiencies of vitamins A or E cause microcytic anemia appear to involve decreased heme synthesis or impaired release of iron from storage tissues. (See Table 14-4, which contains suggestions for mechanisms related to common forms of anemia. Note that most of the nutrition-related microcytic anemias involve defects in either iron release from storage tissue or heme biosynthesis.)

Sickle Cell Anemia and Other Hemoglobinopathies

There are many variants in hemoglobin that result from substitutions of only a single amino acid in one or more of the hemoglobin chains.[11] More than 220 human *hemoglobin variants* are known. Most were discovered during the course of population survey studies and are not the cause of clinical syndromes; however, several hemoglobin variants cause serious anemias. One such variant causes *sickle cell anemia,* which occurs predominantly in blacks. In this form of anemia, the red blood cell takes on a peculiar elongated or sickled shape. With inappropriate amino acid substitutions in hemoglobin, there is abnormal packing of hemoglobin in red blood cells, and the red cell takes on a bizarre shape at low oxygen tension. As the cells sickle, they become ridged and can obstruct capillary blood flow. The cells also are ruptured easily so that there is damage to various organs and tissues. Any organ or system may be involved. Approximately 8 percent of blacks in the United States are *heterozygous* for this variant. The *genetic* or *gene frequency* is as high as 30 percent in parts of Central Africa.

The most important feature of nutritional therapy in sickle cell anemia is to assure that there is not excessive iron storage. The diet should be normally low in iron. Iron-rich foods such as liver and iron-fortified cereals should be excluded from the diet. In addition, the diet should be low in fat (less than 30 percent of the total calories), particularly if liver and gallbladder disease accompany the anemia.

Requirements for water-soluble vitamins, however, are often high, because of the need to continually synthesize large numbers of new red blood cells. It has been suggested that zinc supplementation may be helpful. A considerable quantity of zinc is found in erythrocytes, bound to the enzyme carbonic anhydrase. This zinc is lost as the cells are lysed. In contrast to iron, zinc is readily excreted from the body. Also, the sickle cell patient may suffer from ulcerative lesions; supplements of zinc (20 to 30 mg/day) may help to promote normal wound healing.

Thalassemias are another group of disorders that result in anemia. In the thalassemia syndromes, there usually is an absence of or diminished synthesis of one of the globin chains of hemoglobin. For example, in *alpha-thalassemia,* the alpha chain of hemoglobin is absent or reduced in content in the red blood cell. In beta-thalassemia, the beta chain of hemoglobin is absent or reduced in content.

Of the two forms, beta-thalassemia occurs most often and frequently is seen in people of Mediterranean origin. Similar to the sickled red cell, red blood cells in beta-thalassemia take on abnormal shapes. These red blood cells are fragile and rupture easily. Untreated children with beta-thalassemia usually die at an early age. With blood transfusions, however, many children can survive to their early twenties. The nutritional care in this condition is directed toward provision of a well-balanced diet rich in water-soluble vitamins and, if transfusions are a part of the treatment, low in iron.

Hemolytic Anemia

There are always red blood cells of varying age in circulation and, since the red blood cell has a finite life span, there are always red blood cells undergoing destruction. An increased rate of destruction of red blood cells can occur because of mechanical damage (e.g., that which is a result of an artificial heart valve), the effects of various autoimmune disorders, or alterations in red cell shape.[12] Red blood cell membrane defects also may cause rupture of red cells. Increased lysis may occur owing to defects in certain metabolic pathways within the red blood cell that protect against oxidative damage. When red blood cell lysis or *hemolysis* is increased because of one of these processes, *hemolytic anemia* may occur.

Vitamin E deficiency can result in hemolysis of red blood cells. Hemolysis of red cells

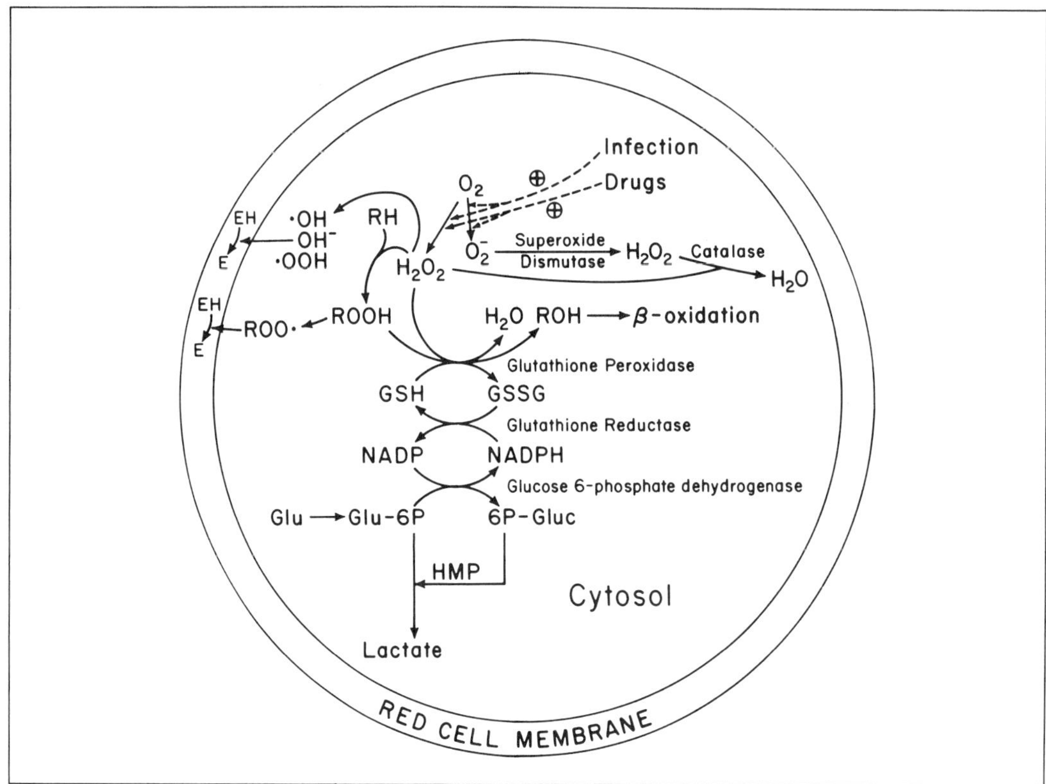

Figure 14-10. Selected steps in the defense against oxidants that alter red blood cell metabolism and membrane integrity. Infections, certain drugs, and some dietary components appear to increase production of peroxides by red blood cells. Superoxide (O_2^-), hydrogen peroxide (H_2O_2), organic and lipid-derived peroxides (ROOH), hydroxyl anions and radicals (OH^-, $\cdot OH$), or hydrogen peroxide radicals ($\cdot OOH$) in high concentration can alter hemoglobin structure and cellular membrane lipids so that hemolysis of the cell may result. Vitamin E (EH) acts within the membrane to protect against the destructive action of oxidants. In the cytosol, superoxide dismutase, glutathione peroxidase (catalyzes the oxidation of glutathione [2GSH → GSSH]), and catalase act to reduce the levels of superoxide and hydrogen peroxides. Essential to these steps is a high cellular concentration of NADPH derived from NADP following the oxidation of glucose-6-phosphate (Glu-6P) to 6-phosphoglucuronic acid (6P-Gluc). These compounds then are metabolized further in the hexose monophosphate shunt pathway (HMP).

is, in fact, one of the few deficiency signs that has been observed consistently in vitamin E–deficient humans. When hemolysis is observed in young infants, vitamin E deficiency may be an underlying cause since infants are born with low stores of vitamin E. In some instances, this appears to result in red blood cell membranes that are more susceptible to oxidative damage and hemolysis. Red cell membranes are composed in part of polyunsaturated lipids. Since unsaturated fats are easily oxidized, the potential for oxidative damage of the red blood cell membrane is high. Hydrogen peroxide and lipid peroxides form when oxygen tension is high. Thus, it is very important for the red blood cell to control the level of peroxide-containing compounds.

Vitamin E works directly within the membrane to protect against oxidative and peroxidative damage (Fig. 14-10). There are also a number of enzymes that act in the cytosol of red blood cells to control the levels of damaging oxidants (see Fig. 14-10). One form of oxygen that is particularly damaging to red blood cells is the *superoxide radical.* The enzyme *superoxide dismutase* functions to limit this form of oxygen to low concentrations. The enzymes *catalase* and *glutathione peroxidase* function to keep cytosol concentrations of hydrogen peroxide low.

Glutathione peroxidase is particularly important in that it reduces both the levels of hydrogen peroxide and lipid peroxides in red blood cells. That glutathione peroxidase is coupled to other enzymes in the red blood cell is also important. An NADPH-synthesizing system is required. NADPH is derived from the production of 6-phosphogluconate from 6-phosphoglucose. The NADPH is used by glutathione reductase to maintain a high level of glutathione, which serves as a cofactor for glutathione peroxidase.

Inherited deficiencies of selected enzymes that result in low levels of NADPH, such as *glucose-6-phosphate dehydrogenase deficiency,* can give rise to increased concentrations of hydrogen peroxide or peroxide-containing compounds within the red blood cell, because of the reduction of NADPH and, subsequently, of glutathione and glutathione peroxidase activity.

The effects of low vitamin E, low NADPH, or low glutathione peroxidase levels, however, usually are not observed until there is a stress on red blood cell metabolism induced by an infection or drugs. It is this type of stress that stimulates peroxide formation. For example, antimalarial drugs, sulfonamides, nitrofurans, and, occasionally, aspirin can precipitate hemolysis in individuals who have a red blood cell deficiency of glucose-6-phosphate dehydrogenase. In patients receiving these drugs, vitamin E has been suggested to be therapeutically helpful in lessening hemolysis.

Dietary factors, too, may be important in precipitating a hemolytic crisis. Signs of acute hemolytic anemia have been observed in individuals (usually of Mediterranean descent) when *fava beans* are consumed as part of the diet. Apparently, components of the fava bean exacerbate peroxidative damage to the red blood cell.

There are a number of nutritional variables to consider when anemia is observed as a secondary response to disease. For each case, good clinical information is needed to determine the anemia classification and the appropriate therapy. The role of the nutritional care specialist is made easier when a good history of the patient is available, since chronic infection, pregnancy, hemorrhage, or large menstrual losses are common underlying causes of anemia. In most instances, the approach to dietary treatment is to establish a well-balanced diet with appropriate supplements. In special instances, however, reduction of intake of selected nutrients such as iron may be indicated.

References

1. Boggs, D.R., and Chervenick, P.A. Hemopoietic stem cells. In T.J. Greenwalt and G.A. Jamieson, Eds., *Formation and Destruction of Blood Cells.* Philadelphia: J.B. Lippincott, 1970.
2. Latjtha, L.G. Haemopoietic stem cells. *Br. J. Haematol.* 29:529, 1975.
3. Goldwasser, E.K. Erythropoietin and the differentiation of red blood cells. *Fed. Proc.* 34:2285, 1975.
4. McIntyre, P.A. The reticuloendothelial system: Organization and physiology. *Johns Hopkins Med. J.* 130:61, 1972.
5. Adamson, J.W., and Finch, C.A. Hemoglobin function, oxygen affinity and erythropoietin. *Annu. Rev. Physiol.* 37:351, 1975.
6. Van Campen, D. Regulation of iron absorption. *Fed. Proc.* 33:100, 1974.
7. National Research Council. *Folic Acid: Biochemistry and Physiology in Relationship to the Human Nutritional Requirement.* Washington, D.C.: National Academy of Sciences, 1975.
8. Scott, J.J., Cartwright, G.E., and Wintrobe, M.M. Acquired aplastic anemia. *Medicine* (Balt.) 37:119, 1959.

9. Beck, W.S. General considerations of megaloblastic anemias. In W.J. Williams, E. Beutler, A.J. Erslev, and R.W. Rundles, Eds., *Hematology,* 2nd ed. New York: McGraw-Hill, 1977, Chapter 34.
10. Pearson, H.A., and Robinson, J.A. The role of iron in host resistance. *Adv. Pediatr.* 23:1, 1976.
11. Bradley, T.B., and Ranney, H.M. Acquired disorders of hemoglobin. *Prog. Hematol.* 8:77, 1973.
12. Machesi, V.T., Furthmayr, H., and Tomita, M. The red cell membrane. *Annu. Rev. Biochem.* 45:667, 1976.

VII. Other Nutrition-Related Problems

15. Disorders of Energy Balance and Body Weight

Increased and decreased body weights are of concern if either is extreme. In terms of numbers of patients, excess body weight is a much more common problem presented to the nutritional care specialist and is considered one of the most prevalent public health problems in the United States. Whereas many people maintain normal body weight with little effort, many others struggle to lose or gain weight to bring their body weights within the limits that are considered desirable in our society. In this chapter, problems characterized by excess or insufficient body weight—that is, obesity and underweight—will be explored first by presenting some general principles and then by a discussion of the etiologies, effects, and various approaches to treatment of obesity and underweight.

Energy intake may consist of food or infused nutrients, and total energy expenditure is the sum of energy used for resting metabolism, physical work, maintenance of body temperature, and thermogenic effects of food. The laws of thermodynamics that govern the universe also apply to human beings and other animals. If a person has an energy intake that is greater than his or her output, he or she is in *positive energy balance* and will store energy and gain weight, primarily as fat. If energy use is greater than energy intake, a person will be in *negative energy balance* and will lose weight. The principle is very simple, but difficulties arise in understanding why some people cannot maintain weight within normal limits.

We do not understand the reasons for the positive energy balance in overweight patients, whether it be the consequence of increased food intake or decreased activity. It is no more helpful to say that a person is fat because he or she eats too much than to say a person is an alcoholic because he or she drinks too much, although we have tended to simplify the problem in this manner. Because our understanding of the control mechanisms is limited, excess body weight can be a problem that is resistant to known methods of treatment.

ADIPOSE TISSUE

Since energy is conserved, that energy which is consumed in excess of requirement will be stored as chemical energy. In the adult, the major storage form of this energy is triglyceride. The tissue that stores body fat is known as *adipose* (fatty) *tissue* and the individual cells are *adipose cells.* In many other chapters of this text, we discussed diseases of a specific organ or organ system. In this chapter, we will consider the adipose tissue as an organ or perhaps as an organ system that is distributed at a number of sites throughout the body, as is the immune system.

There are two types of adipose tissue, white and brown. *Brown adipose tissue* is located between the muscles of the neck and back, in the *axillae* (armpits) and groin, and around the viscera of the abdomen and thorax. In the cells of brown adipose tissue, the fat exists as multiple droplets (*multilocular*). The cells are only approximately 10 percent of the size of white adipose tissue cells, but they have larger mitochondria in greater numbers.

Brown fat is well developed in newborn infants and will oxidize its fat during exposure to cold in order to produce heat (*nonshivering thermogenesis*). The large mitochondria are important in this process. The heat warms nearby tissue and is carried elsewhere in the body by the circulation. The thermogenesis apparently is accomplished via a futile cycle in which triglycerides are hydrolzyed to fatty acids, then to their coenzyme A derivatives, and back to triglycerides. In this process, high-energy phosphate is expended. ATP is hydrolyzed to AMP and inorganic phosphate and then regenerated. The net result is the combustion of fuel that generates heat but accomplishes nothing else.

Nonshivering thermogenesis is easily demonstrated in newborn infants. Some brown adipose tissue has also been shown, by histologic methods, to be present in adult men and women.[1] Its metabolism in the adult is under investigation.

White adipose tissue differentiates at 3 to 4 months of gestation from mesoderm and is a form of connective tissue (see Fig. 1-2). It is located predominantly around the kidneys and in the abdominal cavity (omental fat), under the skin, and between skeletal muscle fibers. Its primary function is to store energy.

A 70-kg man contains, on the average, 9 to 13 kg of adipose tissue, of which approximately 80 percent is triglyceride. However, the total weight of adipose tissue has been reported to be capable of varying as much as fiftyfold, a change which is greater than that of any other organ in the body while still being compatible with life. The amount varies normally with sex. In proportion to body weight, it is greater in women than in men. It also varies with age. It comprises approximately 28 percent of body weight at birth and 20 percent at 1 year of age. It then tends to remain constant until puberty when there may be another period of increase in girls. Usually in boys, there is a decrease at puberty.

The increase in adipose tissue can occur, as it does in other organs, by an increase in the number of cells or an increase in the size of the cells or both. However, it currently is believed that a decrease in "adipose organ" size occurs only by a decrease in the size of adipose cells, not by a decrease in the number of cells.

Each cell of white adipose tissue contains a thin layer of cytoplasm surrounding triglyceride in a single droplet (*monolocular*), the size of which determines the size of the cell. The cell nucleus lies in the thin layer of cytoplasm so that a cross section of a lipid-filled cell that passes through the nucleus looks like a signet ring.

At one time, adipose tissue was considered to be a rather static, nonreactive tissue that provided padding and insulation from cold and was a passive recipient of excess calories. It now is appreciated that adipose tissue is in a continuous state of flux and is important in many metabolic processes.

Adipose cells form and store triglycerides and also release fatty acids for energy. When the body is not in a fed state, the supply of carbohydrate for energy is depleted in a matter of hours (see Chapter 9). Thus, adipose tissue serves an important function in making us independent of food intake which otherwise would have to occur every few hours.

Theoretically, the adipose cell can acquire fatty acids by three routes. Fatty acids may by synthesized within the adipose cell from excess glucose. In the presence of insulin, glucose entry into cells and synthesis of fatty acids from glucose are increased. Fatty acids may also be acquired from those circulating in the plasma bound to albumin. Third, they can be acquired following release from lipoproteins, a reaction catalyzed by lipoprotein lipase.

Adipose tissue has two lipase systems, each with its own regulatory system. *Lipoprotein lipase* (LPL) catalyzes the reactions by which plasma triglyceride is metabolized to free fatty acids for triglyceride synthesis within the adipose cell. Lipoprotein lipase activity is increased following food intake, possibly owing to increased insulin levels. Thyroid hormone also increases in activity. In humans, the adipose cell is believed to get most of its fatty acids by esterifying preformed fatty acids, and very little by synthesis from glucose within the cells.

The other lipase, *hormone-sensitive lipase*, catalyzes the metabolism of triglyceride within the adipose cell for release of free fatty acids into the plasma. It is inhibited by insulin. Details of the reactions involving these lipases and their control are given in Chapter 9.

SOME DEFINITIONS OF TERMS

Before we consider body weight control mechanisms, some definitions are necessary. *Hunger* is defined as a craving that arises physiologically from the body's need for food. The sensations usually are unpleasant. *Hunger* occasionally is used to refer to a craving or need for other materials, such as "air hunger," but this use of the term is less common. In contrast to hunger, *appetite* is a natural desire for a specific food that is stimulated by the sight, smell, and thought of food. It is strongly influenced by memory and other associations. *Satiety* refers to the complete absence of hunger. It occurs very rapidly. *Anorexia* is the abnormal absence of a desire for food at a time of need for food and when the desire for food would be expected.

The energy content of food is measured most commonly in *kilocalories,* often loosely called *calories,* particularly in the popular literature. A proposal to convert units of energy from calories or kilocalories to joules and kilojoules has received some attention. To review, the *joule* is the *work* done in moving a mass a distance of 1 m against a force of 1 newton. A newton is the force that will move a mass of 1 kg with an acceleration of 1 m/sec/sec. The *kilocalorie* (kcal) is the amount of *heat* required to raise the temperature of 1 kg of water 1°C. from 14.5° to 15.5°C. There are 1,000 calories in a kilocalorie. The kilojoule is equal to 0.239 kcal, or a kilocalorie equals 4.184 kJ. The conversion can thus be made by applying the formula:

$$\text{kJ} = \text{kcal} \times 4.184$$

In the calculation of the energy of nutrients, then, we have:

Carbohydrate	1 g = 4 kcal = 17 kJ
Protein	1 g = 4 kcal = 17 kJ
Fat	1 g = 9 kcal = 37.6 kJ
Alcohol	1 g = 7 kcal = 29.3 kJ

Most patients will not be familiar with joules but will have some concept of a calorie. Therefore, it is necessary for the nutritional care specialist to continue to use this term in contacts with patients. On the other hand, the joule is increasingly used in the scientific literature, and so the nutritional care specialist must understand its meaning to read the professional literature. Because tables of food values and estimations of energy expenditure useful to the nutritional care specialist give values in kilocalories, that is the term used in this text.

CONTROL OF ENERGY BALANCE

There is evidence that a control mechanism exists for the maintenance of a normal proportion of adipose tissue, estimated to be approximately 120 g/kg of body weight in men and 260 g/kg of body weight in women. Since energy balance relates energy intake to energy use, it is intake and use which, in the final analysis, are the possible points of regulation.

Control of Food Intake

The central nervous system (CNS) integrates the overall control of food intake. To understand the control processes completely, we would have to know three things. First, we would need to know how the central nervous system is informed of the nutrient status. Second, we would need to know how that information is integrated with information on nutrient needs, previously learned knowledge of specific foods, and other related matters. Last, the process by which the decision to eat is translated into eating activity in a given environment would have to be understood. At the present time, we do not have a complete knowledge of any of these phases of food intake control. However, some facts are known, and theories are plentiful.

Central Controls

Experiments with animals have demonstrated that central influences on eating activity involve many areas of the brain. Among these, the hypothalamus, an area at the base of the brain (Fig. 15-1), has been studied extensively. Within the hypothalamus, there is a pair of cell aggregations known as the *ventromedial hypothalami* (VMH). These areas have been considered to act as a center for satiety. Nearby on either side are another pair of centers, the *lateral hypothalami* (LH), which together are thought to act as a "feeding center." Normally, when the VMH is stimulated, it inhibits the LH. The animal will continue to eat unless the VMH turns off the LH system.

If the fiber tracts lateral to the VMH are destroyed, the inhibition of LH is removed and a laboratory rat will overeat (*hyperphagia*).[2] Destruction of the VMH itself is associated with hyperinsulinemia and hypothalamic obesity. Destruction of either the VMH or associated fiber tracts is associated with hyperactivity of the vagus nerve. In contrast, if the LH is destroyed, a rat will stop eating (*aphagia*). In people in whom the VMH or LH has been damaged by a tumor or trauma, the response has been shown to resemble that seen in the rat, with the hypothalamus serving as an integrating and relay station for food intake control.

The question then arises regarding how these impulses are transmitted. Recent investigations of CNS functions in food intake control have centered on the biochemical messengers in impulse transmission. A brief explanation of neurotransmitters is provided in Chapter 11 and should be reviewed if necessary.

Acetylcholine, dopamine, norepinephrine, and serotonin may be involved in the control of food intake. Norepinephrine analyses in the animal brain show the highest concentration in the hypothalamus. As a general rule, injection of alpha-adrenergic drugs have elicited eating responses, whereas satiety responses are provoked by beta-adrenergic agonists.[3] However, the results of manipulation of norepinephrine are complex and contradictory. Both an excess and a deficiency lead to hyperphagia in animal experiments.[4] In addition, the dose of epinephrine required to reduce food intake is exceedingly high.[5] Further research on this

Figure 15-1. Cross section of rat brain showing location of the paired ventromedial hypothalami and lateral hypothalami in relation to the lateral ventricles, the third ventricles, and the thalamus.

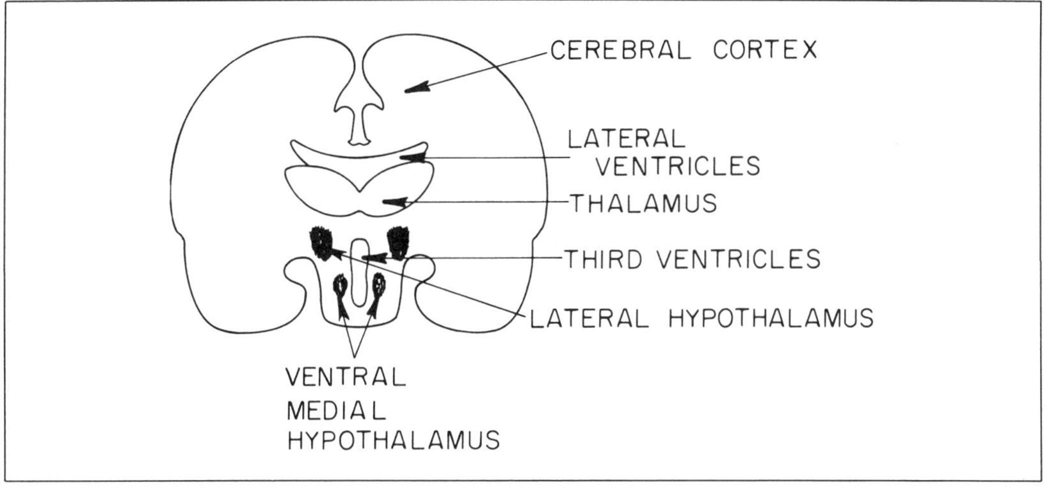

subject should be of great interest to the nutritional care specialist.

Several peptides may also be involved in controlling food intake and are the subject of current research. It has been suggested that *cholecystokinin* (CCK) causes satiety. However, the inhibition is very short-lived. Even if repeated doses are given and meal size is decreased in an animal, meal frequency increases so that the total is constant. Further research in this area is handicapped at present by the lack of a method to measure plasma CCK.

Bombesin, found in the gut and brain, will decrease food intake on injection into brain central ventricles.[6] *Thyrotropin-releasing hormone* and *somatostatin* also are involved in food intake control.[7,8] Satiety may be signaled by an increase in endogenous *endorphins* and *enkephalins* (opioidlike compounds) reacting with opioid receptors in the brain.[9] Morphine and heroin, opioid compounds, would thus be expected to decrease body weight by signalling satiety, and evidence indicates that they do so (see Chapter 16).

Peripheral Control Mechanisms

An important next question is, "What stimulates the hypothalamus?" There are apparently a number of peripheral factors that provide information to the central control. The control produced may be short-term or long-term. It generally is believed that medium-term and long-term controls are more precise. Although food intake may vary greatly from day to day, the long-term control normally will maintain body weight within very narrow limits. Control mechanisms are not well understood but, based on current information, are classified as metabolic, hormonal, gastrointestinal, sensory, and cortical.

Metabolic Factors. Metabolic factors are believed to provide medium-term and long-term control of food intake, but their precise nature is unknown. A number of theories have been proposed.

First, the *glucostatic theory,* proposed for medium-term control of body weight, postulates the existence of receptors in the VMH, LH, and possibly in the liver that are sensitive to the rate of glucose utilization.[10] When blood glucose concentration varies, the blood insulin concentration also changes. Therefore, it now is suggested that both glucose and insulin stimulate the satiety center after a meal.[11] The various factors influencing glucose use and insulin concentration in the blood were reviewed in Chapter 9.

Second, a *lipostatic control* is proposed. For long-term control of body weight, the VMH supposedly stabilizes fat stores by acting as a deterrent to the accumulation of excess fat.[12] The lateral hypothalami, then, conserve fat.[13] It has been postulated that there is a *set point* of adipose tissue cell size (rather than number of cells) that is sensed. Food intake then is regulated to maintain body weight at this set point. The adipose tissue reserves may be monitored by sensing a messenger substance, the identity of which is unknown. Daily fluctuations of free fatty acids are so great that fatty acids are unlikely to be the control messenger. Glycerol may be sensed directly or metabolized to glucose and then sensed by the VMH as a measure of adipose tissue stores.[10] The hypothalamus metabolizes glycerol at a higher rate than do other parts of the brain. Prostaglandins, released during lipolysis, also are candidates for the role of messenger. Hervey[14] proposes that some substance, produced by or dissolved in fat, serves as a sensor to measure storage of energy. According to the theory, this sensor material would decline as more energy was stored, which in turn would signal the hypothalamus to reduce food intake. As the concentration of the sensor increases and fat stores are released, the hypothalamus would receive a signal to increase food intake.

The identities of the proposed regulatory substances are unknown. A steroid, such as progesterone, has been suggested as one reasonable candidate.[15] Another possibility relates to the cell surface. As the adipose cells change in number or size or both, changes may occur in the total cell surface. Since the cell membrane contains hormone receptors and some enzymes occur on or near the cell surface, this surface change may be a crucial control factor. It has been shown, for example, that insulin receptors decrease in number in obese persons. As with other theories of food intake control, the lipostatic theory needs further investigation.

The third theory suggests the existence of an *aminostat.* Laboratory rats have been observed to alter their food intake to meet their protein requirements. In addition, diets that have imbalanced amino acid patterns cause decreases in food intake in both animal and human subjects.[16] Therefore, amino acids may also be related to food intake control. The plasma amino acid pattern may be sensed directly, or an altered supply of amino acids may affect neurotransmitters in the brain.[17,18] This mechanism is still controversial.[18] The concentrations of some neurotransmitters are influenced by diet. For example, high protein intakes increase brain tyrosine and dopamine (see Chapter 11).

Whether the material sensed is the amino acid pattern directly, neurotransmitters derived from amino acids, or some other amino acid derivative, the adjustments in intake are rapid. The receptor system apparently is in the brain,[19] but not necessarily in the hypothalamus.

Finally, the *thermostatic theory* of medium-term or long-term control of food intake is based on the observation that animals eat more when it is cold and less in a warm environment. The *preoptic anterior hypothalamus* (POAH) is thought to be the area responsive to heat. The animal then presumably eats to be warm and stops eating to cool off.[20] The heat produced by the thermogenic effect or specific dynamic action of food may cause an increase in heat production which acts as a satiety signal to the POAH.

Hormonal Factors. Hormones also affect food intake. *Insulin* may be sensed directly[21] or via its effect on blood glucose levels. High plasma insulin levels are found in obese patients, and there is evidence that insulin secretion is stimulated by the LH via the vagus. Yet, the relationship of insulin to the control of food is controversial. Insulin is reported to cause an increase in food intake. In a diabetic patient, for example, excess insulin can cause obesity. Others have suggested, based on animal experiments, that increased insulin reduces food intake. Further research is needed to clarify the role of insulin.[22]

Glucocorticoids tend to increase the food intake if given in large doses. *Thyroid hormones* increase catabolism and decrease adipose tissue stores, leading to increased food intake. *Estrogen* and *gastrointestinal hormones,* including CCK, also may affect food intake.

The overall effect of the hormone balance on food intake is far from clear. Further research is needed to clarify the role of each hormone before the effects of their interaction can be studied.

Gastrointestinal Factors. Chemoreceptors and *stretch receptors* in the pharynx, stomach, intestines, and liver that sense the presence of food and distention may provide clues to satiety. The *liver* may have sensors to monitor lipid absorption. Long-chain fatty acids absorbed directly into the lymphatic system bypass the liver. It has been suggested that animals that become obese when fed a high-fat diet do so because the liver does not sense the fat content of the diet. The use of an equicaloric diet with medium-chain triglycerides, which are absorbed into the portal circulation, in place of long-chain fatty acids, does reduce the tendency to obesity.

Sensory Factors. Taste, smell, and *texture* of food may influence food intake by their effects on the brain, with responses being based on previous experiences. These factors can elevate insulin secretion and intestinal motility in preparation for food intake via the autonomic nervous system.

Cortical Factors. Some emotional reactions also influence food intake. Unpleasant situations may interfere with eating, whereas pleasant sensations can cause a person to eat past the point of satiation. A specific case in point is eating until uncomfortably full on holidays and during other celebrations.

Control of Energy Expenditure

A considerable amount of controversy exists concerning the possibility that excess energy can be dissipated in the form of heat. Therefore, this is an area of active current research.

There is some evidence that mechanisms do exist for maintenance of stable body weight despite differences in food intake. One study, for example, showed that individuals of normal weight who were overfed required more energy per unit of surface area to maintain their weight than did spontaneously obese persons.[23] The data suggested that the overfed subjects had a tendency to "burn off" excess energy.[11] Experiments in rats demonstrated that overfeeding caused a significant increase in heat production.[24] Alternatively, it is suggested that the excess energy was used in synthetic processes for storage, to move the heavier body and to maintain an increased basal metabolic rate (BMR).

If mechanisms for dissipation of energy as heat do exist, we might then question what the nature of these mechanisms is. Brown fat has recently been proposed to have an important role in determining the expenditure of energy. It may serve to dissipate excess energy,[9] in addition to its function of maintaining body temperature. It is hypofunctional in genetically obese animals, but its contribution to obesity in these animals and its significance in humans are unknown. It has been suggested that metabolic efficiency varies in other tissues also by futile cycles and by alterations in protein turnover or sodium pump activity,[11] but the effects of these mechanisms are limited.[25] Increased energy consumption following overfeeding ("Luxuskonsumption") has not been demonstrated according to some investigators,[26] but others suggest that the dissipation of heat via futile cycles occurs after feeding (*thermogenic response* or *specific dynamic action*),[25] following exercise, and during stress.[11] The thermogenic response after feeding arises partly from the increased rate of synthetic reactions, but this does not account for all heat. Following exercise, oxygen is consumed at an accelerated rate. It is proposed that this oxygen is used in replenishing phosphocreatine, reoxygenating myoglobin and hemoglobin, converting lactate to glucose and glycogen, and stimulating futile cycles. This latter might persist for hours and add considerably to the total energy expenditure. Stress is thought to increase the activity of cycles for mobilization and the use of glucose and fatty acids, by pathways involving epinephrine and glucagon. James et al.[25] propose an interaction between dietary fat intake and brown fat metabolism as well as differences in dietary thermogenesis. Current research is investigating the possibility of differences in these metabolic processes in obese and nonobese individuals.[25]

Another question related to the role of energy expenditure in the regulation of energy balance asks whether changes in food intake influence physical activity. There is good evidence that they do in *some* circumstances. Some laboratory animals and humans, when underfed, will reduce their physical activity.[26] On the other hand, underfed rodents increase their activity. It is not known whether overfeeding will stimulate an increase in activity. The insistent demand of small children for physical activity may indicate that such an effect does exist, but there is no concrete supporting evidence.

OBESITY

Obesity can be considered a form of malnutrition. Depending on the definition used, 40 million to 80 million people (or as much as 30 percent of the population of the United States) are considered to be obese.

There are no universally accepted definitions of overweight or obesity, but *overweight* frequently is defined as a body weight from 10 to 20 percent higher than the usual weight for height. It does not always refer to excess fat, since some individuals with above-average muscle development weigh more than usual for their height but do not contain excess fat. This situation sometimes occurs in athletes who are over*weight* but not over*fat.*

Obesity is defined as an excessive accumulation of body fat, but the proportion of fat is difficult to determine. As a consequence, we use body weight to define obesity. On that basis, obesity is defined as body weight 20 percent or more above desirable levels in women and 25 percent or more above desirable levels in men.

Morbid obesity refers to a degree of obesity that clearly correlates with excess morbidity and mortality. Frequently, 45.4 kg (100 lb.) of excess weight is used as a standard, although this definition is arbitrary. Obesity is considered a symptom of disease, not the disease itself. Thus, its status is similar to that of anemia or hypertension.

Diagnosis

Research Methods

The definitions just given suggest that obesity is defined on the basis of body weight compared to a standard. Although that usually is the case, such an approach is limited in that it does not provide a measure of body fat. Methods that provide a basis for estimates of body fat are available for research purposes. These include measurements of body density or specific gravity and the use of soft tissue roentgenography or ultrasound. However, these methods are impractical for general clinical use.

There are a number of simpler methods which do not provide measurement of body fat but are easier to use and provide a practical index of obesity in clinical situations.

Comparison with Tables of Ideal Weight

The most widely used method of determining obesity is to compare body weight with that listed on height-weight tables for a person of the same height and sex. The tables issued by the Metropolitan Life Insurance Company and by the Fogarty International Center (see Appendix B) are widely used. The Metropolitan Life Insurance Company tables are divided by sex, height, and frame size. Since they do not give guidance for determining frame size, a method for frame size estimation has been added to Appendix B. The values given in the tables are for individuals aged 25 years or older. For young women 18 to 24 years old, 1 lb. is subtracted for each year younger than 25. The weights are given assuming that indoor clothing and shoes with 2-in. heels are worn. The Fogarty tables are based on weight without shoes or other clothing.

Separate tables are used for children. The National Center for Health Statistics[27] has issued growth charts for children aged 0 to 36 months and 2 to 18 years. These are divided according to sex. Obesity can be detected using these charts. If a child is in the fiftieth percentile for height and the eightieth percentile for weight, for example, obesity is probable.

A rapid system for estimating ideal weight consists of calculating weight from height:

For men: 106 lb. for the first 5 ft plus 6 lb. for each added inch **(1)**

For women: 100 lb. for the first 5 ft plus 5 lb. for each added inch **(2)**

A somewhat more generous estimate which takes frame size into consideration provides 105 to 110 lb. for the first 5 ft, 5 lb. for each added inch *plus* 5 lb. for medium frame or 10 lb. for heavy frame.

Whether tables of ideal weight or one of these rapid calculations is used, a useful means of expressing overweight is as a percentage above ideal:

$$\frac{\text{Present weight} \times 100}{\text{Ideal weight obtained from a table}} = \text{\% overweight} \quad \textbf{(3)}$$

This is not very exact, but errors are not large, and it has the advantage of being easily understood by most patients.

Triceps Skinfold

The method of diagnosing obesity by measuring the triceps skinfold is described in Chapter 2. Measurements greater than 18.6 mm in men and 25.1 mm in women indicate obesity.

Height-Weight Ratios

Several ratios of height and weight have also been used to diagnose obesity. In order of preference, according to Keys et al.,[28] they are:

Body mass index (obesity index; Quetelet index): $\frac{W\ (kg)}{H^2 (m)}$ **(4)**

Simple ratio: $\frac{W}{H}$ **(5)**

Ponderal index: $\frac{H\ (\text{cm or in.})}{W\ (\text{lb. or kg})}$ **(6)**

where W = weight and H = height. The unit varies with the index in use.

Table 15-1. Minimum Body Mass Index in Obesity[a]

Frame Size	Men	Women
Small	25.4	24.7
Medium	27.5	27.0
Large	29.9	29.9

[a] Based on data from James, W.P.T., Ed., *Research on Obesity.* London: Medical Research Council, 1976; and Stern, J.S., and Kane-Nussen, B., Obesity: Its Assessment, Risks and Treatments. In R.B. Alfin-Slater, D. Kritschevsky, and R.E. Hodges, Eds., *Human Nutrition—A Comprehensive Treatise.* New York: Plenum, 1979. Obtained from dividing weight in kilograms by height in meters squared, without clothes or shoes.

The body mass index, using weight in kilograms and height in meters, indicates obesity if values obtained exceed those given in Table 15-1. Of those ratios given, it correlates best with skinfold measurements. A ponderal index of 12 or less, calculated using height in inches and weight in pounds, is considered to indicate obesity.

A more complex system, the *adiposity index,* uses skinfold measurements as well as height and weight:

Men: $0.34 + 222\frac{W}{H^2} + (0.00740 \times [\text{subscapular} + \text{triceps skinfold in mm}])$ **(7)**

Women: $0.34 + 242\frac{W}{H^2} + (0.00571 \times [\text{subscapular} + \text{triceps skinfold in mm}])$ **(8)**

Rapid Self-Assessment Methods

A number of simple self-assessment methods, which are imprecise but sometimes useful, have been listed by Stern and Kane-Nussen.[29] With these methods, excess fatness is "probably indicated" as follows:

Belt test: Circumference at navel exceeds circumference at nipples.

Broca index: Weight in kilograms is greater

than height in centimeters minus 100. Used extensively in Europe.

"Magic 36" test: Height in inches minus waist circumference in inches equals less than 36.

Ruler test: When lying flat, a ruler parallel to the vertical axis of the body cannot touch both ribs and pubic bone.

Pinch test: A pinch of skin and subcutaneous fat on back of upper arm, side of lower chest, and just below shoulder blade in back exceeds 1 in.

Mirror test: Self-assessment of excess fat while nude before a mirror (except when the person has an abnormal body image, as in anorexia nervosa).

Classification of the Obesities

For many years, obesity was treated as a psychological problem, often with moral overtones. Obese individuals were considered to lack self-control, to be gluttons and social deviants, and to have personality disorders of varying degrees of severity. Although these attitudes still are somewhat common, recent research has indicated the complexity of the problem so that the obesities now are recognized as multiple. They have been classified in several ways, to facilitate understanding of their etiology and pathogenesis.

Classification According to Pathogenesis

Obesity has been classified as *exogenous* (regulatory) or *endogenous* (metabolic). This early classification proposes that exogenous obesity involves an impairment of the central regulation of food intake.[30] Metabolism of other tissues is considered to be normal, but there is evidence that inactivity is characteristic of the individual and often precedes the development of obesity. The inactivity contributes to the positive energy balance by reducing the output of energy.

Metabolic or endogenous obesity has been defined as the type in which overeating is the consequence of abnormal fat and carbohydrate metabolism or some other disorder.[30] A major difficulty with this type of classification is that it tends to obscure the fact that a positive calorie balance is necessary for weight gain in either case.

Etiologic Classification

Classification of obesity according to etiology is more recent and somewhat more useful than pathogenetic classification. Many factors have been shown to be involved in the etiology of obesity.

The involvement of *genetic factors* has been shown clearly in laboratory and farm animals.[31] Genetic effects in most cases of human obesity are less firmly established, but there are five inherited syndromes that involve obesity among their manifestations.

The *Prader-Willi syndrome* is characterized by mental retardation and the onset of obesity at age 2 or 3 years. Nutritional care of Prader-Willi patients is described in more detail in Chapter 16. This syndrome generally is believed to be genetically transmitted, although the evidence is weak.

The evidence is stronger for genetic transmission of the other four syndromes. The manifestations of the *Laurence-Moon-Biedl syndrome* include mental deficiency, obesity, retinal degeneration leading to blindness in adulthood, *polydactyly* (extra fingers and toes), *hypogonadism* (lack of sexual development), and sometimes congenital heart disease and kidney disease. The *Alstrom syndrome* is characterized by obesity, retinal degeneration leading to blindness in childhood, nerve deafness, and diabetes mellitus. This condition is rare.

Hyperostosis frontalis interna (*Morgagni-Stewart-Morel syndrome*) usually first appears in women at age 20 to 60 years. Manifestations include obesity and *virilism* (development of masculine physical and mental traits in a woman). The term *hyperostosis frontalis interna* refers to the formation of new bone that protrudes in patches on the internal surface of the forehead. The condition may be accompanied by mental slowness, loss of memory, headache, irritability, and other neurologic symptoms. The syndrome is exceedingly rare.

The last of the four syndromes discussed here actually may be three syndromes with similar manifestations. Collectively they have been called *triglyceride storage diseases.* Little is known of these conditions since they have been identified in only a few families. On the basis of studies of these patients, the three types may be:[32]

Type 1, resulting from a defect in the activation of adenyl cyclase complex, producing decreased levels of cyclic AMP in adipose tissue
Type 2, resulting from failure of activation of hormone-sensitive lipase by cyclic AMP
Type 3 (also known as *primary familial xanthomatosis*), resulting from a defect of a lipase

In addition to these rare syndromes, increased occurrence of obesity within families and ethnic groups and in identical twins have been documented as examples of the genetic basis for obesity.[33] Although these data support the concept of a genetic contribution to obesity in some patients, there is debate regarding the extent to which environmental influences versus genetic influences cause obesity.

Hypothalamic obesity has been clearly demonstrated in both animals and humans after the hypothalamus has been injured, as in the case of an encroaching tumor. It is very rare.

Endocrine disorders also cause obesity, although perhaps not as often as many would like to believe. Obesity occurs in cases of excess corticosteroids (*Cushing's syndrome*), insulin excess, castration, or alterations in the levels of progesterone or estrogen (*Stein-Leventhal syndrome*). Pregnancy frequently is followed by weight gain.

Physical inactivity is a clear cause of weight gain in patients whose activity is restricted by injury (see Chapter 16). It has also been documented to contribute to other forms of obesity, even though it may not be obvious to the casual observer.

Nutritional factors may play a role in the development of obesity in animals and humans. Variation in protein intake affects the amount of energy storage, although the mechanism is not clear. Thus, it appears that diet composition affects obesity. High-fat diets and high-sucrose diets are used to produce obesity in animal experiments, but the mechanism may be based on palatability.

Overfeeding of children may be especially important in causing childhood obesity. It has been suggested that overfeeding of infants may "program" the child for obesity later.

The use of some *drugs* also can cause obesity. Cyproheptadine, tricyclic antidepressants, and the phenothiazines are those particularly associated with weight gain (see Chapter 3).

Physiologic and psychic trauma can contribute to the etiology of obesity in animals. In humans, the relationship is less obvious; however, emotional stress has been associated with the onset of obesity in some cases.[30]

Environmental factors such as cultural food habits also can contribute to the development of obesity.[30,31]

Two types of obesity sometimes are classified as of a special psychological origin. One results from the *night-eater syndrome* in which the patient has insomnia and hyperphagia in the evening along with anorexia in the morning. It has been associated with stress and has a poor prognosis unless the stress can be removed. The other type of patient, also reacting to stress, is the *binge eater.* This person may be one who progresses to anorexia nervosa.

In the final analysis, all the factors just listed result in an intake of energy in excess of output. Thus, it is necessary to remember that positive energy balance is the only fundamental cause of obesity.

Anatomic Classification of Fat Distribution

There are several means of classifying fat accumulations based on their distribution within the body. This distribution may be generalized or localized.

Localized Fat Accumulations. A number of conditions cause localized fat accumulations. These are not considered obesity but are given here to provide an overall perspective:

Lipomas, associated with other diseases (see Chapter 8)
Dercum's disease (*adiposis dolorosa*), a disease with painful fat accumulations and nerve lesions
Weber-Christian disease, a nodular panniculitis (inflammation of subcutaneous fatty tissue)
Liposarcomas (see Chapter 13)
Lipid storage disease

The nutritional care specialist should be aware of the existence of these conditions, but they will not be discussed further in this chapter.

Generalized Fat Distribution. One descriptive system of generalized fat distribution refers to *somatotype* (body build) which has been related to the incidence of obesity. Body build has been classified into three groups. *Ectomorphs* are described as those individuals who are linear in build, appear fragile, and have a large relative surface area, thin muscles, and a thin layer of subcutaneous fat. *Mesomorphs* have a preponderance of muscle, connective tissue, and bone, with a rectangular outline. *Endomorphs* have large digestive viscera, accumulations of fat, and a soft, rounded appearance with large trunk and thighs and tapering extremities. In a study of adolescent girls, obesity occurred most often in endomorphs, less often in mesomorphs, and least often in ectomorphs. The relationship was less clear-cut in adults, but the trend was similar.[34] These constitutional factors may provide a predisposition to obesity and cause body weight to vary somewhat from the ideal because of heavy bone and muscle structure. Endomorphs have a higher incidence of obesity.

Another system of anatomic classification of obesity uses the terms *gynecoid* and *android.* A gynecoid (femalelike) distribution of fat refers to fat accumulation particularly around the hips and lower abdomen. It also is referred to as *lower body obesity.* The android (malelike) type describes fat accumulation over chest and arms (upper body) rather than the lower trunk.

The relative amounts of adipose tissue deposited in the upper and lower trunk have been quantitated by Vague et al.[35] The method requires measurement of skinfold thickness and circumference (see Chapter 2 for the procedure) of the mid–upper arm over the biceps and of the midthigh (femoral). The *adipomuscular ratio* (*AMR*) then is calculated:

$$\text{AMR} = \frac{\text{Skinfold thickness}}{\text{Circumference}} \qquad \textbf{(9)}$$

Typical gynecoid values are 0.48 for biceps AMR and 0.63 for femoral AMR. Thus, the ratio of biceps AMR to femoral AMR is much less than 1. By contrast, typical android values are 0.21 for biceps AMR and 0.19 for femoral AMR. Thus, the ratio is greater than 1. This calculation, then, provides a quantitative definition of the android and gynecoid fat distributions which may affect the chances for success in weight reduction. The mechanisms are unknown, but the gynecoid type is considered to be more difficult to treat successfully.

Another anatomic classification of the obesities is based on the number and size of adipose cells. Obesity has been classified as *hypercellular* or *hyperplastic* (containing an increased number of cells) or as *hypertrophic* (containing larger fat cells) with a more nearly normal number of fat cells (*normocellular*). It is possible to have a mixture of types. Nevertheless, this classification currently is considered useful since there is some evidence that cellularity is based on age of onset of obesity and has prognostic value.

Classification by Age of Onset

The last classification divides obesities into *adult-onset* and *juvenile-onset* conditions. This is a fairly new concept. Most obese persons (90 to 95 percent) are of the adult-onset type; in them, obesity develops slowly, beginning at approximately age 25 years and progressing until age 55 or so. The adult-onset obese person is expected to have a hypertrophic obesity. There is evidence that the juvenile-onset obese person, in whom obesity began in childhood, has a greater number of fat cells—that is, hyperplastic obesity.[36] The juvenile-onset category has been further subdivided into types 1 and 2. In *type 1,* onset is in infancy and the condition is characterized by hyperphagia. In *type 2,* onset is in childhood and the imbalance results from decreased energy expenditure.

Increased organ or tissue size during growth may be the consequence of an increase in the number of cells, an increase in the size of cells, or both. It is postulated that, in humans of normal weight, there are two periods in which adipose tissue cells multiply: in infancy up to the age of 2 years and during puberty. The stimuli to the increases are unknown but probably are genetic, endocrine, nutritional, and environmental in some combination. In very obese children, the numbers of fat cells may continue to increase between age 2 and puberty, a time when fat cell number is stable in children of normal weight. There is some question on this point. The development of fat cells cannot be studied prior to the time that they contain fat, since we have no satisfactory techniques to identify them. The increase in numbers of cells in obese infants is postulated to stem in part from early overfeeding and the early introduction of solid foods.[37] The possible involvement of genetic factors is debated.

The prognosis for successful weight reduction often is estimated on the basis of the android/gynecoid and age-of-onset classifications. Current opinion holds that juvenile-onset hyperplastic obesity with gynecoid distribution of fat is exceedingly difficult to treat successfully.

Hazards of Obesity

In our society, the obese or overweight individual often is stigmatized, and the psychological effects and social rejection are important among the hazards of obesity. There are many other risks, and it generally is agreed that obesity is detrimental to one's well-being.

In obese persons, mortality and morbidity are increased in heart disease, cerebrovascular accident, cancer, diabetes, accidents, renal disease, gallstone disease, some respiratory diseases, osteoarthritis, endometrial carcinoma, and some skin disorders.[29] Other disturbances associated with extreme obesity include hirsutism, infertility, menstrual irregularities, and edema.[29] In obese surgery patients, anesthesia dosages may be difficult to determine,[38] and the incidence of postoperative sepsis and wound rupture are increased. Life expectancy of an obese person thus is decreased in the presence of these conditions.[15,38,39] The *pickwickian syndrome* (*obesity hypoventilation syndrome*) is the only condition in which excess adipose tissue can lead to death without any other contributing factor (see Chapter 8).

It is not always clear whether obesity is primary in causing development of a disease or whether it tends to increase mortality in existing conditions. It also is not clear whether, once the disease is established, it can be ameliorated by weight reduction. Another important question concerns the relationship of severity of the obesity to the amount of risk of morbidity or mortality. The data relating body weight to morbidity and mortality suggest that those people whose obesity does not exceed 30 percent of ideal weight are actually at *decreased* risk. Risk increases when adiposity reaches more than 30 percent above ideal levels, and risk is clear in the morbidly obese.

Metabolic Alterations in Obesity

Many alterations in metabolism have been observed in the person who is obese. These may be discussed in terms of (1) effects on the adipose cell in particular, (2) effects on metabolism in general, and (3) the response to the energy deficit when the individual is dieting.

Effects of Increased Adipose Cell Size on Its Metabolism

As it enlarges, the adipose cell adapts metabolically, with progressive inhibition of lipogenesis and inhibition of pentose shunt enzymes. As fat cells become larger, they also become insulin-resistant. Among other consequences, they have a decreased number of receptor sites on their cell membranes. Insulin promotes fat storage; therefore, as the cell enlarges and becomes resistant, additional storage becomes more difficult. These reactions may provide a limit to the development of larger cells and also may be a mechanism for maintenance of a set point. The constraint on cell size subsequently restrains food intake.

It formerly was suggested that the number of cells did not increase in adult-onset obesity and that the cells only got larger as they filled with lipid. More recent work on rats has suggested that, in the adult, once fat cells have achieved maximum size, further increase involves an increase in cell number if energy intake continues.[40] Some indirect evidence suggests that a similar phenomenon occurs in obese humans.[41]

In weight reduction, as the cell size is reduced and insulin sensitivity is increased, mobilization of triglyceride could become more difficult. Studies suggest that some regulatory mechanism prevents the decrease of body fat below a certain level related to the size of fat cells.

Weight loss apparently causes a decrease in cell size but not in cell number in either juvenile-onset or adult-onset obesity. This fact may provide an explanation for the difficulty in weight reduction experienced by many individuals. If a person with large numbers of fat cells reduces his or her weight, that person may have symptoms of hunger equivalent to those felt by starving nonobese people.[13]

Although largely speculative, the distinction between hyperplastic and hypertrophic obesity might account for the greater difficulty in weight reduction reported in patients with childhood obesity. Investigation has revealed that the patient with hyperplastic obesity whose weight is reduced will maintain the weight a shorter time and experience a higher relapse rate.

The existence of a messenger between adipose cell size and regulation of energy balance is proposed, but its identity is unknown. Those described earlier in the discussion of the lipostatic theory of weight control (p. 560) are possible candidates.

These theories of the effects of adipose cell size on metabolism require further investigation. However, present knowledge suggests that obesity prevention is greatly preferable to treatment of existing obesity.

Effects on Metabolism in General

A variety of biochemical abnormalities may be present in the severely obese, but none has persisted when body weight was reduced. Therefore, it appears that they are the result, not the cause, of excess body weight. Some of these abnormalities include (1) an abnormal glucose tolerance test, (2) increased fasting levels of plasma glucose and plasma insulin, and (3) increased insulin response to a glucose load and other cues for insulin release. The relationship of insulin to hyperphagia is receiving much attention recently, since it has been shown that the hypothalamus can stimulate increased insulin release from the pancreas via the vagus nerve. Other biochemical abnormalities in the obese include hypertriglyceridemia, elevated fasting levels of free fatty acid, and elevated plasma ketones.

Physiologic Responses to Energy Deficit During Weight Loss

When dietary sources of glucose are inadequate, the body's stored glucose reserves are used up in a few hours. Glucose must then be supplied to those tissues for which it is essential from glucogenic amino acids and from glycerol. If the deficit continues, as it would in an obese person who is dieting successfully, the body adapts to conserve its amino acids. A major energy source is adipose tissue from which the liver produces large amounts of ketones. This adaptive process is described in detail in Chapter 12 and is diagrammed in Fig. 12-2.

Treatment

Treatment of obesity is aimed toward weight loss. It has taken many forms, including primarily diet, drugs, surgery, exercise, and behavior modification. Unfortunately, most individuals using standard treatments do not lose any appreciable amount of weight,[42] much less achieve a permanent cure.[43] Those individuals who do achieve permanent weight loss are generally those in whom the amount of excess weight was small.[44] The successful treatment of obesity presents a major challenge to the nutritional care specialist.

Before treatment is undertaken, careful consideration should be given to whether weight reduction is in the best interests of the patient. At one time, weight loss was recommended almost automatically to every patient who was overweight. More recently, consideration is given to the following questions:

1. Is there a serious health condition that makes weight reduction advisable? How much weight loss is necessary?
2. Is the patient well adjusted to his or her weight? Is he or she motivated to change? If so, are the patient's objectives realistic?
3. Has the patient's weight been stable?
4. Will a reduced weight be compatible with the patient's important relationships with others (spouse, close friends)?

The answers to these questions may reveal that attempts at weight reduction are not the most advisable course. If, however, the decision is made to attempt weight reduction, the following procedures may be considered.

Dietary Treatment

To be successful, any treatment must produce and maintain an intake of energy that is less than output so that the individual must draw on his or her body fat stores to supply his or her energy needs. The various means by which this has been proposed to be accomplished are described here.

Conventional Restricted-Calorie Diet. Many physicians and nutritional care specialists recommend a restricted-calorie diet plan, often based on the same food lists used for planning diabetic diets (see Chapter 9) and planned in such a way as to establish a pattern for lifetime eating behavior. Permanent successful weight reduction is rare with this classic approach, which is regarded as the safest method of reducing. Nevertheless, since the diet is used extensively, its planning will be described.

Step 1. Establish kilocalorie content of the diet. The amount of energy that will maintain weight must be estimated before the caloric deficit can be established. A simple procedure is based on measures of caloric use during starvation. The energy used during starvation is taken as the minimum amount necessary to maintain weight. Bray[15] has found that this quantity exceeds 1,000 kcal in adults. Thus, any patient whose intake is 1,000 kcal or less will lose weight. This procedure is, of course, very imprecise. It makes no allowances for normal differences in body size or differences in activity.

To individualize the kilocalorie prescription, a second, more desirable approach may be used. The basal requirement for weight maintenance may be estimated by assuming 1 kcal/kg of body weight per hour. Thus, a man weighing 90 kg would have a basal requirement of 90 × 1 × 24 or 2,160 kcal. To this figure, an increment for activity is added. Usual additions are 30 percent of basal for sedentary activity, 50 percent for light activity, 75 percent for moderate activity, and 100 percent for the very active person. Thus, our 90-kg man, if he had sedentary activity, would require 2,160 + 648 or 2,808 kcal to maintain his weight.

A somewhat more exact system involves the use of a nomogram by which surface area is obtained from the body weight and height. The surface area, age, and sex then are used on the nomogram to arrive at basal energy expenditure. An increment for activity must again be added to obtain the maintenance energy level.

Once the maintenance energy level has been estimated, an appropriate diet may be established. Commonly used diets for weight reduction for the average adult contain 1,000 or 1,200 kcal/day. Sometimes diets of 800 kcal are used for the patient who has a small surface area, or for an elderly or handicapped person whose activity is limited. Generally, diets containing even fewer calories are not as effective as might be assumed. Some adaptation to conserve energy may occur[44] so that little more fat is catabolized.[45,46] The mechanism for this conservation of energy is unknown, but Bray[15] suggests that if a diet is more severely limited, little additional weight loss results. Some patients can reduce body weight while eating diets containing higher calorie levels, such as 1,500 or 1,800 kcals, if they are active or normally have a large body size. A man 6 ft 6 in. tall who does hard physical labor, for example, would lose weight on an 1,800-kcal diet.

The energy content of body fat is approximately 3,500 kcal/lb. This value may be used to estimate the rate of weight loss. If a patient's intake were 1,000 kcal less per day than his or her need for maintenance, that patient could lose 2 lb./wk for the total deficit of 7,000 kcal. Let us assume that our 90-kg (198-lb.) man has an ideal weight of 70 kg (154 lb.). Since he is 44 lb. overweight, he must maintain his daily 1,000-kcal deficit for 22 weeks to reach ideal weight.

This method for estimating weight loss is useful but tends to oversimplify. As patients lose weight, BMR may decrease. If energy intake is not reduced also, the rate of loss decreases. Our 90-kg man, for example, might begin his diet at 1,800 kcal. When his body weight reaches 80 kg, weight maintenance needs could be 2,500 kcal. Under these circumstances, a 1,000-kcal deficit would require a 1,500-kcal diet. There is some evidence that an even lower figure will be required if the loss is to be maintained. In addition, other physiologic changes may help the obese patient maintain weight. Each 100 g of fat produces 112 g of water when it is oxidized. This water must be excreted before weight loss is observed.

When our patient reaches his ideal weight of 70 kg, his weight maintenance need, if activity has not changed, will be 70 × 1 (maybe) × 24, or 1,680, + 504, or 2,184 kcal. A diet of approximately 2,180 kcal might maintain him at ideal weight, but there is some evidence that his basal requirement falls to less than 1 kcal/kg/hr, although the metabolic basis for this change is unknown. At 2,180 kcal, then, it is possible that he will gain weight. If he returns to his previous diet of 2,800 kcal or more, he will surely regain his lost weight.

In determining kilocalorie levels for control of obesity in children, care must be taken to allow for normal growth and development. Lean body mass must be preserved carefully; therefore, restrictions are moderate. At ages 1 through 5 years, a restriction of 10 percent of kilocalories sometimes is recommended. After age 5, a restriction of 10 to 25 percent may be used to maintain a stable weight while growth in height occurs. Alternatively, weight loss of 0.5 lb./wk may be the objective.

Step 2. Distribute kilocalories among protein, fat, and carbohydrate. Having established the desired energy content of the diet, the nutritional care specialist must distribute those kilocalories among protein, fat, and carbohydrate. As a general guideline, protein is provided generously, usually 0.8 to 1.5 g/kg of body weight, and sometimes more. One objective is to prevent loss of lean body tissue. In addition, animal foods have high satiety value, and their generous use may increase compliance with the diet. The nutritional care specialist must remember, however, that their high cost presents a hardship for some patients.

The remaining energy in the diet is distributed between carbohydrate and fat. The merits of a high-fat, low-carbohydrate diet compared to an equicaloric low-fat, high-carbohydrate diet have been debated for decades. Some studies have shown extra weight loss on the low-carbohydrate diet over the short term, but these effects are believed to be related to changes in water balance.[47] Studies over longer periods have not shown any differences in weight loss between a low-calorie high-fat diet and an equicaloric high-carbohydrate diet.

In summary, weight loss occurs if there is a caloric deficit regardless of the source of the calories contained in the diet. There is no evidence that weight reduction is altered when the source of nonprotein calories is changed. Therefore, plan a diet that is compatible with the patient and to increase compliance, and plan a diet that will help to redefine the patient's eating habits to increase the possibility of long-term maintenance of the weight loss.

Step 3. Establish frequency of meals. The number of meals per day must also be established and has been another area for debate. The effects of meal-eating once or twice daily compared to nibbling at more frequent intervals have been investigated in animals. Rats fed by a stomach tube twice daily had more body fat than those allowed to nibble ad libitum.[48] Epidemiologic and clinical studies have shown that obese individuals tend to eat most of their food in one or two meals per day.[49–51] This pattern of food intake also has a detrimental effect on serum cholesterol and glucose tolerance.[49–52] Nevertheless, the frequency of meals does not affect the overall rate of weight change in subjects on kilcalorie-deficient diets.[53,54] A regimen of three meals or more per day generally is recommended, not for increased weight loss but to modulate serum cholesterol changes and improve glucose tolerance. However, this matter still is the subject of controversy. In planning for the individual patient, it seems logical to use the meal pattern that makes it easiest for the patient to comply with the kilocalorie restriction.

Step 4. Plan for adequate vitamins, minerals, and fluid. The diet is intended to be used for a long period and should be planned carefully to include adequate amounts of vitamins and minerals. Supplements should be considered if the kilocalorie restriction is severe.

Even if the patient adheres carefully to the diet, weight usually is not lost in a straight linear progression. Water balance is influenced by the carbohydrate content of the diet, and water balance may not be reached for approximately 10 days after the diet is instituted. In that time, weight loss may be substantial. At other times, the weight may plateau for 10 days or so because of some fluid retention, even though the amount of adipose tissue is decreasing. Unless the patient has a complicating condition affecting water balance, fluid retention is a transient effect and is not a justification for fluid restriction. If this phenomenon is explained to patients, it may help to prevent a feeling of discouragement and defeat and the use of harmful medications. The use of diuretics for weight reduction should be discouraged.

Step 5. Plan the diet. A common procedure for diet planning is the same as that used in planning the diabetic diet from the exchange lists (see Chapter 9), although a little more flexibility usually is allowed in the calorie distribution. If the patient requires a diet containing 1,000 kcal, the prescription might specify 80 g of protein, 30 g of fat, and 110 g of carbohydrate to provide 1,030 kcal. Using the same method described in Chapter 9, this diet, which is an example of a low-fat diet, might contain the following exchanges:

Food	*Exchanges*
Milk, skim	2
Vegetables	2
Fruit	3
Bread	3
Meat, lean	8
Fat	1

With these exchanges, the diet would contain 78 g of protein, 29 g of fat, and 109 g of carbohydrate, for a total of 1,009 kcal.

Alternatively, a more generous fat allowance could be provided at the expense of carbohydrate by providing 78 g of protein, 39 g of fat, 89 g of carbohydrate, and 1,019 kcal, as follows:

Food	*Exchanges*
Milk, skim	2
Vegetables	2
Fruit	3
Bread	1
Meat, lean	8
Fat	3

Patients are advised to distribute all the foods in somewhat equal proportion among the three meals.

As is true with the diabetic diet, the patient needs information on the use of "free" foods, methods for accurate determination of portion size, and, sometimes, the energy content of alcoholic beverages and snack foods. Practice in estimating portion size is especially important for obese patients, many of whom tend to underestimate portions and thus continue to overeat even though they are attempting to comply with the diet.

Formula Diets. Formula diets, in the form of liquids, powders, wafers, or bars, become popular at regular intervals. They generally supply approximately 900 kcal from 20 percent protein (45 g) and 50 percent carbohydrate. For long-term use, they do nothing to retrain the patient in his or her eating habits. It sometimes is necessary to explain to a patient that the formula is to be taken *in place of,* not in addition to, a meal.

These diets may be useful for a person who wishes to lose just a few pounds or for the person who needs to lose weight quickly in anticipation of surgery. They may be convenient for one meal per day, usually breakfast or lunch, for the long-term dieter. The formula diets do not provide the "miracle cures" for which many patients are looking and may actually contribute to defeat because of their monotony.

Fasting or Starvation. A third type of dietary treatment of obesity involves fasting. This is a severe treatment which should be used only if the patient is hospitalized. It should not be used if the patient has a history of gout or of cardiovascular, renal, or hepatic disease.

In some institutions where this type of treatment is employed, the patients are allowed small amounts of black coffee, tea, or fruit juices and raw vegetables with high water content such as lettuce and tomatoes. The patient receives a liberal amount of water and vitamin supplements and is encouraged to exercise normally. It is claimed that a major advantage of this method is that the patient becomes ketotic and feelings of hunger subside; however, there is some evidence that this is not true.[55]

Other effects of fasting are summarized in Figs. 12-1 and 12-2. As these figures indicate, fasting is accompanied by a rapid nitrogen loss at first, followed by an adaptation to a slower, steady rate of loss.

A variation of the starvation regimen is the *protein-sparing modified fast.*[56] Protein foods of high biologic value to provide 1.5 g of protein per kilogram of body weight per day are given in two to three meals per day. The purpose is to replace the protein that is metabolized. The Recommended Dietary Allowances of vitamins and minerals, 500 mg of calcium, 5 g of sodium chloride, and 25 mEq of potassium, also are prescribed. Fluids, at least 1,500 ml/day, are given as desired.[57] In the program recommended by Bistrian,[58] the patient also is taught principles of nutrition and exercise management, assertiveness techniques, and relaxation techniques, receives behavior therapy, and is monitored carefully throughout. The patient is weaned carefully from the diet and given a weight maintenance diet when treatment is ended.

Side effects can include decreased gut motility and constipation, fluid and electrolyte imbalance, cardiac arrhythmia, hyperuricemia and gout, amenorrhea, and temporary hair loss. The diet obviously is hazardous and should *never* be used without the close supervision of a physician. It should not be used by pregnant women under any circumstances.

The patient can lose 1 lb. every 2 to 3 days on this regimen and thus lose more weight than when adhering to a conventional diet. However, the use of the protein-sparing modified fast has been questioned, since it does nothing to correct the patient's eating habits. Also, the general principle of this fast has been applied with the use of hydrolysates of incomplete protein and without adequate monitoring; such misuse has had disastrous results (see the next section).

Fad Diets. A variety of fad diets have succeeded one another over the years and probably will continue to do so. Many promise miracle cures and easy weight loss without dieting. In fact, any success achieved is usually the consequence of reduced energy intake because the diet is boring or unpalatable.

One type that is regularly resurrected is the *no-carbohydrate* or *low-carbohydrate diet,* which contains high protein plus high or moderate amounts of fat. Like the starvation diet, it tends to cause ketosis. The diet may cause rapid weight loss for a week or so, largely as a result of water loss. In addition, the diet usually is low in calories because of the difficulty in planning for enough calories from protein and fat alone. However, this is yet another diet that does nothing to change faulty eating habits, and the patient usually regains the weight lost.

Another type of diet often presented with great fervor is the one that *emphasizes one or a few foods* that are proposed to have miraculous properties—for example, the grapefruit, or bananas-and-milk, or lecithin/B_6/apple cider vinegar/kelp diets. Unfortunately, many are inadequate and most do little to establish better food habits. Some may be downright dangerous. Table 15-2 lists some of the better-known popular diets and discusses their properties.

Very-low-energy formula diets containing only incomplete protein from hydrolyzed collagen or gelatin were found to be a very hazardous form of weight control. In 1977 and 1978, fifty-eight persons were reported to have died after using a "liquid protein diet" to lose weight. In sixteen of these patients, sudden cardiogenic death was documented even though none had prior history of cardiovascular disease.[59] Death was caused by ventricular arrhythmia, but the underlying pathology is unknown.

At intervals, a weight reduction scheme is promoted in which it is claimed that some substance will interfere with digestion, absorption, or metabolism of food, thus causing weight loss without calorie restriction.

Table 15-2. Evaluation of Some Diets for Weight Reduction

Diet	Description
Anticellulite Diet	This is basically a good diet. It emphasizes raw vegetables, freshly prepared vegetable juices, and plenty of water, and limits meat, fish, and poultry to broiled lean cuts. It is important to remember that cellulite is just a fancy name for ordinary fat.
Dr. Atkins' Diet Revolution	This is a low-carbohydrate, high-protein diet containing an unlimited supply of protein and fat while severely restricting carbohydrates. Weight loss may be 8 lb. in the first week but will be mostly water. When carbohydrates are added to the diet, the lost water and lost weight will be regained. The diet may also result in extreme fatigue, irregular heartbeat, nausea, syncope, and calcium depletion. It is deficient in iron. In pregnant women, the resulting ketosis may harm the unborn child.
Banana–Skim Milk Diet	This diet contains four bananas plus five 8-oz. glasses of skim milk per day. It is deficient in vitamin A, niacin, thiamine, and iron unless vitamins and minerals are supplemented. It provides less than 1,000 kcal/day. The diet is very boring, and weight loss obviously occurs because of the calorie restriction, not from any particular properties of bananas and milk. Vitamin and mineral supplements are essential.
Calories Don't Count	This is a low-carbohydrate diet. It is claimed that if you eat the "right" amount of polyunsaturated fats, the pituitary gland will be stimulated and body fat will be burned at a higher rate. The only proved effect of the polyunsaturated fat (safflower oil) is to add 124 kcal/tbsp. The diet is low in calcium and riboflavin. It could be low in vitamin C unless the vegetables are selected carefully.
Lecithin B_6 Apple Cider Vinegar Kelp Diet	This diet calls for lecithin (2 tbsp./day) to "help emulsify your fat," vitamin B_6 to "help metabolize your fat," apple cider vinegar (1 tsp. following each meal) for potassium and because "vinegar and fat do not mix," and 6 tablets of kelp after each meal for iodine to "make your thyroid gland speed up your metabolism." No evidence indicates that the diet increases weight loss.
The Magic Mayo Diet or Grapefruit Diet	This diet recommends one-half grapefruit or grapefruit juice with every meal. It allows all the meat, fish, and eggs you can eat, and limits sugars and starches. The grapefruit is supposed to act as a "catalyst that activates fat burning." The Mayo Clinic does not recommend this diet.

Compiled from Stern, J.S., Weight control programs. In M. Winick, Ed., *Nutritional Disorders of American Women.* New York: John Wiley and Sons, 1977; Berland, T., *Rating the Diets. New Ways to Lose Weight.* New York: Consumers Union, 1977; and California Dietetic Association, *A Dozen Diets for Better or Worse.* Los Angeles: California Dietetic Association, 1973.

One of the more recent is the promotion of a so-called starch blocker. It is claimed that this substance, a protein from kidney, northern, or other beans, blocks the action of alpha-amylase and thus interferes with the digestion of starch. Each pill was advertised as interfering with the digestion of 400 to 750 starch calories, depending on the brand. One of its leading proponents advocated that the starch blocker be taken with a diet providing 700 kcal of starch and 500 kcal from other sources. With a 1,200-kcal diet, most patients would lose weight, and attributing the loss to the starch blocker would be unjustified. Nevertheless, starch blockers were selling very well at $10 to $20 per bottle (in 1982) until further sales were banned in the United States by the Food and Drug Administration (FDA) pending evidence that the product was safe and effective. The FDA had received complaints from users of nausea, vomiting, diarrhea, flatulence, and abdominal pain. If starch blockers worked as advertised and undigested starch reached the colon, microbial metabolism of starch could cause flatulence, abdominal cramps, and diarrhea. Further research is needed to clarify these issues. In the future, if approved for use, the product will probably be classified as a drug, although the vendors have insisted it is a food. Related compounds, currently under investigation, are discussed in the section on drug treatments for obesity (p. 579).

Other Aids to Weight Reduction

It has been obvious to nutritional care specialists for many years that simply teaching an obese patient the mechanics of an energy-restricted diet often does not lead to permanent weight reduction. In view of this fact, a number of other procedures are used in combination with or as a substitute for calorie restriction. Primary among these are exercise programs, behavior modification, group therapy, drugs, and surgery.

Exercise. The amount of exercise required to use excess kilocalories generally is regarded to be very great. Examples of common snack foods and their caloric equivalents in exercise as usually stated are given in Table 15-3. There is some evidence, however, that exercise increases resting and basal metabolic rate for a period of time that exceeds the duration of the exercise itself. This still is controversial, but if true, the energy cost of exercise would be greater than the values indicated by Table 15-3 and thus exercise would be recognized as being of greater value in weight reduction than has commonly been believed. Still, the amount of time required to "work off" the effects of a single milk shake in excess of need, for example, should make clear the advantage of prevention of excess intake.

Given the existence of obesity, though, exercise should be a part of any obesity treatment program, since exercise reduces body fat, regardless of weight. Studies of obese infants,[60] adolescent girls,[61] and adult women[62] indicate that, in all three groups, activity was less even though their food intake was not necessarily greater than that of their lean counterparts. It is difficult to motivate obese individuals to exercise, and careful monitoring or a structured program of exercises may be helpful.

Exercise may help to decrease food intake, even though many individuals believe that it will increase appetite.[63,64] On the contrary, Mayer[65] has shown that, in both rats and humans, food intake actually is increased when the body is very *in*active. Food intake decreases with light activity and rises in those with greater activity. The increase with heavy activity was proportionate to expenditure and did not lead to obesity.[65]

The amount and type of exercise should be chosen with care. Complicating conditions, such as cardiovascular disease and degenerative joint disease, must be taken into consideration, especially in the morbidly obese. The nutritional care specialist should work with others (the physician and physical therapist) on the health care team in coordinating kilocalorie intake with an exercise program.

Table 15-3. Energy Equivalents of Selected Snack Foods and Activities

		Activity				
Snack Food	Kcal	Walking (min.)	Bicycling (min.)	Swimming (min.)	Running (min.)	Reclining (min.)
Beer, 1 glass	114	22	14	10	6	88
Cake, two-layer, 1/12	356	68	43	32	18	274
Carbonated beverage, 1 glass	106	20	13	9	5	82
Doughnut	151	29	18	13	8	116
Ice cream, 1/6 qt	193	37	24	17	10	148
Ice cream soda	255	49	31	23	13	196
Malted milk shake	502	97	61	45	26	386
Milk shake	421	81	51	38	22	324

Based on data in Konishi, F., Food and energy equivalents of various activities. *J. Am. Diet. Assoc.* 46:187, 1965.

The energy cost of exercise varies with the type of activity, the amount of participation, duration of activity, and the body weight of the individual.[29] According to many tables, a person who weighs 200 lb. might expend only 350 kcal playing golf or as much as 1,042 kcal in judo or karate in 1 hour. Some activities lend themselves to great variation in the amount of effort expended. Our 200-lb. obese individual might expend, in 1 hour, 304 kcal bicycling at 5 miles per hour, 600 kcal at 10 miles per hour, and 868 kcal at 13 miles per hour. These expenditures would double if he or she continued the activity at the same pace for another hour. The heavier the individual, the greater the weight loss for a given activity. For example, if a man were swimming at a moderate pace of 45 yd/min., approximate expenditure might be 522 kcal/hr if he weighed 150 lb., 696 kcal/hr at 200 lb., and 870 kcal/hr at 250 lb. It is important to remember that these examples are estimations only and are influenced by an individual's skill in a given activity as well as the environmental temperature and consequent need to maintain body temperature.

There is no evidence that exercise is useful in "spot reducing" of subcutaneous fat. It may, in certain activities, lead to muscle development in some areas of the body.[66]

Behavior Modification. The procedures used in modifying eating behavior may vary with the concept of the problem as perceived by the nutritional therapist. One view is to consider problem eating as a sign of personality dysfunction. A more recent concept holds that eating behavior is learned and that poor eating practices can be unlearned. Problem eating is seen as the problem itself, not as a sign of another problem.

The theory behind behavior modification is based on principles of learning that are applied to normal behavior. Three types of learning principles will be described.

Observational or imitation learning requires observation of the behavior of another person who serves as a model. It can be very effective in children, for example, particularly if their behavior is reinforced.

Conditioning (*classic conditioning, pavlovian conditioning, or stimulus-response learning*) has also been attempted to modify eating behavior. In general principle, the method involves pairing a stimulus that elicits a given response with a neutral stimulus that does not elicit the response. Eventually, the neutral stimulus alone will elicit the response. It may be used in combination with the third method.

Operant conditioning or *trial-and-error learning* is, to a large extent, the basis for behavior modification techniques used in nutritional counseling and will therefore be described in more detail. It is based primarily on the assumption that behavior is controlled by the consequences that follow it. The behavior to be modified, the *target behavior,* is followed by a consequence known as a *reinforcer.* Reinforcers that increase the frequency of a target behavior are called *positive reinforcers* or *rewards,* whereas those that increase the behavior when removed are *negative reinforcers* or *aversive stimuli.* Negative reinforcers are presented before the desired response begins and are removed when it does begin. Negative reinforcement has been used in obesity therapy by subjecting the patient to unpleasant stimuli such as foul-smelling odors or electric shock prior to presenting problem foods. The method has suffered from a high dropout rate and has been successful primarily only over a short term.[67]

Another aspect of operant conditioning involves the process of *extinction.* It is based on the principle that if reinforcement of behavior is removed, the behavior will decrease. It requires the identification of and removal of reinforcers, processes that may be difficult.

Difficulty in therapy also arises if the desired behavior does not occur and therefore cannot be reinforced. Under these circumstances, a process known as *shaping* can be used. Some part or approximation of the desired behavior can be reinforced and then changed, at intervals, to approach the desired behavior. A patient might first decrease the intake of only one food, or agree to forego one part of a meal, for example. The desired diet might then be approached and reinforced in stepwise fashion.

In behavior modification programs for weight reduction, a variety of procedures based on the previously listed learning principles has been used. In general, the program begins with a diagnostic period to attempt to identify the factors that cause the maladaptive eating behavior. The patient is asked first to keep a diary of the type and amount of foods eaten and the circumstances of eating such as time, place, position, associated activities, others present, degree of hunger, and emotional state. From this record, the patient and therapist identify problem areas leading to overeating. Some problem areas might include eating leftovers from family meals to avoid waste, snacking while watching television, or eating very rapidly. Once problem areas are identified, the patient and nutritional care specialist together initiate desired changes. The shaping process might be very appropriate here.

Techniques for modification of eating behaviors include the following:

1. *Contingency contracting* consists of a signed agreement between the patient and therapist, which specifies behaviors to be changed and the rewards or penalties to be applied. One example required the patient to deposit specified valuables with the therapist to be "earned" back by weight loss.

2. *Positive reinforcement* can involve earning a reward for certain behaviors — that is, specified weight loss. Spouses have been enlisted to provide rewards in the form of encouragement and approval.

3. *Stimulus control and environmental management* procedures have received a great deal of attention. They seek to modify the environment that supports the overeating behavior.[68] This must be a cooperative procedure, involving both the therapist and patient, and requires imagination. Stuart[69] has suggested some procedures that he found to be useful in suppressing cues to eating:

Eat in one room only.
Do nothing else while eating.
Clear dishes from a meal directly into the garbage.
Make only the proper foods available by shopping from a list and only after a meal.
Prepare and serve small quantities only.
Eat only with utensils.
Chew food slowly.
Set utensils down between bites of food.

4. *Self-monitoring* includes calorie-counting from a chart, keeping a weight chart on a line graph, and writing down the amount of everything eaten. It provides the patient feedback on progress but has not been successful unless combined with other techniques.

Behavior modification was reported to be very successful when first presented,[70] but subsequent investigation has moderated the original enthusiasm for the method.[71] The weight loss 5 years after treatment was not significantly better than that seen in patients treated by traditional methods.[71] Nevertheless, if weight loss is to be maintained, eating behavior must be modified; therefore, it is logical to continue to attempt modification by some method.

Group Counseling. Sometimes obese patients are treated in groups rather than individually. Some studies have indicated little or no difference in the effectiveness of long-term group therapy, individual therapy, and no therapy,[72,73] but others report better results with group therapy.[74] For short-term use, at least, group treatment appears to be more effective than individual treatment.

A number of self-help groups have been established, often using behavior modification as part of their program. Examples of this type of program include Weight

Watchers, Inc., TOPS (Take Off Pounds Sensibly), Diet Workshop, and Overeaters Anonymous. Little data are available on the effectiveness of these groups. A few limited studies suggest that they are not helpful in the long term for the vast majority of patients.[15] The dropout rate has been reported to be 95 percent, but the groups may be successful in the remaining 5 percent.

Summer camps for obese children are numerous, providing programs for kilocalorie restriction, exercise, and nutrition education. Their effectiveness has not been evaluated.

Drugs. The lack of success in treatment of obesity by dieting had led to a search for drugs that might be helpful. According to Bray,[15] the ideal drug for weight reduction must be nontoxic, well tolerated, allow titration of body weight to the desired level, exert no deleterious metabolic effects, and be inexpensive. Although no drug meets all these criteria, a number of drugs have been used. They focus primarily on reducing energy intake.

The most commonly used drugs for obesity are *appetite depressants* or *anorectics.* Most are *phenylethylamines,* except for *mazindol* (Table 15-4). Phenylethylamines are similar in structure to the catecholamines dopamine, norepinephrine, and epinephrine. Most have many of the same effects—that is, increased energy, euphoria, wakefulness, decreased fatigue, tachycardia, and increased blood pressure. In attempts to avoid these side effects, substitutions on basic molecule have been made. In the molecule

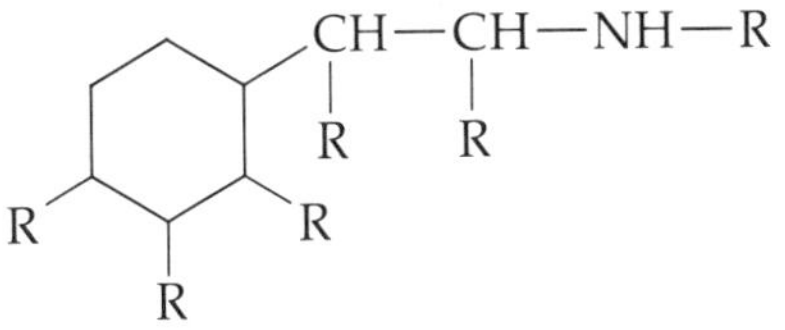

CH—CH—NH—R
R R
R R
R

substitutions have been made at all points indicated by R, most often by $-H$, $-OH$, $-CH_3$, $-Cl$, $=O$, $-C_2H_5$, or combinations of these. As a result, a number of similar but slightly different proprietary drugs

Table 15-4. Anorectic Agents Used in Weight Reduction

	Nutrition-Related Side Effects				
Drugs	Dry Mouth	Nausea	Abdominal Discomfort	Constipation	Diarrhea
Phenylethylamines					
Amphetamine sulfate (Delcobese, Benzedrine, etc.)	×	×	—	×	×
Benzphetamine hydrochloride (Didrex)	×	×	×	—	—
Chlorphentermine hydrochloride (Pre-Sate)	×	×	—	×	—
Clortermine hydrochloride (Voranil)	×	×	—	×	—
Diethylpropion hydrochloride (Tenuate, Tepanil)	×	×	×	×	—
Fenfluramine hydrochloride (Pondimin)	×	×	—	—	×
Metamphetamine hydrochloride (Desoxyn)	×	×	—	×	—
Phendimetrazine tartrate (Plegine, Bacarate, Bontril PDM, Melfat, Obe-Nil, Statobex, Trimtabs)	×	—	×	×	—
Phenmetrazine hydrochloride (Preludin)	×	×	—	×	—
Phentermine (Fastin, Ionamin, Wilpo, Adipex-P)	—	×	—	—	—
Phenylpropanolamine hydrochloride (nonprescription)	—	—	—	—	—
Nonphenylethylamine					
Mazindol (Sanorex)	×	×	—	—	—

× = present; — = incidence less than with placebo.

are available. Their modes of action are not all identical. Their side effects also vary. *Amphetamine,* which might be considered the parent compound, may act by an effect on the lateral hypothalamus.[75] It has been suggested that amphetamine causes a stimulation of dopaminergic and beta-adrenergic receptors by causing a release of dopamine and norepinephrine in the LH.[76] By contrast, fenfluramine is postulated to cause the release of serotonin from other central sites.[77] In addition to their modification of central systems in the brain involved with food impulse regulation, some anorectics (e.g., fenfluramine, and mazindol) also produce changes in energy metabolism.[78] In animals, triglyceride absorption was reduced and glucose uptake by human muscle and adipose tissue was increased. It is not known yet whether these changes are involved in the production of anorexia or are side effects.

Over the short term, anorectics increase weight loss, but long-term follow-up indicates that patients treated with drugs lose less. The effectiveness of these drugs is difficult to evaluate because of a high dropout rate in the subjects of the studies. As a result, the use of anorectics is controversial and is complicated by their involvement in drug abuse.

There are a number of new drugs under investigation that apparently function at sites in the gastrointestinal tract. Three of these are analogues of citric acid and act as anorectics.[79]

Other drugs believed to have potential to promote weight loss interfere with intestinal absorption of lipid or carbohydrate. Some *surface active agents* may reduce lipid absorption by inhibiting pancreatic lipase. *Neomycin* reduces intestinal flora and produces steatorrhea (see Chapters 3 and 5). *Carbohydrate absorption inhibitors* include the alpha-amylase inhibitors or starch blockers previously described. Other materials under investigation include additional alpha-amylase inhibitors and sucrase inhibitors.[79] Long-term studies of their effects are needed before they are made available for human use.

Bulking agents are intended to reduce food intake by a different mechanism than that of anorectics. Materials such as methylcellulose and guar gum have been added to food or dietetic candy with the intent to fill the stomach with inert, nondigestible material. The hope is that the obese person then will eat less. Unfortunately, clinical trials do not indicate that the method is effective, and flatulence is a problem.[80]

The third category of drugs used as weight-reducing aids have been categorized as *metabolic affectors.* Some deserve particular mention. *Thyroid hormone* has been used for many years on the assumption that it would stimulate oxygen consumption and increase fuel use. Unfortunately, in addition to fat consumption, protein loss increases.[81] These protein losses can be minimized by increasing dietary protein,[82] but the results of thyroid medication are no better than with diet alone.[15] The use of exogenous thyroid hormone also causes side effects including increased myocardial irritability; therefore, its use rarely is indicated.

Injections of *human chorionic gonadotropin* (HCG) are used in many clinics along with a very-low-calorie (500-kcal), low-fat diet. The originator of this treatment method claims that it "melts away" fat and reduces hunger.[83] Carefully controlled clinical trials indicate that HCG neither reduces hunger nor promotes weight loss beyond that which would be obtained by diet alone.[84–86]

Human growth hormone, another metabolic affector, has been used recently in the treatment of obesity. It depletes body fat, and limited trials indicate that it may be effective. However, the hormone is in short supply. If more becomes available, additional research may be possible.

Other possible approaches to drug therapy include inhibition of pancreatic amylase, replacement of dietary fat with a noncaloric synthetic fat, such as sucrose polyester, that is not absorbed, decreasing the efficiency of lipid and carbohydrate oxidation, and normalizing hormone changes typical of the obese.[57]

On the whole, it appears that treatment of obesity with presently available drugs has little to offer. An ideal drug to promote weight loss is not available yet.

Surgery. Surgical treatments for obesity have been developed largely because of the poor response to less drastic measures. The methods that have been used will be described briefly, with emphasis on nutritional consequences.

Lipectomy. It might seem logical to ask why obesity could not be treated by *adipectomy* or *lipectomy* (surgical removal of adipose tissue). Since the number of fat cells is thought to be reduced during weight loss, the surgical removal of numbers of cells might be postulated to make it easier for patients to maintain their loss. There are few studies of the effects of such treatment. However, the little evidence available demonstrated in three patients that lipectomy did not prevent regaining lost weight, although the adiposity did not recur at the same sites.[87] These results suggest that it is the mass of adipose tissues or cell size that is controlled rather than the number of cells. This type of surgery sometimes is undertaken for cosmetic reasons, but it is not considered a primary treatment. In addition, *panniculectomy* (surgical removal of excess abdominal skin and fat) following large weight losses sometimes is done for cosmetic purposes.

Jejunoileal bypass. Jejunoileal bypass surgery causes weight loss by producing malabsorption and also by reducing food intake. The procedure is major surgery and is not undertaken lightly. The criteria for selection of a patient for this type of surgery include:[29,87]

Massive obesity, with body weight at least 50 percent more than ideal weight in men or 80 percent more than ideal weight in women
Failure to reduce and maintain reduced weight with other forms of treatment for at least 3 years
Absence of endocrine disease that causes the obesity
Absence of diseases increasing surgical risk, such as liver disease
Presence of diseases the prognosis of which improves with weight loss, such as diabetes mellitus or congestive heart failure
Age between 14 and 55 years

The surgical procedure consists of establishing the continuity of the gastrointestinal tract so that approximately 30 to 50 cm of the proximal small intestine is attached to 10 to 15 cm of distal ileum (Fig. 15-2). The anastamosis may be end-to-end or end-to-side with similar results. The appendix is removed. The stomach and large intestine are intact. The bypassed portion of the intestine, approximately 20 ft or 6 m, is left in place. Thus, the procedure can be reversed if necessary. The net result is similar to the short bowel syndrome described in Chapter 6.

Diarrhea occurs in all patients postoperatively, with fifteen to twenty bowel movements daily at first and decreasing to approximately five per day after 6 months.[88] It is important, especially during the first month, to prevent excessive food intake for the size of the remaining bowel or the patient will vomit, causing loss of protein, electrolytes, and fluid. Approximately 30 percent of weight is lost in the first year,[89] and the weight stabilizes after approximately 2 years with weight maintenance at approximately 62 percent of maximum.

A number of serious side effects may occur. Patients may develop such severe electrolyte imbalances as to require hospitalization. Serum concentrations of calcium, magnesium, and potassium may be low. Some patients also develop deficiencies of vitamin B_{12} and fat-soluble vitamins.

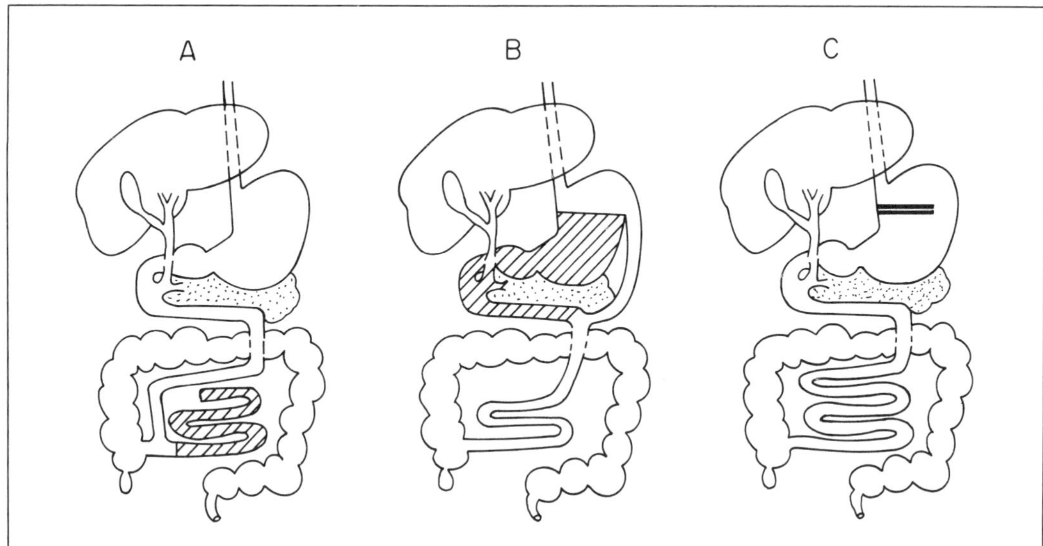

Figure 15-2. Surgical treatment of obesity. (**A**). *Jejunoileal bypass. Anastomosis of jejunoileal bypass may be end-to-end or end-to-side.* (**B**). *Gastric bypass.* (**C**). *Gastroplasty.*

Progressive liver disease occurs in some intestinal bypass patients, with inflammation and fibrosis, sometimes progressing to cirrhosis. The etiology of the liver condition is not clear. Experiments with animals suggest that the hepatic lesion is caused by toxins produced by bacterial overgrowth in the bypassed intestine.[90] Others have suggested that liver failure may be the result of nutritional deficiency.[91]

Other complications include death in 0 to 6 percent of patients, wound infection in 2 to 5 percent, thromboembolism in 1 to 5 percent, and renal failure in 3 percent.[87] A small number of patients develop severe psychiatric problems. Complications are life-threatening in approximately 4 percent of patients, and the normal intestinal continuity must be reestablished. It is important that patients having their bypass surgery reversed have good protein nutrition prior to surgery. Ideally, restoration is done before the patient is seriously protein-depleted. For protein-depleted patients, Mason[92] recommends the use of hyperosmotic amino acid and glucose infusions via a central vein (see Chapter 12). The patient is given 3 to 4 L/day. One of these infusions is glucose-free to mobilize fat from the liver. The central line is left in place for feeding after surgery, since these patients have a prolonged ileus. Most patients return to their original obese weight after bypass reversal. The most commonly held current opinion is that the risks of this type of surgery are not justified by the benefits.

Jejunoileal bypass has been done extensively in the past, and some of these patients may come to the attention of the nutritional care specialist postoperatively. The patients should receive potassium supplements, particularly when diarrhea is severe. Potassium-rich fruits and vegetables should be emphasized when the postoperative patient recovers sufficiently to eat them. Supplements of calcium, magnesium, and all vitamins may be required.

A *high-protein* diet to protect the liver and *low fat* to reduce steatorrhea, provided in *small meals,* may be helpful. Alcohol should be avoided for at least 1 year and preferably permanently to avoid overtaxing the liver. Pregnancy should be avoided while weight loss is occurring.

Gastric bypass. Gastric bypass has been offered as an alternative to intestinal bypass. It causes weight loss by reducing food intake and delaying stomach emptying. There may be a small amount of malabsorption.

The surgery consists of creation of a gastroenterostomy, thereby reducing the reservoir function of the stomach by as much as 90 percent (Fig. 15-2B). The bypassed portion of the stomach can be restored to continuity if necessary. There are fewer complications but weight loss is less than that following intestinal bypass. The loss is greatest in young patients. Dumping syndrome, steatorrhea, and gallstones sometimes are complications,[93] and the patient may require counseling on diet for dumping syndrome (see Chapter 6). A low-fat diet helps in reducing steatorrhea.

A variation of gastric bypass is *gastroplasty* or *gastric stapling.* The procedure consists of a partial division of the stomach (Fig. 15-2C), leaving a passageway approximately 1.5 cm in diameter. Weight loss is even less than with gastric bypass, but complications are greatly reduced. This is a newer procedure the long-term effects of which have not been totally evaluated yet.

The diet following gastric partitioning must be progressed with caution. Throughout, kilocalories are maintained at 600 or less plus vitamin and mineral supplements during the period of weight loss. A protocol from the University of Utah suggests the following:

Week 1: 90 ml/hr or less of clear liquids—water, clear fruit juice, weak coffee or tea, dessert gelatin, popsicles, salty broth, soda pop (allow to go flat).

Week 2: Up to 120 ml/hr of full liquids (see Chapter 2) with caution to assure that high-calorie fluids are not provided.

Weeks 3 through 6: Gradually add puréed foods: soups, soft eggs, cottage cheese, mashed potatoes, followed by puréed cooked fruits and vegetables, mashed banana, puréed poultry, mashed fish, processed cheese. Increase to a *maximum* of 150 ml/hr in week 6.

A crucial question is does the mortality improve in these surgery patients compared to that of untreated morbidly obese patients? Until this question is answered, surgical procedures for treatment of obesity will be used with caution by most surgeons.

Jaw wiring. Jaw wiring or jaw fixation consists of wiring the upper and lower jaws together so that intake of liquids is possible but eating solid foods is almost impossible. Weight loss, in one study, averaged 25.3 kg in 6 months, an amount similar to that seen in intestinal bypass patients.[94] Most regained some of the weight once the wires were removed. Possible complications include dental caries and deterioration of muscle function in the jaw. Patients are advised to carry wire clippers to remove the wire in case of vomiting to avoid choking.

Nutritional care should include counseling on the variety of liquid and semiliquid food that can make up the diet. Particular attention should be paid to ensure that the diet is adequate in protein, minerals, and vitamins without providing excess calories.

Hypothalamic stereotoxy. Hypothalamic stereotoxy is a procedure used primarily in animal experiments in which electrolytic lesions are created in the LH. It can result in diminished food intake and a consequent decrease in body weight. The procedure has been used on only a few morbidly obese human subjects and produced only a small, temporary decrease in body weight.[95] This technique is considered experimental for use on animals only.

Truncal vagotomy. Truncal vagotomy is an experimental procedure which has been used on a limited number of patients. There are no serious side effects. The vagotomy interferes with the pathway from the hypothalamus to the pancreas which stimulates insulin production. As plasma insulin levels fall, food intake decreases. In some patients, body weights improved, whereas the results in others were unqualified failures.

Acupuncture. Acupuncture also has been tried as a treatment for obesity. In a controlled study,[96] no significant weight reduction was achieved with this treatment.

Psychotherapy. Psychiatric treatment is not often successful in the treatment of obesity unless the patient has a treatable psychiatric disorder and the obesity is of recent development as a consequence. Some cases of depression are associated with weight gain. Unfortunately, the tricyclic antidepressants also cause weight gain.

Hypnosis. Hypnosis has been used only occasionally, and its long-term effectiveness is unknown. Some techniques reported include posthypnotic suggestion, substitution of gum chewing for eating, substitution of physical activity for eating, and hypnotic anesthesia to control hunger pangs.

Most Highly Recommended Therapy for Obesity

It must be recognized that the causes of obesity are poorly understood and the treatments available at present are largely ineffective and sometimes hazardous. However, almost any treatment will give some short-term results. Given these limitations, the most highly recommended therapy consists of individualized treatment coupled with group counseling, using restriction of calorie intake, increased physical activity, and instruction in behavior modification to change eating behavior permanently. For maintenance of weight loss, the patient may need to remain in treatment almost indefinitely. Successful weight reduction remains a challenge and a source of frustration to the nutritional care specialist. One should remember that a great service is being performed for the patient if he or she is helped to achieve a stable weight and prevent further weight gain.

Psychological Factors in Obesity

The nutritional care specialist must be sensitive to the psychological factors involved in treating obesity, which can be divided into (1) factors causing obesity, (2) those that result from the existence of the obesity, (3) those that arise from attempts to lose weight, and, occasionally, (4) factors that arise from successful weight loss.

Some, but by no means all, patients become obese as a consequence of a psychiatric disorder. No single disorder has been identified as being involved in the etiology of obesity, but when one does exist, it must be treated before nutritional treatment for weight reduction can be undertaken.

The stigma attached to obesity in our society may be the cause of emotional disturbance. The obese person can develop a syndrome of low self-esteem, depression, and hostility.[97] Treatment is thought to require raising the self-esteem. The attitude of health professionals toward the obese can be very important in this regard. Health professionals whose attitude toward the obese is to stigmatize them are unlikely to be helpful.

Other obese patients have problems that are not severe enough to be classified as psychiatric problems but for which their overeating compensates, including emotional problems such as depression, frustration, worry, hopelessness, isolation, guilt, or shame. Food may relieve tension in such patients. A person who gains weight after giving up smoking may be substituting one method of relieving tension for another. It has been suggested that the effect is mediated via corticosteroid hormones. On the whole, however, the mechanisms relating emotional factors and obesity are unknown.

Emotional problems sometimes arise during or following weight loss. The reasons for this are not always clear. Patients with juvenile-onset obesity in one study showed frequent symptoms of anxiety and depression and viewed the process of weight loss as severe starvation.[98] They had disturbances in body image and continued to see themselves as fat even after weight loss.

Problems may arise for the occasional patient who successfully loses weight. Some patients adjust to the stigma of obesity by developing friendships with other obese individuals. For others, obesity is an important component in maintaining their relationships with spouses. Weight loss sometimes can disrupt these relationships.

Prevention of Obesity

The best "treatment" for obesity is prevention. In contacts with obese patients, the nutritional care specialist sometimes will have an opportunity to influence the parents to prevent obesity in their children. Fomon[99] has suggested some procedures:

1. Encourage mothers to breast-feed their infants.
2. Educate parents on the dangers and problems of overfeeding and on the influence of childhood eating patterns on later nutritional status.
3. Instruct parents to delay introduction of solid food in their child's diet until the child is 4 to 6 months old.
4. Promote physical exercise.
5. Encourage parents to develop facilities for year-round physical activity.
6. Instruct parents to use more smaller meals rather than fewer larger meals, but do not increase kilocalories in the process.
7. Give special help and counseling to parents who are obese.

UNDERWEIGHT

A much smaller number of people have a problem in gaining weight rather than in losing weight. These patients are classified as *underweight* (15 to 20 percent or more below ideal weight).

Underweight in General

Etiology

A number of conditions can cause a person to be underweight. Poor absorption and utilization of food was discussed in Chapter 6. Some patients are underweight because they have a wasting disease such as cancer (see Chapter 13). Others are underweight because of psychological or emotional stress or abnormality. Others take in an inadequate quantity or quality of food. If the patient has a disease that causes the underweight condition, the nutritional needs relevant to that disease must also be considered when planning the diet. Thus, combinations of several diet modifications may be necessary.

General Effects

Underweight patients have decreased resistance to infection, increased sensitivity to cold, and weakness. Undernutrition can cause depressed function of the pituitary, adrenal, and thyroid glands and the gonads. Growth is retarded in children.

Treatment

Although obese patients may find it hard to believe, it frequently is very difficult for an underweight person to gain weight. In order to increase his or her weight, a person must have an energy intake that is in excess of output. The basic need for the underweight patient is, therefore, a high-calorie diet. Current energy needs must be met plus an additional 500 to 1,000 kcal. Food intake may be increased gradually to prevent gastrointestinal disorders. The additional kilocalories may be provided in any of three ways: (1) extra portions of usual foods at regular meals, (2) more concentrated foods, or (3) between-meal snacks. The procedures used should conform to the patient's preferences.

The protein allowance is maintained at a generous or high level, 100 g or more. Protein will be needed for repair and replacement. As the energy level of the diet increases, protein also increases if the planned diet is to contain normal foods since most high-carbohydrate foods contain some protein.

The carbohydrate and fat content of the diet must, of course, be increased to achieve the positive calorie balance. The distribution between the two can be made largely on the basis of the patient's preferences. More concentrated sources of kilocalories are advised to reduce the total bulk of the diet.

Vitamins and minerals should be provided at optimal levels. Increased intake of food will increase intake of micronutrients, but supplementation of B vitamins sometimes is needed as kilocalorie intake is increased. Their appetite-stimulating effect may also be helpful.

The patient should be involved in planning the diet. Behavior modification techniques are used as they are for changing the eating habits of obese patients.

Anorexia Nervosa

Anorexia nervosa is a disorder in which underweight can become severe to the point of being life-threatening. It represents a special form of undernutrition. The patient becomes extremely emaciated as a result of self-starvation. Weight loss is at least 25 percent and often is more severe.

More than 90 percent of anorexia nervosa patients are adolescent girls at onset of the disease. The condition usually first appears shortly after puberty, but occasionally there is prepubertal or late adolescent onset. It is found in the middle and upper classes of affluent societies and is not seen in underdeveloped countries. It was first described in 1868 and was long considered a very rare condition. In recent years, however, the incidence is believed to be increasing, although little epidemiologic data are available.

Etiology

Anorexia nervosa has been classified as *primary* or *atypical.* Atypical forms may be secondary to other conditions such as schizophrenia, depression, or hysteria.

The cause of primary anorexia nervosa is uncertain, but the opinion held by most of those who have studied the disease is that anorexia nervosa is psychological in origin. The typical patient is described as highly intelligent, introverted, overly sensitive, perfectionist, and compulsive, with serious deficits in personal development. A deep-seated feeling of ineffectiveness and inadequacy is a common finding. The disease has been proposed to arise from disturbed family relationships in which the patient does not develop a sense of autonomy and effectiveness.[100] There are, however, other opinions.

As an alternative, it has been proposed that anorexia nervosa is a disease in which there is an immature functioning of the hypothalamus that interferes with normal maturation at puberty.[101] However, this theory does not explain the occurrence of the disease only in developed countries, nor does it explain the class distinction in developed countries.

It has also been suggested that the pathologic family situations are not the cause of the disease. Rather, they may arise as a result of the stresses created by the disease in one of its members.

Clinical Manifestations

The outstanding feature of anorexia nervosa is severe weight loss that occurs in the absence of organic disease. A weight loss of at least 25 percent of normal body weight is considered a prerequisite for diagnosis. The patient who loses weight from organic disease typically is aware of the loss, worries about it, and regards it as undesirable. By contrast, the anorexia nervosa patient defends her right to lose weight and complains of being too fat, even when she is seriously emaciated. Only a few known cases were obese before they began dieting. The patients have a *distorted body image* and seem to enjoy and take pride in the progressive weight loss. They often will claim that they do not need to eat and seem to regard their bodies as not their own.

The anorexia nervosa patient *refuses to eat* or eats only a minuscule amount. Bruch[100] tells of one patient who described breakfast saying, "I ate my Cheerio." Patients have been described as spending several hours eating minute amounts of food and complaining of feeling full after only a bite or two. Others have occasional *eating binges* which are *followed by self-induced vomiting* or the use of diuretics, enemas, or large doses of laxatives. There is a great feeling of guilt for losing control.

Many patients are reported to have been somewhat athletic prior to their illness. However, as the disease progresses, the activity tends to change from team sports to those activities that can be performed alone, such as jogging, running, swimming, or calisthenics. The activity takes on a frantic character. Along with the *hyperactivity*, the patient often becomes obsessed with attaining perfection in academic performance. She denies feelings of fatigue despite her various activities and little sleep. Social contact becomes less frequent until the patient is well isolated.

The name of the disease indicates loss of appetite; however, this is apparently a misnomer. Recovered anorexics have reported that they suffered greatly from hunger but somehow obtained great satisfaction from not "giving in." Some patients spend much time preparing foods for others to eat, although they refuse to partake themselves. Some collect recipes, walk around food stores, and spend much time in other activities that indicate their minds are consumed with thoughts of food.

As the weight loss progresses, other clinical manifestations appear. They are thought to be the consequence of the malnutrition, since many of these same manifestations have been seen in victims of famine.

There are no definitive laboratory tests for diagnosis. There are a variety of hormone imbalances. Amenorrhea (failure to menstruate) is invariable in girls. Reduction in gonadotropic hormone levels (luteinizing hormone [LH] and follicle-stimulating hormone [FSH]) and alterations in growth hormone and insulin also are found. Neurohormones affecting eating behavior—norepinephrine, dopamine, and serotonin—also regulate insulin, growth hormone, LH, and FSH, and it has been suggested that an alteration of hormone balance in these patients constitutes a biologic predisposition to the disease.[102] However, these changes usually are regarded as the consequence rather than the cause of anorexia nervosa. It is not known whether they precede or follow the onset. Hormone levels do not necessarily return to normal when weight is normalized.

Other manifestations include lowered basal metabolic rate, poor thermoregulation, cold intolerance, anemia, pallor, dry skin, constipation, abdominal pain, hypotension, bradycardia, growth of downy hair (*lanugo*) over the body, and sleep disturbances. Laxative and diuretic abuse can cause electrolyte imbalances and dehydration. The dehydration can produce a reduced production of saliva which is also more viscid. The mouth may be very acidic, caused by vomiting or the use of acid fluids such as fruit juice for thirst. The changes in saliva and the acid pH cause an erosion of the teeth called *perimolysis*, in which the substance of the teeth is lost and many caries appear at atypical locations.[103,104] The anatomy of the oral cavity and teeth and nutritional care of oral cavity problems are described in Chapter 5.

As the disease and its attendant weight loss progresses, the psychological effects of starvation appear, making the illness even more difficult to treat. The weight lost includes not only body fat but also muscle protein. The biologic effects are those of starvation. Mortality has been reported to vary from 5 to 20 percent.

Treatment

The anorexia nervosa patient is very ill and treatment is urgent. Sometimes, fluid and electrolyte therapy and total parenteral nutrition (TPN) (see Chapter 12) are needed as life-saving measures. Longer-term treatment designed to get at the root of the problem consists of a combination of psychotherapy and nutritional rehabilitation. Hospitalization often is recommended, and the patient is placed in a nonstress environment. Psychotherapy is the most important aspect of treatment to address the central problems, but some weight gain prior to the initiation of psychotherapy often is desirable.

Various procedures have been recommended to increase food intake. The role of the nutritional care specialist is supportive and varies with the treatment protocol in a particular center. The anorexia nervosa patient is not given a selective menu as is often provided to other patients. Instead, the decision is made for her. If the patient refuses solid food, high-protein high-calorie liquids (see Appendix L) can be provided instead. If the patient absolutely refuses to eat, tube feeding or TPN may be required, although some patients will manage to discontinue this type of feeding also.

Behavior modification, based on a reward system for eating, sometimes is used with good results, but in some patients these methods are ineffective and may be harmful. Bruch[105] warns against the use of punitive behavior modification methods. Patients may feel tricked into loss of control and have a sense of personal ineffectiveness, the proposed cause of the problem in the first place.

Patients often require several years of treatment. They are considered recovered if they eat a reasonable diet that maintains a stable weight within reasonable limits, menstruate regularly, and have interpersonal relationships appropriate for age.

Bulimia Nervosa

Bulimia nervosa, also known as *bulimarexia* or *gorge-and-purge syndrome,* has only recently been recognized as a separate and definable disease. There are some similarities to anorexia nervosa and also some important differences.

Bulimia is defined as an abnormal increase in hunger sensations. The bulimia patient, generally female, has episodes of insatiable appetite in which she goes on an eating binge and can consume 10,000 to 20,000 kcal/day. This is followed by purging by self-induced vomiting and use of laxatives and diuretics. While the anorexia nervosa patient may break off fasting with an occasional binge, the bulimia patient has repeated binges.

Bulimia is more likely to develop in adults than in adolescents. The typical patient, as in anorexia nervosa, is a perfectionist with low self-esteem and a distorted body image. She is digusted by fat but preoccupied with food. The bulimia patient, however, may be of normal weight and described as slim. She often is attractive, successful, and extroverted. The food binges and purges are hidden and eventually interfere with other aspects of her life, leading to isolation.

The incidence of the disease is apparently high, although few data are available. It has been estimated, for example, that 20 percent or more of female college students are bulimic.

Hazards include electrolyte and fluid imbalances, anemia, tears in the lower esophagus, difficulty in swallowing, swollen and infected salivary glands, and dental problems.

Treatment consists of psychotherapy, often in groups. Nutritional care is supportive. The nutritional care specialist sometimes can help the patient control the binges. Many of the techniques of behavior modification have been used. For example, patients can be advised to keep a diary to identify and then avoid circumstances that precipitate a binge. Another technique is to set time limits on binges with a kitchen timer. The clock can be set for 5 minutes for the binge period and then reset for an hour later when another 5-minute binge is allowed. This procedure may help the patient achieve some measure of control. Food should not be eaten out of the original container, but a small portion should be put on a plate and eaten in a dining room, a procedure that might interfere with eating whole bags of cookies, gallons of ice cream, loaves of bread, and similar amounts of food. These techniques at least may help to reduce the number of binges and amounts of food consumed and thus reduce the necessity for purging. The potential for cure is unknown.

References

1. Heaton, J.M. The distribution of brown adipose tissue in the human. *J. Anat.* 112:35, 1972.
2. Sclafani, A., and Berner, C.N. Hyperphagia and obesity produced by parasagittal and coronal hypothalamic knife cuts: Further evidence for a longitudinal feeding inhibitory pathway. *J. Comp. Physiol. Psychol.* 91:1000, 1977.
3. Leibowitz, S.F. Central adrenergic receptors and the regulation of hunger and thirst. In I.J. Kopin, Ed., *Neurotransmitters.* Proceedings of the Association for Research in Nervous and Mental Disease, vol. 50. Baltimore: Williams and Wilkins, 1972.
4. Marshall, J.F. The role of catecholamine-containing neurons in food intake. In G.A. Bray, Ed., *Recent Advances in Obesity Research: II.* London: Newman Publishing, 1978.
5. Leibowitz, S.F. Ingestion in the satiated rat: Role of alpha and beta receptors in mediating effects of hypothalamic adrenergic stimulation. *Physiol. Behav.* 14:743, 1975.
6. Gibbs, J., Fauser, D.J., Rowe, E.A., et al. Bombesin suppresses feeding in rats. *Nature* 282:208, 1979.
7. Vijayan, E., and McCann, S.M. Suppression of feeding and drinking activity in rats following intraventricular injection of thyrotropin-releasing hormone (TRH). *Endocrinology* 100:1727, 1977.
8. Lotter, E.C., Krinski, R., McKay, J.M., et al. Somatostatin decreases food intake of rats and baboons. *J. Comp. Physiol. Psychol.* 95:278, 1981.
9. Bray, G.A. Regulation of energy balance: Studies on genetic, hypothalamic and dietary obesity. *Proc. Nutr. Soc.* 41:95, 1982.
10. Bray, G.A., and Campfield, L.A. Metabolic factors in the control of energy stores. *Metabolism* 24:99, 1975.
11. Newsholme, E.A. The interrelationship between metabolic regulation, weight control and obesity. *Proc. Nutr. Soc.* 41:183, 1982.
12. Kennedy, G.C. The role of depot fat in the hypothalamic control of food intake in the rat. *Proc. R. Soc.* (Lond.) 140:578, 1953.
13. Nisbett, R.E. Hunger, obesity and the ventromedial hypothalamus. *Psychol. Rev.* 79:433, 1972.
14. Hervey, G.R. Physiological mechanisms for the regulation of energy balance. *Proc. Nutr. Soc.* 30:109, 1971.
15. Bray, G.A. *The Obese Patient.* Major Problems in Internal Medicine, vol. 9. Philadelphia: W.B. Saunders, 1976.
16. Harper, A.E., Benevenga, N.J., and Wohlhueter, R.M. Effects of ingestion of disproportionate amounts of amino acids. *Physiol. Rev.* 50:428, 1970.
17. Lytle, L.D., and Messing, R.B. Appetite in the regulation of food intake for energy (animal and man). *Prog. Food Nutr. Sci.* 2:49, 1976.
18. Liebowitz, S.F. Reciprocal hunger-regulating circuits involving alpha- and beta-adrenergic receptors located respectively in the ventromedial and lateral hypothalamus. *Proc. Natl. Acad. Sci. U.S.A.* 2:49, 1976.
19. Rogers, Q.R., and Leung, P.M.B. The influence of amino acids on the neuroregulation of food intake. *Fed. Proc.* 32:1709, 1973.
20. Brobeck, J.R. Food intake as a mechanism of temperature regulation. *Yale J. Biol. Med.* 20:545, 1948.
21. Oomura, Y. Effects of glucose and free fatty acid in chemosensitive neurons in the rat hypothalamus. In D. Novin, W. Wyrwicka, and G. Bray, Eds., *Hunger: Basic Mechanisms and Clinical Implications.* New York: Raven Press, 1975.
22. Woods, S., Lotter, E.C., McKay, L.D., and Porte, D., Jr. Chronic intracerebroventricular infusion of insulin reduces food intake and body weight of baboons. *Nature* 282:503, 1979.
23. Sims, E.A.H., Danforth, E., Jr., Horton, E.S.,

et al. Endocrine and metabolic effects of experimental obesity in man. *Recent Prog. Horm. Res.* 29:457, 1973.
24. Rothwell, N.J., and Stock, M.J. A role for brown adipose tissue in diet-induced thermogenesis. *Nature* 281:31, 1979.
25. James, W.P.T., Trayhurn, P., and Garlick, P. The metabolic basis of subnormal thermogenesis in obesity. In P. Björntorp, M. Cairella, and A.N. Howard, Eds., *Recent Advances in Obesity Research: III.* London: John Libbey, 1981.
26. Hervey, G.R., and Tobin, G. The part played by variation in energy expenditure in the regulation of energy balance. *Proc. Nutr. Soc.* 41:137, 1972.
27. National Center for Health Statistics. NCHS Growth Charts, 1976. *Monthly Vital Statistics Report* 25(3), Suppl. (HRA) 76-1120. Rockville, Md.: Health Resources Administration, 1976.
28. Keys, A., Fidanza, F., Karvonen, M.J., et al. Indices of relative weight and obesity. *J. Chronic Dis.* 25:329, 1972.
29. Stern, J.S., and Kane-Nussen, B. Obesity: Its assessment, risks and treatments. In R.B. Alfin-Slater, D. Kritschevsky, and R.E. Hodges, Eds., *Human Nutrition—A Comprehensive Treatise,* vol. 4. New York: Plenum, 1979.
30. Mayer, J. *Overweight: Causes, Cost and Control.* New York: Prentice-Hall, 1968.
31. Mayer, J. Genetic, traumatic and environmental factors in the etiology of obesity. *Physiol. Rev.* 33:472, 1953.
32. Galton, O.J., Gilbert, C., Reekless, J.P.D., and Kaye, J. Triglyceride-storage disease. A group of inborn errors of triglyceride metabolism. *Q.J. Med.* 43:63, 1974.
33. Gurney, R. The hereditary factor in obesity. *Arch. Intern. Med.* 47:557, 1936.
34. Seltzer, C.C., and Mayer, J. Body build (somatotype) distinctiveness in obese women. *J. Am. Diet. Assoc.* 55:457, 1969.
35. Vague, J., Rubin, P., Jubelin, J., et al. Regulation of the adipose tissue mass: histometric and anthropometric aspects. In J. Vague and J. Boyer, Eds., *The Regulation of Adipose Tissue Mass.* Amsterdam: Excerpta Medica, 1974.
36. Iverson, F. Psychogenic obesity in children. I. *Acta Paediatr. Scand.* 42:8, 1953.
37. Sonne-Holm, S., and Sorensen, T.I.A. Postwar course of the prevalence of extreme overweight among Danish young men. *J. Chronic Dis.* 30:351, 1977.
38. Warner, W.A., and Garrett, L.P. The obese patient and anesthesia. *J.A.M.A.* 205:102, 1968.
39. James, W.P.T., Ed. *Research on Obesity.* London: Medical Research Council, 1976.
40. Faust, I.M., Johnson, P.R., Stern, J.S., and Hirsch, J. Diet induced adipocyte cell number increase in adult rats: A new model of obesity. *Am. J. Physiol.* 235:E279, 1978.
41. Hirsch, J., and Batchelor, P.R. Adipose tissue cellularity in human obesity. *Clin. Endocrinol. Metab.* 5:299, 1976.
42. Stunkard, A.J., and McLaren-Hume, N. The results of treatment of obesity: A review of the literature and report of a series. *Arch. Intern. Med.* 103:79, 1959.
43. Hollenberg, C.H. The fat cell and the fat patient. *R. Coll. Phys. Surg. Can.* 8:119, 1975.
44. Bray, G.A. The myth of diet in the management of obesity. *Am. J. Clin. Nutr.* 23:1141, 1970.
45. Buskirk, E.R., Thompson, R.H., Lutwak, L., and Whedon, G.D. Energy balance of obese patients during weight reduction: Influence of diet restriction and exercise. *Ann. N.Y. Acad. Sci.* 110:1918, 1963.
46. Blondheim, S.H., Kaufman, N.A., and Stein, M. Comparison of fasting and 800–1000 calorie diet in obesity. *Lancet* 1:250, 1965.
47. Russell, G.F.M. The effects of diets of different composition on weight loss and sodium balance in obese patients. *Clin. Sci.* 22:269, 1962.
48. Cohn, C., Joseph, D., Bell, L., and Allweiss, M.D. Studies on the effects of feeding frequency and dietary composition on fat deposition. *Ann. N.Y. Acad. Sci.* 131:507, 1965.
49. Fabry, P., Fodor, J., Hejl, Z., et al. The frequency of meals: Its relationship to overweight, hypercholesterolemia and decreased glucose-tolerance. *Lancet* 2:614, 1964.
50. Huenemann, R.L. Food habits of obese and non-obese adolescents. *Postgrad. Med.* 51:99, 1972.
51. Young, C.M., Scanlan, S.S., Topping, C.M., et al. Frequency of feeding, weight reduction and body composition. *J. Am. Diet. Assoc.* 59:466, 1971.
52. Young, C.M., Hutter, L.F., Scanlan, S.S., et al. Metabolic effects of meal frequency on normal young men. *J. Am. Diet. Assoc.* 61:391, 1972.
53. Bortz, W.M., Wroldsen, A., Issekutz, B., and Rodahl, K. Weight loss and frequency of feeding. *N. Engl. J. Med.* 274:376, 1966.

54. Finkelstein, B., and Fryer, B.A. Meal frequency and weight reduction in young women. *Am. J. Clin. Nutr.* 24:465, 1971.
55. Silverstone, J.T., Stark, J.E., and Buckle, R.M. Hunger during total starvation. *Lancet* 1:1343, 1966.
56. Blackburn, G.L., Bistrian, B.R., and Flatt, J.P. Role of protein-sparing modified fast in a comprehensive weight reduction program. In A. Howard, Ed., *Recent Advances in Obesity Research: I.* London: Newman Publishing, 1975.
57. Blackburn, G.L., and Greenberg, I. Multidisciplinary approach to adult obesity therapy. In G. Bray, Ed., *Obesity: Comparative Methods of Weight Control.* Westport, Conn.: Technomic Publishing, 1980.
58. Bistrian, B.R. Clinical use of the protein-sparing modified fast. *J.A.M.A.* 21:2299, 1978.
59. Bray, G.A. An evaluation of treatments for obesity. In G. Enzi, G. Crepaldi, G. Pozza, and A.E. Renold, Eds., *Obesity: Pathogenesis and Treatment.* London: Academic, 1981.
60. Rose, H.E., and Mayer, J. Activity, caloric intake, fat storage and the energy balance of infants. *Pediatrics* 41:18, 1968.
61. Bullen, B.A., Reed, R.B., and Mayer, J. Physical activity of obese and non-obese adolescent girls appraised by motion picture sampling. *Am. J. Clin. Nutr.* 4:211, 1964.
62. Stunkard, A. Physical activity, emotions and human obesity. *Psychosom. Med.* 20:366, 1958.
63. Edholm, O.G., Fletcher, J.G., Widdowson, E.M., and McCance, R.A. The energy expenditure and food intake of individual man. *Br. J. Nutr.* 9:286, 1955.
64. Crews, E.L., III, Fuge, K.W., Oscai, L.B., et al. Weight, food intake and body composition: Effects of exercise and protein deficiency. *Am. J. Physiol.* 216:359, 1969.
65. Mayer, J. Why people get hungry. *Nutrition Today* 1:2, 1966.
66. Gwinup, G., Chelvam, R., and Steinberg, T. Thickness of subcutaneous fat and activity of underlying muscle. *Ann. Intern. Med.* 74:408, 1971.
67. Ley, P., Bradshaw, P.W., Kincey, J.A., et al. Psychological variables in the control of obesity. In W.L. Burland, P.D. Samuel, and J. Yudkin, Eds., *Obesity Symposium.* Edinburgh: Churchill Livingstone, 1974.
68. Bernard, J.L. Rapid treatment of gross obesity by operant techniques. *Psychol. Rep.* 23:663, 1968.
69. Stuart, R.B. A three-dimensional program for the treatment of obesity. *Behav. Res. Ther.* 9:177, 1971.
70. Stuart, R.B. Behavior control of overeating. *Behav. Res. Ther.* 5:357, 1967.
71. Levitz, L.S., and Stunkard, A.J. A therapeutic coalition for obesity: Behavior modification and patient self-help. *Am. J. Psychiatry* 131:423, 1974.
72. Bowser, L.J., Trulson, M.F., Bowling, R.C., and Stare, F.J. Methods of reducing. Group therapy vs. individual clinic interview. *J. Am. Diet. Assoc.* 29:1193, 1953.
73. Munves, E.D. Dietetic interview or group discussion-decision in reducing. *J. Am. Diet. Assoc.* 29:1197, 1953.
74. Howard, A.N. Dietary treatment of obesity. In I. McLean-Baird and A.N. Howard, Eds., *Obesity: Medical and Scientific Aspects.* Edinburgh: E. and S. Livingstone, 1969.
75. Blundell, J.E., and Leshem, M.B. Central action of anorexic agents: Effects of amphetamine and fenfluramine in rats with lateral hypothalamic lesions. *Eur. J. Pharmacol.* 28:81, 1974.
76. Leibowitz, S.F. Amphetamine: Possible site and mode of action for producing anorexia in the rat. *Brain Res.* 84:160, 1975.
77. Sullivan, A.C., and Cheng, L. Appetite regulation and its modulation by drugs. In J.N. Hathcock and J. Coon, Eds., *Nutrition and Drug Interrelationships.* New York: Academic, 1978.
78. Sullivan, A.C., and Comai, K. Pharmacological treatment of obesity. In G.A. Bray, Ed., *Obesity: Comparative Methods of Weight Control.* Westport, Conn.: Technomic Publishing, 1980.
79. Sullivan, A.C., Comai, K., and Triscari, J. Novel antiobesity agents whose primary site of action is the gastrointestinal tract. In P. Björntorp, M. Cairella, and A.N. Howard, Eds., *Recent Advances in Obesity Research: III.* London: John Libbey, 1981.
80. Duncan, L.J.P., Rose, K., and Meiklejohn, A.P. Phenmetrazine hydrochloride and methylcellulose in the treatment of refractory obesity. *Lancet* 1:1262, 1960.
81. Bray, G.A., Melvin, K.E.W., and Chopra, J.J. Effect of triiodothyronine on some metabolic responses of obese patients. *Am. J. Clin. Nutr.* 26:715, 1973.
82. Lamki, L., Ezrin, C., Koven, I., and Steiner, F. 1-Thyroxine in the treatment of obesity without increase in the loss of lean body mass. *Metabolism* 22:617, 1973.
83. Simeons, A.T.W. The action of chorionic

gonadotropin in the obese. *Lancet* 2:946, 1954.
84. Hastrup, F., Nielson, F., and Skouby, A.P. Chorionic gonadotropin and the treatment of obesity. *Acta Med. Scand.* 168:25, 1960.
85. Young, R.L., Fuchs, R.J., and Woltjen, M.J. Chorionic gonadotropin in weight control. A double-blind cross-over study. *J.A.M.A.* 236:2495, 1976.
86. Carne, S. The action of chorionic gonadotropin in the obese. *Lancet* 2:1282, 1961.
87. Montorsi, W., and Doldi, S.B. Surgical treatment of obesity. In G. Enzi, G. Crepaldi, G. Pozza, and A.E. Renold, Eds., *Obesity: Pathogenesis and Treatment.* London: Academic Press, 1981.
88. MacLean, L.D., and Shibata, H.R. The present status of bypass operations for obesity. *Surg. Ann.* 9:213, 1977.
89. Bleicher, J.E., Cegielski, M., and Saporta, J.A. Intestinal bypass operation for massive obesity. *Postgrad. Med.* 55(4):65, 1974.
90. Hollenbeck, J.I., O'Leary, J.P., Maher, J.W., and Woodward, E.R. An aetiological basis for fatty liver after jejunoileal bypass. *J. Surg. Res.* 18:83, 1975.
91. Moxley, R.T., Pozefoky, T., and Lockwood, D.H. Protein nutrition and liver disease after jejunoileal bypass for morbid obesity. *N. Engl. J. Med.* 290:921, 1974.
92. Mason, E.E. *Surgical Treatment of Obesity.* Philadelphia: W.B. Saunders, 1981.
93. Mason, E.E. From giant hernias to gastric bypass. In W.L. Asher, Ed., *Treating the Obese.* New York: Medcom Press, 1974.
94. Rodgers, S., Burnet, R., Goss, A., et al. Jaw-wiring in the treatment of obesity. *Lancet* 2:1221, 1977.
95. Quaade, F., Vaernet, K., and Larsson, S. Stereotaxic stimulation and electrocoagulation of the lateral hypothalamus in obese humans. *Acta Neurochir.* (Wien) 30:111, 1974.
96. Mok, M.S., Parker, L.N., Voina, S., and Bray, G.A. Treatment of obesity by acupuncture. *Am. J. Clin. Nutr.* 29:832, 1976.
97. Flack, R., and Grayer, E.A. Consciousness-raising group for obese women. *Soc. Work Health Care* 20:484:1975.
98. Grinker, J. Behavioral and metabolic consequences of weight reduction. *J. Am. Diet. Assoc.* 62:30, 1973.
99. Fomon, S.J. *Nutritional Disorders of Children: Prevention, Screening, and Follow-up.* D.H.E.W. Publication No. (HSA) 77-5104. Washington, D.C.: U.S. Department of Health, Education and Welfare, 1977.
100. Bruch, H. *Eating Disorders.* New York: Basic Books, 1973.
101. Katz, J.L., and Weiner, H. A functional anterior hypothalamic defect in primary anorexia nervosa? *Psychosom. Med.* 37:103, 1975.
102. Halmi, K.A. Anorexia nervosa: Recent investigations. *Annu. Rev. Med.* 29:137, 1978.
103. Hellstrom, I. Oral complications in anorexia nervosa. *Scand. J. Dent. Res.* 85:71, 1977.
104. Schleimer, K. Anorexia nervosa. *Nutr. Rev.* 39:99, 1981.
105. Bruch, H. Perils of behavior modification in treatment of anorexia nervosa. *J.A.M.A.* 230:1419, 1974.

Bibliography

Berland, T. *Rating the Diets: New Ways to Lose Weight.* New York: Consumers Union, 1977.

Björntorp, P., Cairella, M., and Howard, A.N. *Recent Advances in Obesity Research: III.* London: John Libbey, 1981.

Blonz, E.R., and Stern, J.S. Obesity and Fad Diets. In L. Ellenbogen, Ed., *Controversies in Nutrition.* New York: Churchill Livingstone, 1981.

Bray, G.A., Ed. *Obesity in Perspective.* Fogarty International Center Series on Preventive Medicine, D.H.E.W. Publication No. (NIH) 75-708. Washington, D.C.: U.S. Department of Health, Education and Welfare, 1975.

Bray, G.A., Ed. *Recent Advances in Obesity Research: II.* London: Newman Publishing, 1978.

Bruch, H. *Eating Disorders.* New York: Basic Books, 1973.

Bruch, H. *The Golden Cage: The Enigma of Anorexia Nervosa.* Cambridge, Mass.: Harvard University Press, 1978.

Buchwald, H., Ed. Symposium on morbid obesity. *Surg. Clin. North Am.* 59(6):961, 1152, 1979.

Collipp, P.J., Ed. *Childhood Obesity,* 2nd ed. Littleton, Mass.: PSG Publishing, 1980.

Enzi, G., Crepaldi, G., Pozza, G., and Renold, A.E., Eds. *Obesity: Pathogenesis and Treatment.* London: Academic, 1981.

Howard, A., Ed. *Recent Advances in Obesity Research: I.* London: Newman Publishing, 1975.

Mancini, M., Lewis, B., and Contaldo, F. *Medical Complications of Obesity.* London: Academic, 1979.

Mason, E.E. *Surgical Treatment of Obesity.* Philadelphia: W.B. Saunders, 1981.

Maxwell, J.D., Gazet, J.C., and Pilkington, T.R.E. *Surgical Management of Obesity.* London: Academic, 1980.

Vigersky, R.A. *Anorexia Nervosa.* New York: Raven Press, 1977.

Sources of Current Information

International Journal of Obesity
Obesity and Bariatric Medicine

16. Nutrition in Handicapping Conditions

A number of conditions involving the nervous system, muscles, skeleton, or a combination of these tissues affect nutritional status. Since many of these disorders lead to permanent handicaps with features in common and since many require similar nutritional care, they are included in this one chapter. For convenience, other conditions involving the neuromuscular and musculoskeletal systems also are described in this chapter.

CLEFT LIP AND PALATE

In normal prenatal development, at approximately 4 to 6 weeks' gestation, the upper lip is formed from a central flap and two side flaps which grow toward each other and fuse. If the fusion fails to take place, the child is born with a *cleft lip* which may be unilateral or bilateral, complete or incomplete. At the same time, the infant may have a *cleft palate.* Normally, the palate develops as tissue grows in from the sides and joins in the middle. If this fusion does not occur, an opening exists between the mouth and nose. The cleft may be in the soft palate alone or in both soft and hard palate. Hard palate clefts may be partial or total. The width of the cleft also varies. These conditions cause feeding and respiratory problems. The infant cannot create an airtight seal necessary for the production of negative pressure and therefore has difficulty in sucking. Swallowing sometimes is affected also. Body length and weight may be subnormal, probably related to feeding difficulties. Yet, good nutritional status must be carefully maintained in preparation for surgical repair of the deformity.

The infant who has a cleft of only the soft palate can be fed in the normal manner but must be held upright to prevent the feeding from entering the nose. Because of the lack of suction in all other types of cleft, special equipment for feeding is necessary. Two types are available. The *Brecht feeder* consists of a bulb-type syringe with a rubber or plastic tube. The *Beniflex feeder* has a cross-cut nipple. It is used for soft palate or partial hard palate clefts.

Another problem is excessive air intake. Feeding in an upright position with frequent burping is necessary. Acidic and spicy foods should be avoided, since they tend to cause irritation of the mouth and nose. Other foods to avoid for some children are nuts, peanut butter, leafy vegetables, peelings of raw fruit, and creamed dishes, all of which are reported to get caught in the cleft.[1] The child may be fed puréed foods thickened with graham crackers or vanilla wafers. Other problems include dental decay or malocclusion which interfere with sufficient food intake. Some children eat very slowly and tire before the meal is complete. To assure adequate calorie intake, smaller more frequent meals of high caloric density (low fluid content) may be necessary.

A cleft lip often is repaired when the infant reaches a weight of 10 lb. or at approximately 6 to 8 weeks of age. A Brecht feeder is used before surgery. It may also be used postoperatively with care not to press on the suture line. Clear liquids are given for 2 days, after which formula feeding may begin. Each formula feeding is followed by some water to prevent contamination of the suture line. The Brecht feeder may be abandoned in 1 to 1½ months.

Repair of a cleft palate is not done until the infant is 12 to 14 months old. The child is weaned from the feeder at the age of 4 to 6 months and accustomed to the use of a cup and spoon for feeding. Prior to surgery, clear liquids are given occasionally so the infant becomes accustomed to them. In addition, the child should also become accustomed preoperatively to arm restraints which prevent the child's putting the hands in the mouth. Postoperatively, the child is fed from a cup only, not with a spoon or through a straw, to avoid injuring the repair site. A common protocol for postoperative feeding consists of clear liquids for 5 days, then full liquids for 10 days, followed by progression for 10 to 20 days to a soft, finely puréed, or mashed diet. The normal diet for age may then be resumed, except that very hard foods such as crackers and zwieback should be avoided for up to 2 months.

NEUROMUSCULAR AND NERVOUS SYSTEM DISORDERS

Neuromuscular and nervous system disorders accompanied by nutritional problems can occur in children or adults. Disabilities are seen in individuals of various ages who have had head injuries or cerebrovascular accidents or who become senile. Accompanying eating problems vary in severity. Enlarged tonsils and throat infections may cause minor problems that require correction. Other individuals have disorders of the skeleton, nervous system, or muscles that are very serious.

Approximately 3 percent of the population in the United States are mentally retarded or have other developmental problems. Nearly half of these are children or adolescents, many of whom survive to adulthood. Impairments in some cases are minimal but may be moderate or, sometimes, very severe. Many have multiple handicaps. These conditions, collectively known as *developmental disability* or *developmental delay,* are described as "significant physical, mental, or sensory impairment often accompanied by associated disabilities found in various combinations of a visual-perceptual-motor, language, or behavioral nature that can affect major life activities."[2]

Many factors may cause brain damage during the course of development. Some genetic abnormalities, such as phenylketonuria, may lead to hereditary metabolic disorders with effects on the brain (see Chapter 10). Chromosomal abnormalities cause conditions such as Down's syndrome, described later in this chapter (p. 606). Later in pregnancy, maternal drug addiction, toxemia, and conditions causing fetal malnutrition may cause brain damage. In the perinatal period, prematurity, trauma during the birth process, hypoglycemia, and hyperbilirubinemia contribute to brain damage, and in early childhood, infections, tumors and trauma may damage the brain. In a child who is normal at birth, disability may be the result of environmental deprivation. Children who survive drowning accidents or other incidents causing anoxia sometimes are permanently brain-damaged. At the same time, it is important to remember that, although many brain-damaged children are mentally retarded, this is not invariably the case. Some children have motor dysfunction without a decrease in intelligence. In either case, problems associated with feeding often provide the first clue to the existence of central nervous system deficit.

Anatomy and Physiology of Food Intake

As in other parts of the body, the bones provide the foundation and the muscles, controlled by the nerves, provide power for movement involved in food intake. The *skeletal structure* involved in eating consists of three bones. The *mandible* (lower jaw bone) is important in eating since it is the only bone in the face that is free to move. The muscles attached to the mandible are under voluntary control and, when normally coordinated, make it possible for a person to elevate and lower the mandible to close and open the mouth. The muscles also make it possible to protrude and retract the mandible, to move it laterally, and to maintain it in a position so that the mouth is closed at rest. The *maxillae* are actually two bones that form the upper jaw and hard palate. They are stationary, and so the mandible must rise to meet the upper jaw for chewing. The *hyoid bone* is suspended from the temporal bone by ligaments but is not attached to any other bone. Some muscles of the tongue and floor of the mouth are attached to the hyoid bone, which moves up involuntarily during swallowing to aid in sealing off the epiglottis.

Using the bones as levers, the *muscles* contract to cause movement if stimulated by the nerves. Muscles can only pull by *contracting* (shortening). They return to their original length by relaxing, but there is no mechanism by which a muscle can push. A muscle's potential for work is related to its *tone* or *tension* (degree of firmness). In general, three possible categories of tone are described: *hypotonic, flaccid,* or *floppy* and *atonic* muscles are soft and flabby; *hypertonic, spastic,* or *stiff* muscles are rigid and hard in a continuous contraction or convulsion; and muscles with *normal tone* have some resilience when at rest. The muscle must have sufficient tone to perform its function but not so much that further contraction is difficult.

The amount of muscle tension is influenced by the number of muscle fibers stimulated by the *nerves.* When there is a disturbance in the impulses from the central nervous system, there will be a disturbance in the related muscles. Depending on the nature of the disorder in the nervous system, the muscle may be hypertonic, weak, paralyzed, or have alternating tone. If the nerve supply to the muscle is severed, the fibers of the muscle atrophy so that the muscle will be much smaller than its normal size. The degenerated fibers are replaced by fibrous tissue. Therefore, it is important that the muscles used in eating not be allowed to atrophy from disuse. Loss of function from disuse is difficult, sometimes impossible, to correct. An equally important consideration is that many muscles for eating are used also for speech. If these muscles are allowed to atrophy, speech will be affected.

The brain and many nerves are involved in the eating process. When the nervous system malfunctions, either in the brain itself or in peripheral nerves, a variety of problems is possible. In addition to the problems related to the muscles, nerve disorders can cause loss of sensation in the face, mouth, or soft palate, thereby causing loss of taste perception and inability to locate, and thus control, food in the mouth. Nerve disorders can affect salivary gland function as well.

There are a number of reflexes that are important functional components of the eating process. Eating disorders may involve hyperactive, hypoactive, absent, or abnormal reflexes. Sometimes, a normal reflex may persist beyond the age at which it usually comes under voluntary control. In other cases, feeding difficulties arise because of lack of control of total body posture.

Nutritional Care in Developmentally Delayed Patients

Nutritional problems in developmentally delayed children may be classified as those related to (1) feeding skills, (2) nutrient intake and function, and (3) behavior.

Feeding Skills and Food Intake

The normal infant develops feeding skills in a specific sequence. In a developmentally delayed child, this same sequence often is followed, but the rate at which progress occurs may be slowed to varying degrees. In other cases, these developmental landmarks are abnormal. Thus, it is important to be familiar with normal development and to be able to relate these to nutritional needs in handicapped children.

A child exhibits typical patterns of posture and movement as he or she develops. In motor development, reflex contraction is followed by voluntary contraction and muscle control develops *cephalocaudally* (from the head downward). Large muscle movement precedes fine motions.

The infant begins with certain simple reflexes which are modified and inhibited (controlled) as he or she develops. Although these reflexes are significant in their relation to each other, they are described separately for clarity.

Total Body Reflexes. The total body reflexes are present in the normal infant for a few months and then fade, but they can interfere with development of eating if they persist beyond the age at which they normally are brought under control.[3] Children with *persistent flexor reflexes* are hard to position for feeding. They tend to be bent in a fetal position, making feeding or eating difficult. Poor equilibrium and poor head control make chewing and swallowing difficult. Tongue control and hand-to-mouth coordination are poor.

Extensor thrusting (extension reflexes) can be initiated in some brain-damaged patients by stimulation or pressure in the occipital area of the skull or on the balls of the feet. The arms and legs become extended with a stiff trunk and with the head and neck thrown back. Hand-to-mouth movements or movements across the midline of the body are inhibited.

Moro's reflex is elicited if the head drops back suddenly. There is a rapid extension and then flexion of the limbs as if embracing something. It occurs normally in an infant to the age of approximately 4 months. If it persists beyond that age, it interferes with sitting balance and hand-to-mouth movement.

The *asymmetric tonic neck reflex* occurs normally in infants from birth to 4 to 7 months of age.[4–7] When the face is turned to one side, the arm and leg on that side will become extended and the opposite side will become flexed. This sometimes is referred to as the "fencing position." The normal infant can move away from this position and bring a hand to his or her mouth to suck on the fingers. The developmentally disabled infant who has a dominant asymmetric tonic neck reflex cannot bring food to his or her mouth while looking at the food. The reflex interferes with head and trunk control and with normal arm and head movements in feeding.

A strong *tonic labyrinthine reflex* can force a child into an extensor position, holding his or her head and neck in extension. This posture makes swallowing difficult.[3]

Normal muscle tone makes possible the sitting position, arm and head movement, and mouth movements for eating. An infant with increased muscle tone may be unable to bend at the hips in order to sit or to control the head and neck to stay in a sitting position. Increased tonus sometimes prevents movement of the lips, tongue, and jaw for chewing. The hypotonic infant may have difficulty in maintaining a sitting posture and in maintaining lip closure or jaw movement.

Suckling infants are fed in a semirecumbent, flexed position, allowing the baby to swallow easily. Normally, at approximately 6 months of age, a child may be placed in a high chair for eating. At approximately 18 to 24 months, the normal child is sufficiently coordinated that a baby high chair is no longer needed.

If the child has no head and trunk control, support must be provided with the trunk and head flexed forward. If the head is extended, the child will gag. His or her head, trunk, and feet should be supported in an upright symmetric position for feeding.

Oropharyngeal Reflexes. Other reflexes, classified as oropharyngeal reflexes, are involved in eating. These will be described individually for the sake of clarity, but it is important to remember that the sequence of action is crucial. Table 16-1 summarizes normal developmental landmarks related to feeding.

Rooting reflex. The rooting reflex is present at birth or appears soon after birth except when urinating and for 2 hours or so after eating. It fades at approximately 3 months of age. It is a food-seeking behavior in which the infant will turn its head toward the stimulus if the cheek or corner of the mouth is touched with a nipple or a finger. If rooting movement continues after the food source is located, it may interfere with the development of sucking.

Suckling and sucking-swallowing reflex. There is a difference between suckling and sucking. From birth to approximately 5 months, *suckling* can be seen. At first, it can be elicited by stimulating almost any body part but, within a few days, only the lips, cheeks, and inside of the mouth are responsive. Suckling is a continuous process in which the passage from the nose is open so that nose breathing and swallowing occur simultaneously. It occurs with the body in a flexed position and will not take place when the infant's body is extended.

Sucking follows the more primitive suckling. It is a discontinuous process in which liquid accumulates in the mouth. Before swallowing, there must be a pause in breathing. The sucking-swallowing reflex begins soon after birth, but becomes a voluntary activity by 6 months of age. The reflex consists of opening the mouth to accept a nipple followed by sucking whenever the corners or center of the upper lip are touched.

Some premature or retarded infants do not have the ability to suck and must be assisted. They must be able to create a seal with the lips and closure of the soft palate to create a negative pressure. The posterior tongue provides the pumping action.

In the sucking reflex, when the mouth has moved to the stimulus, the tongue retracts and the lips close. The movement of the hyoid bone shows that swallowing occurs. The sucking-swallowing reflex is replaced after approximately 1 year with a mature swallowing pattern.

Table 16-1. Normal Development of Reflexes and Feeding Skills

Approximate Age[a]	Reflexes and Skills
Newborn	Lack of head and trunk control; must have total support Rooting reflex; sucking-swallowing primarily through up-and-down jaw movement Palm-chin reflex Extrusion reflex (pushes out solid food placed on tongue)
1–2 months	Palm-chin reflex diminished Begins head control but still requires support Some hand-to-mouth skill Protraction-retraction tongue movement Solid foods involuntarily ejected
2½–3 months	Mature sucking Reflexive palmar grasp disappears at approximately 12 weeks
4–5 months	Asymmetric tonic neck reflex disappears at 4–7 months Extrusion reflex disappears at approximately 4 months Head and upper trunk control—may sit in infant seat or high chair Frequently puts hands to mouth Elevation tongue movement; negative pressure sucking
5 months	Sits in high chair with support Up-and-down chewing movement Tongue lateralization begins Can drink from cup if it is held by others
6 months	Good head control Some independent sitting Bites on soft food; chews Can hold bottle, hold and eat biscuit Can reach for and grasp objects
6–8 months	Sits well in high chair Holds bottle alone Reaches for dish, spoon Begins up-and-down chewing if given chewable foods Transfers objects between hands Can grasp large pieces of food Chews easily dissolved foods Finger-feeds Uses fingers in grasping
8–9 months	Sits independently Bite reflex disappears Finger-feeds bite-size pieces of food Can grasp small pieces Lips close when swallowing
9–11 months	Good eye-hand-mouth coordination Can pick up small pieces of food Finger-feeds easily Bites off correct amount Lateral tongue movement Rotary chewing begins at approximately 10 months
12–18 months	Finger-feeds much of meal, but messy Uses spoon at approximately 15 months; may rotate spoon near mouth Drinks from cup with moderate spillage
18 months	Drinks from glass or cup with little spillage Uses spoon without rotation
24 months	Good rotary chewing Competent spoon feeding
30 months	Straw sucking complete Chews well
36 months	Uses utensils Feeds self well

[a] The range of normal variability is wide and the ages given are merely approximations.

Bite reflex. The bite reflex is present at birth and normally comes under voluntary control in 3 to 6 months. It consists of a sudden, snapping viselike closure of the mandible elicited by touching the lips, teeth, gums, or tongue.[6] If it persists past 5 to 6 months of age or if it is oversensitive, it interferes with other developmental activities such as taking food from a cup or spoon, chewing, and speaking. In addition, it can cause damage to the lips, tongue, or cheeks. The patient may need help in overcoming this reflex.

Drooling. Drooling, although not a reflex, begins in the normal infant at approximately 3 months and subsides before 12 months. The child with poor lip closure and weak swallowing almost always drools excessively. It is associated with wet clothing, unpleasant odors, and social stigma. Development of strong lip closure controls drooling.

Gag reflex. The gag reflex normally is present at birth and is located at the tip of the tongue. It moves to the back of the mouth in the ensuing 6 to 8 months. It is not a normal part of taking food but is a protective mechanism. It consists of contraction of the constrictor muscles of the pharynx[6] and is elicited by pressure at the middle of the tongue and areas back to the *uvula* (the fleshy mass that descends from the back of the soft palate above the root of the tongue). Its decrease is associated with the development of chewing, but it never disappears completely, even in the adult.

A *hypoactive gag reflex* is a serious problem since the child is unable to sense choking. It is seen in Down's syndrome (see p. 606), and also is present in floppy infant syndrome and pseudobulbar palsy, conditions in which hypotonia is prominent.

The *hyperactive gag reflex* is elicited by stimulation of other areas of the mouth. It interferes with eating and can make the swallowing of solid food difficult or impossible. In swallowing, it may be helpful to have the head tilted back slightly. This causes the tongue to drop down and back, reducing its stimulation. Parents may be counseled to feed the child from straight ahead to avoid triggering abnormal reflexes.

Arm and Hand Control and Eye-Hand Coordination. The normal child also develops controlled arm and hand movements and eye-hand coordination at appropriate ages. The newborn infant usually can bring its hand to its mouth for sucking. The ability to reach and grasp large objects usually develops at 3 to 4 months, and a pincer movement to pick up tiny objects at approximately 6 months. In central nervous system dysfunction, the hand-to-mouth movement may be abnormal. Persistent asymmetric tonic neck reflex causes the head to turn away as the hand comes to the mouth. A persistent primitive grasp interferes with handling of utensils. The child's grasp and movement to the mouth may need to be guided at first. Adaptive equipment may be necessary.

In evaluation of arm and hand movement for self-feeding, factors that should be observed include finger grasp, palmar grasp, wrist and elbow flexion, wrist rotation, hand and arm steadiness, and coordination of hand-to-mouth movement. A normal infant has a reflexive *palmar grasp* at 1 to 2 days of age which persists for approximately 3 months.[8] If it persists beyond the time when the child is ready for independent use of his or her hands, as for finger feeding, the child will not be able to voluntarily grasp or release objects.[9]

The normal infant regards the feeding bottle and may touch it at approximately 5 months. He or she can hold or stabilize it with a palmar grasp at 7 months or so.[10] This visual coordination is a necessary development in normal feeding.

The *palm-chin reflex* is present in premature and some newborn infants but disappears by 3 to 4 months.[6] As a result of this reflex, the jaw is open as long as any pressure is applied to the *thenar eminence* (the bulge on the palm at the base of the thumb). If the reflex persists, a child cannot hold food in his or her mouth when the palms are stimulated.

Learned Eating Skills. To progress in eating skills, the child must develop jaw stability and tongue and lip control. He or she also must know how to chew and swallow. These are learned eating skills, not reflexes. Swallowing is a reflex only after the bolus of food reaches a critical point.

Jaw stability. Jaw stability is indicated by the position of the lower jaw. Normally, when a child is at rest, the mandible is elevated or closed. Treatment is indicated if the mandible is (1) open or depressed, (2) protracted or jutting outward, (3) retracted or drawn inward, or (4) closed and cannot be voluntarily opened.

Lip closure. Some patients require treatment to achieve adequate closure and control of the lips when they are at rest or while eating.

Tongue control. Tongue control is important in eating and is a prerequisite for speech. It positions food for both chewing and swallowing. Normally, at 6 months, the child is capable of elevation, depression, lateralization, retraction, and protraction of the tongue. The protraction or forward thrust is the most common action of the tongue.

Some children have abnormal *tongue thrust* in which the tongue extends forward or laterally between or against the teeth. It can be the result of tonsillitis, early thumb sucking, or early loss of primary incisors. Often the child has a hypersensitive mouth, and tongue movement occurs on stimulation of the lips, tongue, or palate. If the child has a minor problem, it may correct itself in time, but correction without treatment is unlikely if the condition persists after the age of 10 years.[11] Tongue thrust prevents getting food in the mouth or keeping it there. It also interferes with swallowing. The objective of treatment, then, is for the tongue to remain in an appropriate position in the mouth.

Chewing. If chewing is to develop, the diet must be progressed appropriately from liquid to purêed to chopped foods as the child matures. Normally, all food is liquid for 3 months, with soft purêed food used in the next 2 months. Chopped foods are introduced at approximately 7 months.

Rotary chewing, a process distinct from biting, begins at 9 months or slightly later. At that time, usual table foods may be used, adjusted for the eruption of the molars for grinding. At first, chewing occurs in an up-and-down motion, but gradually, the side-to-side motion develops.

The incisors erupt at 6 to 9 months to provide for biting. Molars erupt between 12 and 24 months, at which time lateral jaw movements for chewing occur. The first permanent molars erupt at 6 years.[12] Tongue movements must be coordinated and controlled to keep food between the molars for chewing, and the lips must remain closed.

Mature swallowing. To develop the normal mature swallowing pattern, the child must have jaw stability, contracted masseter muscles but relaxed muscles in the floor of the mouth, and tongue control. It is a complex combination of voluntary and involuntary actions involving twenty-two muscles and is learned over a period of time. In the handicapped child, jaw closure, tongue placement, and lip closure may have to be taught separately and then coordinated.

Self-Feeding Skills. Self-feeding skills are important objectives in correcting eating handicaps. The techniques progress from bottle or breast feeding to assisted spoon feeding and finger self-feeding and, finally, to the use of utensils.

Drinking from a cup or glass. The normal infant can sip liquids from a cup or glass at the age of 8 to 10 months, drink with help at 12 to 14 months, and drink with little help at approximately 18 months. For developmentally disabled children, teaching this technique may begin with the use of thin liquids, advancing to thicker liquids as ability increases. Some children, however, have greatest difficulty with thin liquids and so teaching must begin with thicker mixtures.

Finger self-feeding. A child may begin self-feeding with his or her fingers as soon as he or she can pick up objects and put the hands to the mouth. Foods that are suitable for this purpose include pieces of fruit or vegetables, crackers, cheese, or dry cereals. A child with an eating handicap may need help in learning to finger-feed, a skill that must precede self-feeding with a spoon. The piece of food may be placed in the child's hand and guided to his or her mouth at first. As skill develops, self-feeding as much as possible should be encouraged.

Self-feeding with a spoon. When a child can pick up food with his or her fingers and bring it to the mouth, he or she can begin to practice with a spoon. The child should begin with a *pronated grasp* (with the palm down). The normal child learns to hold the spoon with the hand in the *supinated* (palm upward) position at 18 to 24 months. At the same age, a normal child will begin to stab with a fork, but this maneuver is not well established until approximately 4 years of age. A normal child of 8 can cut with a knife.[9,13,14]

Sometimes special equipment for eating is helpful. Depending on specific need, special utensils may be provided with padded, extended, or bent handles or with a ring or cuff on the handle to facilitate holding. The plate on which the food is placed may be anchored and have sides so the food can be "trapped." At first, food that tends to stick to the spoon should be used. Very liquid or slippery foods should be avoided until the child has developed some skill in the use of utensils.

Diet Texture. Many of the problems of nutrient intake in developmentally delayed patients are avoidable if guidance is provided to parents or other caretakers on food texture changes and appropriate expectations of feeding skills.

The texture of the diet must be varied as eating skill advances. If the texture is not appropriate, there is risk of choking or gagging, or of aspirating food into the lungs. If appropriately textured foods are not provided at the time that the patient is developmentally ready to advance to the next stage, his or her development may be further delayed and may be irreparably damaged. Table 16-2 lists various feeding skills and the

Table 16-2. Procedures in Development of Feeding Behaviors

Skill Developed	Procedure Indicated	Examples
Sucking	Use fluids	Milk
Elevation of tongue moves food to back of mouth	Continue using liquids	Milk
Swallowing (with head forward and no gagging); elevation of back of tongue	Introduce blended diet	Baby food; thick purees; mashed potatoes; applesauce; custards; ice cream; yogurt; mashed banana
Up-and-down chewing with jaw control and minimal drooling	Start finely ground foods	Oatmeal; cottage cheese; finely ground meat; scrambled egg; well-mashed cooked vegetables; egg salad; peanut butter if no tongue thrust
Lateral tongue movement	Begin coarsely ground foods	Ground meats in gravy; tuna fish; chopped fruits and vegetables; fine coleslaw; cheese; rice; liverwurst; banana slices; flavored yogurt
Rotary chewing	Use chopped foods	Crackers; finely chopped meats; fruits and vegetables; salad greens; coleslaw; macaroni; dry cereal
Reaches for and grasps objects; brings hands to mouth	Begin finger feeding with large pieces	Crackers; teething biscuit; oven-dried toast; cheese sticks
Voluntary release	Finger feeding with small pieces	Dry cereals; small pieces of meat; cottage cheese
Put lips on cup rim	Begin cup feeding	
Reaches for spoon; ulnar deviation of wrist	Self-feeding	Foods that adhere to spoon; cooked cereal; mashed potato; applesauce; cottage cheese
Increased rotary movement of jaw	Increase texture and variety	Chopped meats; raw vegetables and fruits

feeding procedures indicated. Incoordination during feeding often precedes abnormal speech development; therefore, it is important that therapy begin early.

Behavioral Problems

Some feeding problems are primarily behavioral in nature. They may occur in developmentally delayed children and in children who are able to eat but who are considered problem eaters. There are several types of behavioral problems.

In some cases, eating is associated with unpleasant consequences. This can occur in patients for whom food intake must be frequent, is time-consuming, or is associated with discomfort. Additional incentives must be offered to offset these negative factors.

Some patients use the feeding situation to manipulate the environment, including the parents. The parents often profit from counseling to regain control in such cases. Sometimes, however, it is the parent who institutes the inappropriate feeding programs. Some stressed families need professional family counseling to help them to cope with these situations. It is in circumstances such as these that the cooperation of members of the health care team other than the nutritional care specialist is invaluable.

Nutritional Needs and Problems

The developmentally disabled child needs the same nutrients as the normal child. In some cases, however, the quantities required are different. There are several problems that are seen frequently.

Growth Retardation. Many brain-damaged children are retarded in growth. In many cases, the reason for this is unknown, but since eating handicaps are common, it is important to assure that malnutrition does not contribute to the growth deficit. When a child is shorter than normal, age should not be used as a basis for estimation of energy need or the child will become overweight. The kilocalorie ration should be provided in proportion to the child's height and activity to maintain normal body weight.

Overweight. Handicapped patients whose capacity for activity is limited often are obese. Nutritional management in obesity is described in Chapter 15. The therapist should not reward progress in the obese handicapped child with food. Exercise should be increased if possible.

Underweight. Patients with eating and swallowing problems or who fall asleep during meals may be underweight. Some patients have increased muscle tone, increasing their caloric need at the same time that food intake is decreased. In addition to the development of self-feeding skills, an increase in the number of meals per day and the use of liquid supplements and foods of high caloric density are helpful. Some patients apparently are unable to sense hunger and are anorexic. They, too, may be given a high-density diet.

Constipation. Constipation is a commonly occurring problem, particularly in patients receiving soft low-fiber foods or inadequate fluid and in those whose activity is limited. Some developmentally delayed patients may have decreased muscle tone in the intestinal tract. Suggestions for diet modifications for chronic constipation are provided in Chapter 6. These must be altered as necessary for age and the nature of the handicap. In general, increased fluid and fiber are helpful. If the patient is unable to chew raw fruits and vegetables, prunes and soaked bran in the diet may be beneficial.

Fluid Intake. Fluid intake must be carefully monitored in the patient who cannot respond to thirst or who is unable to express a desire for fluid.

Drug-Related Problems. A number of drugs useful in the management of patients with developmental disabilities or behavioral problems have effects that have nutritional implications. *Amphetamine* causes alterations in taste, extreme drowsiness, and depressed appetite. Steroids, on the other hand, increase appetite and can cause obesity.

Many developmentally disabled children are seizure-prone and receive medications for this reason. *Anticonvulsants* can cause folate deficiency. Use of phenytoin sodium (Dilantin), phenobarbital, valproic acid (Depakene), or primidone (Mysoline) results in low serum folate and may cause megaloblastic anemia if the patient becomes very deficient, since anticonvulsants alter folate metabolism.[15] On the other hand, *folate supplements* may precipitate a seizure and should be provided cautiously.[16,17]

Anticonvulsants also increase the need for vitamin D,[18,19] possibly by inducing vitamin D–degrading enzymes. The serum calcium, phosphorus, and alkaline phosphates should be monitored in these patients. Other effects of anticonvulsant therapy include neonatal coagulation defects, gingival hyperplasia, effects on pituitary, insulin, thyroid, and adrenal function, congenital malformations in infants of mothers taking these drugs, and possibly deficiencies of copper, zinc, and pyridoxine. Patients receiving anticonvulsants are given routine vitamin-mineral supplements.

Nutritional Assessment of the Handicapped Child

The assessment of the handicapped child must include nutritional assessment and evaluation of feeding skills. It sometimes requires the effort of a health care team composed of individuals from many areas of expertise. The nutritional care specialist on the team can provide a large part of the nutritional assessment, whereas the assessment of the current level of eating skills sometimes is done by an occupational therapist. Since many of the same structures and functions are involved in both eating and speaking, the participation of a speech therapist is important in some cases. Table 16-3 provides a list of nutrition-related factors that may be observed.

Alterations in the standard procedures for anthropometric measurements given in Chapter 2 may be necessary. In children less than 2 years of age or those incapable of standing upright, *recumbent* length may be substituted for height. If a child's legs are deformed, *sitting height* is used as an alternative to total height. *Crown-rump length* is an equivalent measure in infants. *Serial head circumferences* sometimes are recorded also. The child's weight-to-height ratio should be used to evaluate weight control since many of these children are below normal height for age.

Skeletal maturity is not always related to height in handicapped children. For these individuals, estimates of bone age may be obtained from roentgenograms. This procedure requires a pediatrician or radiologist with skill in interpretation. Similarly, *dental roentgenograms* can be used as an index of development, requiring the services of a dentist. Scoring methods for deciduous teeth have not been developed; therefore, this procedure is not useful for very young children.

The nutrition of handicapped children should be assessed at frequent intervals and followed closely. After infancy, the handicapped child should be evaluated at 6-month intervals. If nutritional problems develop, assessment should occur more frequently to evaluate progress under treatment.

Some Specific Conditions Associated with Developmental Disability

Several of the more common conditions associated with developmental disability are described in some detail here to illustrate

Table 16-3. Feeding Evaluation Observations

- Oral ability
  - Sucking
  - Oral prehension
  - Swallowing
  - Breathing and swallowing coordinated
  - Drooling
  - Lips
  - Tongue size
  - Tongue thrust
  - Tongue mobility
  - Biting
  - Munching
  - Chewing
  - Drinking
- Oral structure
  - Occlusion
  - Teeth
  - Caries
  - Gingiva
  - Oral hygiene
  - Palate
  - Pain on examination
  - Hypersensitivity
  - Teething stage
- Body position
  - Head control
  - Sitting balance
  - Placement of feet
  - Usual feeding position
- Hand use
  - Palmar grasp
  - Pincer grasp
  - Opposition of finger and thumb
  - Hand-to-mouth control
- Developmental feeding
  - Breast ____ bottle ____ weaned ____
  - Baby food ____ junior food ____ mashed table food ____ minced foods ____
  - Cut table foods ____ regular table foods ____
  - Closes hands in on bottle
  - Hand to mouth/sucks on fingers
  - Teething biscuit/holds and brings to mouth
  - Finger-feeds
  - Opposes lips to rim of cup
  - Attempts to grasp spoon
  - Grasps spoon
  - Dips spoon in dish
  - Brings spoon to mouth
  - Holds bottle and drinks independently
  - Grasps cup
  - Raises cup to mouth
  - Cup-lifting, drinking, replacing
  - Scoops well with spoon
  - Feeds independently with spoon
  - Straw drinking
  - Spears with fork
  - Spreads with knife
- Feeding environment
  - Time of feedings (note how long feeding takes)
  - Atmosphere of feedings (tense, pleasant, unpleasant)
  - Person responsible for feeding
  - Parent's or caretaker's attitude toward feeding
  - Past successful and unsuccessful methods
  - Identify positive and negative reinforcing behaviors
- Usual food intake: 24-hour recall or 1-day or 3-day food diaries, depending on the situation
- Total fluid intake
- Medications
  - Type
  - Dosage
  - Time given
- Bowel concerns
  - Regular
  - Constipation
  - Diarrhea
- Anthropometric data
- Clinical findings
- Laboratory findings

Courtesy of Feeding Team, Developmental Evaluation Clinic, Children's Hospital Medical Center, Boston, Massachusetts.
Reprinted with permission from Howard, R.B., Nutritional support of the developmentally disabled child. In R.M. Suskind, Ed., *Textbook of Pediatric Nutrition.* New York: Raven Press, 1981, p. 581.

a number of the problems previously described.

Down's Syndrome

A patient with Down's syndrome (mongolism) has an extra chromosome 21 and thus the disorder is known also as *trisomy 21.* It occurs in approximately 1 in 600 live births. There is a mild to moderate degree of mental retardation, growth retardation, and hypotonicity which may lead to obesity and constipation. Hypotonicity also frequently causes a protruding tongue. The tongue thrust reflex often persists. The patients have narrow nasal passages and tend to be mouth breathers. Development of oral reflexes is delayed, and swallowing is poor. A narrow palate interferes with a proper seal when sucking. Tooth eruption is delayed and chewing difficulties are common. Other dental problems include periodontal disease, malocclusion, hypocalcification, and caries. These add to the chewing problems. There is a high incidence of tracheoesophageal fistulas, pyloric stenosis, and heart defects.

Nutritional care involves development of feeding skills, prevention of obesity, and prevention of nutritional deficiency. Energy content of the diet should be provided in proportion to the patient's height and activity, approximately 16.1 kcal/cm for male patients and 14.3 kcal/cm for female patients. Training must be provided to help the patient control the tongue and keep the mouth closed when eating. As the child becomes older, fiber and fluid in the diet may be increased to avoid constipation. To reduce dental problems, foods high in sucrose, including sweet sticky snacks, should be eliminated. A soft diet may be necessary because of lack of malocclusion and tooth loss, but intake of fresh fruits and vegetables should be increased if possible.

Cerebral Palsy

Cerebral palsy, occurring in 1 or 2 in 1,000 live births, is a group of disorders caused by damage to the brain centers for motor control. The damage usually occurs in the prenatal or perinatal period or occasionally in infancy. Approximately 50 percent of these patients have subnormal intelligence, but others have normal intelligence and some may be gifted. Sometimes sight, hearing, or speech are impaired. Approximately one-third experience seizures. The physical handicaps may be mild or severe. There are several different forms of the condition:

1. In *spasticity,* the patient has hyperactive stretch reflexes, increased muscle tone, and muscle weakness. Movement is blocked by antagonist muscles, and freedom of movement is limited. It may affect the arm and leg on one side only (*hemiparesis*), all four extremities (*tetraparesis*), the legs more than the arms (*spastic diplegia*), or both legs but not the arms (*paraparesis*). Spasticity occurs in 70 percent of cerebral palsy patients.

2. *Dyskinesia* is indicated by many involuntary, uncontrolled, and purposeless movements, which disappear during sleep. The most common form (15 percent of patients) is *athetosis,* in which the patient has slow writhing movements, usually involving the face, neck, trunk, and all four extremities. Athetosis and spasticity can occur in the same patient.

3. *Ataxia* produces incoordination and balance problems. The patient has difficulty in turning and falls frequently. This form is the least common.

4. *Flaccidity* is demonstrated by decreased muscle tone.

Growth retardation, the cause of which is not always known, may be significant in cerebral palsy patients. Since feeding difficulties occur frequently, malnutrition is common[20–22] and probably contributes to the growth retardation. Special efforts must be made to provide energy to maintain normal growth and body weight. The energy content of the diet must be adjusted for the type of motor dysfunction. The patient with athetosis may require as many as 6,000 kcal/day by the time adolescence is reached.[23,24] In the spastic child, caloric needs are lower because of the limitation of movement. In moderate spasticity, 13.9 kcal/cm has been recommended, and in severe cases, approximately 11.1 kcal/cm.[25] Obesity should be carefully avoided. Patients with low caloric intake often need vitamin and mineral supplements. Protein nutrition should be monitored. Requirements of ataxic patients are similar to those of spastics. Since they fall easily, their activity is limited.

Feeding problems commonly seen include almost all those previously described. Muscle incoordination in the lips, tongue, and palate can lead to difficulties in sucking and swallowing and persistent drooling. Persistent bite reflex and asymmetric tonic neck reflex, tongue thrust, and hyperactive gag also are seen. A high arched palate, small lower jaw, and lack of lateral jaw movement cause chewing problems. Hand-to-mouth coordination often is delayed. Dental problems, contributing to self-feeding difficulties, include caries, gingivitis, malocclusion, and tooth loss.

Fetal Alcohol Syndrome

Fetal alcohol syndrome (FAS) has been generally recognized only recently. Alcohol crosses the placenta and enters the fetal circulation very rapidly. It reaches the fetus within 30 minutes. The fetal blood alcohol level becomes equal to the amount in the maternal blood but is cleared more slowly. Alcohol persists in the amniotic fluid.

Fetal alcohol syndrome apparently can vary in severity. The major features of the condition consist of brain injury, growth deficiency, delayed development, and alterations in the structure of the face. The facial characteristics are most easily observed. The head is small, the bridge of the nose is flat, and the eyes have epicanthic folds which obscure the inner corners. The groove between the upper lip and nose is indistinct, and the upper lip is thin and reddish. The severely affected infant may have a significant reduction in height and weight. Mental retardation and irritability also are seen. The condition is permanent, and older children may be hyperactive and have poor coordination.

An important unanswered question is whether there is a safe level of alcohol intake for the pregnant woman. It has been suggested that low levels of intake, in which all absorbed alcohol is detoxified by the liver and does not flow into the general circulation, may be safe. However, the safe level has not been specified. Even very moderate social drinking may cause some abnormalities. Pending further information, the most prudent course probably is to recommend to pregnant women that no alcohol be used.

Maternal alcohol intake can damage the fetus, but the mechanisms are not understood. Alcohol may act directly, possibly by its dehydrating effect on fetal cells. It may affect protein synthesis or formation of neurotransmitters. Acetaldehyde is very toxic and crosses the placenta. This, therefore, may be the toxic agent. Alternatively, increased ethanol-metabolizing enzymes may have a role in the production of anomalies.[26]

The incidence of hypoglycemia and malnutrition, including amino acid, vitamin, and trace element deficiencies, is increased in alcoholics. However, the evidence does not suggest that malnutrition is the sole cause of FAS. Smoking, increased caffeine intake, and drug abuse occur with greater frequency in those who are heavy drinkers. The relative effects of these factors on the incidence of FAS is unknown.

Prader-Willi Syndrome

Prader-Willi syndrome is a congenital disorder the cause of which is unknown. A disturbance in brain development may account for all the symptoms.[27] The clinical manifestations include central nervous system dysfunction, particularly hypotonia and mental retardation. Many patients have craniofacial and limb abnormalities. Of great interest to nutritional care specialists is the tendency to excessive weight gain.

The patients have a severe food-seeking behavior and tend to gorge themselves with any available food. The resulting obesity can be so severe as to result in early death. Although ketogenic diets and anorectic drugs have been used, it appears that the best treatment of the obesity is careful control of food intake. This may require locks on refrigerators, food cupboards, and even garbage cans. If this is done and food intake is controlled with weighed portions, weight control is possible.[28]

Myelomeningocele

Spina bifida is a group of congenital disorders in which there is a defect in the bone encasement of the spinal cord. In *myelomeningocele,* the cord herniates through the defect. A sac filled with cerebrospinal fluid protrudes from the midline of the back. It is covered with a membrane to which nerve roots adhere. The patient has bladder and bowel incontinence and variable weakness to flaccid paralysis in the lower extremities. Many have decreased intelligence, and a large proportion are hydrocephalic.

Among the survivors, obesity is common. Muscle structure is decreased in the denervated area and the proportion of fat is increased. The energy need may be as low as 50 percent of normal and should be provided in proportion to height to maintain normal weight.

The patients may have disorders of ascorbic acid metabolism and often have spontaneous fractures similar to those seen in scurvy. Blood analysis indicates ascorbic acid unsaturation. Vitamin supplementation often is indicated.

An acid-ash diet occasionally is used to maintain an acid urine for prevention of bladder infections. The fluid intake should be monitored and should be generous. A high-fiber diet is helpful to avoid constipation.

Other Feeding Problems

Obstructive lesions or psychological factors may lead to feeding problems even though the child is neurologically normal. Other cases of feeding difficulties are the result of *mismanagement of behavior,* resulting in multiple food dislikes, bizarre food habits, and mealtime tantrums. Provision of information to the parents on normal feeding behavior may be helpful in avoiding the development of such problems. Behavioral problems, once they do develop, may become the responsibility of psychologists, although nutritional care specialists may have a cooperative role.

Failure to thrive is a syndrome occurring in infancy and childhood in which there is growth failure and developmental retardation. It has been linked to environmental deprivation from parental neglect and lack of loving care, sensory stimulation, social contact, and physical handling. Nevertheless, the physiologic effects of failure to thrive are believed to be derived most often from malnutrition, since most children under treatment do gain weight when fed a generous diet.[29] The infant may have poor feeding habits, vomiting, large fecal losses, or high energy requirements. Other suggested mechanisms of the malnutrition are alterations in mineral metabolism, central nervous system disturbances, or constipation.[30]

If the infant does not gain weight when adequate amounts of nutrients for rehabilitation are provided, other factors may be investigated. These include the possible presence of neurologic dysfunction, mechanical obstruction, or malabsorption. Nutritional rehabilitation should be accompanied by long-term follow-up by various members of the health care team.

Neurologic and Neuromuscular Problems in the Older Child or Adult

In addition to the developmentally disabled child who becomes an adult, some normal adults become handicapped. There are a variety of reasons for this. Some patients have progressive neurologic diseases such as multiple sclerosis, parkinsonism, or muscular dystrophy. Some patients have brain damage or spinal cord injuries as a result of trauma or of surgery for tumors. Some patients are handicapped by cerebrovascular accidents.

Nutrition in Rehabilitation Following Traumatic Injury

Techniques for patient rehabilitation following traumatic injury are designed to prevent further disability and to restore function to the maximum extent possible. The nutritional care specialist has an important place in the rehabilitation of many patients in conjunction with the efforts of other health care team members such as occupational, physical, and speech therapists.

The patient's nutritional needs must, of course, be met. Energy content must be individually adjusted to avoid obesity, high enough to provide sufficient energy for physical therapy but decreased for those patients whose activities are reduced. Bowel and bladder problems are frequent in patients with disabling injuries. A high-fiber diet with 2 to 3 liters of fluid per day are recommended for prevention of constipation if renal function is normal. Patients with spinal cord injuries have decreased bladder control and an increased incidence of urinary tract infections. The patient who is immobilized for a long period loses calcium from the bones, raising urinary calcium levels and increasing the risk of renal calculi. Physical therapy providing for muscle tension and weight bearing may be a preventive measure; however, if this is not possible, a low-calcium diet may be necessary.

Many patients need assistance in learning to manage the activities of daily living. For those with disabilities involving the upper body, arms, and hands, some of the same devices used to help the developmentally disabled child to self-feed may be useful (see p. 603). Tables, beds, or trays over wheelchairs may have to be adapted to provide a convenient place to eat.

The adult patient also may need suggestions on methods for food preparation. Detailed information on equipment and techniques is available in *Mealtime Manual for the Aged and Handicapped.*[31] This volume is divided into sections for patients with only one hand, those with weakness in the upper extremities, those with incoordination, loss of sensation, and limited vision, those in wheelchairs, and other handicaps.

Patients often also have serious financial problems as a result of the medical cost of their injuries. They may need help in finding social programs to assist with the cost of food and special equipment.

Parkinson's Disease

Parkinson's disease is a progressive neuromuscular disease in which there is a decreased concentration of dopamine in the basal ganglia of the brain. It is treated with levodopa (L-dopa), a precursor of dopamine. A high-protein diet reduces the effectiveness of this drug, and alcohol antagonizes its action. Advice to patients should include the following:

1. Reduce protein intake to moderate levels and distribute protein evenly among four meals.[32]
2. Do not take the drug at meal time.
3. Maintain normal weight.
4. Avoid alcohol.
5. Do not take vitamin supplements containing pyridoxine or use foods fortified with pyridoxine, since this vitamin may increase the transformation of L-dopa to dopamine before it reaches the brain.[33]

Epilepsy and Other Seizure Disorders

Epilepsy is a chronic nervous disease with periodic excessive neuronal discharges in the brain during which the patient may have loss of consciousness with convulsions. Convulsive seizures may occur in children or in adults. The seizures vary in frequency and severity. *Grand mal* seizures are very severe, whereas *petit mal* seizures are mild.

The most common treatment of epilepsy and other seizure disorders is anticonvulsant drugs. The use of these drugs has many nutritional implications which were described earlier (see p. 605). Alcohol reduces the effectiveness of these drugs and should be avoided.

If anticonvulsant drugs are ineffective, a *ketogenic diet* may be useful to control some types of seizures.[34] The diet is planned using a system similar in principle to the diabetic exchange list, with three-quarters of the energy obtained from fat and one-quarter from protein and carbohydrates combined. It has been reported that a greater ketogenic effect is obtained if 50 to 70 percent of the kilocalories are obtained from medium-chain triglycerides.[35-37] Medium-chain triglycerides can then be used as a smaller proportion of the diet. The diet is relatively unpalatable, and long-term patient compliance is difficult. The diet should be supplemented with water-soluble vitamins, calcium, and iron.

Multiple Sclerosis

Multiple sclerosis is a nervous system disease of unknown etiology. It occurs primarily in adults 20 to 40 years of age at onset. It runs a course of many years, during which the myelin sheaths around nerves degenerate and are replaced by scar tissue. The cause of the disease is unknown, but it may be an autoimmune disease, a slow-acting virus, or a disease of fat metabolism.

Serum linoleate levels are subnormal, particularly when symptoms are severe. A linoleate supplement was reported to ameliorate the symptoms.[38] A low-fat diet containing 10 g of saturated fat, 40 to 50 g of polyunsaturated fat, and 1 tsp. of cod liver oil has also been suggested for treatment.[39,40] It was claimed that the diet retarded the progress of the disease, but its effectiveness is considered by most authorities to be unproved.

Nutritional care usually consists of an adequate diet with attention to maintaining normal weight as activity decreases. Feeding aids are needed as the disease progresses.

Myasthenia Gravis

Myasthenia gravis is a disease in which nerve impulses are not carried normally across the *myoneural junction* (from the nerve ending to the muscle). As a consequence, muscle contraction is poor with easy fatigability, weakness, and paralysis. The disease commonly affects muscles innervated by the bulbar nuclei of the brain and therefore affects the face, lips, tongue, and throat. It may, however, affect almost any muscle.

Soft, easily chewed foods with high caloric density may be helpful to these patients. They eat slowly, so extra time for eating must be allowed and equipment provided to keep food warm. As the disease progresses, tube feedings may be required.

MENTAL ILLNESS

Almost half of the hospital beds in the United States are occupied by patients with mental illness. Many of these patients are malnourished, even though mental illness rarely increases nutrient requirements. There are many reasons for this high incidence of malnutrition. The diet of the patient may have been neglected during a period of emotional stress. Some patients are depressed, disinterested, forgetful, confused, and anxious, all of which can cause a decrease in food intake and lead to nutritional deficiency. Others are compulsive eaters and become obese. Unfortunately, conditions in the hospital also may contribute to poor nutrition in the patient. Although, ideally, the hospital should provide a therapeutic environment, patients are "warehoused" in some institutions where funds are inadequate. A poor diet is provided in some hospitals, and patients with eating problems can be neglected because of a shortage of adequately trained personnel.

The objectives of nutritional care of the hospitalized mental patient are (1) prevention or correction of malnutrition, (2) correction of feeding problems, and (3) restoration of the patient's ability to eat with emotional satisfaction.

A variety of feeding problems are found in mental patients. For example, some patients refuse to eat from a fear of poisoning, a hallucination that they have no stomach, a feeling of guilt, or a desire for suicide. These patients may require tube feeding. Care must be taken to assure that suicidal patients are not provided with implements that can be used for self-destruction. Paper dishes and plastic implements may be needed. Other patients have bizarre, destructive, or disruptive behaviors related to food and may profit from eating in isolation. The anxious patient has difficulty in deciding where and what to eat. Those patients incapable of making a decision may need to be fed one food at a time and given one implement with which to eat. During retraining, cafeteria-style service is helpful to give practice in making choices.

Some patients are hyperactive and are unable to sit still long enough for normal food intake, yet their needs may be increased. These patients should be provided with supplemental foods that can be eaten during activity. Fluid intake of these patients should be monitored carefully.

It must also be remembered that food has symbolic meanings for everyone. In mental illness, these become exaggerated. Good food and a pleasant environment are important in therapy.

Large doses of vitamins have been suggested for treatment of mental illness, based on claims that some people need large quantities of some vitamins for optimal mental function. The procedure is known as *orthomolecular psychiatry*. The American Psychiatric Association does not advocate this treatment, stating that it is unsupported by scientific evidence and that results are not reproducible.[41] The matter remains somewhat controversial, since brain metabolism is not entirely understood. If the psychiatrist prescribes large doses of vitamins, the patient should be observed for signs of vitamin toxicity.

The mentally ill patient who is being treated as an outpatient or the former mentally ill patient who has been discharged from the hospital may have many problems. They often are inexperienced, poor, and have been abandoned by their families. There are many stigmas attached to mental illness by society, and patients have difficulty finding employment. Some of the patients live in halfway houses after discharge from the mental hospital. These facilities should employ a nutritional consultant to assure an adequate diet for residents, but a consultant is not always provided. Some day-care centers also exist to help mentally ill patients. A nutritional care specialist in this setting can teach skills in food shopping and preparation, cleanliness and safety, as well as social skills. Teaching of mentally ill patients requires careful planning, since the patients' attention spans often are short.

DRUG ADDICTION

There is limited information on the nutritional status of and procedures for nutritional care of drug addicts. Nutritional assessment of those addicted to commonly abused narcotics (heroin, cocaine, or lysergic acid diethylamide [LSD]) showed that malnutrition is common; the addict develops a craving for sweets, and the diet generally is high in carbohydrate and may be low in vitamins A, B_{12}, and other B vitamins.[42] Fatty acid composition was altered. Consumption of alcohol was high, and hepatitis, hypertension, and infections were common.

The access of nutritional care specialists to drug addicts is limited until the addicts are associated with some form of residential institutional care or a clinic. Addicts or former addicts in clinics or halfway houses need nutritional counseling and assistance with psychosocial development. The nutritional care specialist skilled in interpersonal relationships could make an important contribution to the rehabilitation of the drug addict if the opportunity develops.

DISEASES OF THE MUSCULOSKELETAL SYSTEM

Musculoskeletal diseases are those that affect the bones, joints, and muscles. Some also affect the internal organs and skin. They may be classified into four broad categories:[43]

1. Diseases that usually affect only the joints (e.g., osteoarthritis)
2. Systemic diseases affecting primarily the musculoskeletal system but also affecting other tissues (e.g., rheumatoid arthritis)
3. Systemic diseases with pain in joints or

muscles but without structural changes (e.g., polymyalgia rheumatica)
4. Diffuse connective tissue disease involving skin, internal organs, and the musculoskeletal system (e.g., systemic lupus erythematosus)

The term *arthritis* is used to designate the diseases in these categories in which there is inflammation of the joints. It occurs in more than 17 million people, and may be acute or chronic and primary or secondary to other diseases. The two most common forms are rheumatoid arthritis and osteoarthritis. Gout also is a form of arthritis but, because it is genetic in origin, it is described in Chapter 10.

Rheumatoid Arthritis

Rheumatoid (atrophic) arthritis is a progressive chronic debilitating disease of unknown etiology occurring in approximately 3 percent of the adult population. Average age at onset is 35 years, but the disease does occur in children. The *synovium* (joint lining) is inflamed and painful. Fibroblasts, blood vessels, and inflammatory cells proliferate. The disease may affect any joint but is seen most often in the hands, knees, ankles, and feet. The patient is in negative nitrogen and calcium balance, with muscle atrophy and bone decalcification. The patient frequently is underweight and anemic. The anemia is hemolytic in origin and is not related to iron intake.

The patient may have fever, rash, and extreme fatigue. A *rheumatoid factor* is found in the blood and synovial fluid but is not specific for this disease; rheumatoid factor is found in other conditions as well. The disease probably occurs in a genetically susceptible individual after an infection that probably is viral. An immune mechanism is believed to perpetuate the joint inflammation.

There is no known cure, and treatment is not very successful. As a result, patients are prone, in desperation, to adopt unproved treatments, including fad diets. Among the so-called remedies suggested are the following:[44]

Take large doses of calcium, riboflavin, pantothenic acid, and vitamins D and E.
Eat only fresh fruit and honey for 3 days.
Eliminate potatoes, tomatoes, eggplant, and red or green peppers from the diet.
Eliminate dairy products, meat, fruit, egg yolk, vinegar, pepper, "hot spices," chocolate, dry toasted nuts, alcoholic beverages, soft drinks, additives, preservatives, and "chemicals" from the diet.
Drink 1 c. of burdock root or burdock burr tea three times daily for 1½ months and drink ginger tea while sitting in a ginger root or apple cider vinegar bath.
Eat watercress, cherries, raw liver, parsley, fish liver oil, or bone meal or drink alfalfa tea or lemon juice.
Drink 6 oz. of celery juice daily and eliminate bread.

Nutritional care actually is focused on:

Provision of an adequate diet. (Patients may have poor food intake, especially if hands and legs are affected.)
Achievement and maintenance of normal weight.
Help with problems of daily living, including preparation of meals.

Patients are given antiinflammatory drugs such as aspirin or indomethacin. If these are ineffective, steroid drugs sometimes are used to reduce pain and stiffness. Among the agents that may be used are adrenocorticotropic hormone (ACTH), cortisone, prednisone, hydrocortisone, and dexamethasone. Side effects of these drugs and related nutritional care are discussed in Chapter 7. Medications should be taken after meals to reduce gastric irritation.

The diet for the juvenile arthritis patient must be adjusted for age. Nutrient levels must be reduced for the decrease in activity but remain sufficient to permit growth. Growth disturbances are common. More than one-half of juvenile patients recover in 1 to 2 years.

Osteoarthritis

Osteoarthritis is known also as *degenerative* or *hypertrophic arthritis.* It occurs almost universally in the elderly. The cause is unknown, but it may develop from stress on the joints. As such, it occasionally develops in younger persons following athletic and other injuries.

The primary lesion is degeneration of the articular cartilage in the joints. It affects the thumb particularly, and also fingers, hips, knees, ankles, and spine. It begins with a feeling of stiffness, particularly in the morning or following a long period of immobilization. Soreness subsides after a warm-up. The disease usually involves only a few joints, but general involvement is possible. The severity of the degenerative lesion may vary from asymptomatic to widespread involvement and disability.

The primary feature of nutritional care is weight reduction if the patient is overweight. This is particularly important if arthritis is present in the spine or weight-bearing joints. Because arthritis tends to limit exercise, weight reduction may be very difficult.

COMMENT

Nutritional care specialists can make important contributions to the care of the handicapped. Although they often are not involved in long-term direct training programs, they may take part in program planning, consultation on normal nutrition and feeding techniques, and direct evaluation, diagnosis, treatment, and rehabilitation of patients.[45]

References

1. Zickefoose, M. Feeding the child with a cleft palate. *J. Am. Diet. Assoc.* 36:129, 1960.
2. Denhoff, E., and Feldman, S.A. *Developmental Disabilities. Management through Diet and Medication.* New York: Marcel Dekker, 1981.
3. Mueller, H.A. Facilitating feeding and prespeech. In P.H. Pearson and C.E. Williams, Eds., *Physical Therapy Services in Developmental Disabilities.* Springfield, Ill.: Charles C Thomas, 1972.
4. Fiorentino, M.R. *Reflex Testing Methods for Evaluating Central Nervous System Development.* Springfield, Ill.: Charles C Thomas, 1973.
5. Bobath, K., and Bobath, B. *The Motor Deficit in Patients with Cerebral Palsy.* London: Spastics Society Medical Education and Information Unit, in association with Heinemann Medical, 1966.
6. Peiper, A. *Cerebral Function in Infancy and Childhood.* New York: Consultants Bureau, 1963.
7. Paine, R.S., and Oppe, T.E. *Neurological Examination of Children.* London: Suffolk Lavenham Press, 1966.
8. Ingram, T.T.S. Clinical significance of the infantile feeding reflexes. *Dev. Med. Child. Neurol.* 4:159, 1962.
9. Twitchell, T.E. Normal motor development. *Phys. Ther.* 45:419, 1965.
10. Campbell, S.K. Facilitation of cognitive and motor development in infants with central nervous system dysfunction. *Phys. Ther.* 54:346, 1974.
11. Gallender, D. *Eating Handicaps. Illustrated Techniques for Feeding Disorders.* Springfield, Ill.: Charles C Thomas, 1979.
12. McDonald, R.E. *Dentistry for the Child and Adolescent.* St. Louis: C.V. Mosby, 1969.
13. Freud, A. *Normality and Pathology in Childhood.* New York: International Universities Press, 1966.
14. Illingworth, R.S. *The Development of the Infant and Young Child,* 5th ed. Baltimore: Williams and Wilkins, 1972.
15. Reynolds, E.H. Folate metabolism and anticonvulsant therapy. *Proc. R. Soc. Med.* 67:68, 1974.
16. Norris, J.W., and Pratt, R.F. Folic acid deficiency and epilepsy. *Drugs* 8:366, 1974.
17. Ch'ien, L.T., Krumdieck, C.L., Scott, C.W., Jr., and Butterworth, C.E., Jr. Harmful effects of megadoses of vitamins: Electroencephalogram abnormalities and seizures induced by intravenous folate in drug-treated epileptics. *Am. J. Clin. Nutr.* 28:51, 1975.

18. Deluca, K., Masotti, R.E., and Partington, N.W. Altered calcium metabolism due to anticonvulsant drugs. *Dev. Med. Child. Neurol.* 14:318, 1973.
19. Lifshitz, F., and Maclaren, N. Vitamin D–dependent rickets in institutionalized, mentally retarded children receiving long-term anticonvulsant therapy: I. A survey of 288 patients. *J. Pediatr.* 83:612, 1973.
20. Hammond, M.I., Lewis, M.N., and Johnson, E.W. A nutritional study of cerebral palsied children. *J. Am. Diet. Assoc.* 49:196, 1966.
21. Gourge, A.L., and Ekvall, S.W. Diets of handicapped children: Physical, psychological and socioeconomic correlations. *Am. J. Ment. Defic.* 80:149, 1975.
22. Pecks, S., and Lamb, M.W. Comments on the dietary practices of cerebral palsied children. *J. Am. Diet. Assoc.* 27:870, 1951.
23. Phelps, W.M. Dietary requirements in cerebral palsy. *J. Am. Diet. Assoc.* 27:869, 1951.
24. Eddy, T.P., Nicholson, A.L., and Wheeler, E.F. Energy expenditures and dietary intakes in cerebral palsy. *Dev. Med. Child. Neurol.* 7:377, 1965.
25. Culley, W.J., and Middleton, T. Caloric requirement of mentally retarded children with and without motor dysfunction. *J. Pediatr.* 75:380, 1969.
26. Ouellette, E. The fetal alcohol syndrome. In J.J. Vitale and S.A. Broitman, Eds., *Advances in Human Clinical Nutrition.* Boston: John Wright-PSG, 1982.
27. Hanson, J.W. A view of the etiology and pathogenesis of Prader-Willi syndrome. In V.A. Holm, S. Sulzbacher, and P.L. Pipes, *The Prader-Willi Syndrome.* Baltimore: University Park Press, 1981.
28. Pipes, P.L. Nutritional management of children with Prader-Willi syndrome. In V.A. Holm, S. Sulzbacher, and P.L. Pipes, *The Prader-Willi Syndrome.* Baltimore: University Park Press, 1982.
29. Kohler, E.E., and Good, T.A. The infant who fails to thrive. *Hosp. Pract.* 4:54, 1969.
30. Fiser, R.H., Jr., Meredith, P.D., and Elders, J.M. The child who fails to grow. *Am. Fam. Physician* 11(6):108, 1975.
31. Institute of Rehabilitative Medicine, New York University Medical Center. *Mealtime Manual for the Aged and Handicapped.* New York: Essandess Special Edition, 1970.
32. Langan, R.J., and Cotzias, G.C. Do's and don't's for the patient on levodopa therapy. *Am. J. Nurs.* 76:917, 1976.
33. Visconti, J.A. *Drug-Food Interaction.* Nutrition in Disease series. Columbus: Ross Laboratories, 1977.
34. Mike, E.M. Practical guide and dietary management of children with seizures using the ketogenic diet. *Am. J. Clin. Nutr.* 17:399, 1965.
35. Huttenlocher, P.R., Wilbourn, A.J., and Signore, J.M. Medium-chain triglycerides for intractable childhood epilepsy. *Neurology* (N.Y.) 21:1097, 1971.
36. Signore, J.M. Ketogenic diet containing medium chain triglycerides. *J. Am. Diet. Assoc.* 62:285, 1973.
37. Huttenlocher, P.R. Ketonemia and seizures: Metabolic and anticonvulsant effects of two ketogenic diets in childhood epilepsy. *Pediatr. Res.* 10:536, 1976.
38. Millar, J.H.D., Zilkha, K.J., Langman, M.J.S., et al. Double-blind trial of linoleate supplementation of the diet in multiple sclerosis. *Br. Med. J.* 1:765, 1973.
39. Swank, R.L., and Bourdillon, R.D. Multiple sclerosis: Assessment of treatment with a modified low fat diet. *J. Nerv. Ment. Dis.* 131:486, 1960.
40. Swank, R.L. Multiple sclerosis: Twenty years on a low fat diet. *Arch. Neurol.* 23:460, 1970.
41. American Psychiatric Association Task Force on Vitamin Therapy in Psychiatry. Megavitamin and orthomolecular therapy in psychiatry (excerpts from a report). *Nutr. Rev.* (Suppl. 1)32:44, 1975.
42. Frankle, R.T., and Christakis, G. Some nutritional aspects of "hard" drug addiction. *Dietetic Currents* 2(3):1, 1975.
43. Houpt, J. Arthritic and Rheumatic Disorders. In A.G. Gornall, Ed., *Applied Biochemistry of Clinical Disorders.* Hagerstown, Md.: Harper and Row, 1980.
44. Meister, K.A. Can diet cure arthritis? *ACSH News and Views* 1:10, 1980.
45. Wallace, H.M. Nutrition and handicapped children. *J. Am. Diet. Assoc.* 61:127, 1972.

Bibliography

Culley, W.J., Goyal, K., Jolly, D.H., and Mertz, E.T. Caloric intake of children with Down's syndrome (mongolism). *J. Pediatr.* 66:772, 1965.

Hargrave, M. *Nutritional Care of the Physically Disabled.* Minneapolis: Sister Kenney Institute, 1979.

Martin, H. Nutrition: Its relationship to children's physical, mental and emotional development. *Am. J. Clin. Nutr.* 26:766, 1973.

Ogg, H.L. Oral-pharyngeal development and evaluation. *Phys. Ther.* 55:235, 1975.

Perlstein, M.A. Drug therapy of cerebral palsy.

In R.S. Illingworth, Ed., *Recent Advances in Cerebral Palsy.* Boston: Little, Brown, 1958.

Pipes, P.L. *Nutrition in Infancy and Childhood,* 2nd ed. St. Louis: C.V. Mosby, 1981.

Reynolds, E.H. Iatrogenic nutritional effects of anticonvulsants. *Proc. Nutr. Soc.* 33:225, 1974.

Strain, G.W. Nutrition, brain function and behavior. *Psychiatr. Clin. North Am.* 4:253, 1981.

Wurtman, R.J., and Wurtman, J.J. *Disorders of Eating and Nutrients in Treatment of Brain Diseases.* Nutrition and the Brain, vol. 3. New York: Raven Press, 1979.

Sources of Current Information

American Journal of Clinical Nutrition
Journal of the American Dietetic Association
Journal of Pediatrics
Pediatric Research

Appendixes

Appendix A. Vocabulary

COMBINING FORMS

Many medical terms are taken from the Greek or Latin, and some words are combinations of the two. The terms listed here are divided into two sections. The *root words* usually refer to the part of the body or tissue, whereas prefixes and suffixes are *modifiers* that describe the variation from normal or the action on the root word.

Root Words

Adeno-	Gland
Andro-	Men
Ano-	Anus
Antr-	Cavity, cave
Arthro-	Joint
-blast	Immature form, sprout, germ
Broncho-	Bronchus
Canc-, carc-	Malignant tumor
Cardi-, cardio-	Heart
Chole-	Bile
Cholecysto-	Gallbladder
Choledocho-	Bile duct
Chondro-	Cartilage
Col-	Colon
Corp-	Body, mass
Crani-, cranio-	Skull
Cyano-	Blue
Cysto-	Bladder; any fluid-filled sac
Cyto-	Cell
Derm-, dermato-	Skin
Duodeno-	Duodenum
Em-	Blood
Encephalo-	Brain, skull
Entero-	Intestine
Erythro-	Red
Esophago-	Esophagus
Esthe-	Feeling, sensation
Fis-	Cleavage, split
For-	Opening, aperture
Forn-	Arch, vault
Gastr-	Stomach
Glosso-	Tongue
Gynec-	Women (especially women's reproductive organs)
Hem-, hemat-	Blood
Hepato-	Liver
Hist-	Tissue
Hydr-	Water
Hyster-, hystero-	Uterus
Idio-	Unknown, strange, peculiar
Ileo-	Ileum
Jejuno-	Jejunum
Laryngo-	Larynx
Leuc-, leuk-	White
Lipo-	Fat
Lith-	Stone
Lymph-	Waterlike
Malac-	Softening
Mea-	Passage
Meg-	Large, great, strong
Menin-	Membrane
Morph-	Form, shape
My-, myo-	Muscle
Myelo-	Marrow
Naso-	Nose
Necro-	Dead
Neph-, nephro-	Kidney
Neuro-	Nerve
Oligo-	Few, scant
Oophor-	Ovary
Ophthalm-	Eye
Os-, oss-, ost-, osteo-	Bone
-osis	Disease
Ot-	Ear
Ovar-	Ovary
Pancreato-	Pancreas
Parieto-	Wall
Path-	Disease
Ped-	Child, feet
Pneumo-, Pneumon-	Lung
Poly-	Many, much

Proct-	Anus, rectum
Pseud-	False
Pulm-	Lung
Pyel-, pyelo-	Pelvis
Py-, pyo-	Pus
Pyr-	Fever, fire
Recto-	Rectum
Reni-, reno-	Kidney
Retic-, reticulo-	Netlike
Rhino-	Nose
Salping-	Tube
Sang-	Blood
Sclero-	Hard
Seb-	Hard fat
Sept-	Thin wall
Septic-	Poison
Sinu-	Curved, hollow
Sta-	Stand
Stomato-	Mouth
Tox-, toxic-	Poison
Tracheo-	Trachea
Uretero-	Ureter
Urethro-	Urethra
Utero-	Uterus
Vari-	Bent, stretched
Veni-, veno-	Vein

Modifiers

A-	Without, from
Ab-, abs-	From
Ad-	To, toward, at
-algia	Pain in
Am-, ambi-, amphi-	Around
-asis	Affected with, disease
Ante-	Before, forward
Anti-	Against, opposite
Brachy-	Short
Brady-	Slow
-cele	Hernia of
Circum-	Around
-cleisis	Closure of
Con-	With
-cyte	Cell
De-	Down, from, away
Demi-	Half
Dextro-	Right
Dia-	Through
Dis-	Apart
-duct	Lead, guide
-dynia	Pain in
Dys-	Difficult, painful
E-	From, out of, without
Ec-	Out
-ectasis	Deletion of
Ecto-	Without, outside, external
-ectomy	Excision of
-ectopy	Displacement of
Ek-	From, out of, without
Em-	In
-emesis	Vomiting
-emia	In blood
En-	In
Endo-, ento-	Within
Epi-	On, against
-esthesia	Feeling, sensation
Eu-	Well, abundant, easy
Ex-	From, out of, without
Exo-	Outside, beyond
Extra-	Outside, beyond
-genesis, -genic	Producing, forming
Hemi-	Half
Hyper-	Over, above, beyond, excessive
Hypo-	Under, deficiency of
Im-, in-	In, into, not
Infra-	Below, beneath
Inter-	Between
Intra-	Within, during
-itis	Inflammation of
Lev-, levo-	Left
-lith	Stone
-lysis, -lytic	Destructive
Mal-	Bad
Meso-	Middle, between
-oid	Formed like
-oma	Tumor
-osis	Disease
Pan-	All, every
Para-	Beside
-pathy	Disease
-penia	Without, lack of
Peri-	Around
-phagia	To eat
-phobia	Fear of
-pnea	Breathing air
-poiesis	To produce
Poly-	Many
Post-	After
Pre-, pro-	Before
Privia-	Without, lack of
-ptosis	Falling of
Quad-, quar-	Four
Re-	Again
Retro-	Backward
-rrhagia	Bursting from
-rrhaphy	Sewing of
-rrhea	Flowing
-rrhexis	Rupture of
-scopy	Viewing of
Semi-	Half
-spasm	Spasm of
-stenosis	Narrowing of

-stomy	Making a mouth
Sub-	Under, below
Super-	Over, above
Supra-	Above
Tachy-	Swift, fast
-tomy	Cutting of
Trans-	Above, beyond, through, across
-trismus	Spasm of
-trophy	Growth or mutation

ABBREVIATIONS USED IN MEDICAL RECORDS

a	Before
A, Asmt	Assessment
ABG	Arterial blood gases
a.c.	Before meals, *ante cibum*
ad lib	As needed or desired
ADL	Activities of daily living
A/G	Albumin/globulin ratio
AODM	Adult-onset diabetes mellitus
AP	Angina pectoris
ARF	Acute renal failure
ASHD	Arteriosclerotic heart disease
a&w	Alive and well
b.i.d., b.d.	Twice daily
b.m.	Bowel movement
BMR	Basal metabolic rate
BP, b.p.	blood pressure
B.S.	Bowel sounds
B.T.	Bed-time
BUN	Blood urea nitrogen
Bx	Biopsy
c̄, c	With
ca	Approximately
Ca	Calcium
CA	Cancer
CAD	Coronary artery disease
CBC	Complete blood [cell] count
CC	Chief complaint
CCU	Coronary care unit
CHD	Coronary heart disease
CHF	Congestive heart failure
CNS	Central nervous system
C/O	Complains of
CRF	Chronic renal failure
CSF	Cerebrospinal fluid
c.v.	Cardiovascular
CVA	Cerebrovascular accident
CVR	Cardiovascular-renal
D/C	Discontinue
dil	Dilate
DKA	Diabetic ketoacidosis
DM	Diabetes mellitus
DOE	Dyspnea on exertion
Dx	Diagnosis
ECG, EKG	Electrocardiogram
EEG	Electroencephalogram
ENT	Ear, nose, and throat
EENT	Eye, ear, nose, and throat
FBS	Fasting blood sugar
FFA	Free fatty acids
FH	Family history
fl	Fluid
FMH	Family medical history
F/U	Follow-up
FUO	Fever of unknown origin
Fx	Fracture
GA	General appearance
GB	Gallbladder
GI	Gastrointestinal
gt	A drop
GTT	Glucose tolerance test
GU	Genitourinary
GYN	Gynecology
Hb, Hgb	Hemoglobin
HBP	High blood pressure
H.C.	High calorie
Hct	Hematocrit
HCVD	Hypertensive cardiovascular disease
H/O	History of
H&P	History and physical
HPI	History of present illness
h.s.	at bedtime, *hora somni*
HTN	Hyptertension
Hx	History
ICU	Intensive care unit
IHD	Ischemic heart disease
IM, i.m.	Intramuscular
IMP	Impression
I&O	Intake and output
I.P.	Intraperitoneal
IV, i.v.	Intravenous
LDH	Lactic dehydrogenase
LE	Lupus erythematosus
LMD	Local medical doctor
L&W	Living and well
mEq	Milliequivalent
MH	Menstrual history
MI	Mitral insufficiency *or* myocardial infarction
mOsm	Milliosmol
MS	Mitral stenosis *or* multiple sclerosis *or* morphine sulfate
N, NML	Normal
NAD	No apparent distress

NCD	Normal childhood disease	RO	Rule out
NG	Nasogastric	ROS	Review of systems
NKA	No known allergies	rx	Take
NPN	Nonprotein nitrogen	Rx	Prescription, treatment
NPO	Nothing by mouth, *non per os*	s	Without
NR	Not Remarkable	SGOT	Serum glutamic oxaloacetic transaminase
N&V	Nausea and vomiting	SGPT	Serum glutamic pyruvic transaminase
OB	Obstetrics	SH	Social history
para	Pregnancies	SOB	Short of breath
p.c.	After eating, *post cibum*	SOBOE	Short of breath on exertion
P.C.	Present complaint	sos	If necessary
PCM	Protein-calorie malnutrition	S/P	Status postoperatively
PH	Past history	S&S	Signs and symptoms
PI	Present illness	stat	At once
PMH	Past medical history	Sx	symptoms
P.O.	Post operative *or* by mouth (*per os*)	T.&A.	Tonsillectomy and adenoidectomy
PP	Patient profile	TG	Triglycerides
PR	Pulse rate	tid	Three times daily
p.r.n.	Whenever necessary	TPN	Total parenteral nutrition
Pt	Patient	TPR	Temperature, pulse, and respiration
PT	Physical therapy *or* prothrombin time	U/A, U.A.	Urine analysis
PTA	Prior to admission	UCD	Usual childhood diseases
PTT	Partial thromboplastin time	UGI	Upper gastrointestinal
PU(D)	Peptic ulcer (disease)	URI	Upper respiratory [tract] infection
PZI	Protamine zinc insulin	V&P	Vagotomy and pyloroplasty
q	Every	VS	Vital signs
q.d.	Every day	w.b.c.	White blood cells
qh	Every hour	WBC	White blood [cell] count
q.i.d.	Four times daily	WDWN	Well developed, well nourished
q.o.d.	Every other day	WNL	Within normal limits
q2h, q3h	Every 2 hours, every 3 hours	W/U	Workup
r.b.c.	Red blood cells		
RBC	Red blood [cell] count		

Appendix B. Standards for Evaluation of Body Weight

FOGARTY INTERNATIONAL CENTER CONFERENCE ON OBESITY RECOMMENDED WEIGHT IN RELATION TO HEIGHT

Height[a]		Recommended Weight for Men[b] (lb.)		Recommended Weight for Women[b] (lb.)	
Feet	Inches	Average	Range	Average	Range
4	10			102	92–119
4	11			104	94–122
5	0			107	96–125
5	1			110	99–128
5	2	123	112–141	113	102–131
5	3	127	115–144	116	105–134
5	4	130	118–148	120	108–138
5	5	133	121–152	123	111–142
5	6	136	124–156	128	114–146
5	7	140	128–161	132	118–150
5	8	145	132–166	136	122–154
5	9	149	136–170	140	126–158
5	10	153	140–174	144	130–163
5	11	158	144–179	148	134–168
6	0	162	148–184	152	138–173
6	1	166	152–189		
6	2	171	156–194		
6	3	176	160–199		
6	4	181	164–204		

From Bray, G.A., Ed., *Obesity in Perspective.* Fogarty International Center Series on Preventive Medicine, vol. 2, part 1. D.H.E.W. Publication No. (NIH) 75-705. Washington, D.C.: Department of Health, Education and Welfare, 1975.

[a] Height without shoes.

[b] Weight without clothes.

ESTIMATES OF FRAME SIZE*

Measure the wrist circumference just distal (toward the hand) to the styloid process at the wrist crease of the right hand.

Calculate the ratio (r) of body frame size to wrist circumference with the formula:

$$r = \frac{H}{C}$$

where H = height in centimeters; C = wrist circumference in centimeters.

Determine the frame size from the following table:

	r Value	
Frame Size	Men	Women
Small	>10.4	>10.9
Medium	10.4–9.6	10.9–9.9
Large	<9.6	<9.9

* Based on information provided in J.P. Grant, P.B. Custer, and J. Thurlow. Current techniques of nutritional assessment. *Surg. Clin. North Am.* 61:437, 1981.

Appendix C. Conversion Factors

1 kilogram = 2.2 pounds
1 liter = 1.06 quarts
2.54 centimeters = 1 inch
1 deciliter = 100 milliliters

To convert milligrams (mg) to milliequivalents (mEq):

$$\frac{\text{mg}}{\text{atomic weight}} \times \text{valence} = \text{mEq}$$

Example: $\dfrac{\text{460 mg sodium}}{23} \times 1$

$= \text{20 mEq sodium}$

To convert milliequivalents to milligrams:

$$\frac{\text{mEq} \times \text{atomic weight}}{\text{valence}} = \text{mg}$$

Example: $\dfrac{\text{38 mEq potassium} \times 39}{1}$

$= \text{1,482 mg potassium}$

To convert the weight of salt to the weight of sodium:

mg salt × 0.4 = mg sodium

Mineral	*Symbol*	*Atomic Weight*	*Valence*
Calcium	Ca	40	2
Chlorine	Cl	35.4	1
Magnesium	Mg	24.3	2
Phosphorus	P	31	2
Potassium	K	39	1
Sodium	Na	23	1
Sulfur	S	32	2
Zinc	Zn	65.37	2

Appendix D. Normal Laboratory Values: Whole Blood, Serum, and Plasma

Test	Material	Normal Value
Acetone	Serum	0.3–2.0 mg/dl
Albumin	Serum	3.2–5.5 g/dl
Ammonia	Plasma	20–150 μg/dl
Amylase	Serum	50–200 Somogyi units/dl
Ascorbic acid (vitamin C)	Plasma	0.6–1.6 mg/dl
	Whole blood	0.7–2.0 mg/dl
Bicarbonate	Plasma	21–28 mEq/L
Bile acids	Serum	<1.0 mg/dl
Bilirubin	Serum	Up to 0.2 mg/dl (direct or conjugated) 0.1–1.0 mg/dl (indirect or unconjugated) Total: 0.5–1.2 mg/dl
Blood gases	Whole blood	
pH		Arterial: 7.35–7.45 Venous: 7.36–7.41
Pco_2		Arterial: 35–45 mm Hg Venous: 35–50 mm Hg
Po_2		Arterial: 50–100 mm Hg
BSP (Bromsulphalein) (5 mg/kg)	Serum	<5% retention after 45 min. or <4 mg/dl
Calcium	Serum	Total: 8.5–10.5 mg/dl 4.3–5.3 mEq/L Ionized: 4.2–5.2 mg/dl 2.1–2.6 mEq/L
Carbon dioxide	Whole blood	Arterial: 19–24 mEq/L Venous: 22–26 mEq/L
	Plasma	Arterial: 21–30 mEq/L Venous: 22–34 mEq/L
Carotene, beta	Serum	60–200 μg/dl
Chloride	Serum	95–108 mEq/L
Cholesterol, esters	Serum	50–70% of total cholesterol (<210 mg/dl)
Cholesterol, total	Serum	150–300 mg/dl (varies with age and diet)
Copper	Serum	110–160 μg/dl
Creatine	Serum or plasma	Men: 0.2–0.6 mg/dl Women: 0.6–1.0 mg/dl
Creatine phosphokinase (CPK)	Serum	Men: 5–35 units/ml Women: 5–25 units/ml
Creatinine	Serum or plasma	0.6–1.5 mg/dl

Test	Material	Normal Value
Creatinine clearance (endogenous)	Serum or plasma and urine	Men: 107–141 ml/min. Women: 87–132 ml/min.
Electrophoresis, lipoprotein	Serum	Alpha: 12–18%, 80–310 mg/dl Beta: 50–70%, 160–400 mg/dl Pre-beta: 11–29%, 50–180 mg/dl Chylomicrons: 0–1%, 0–50 mg/dl
Electrophoresis, protein	Serum	Albumin: 53–68%, 3.5–5.5 g/dl Alpha-1: 2.0–5.0%, 0.1–0.4 g/dl Alpha-2: 8.0–13.0%, 0.4–1.0 g/dl Beta: 11.0–17.0%, 0.5–1.1 g/dl Gamma: 15.0–25.0%, 0.5–1.6 g/dl
Ferritin (adults)	Serum	12–250 μg/dl
Folate	Serum Erythrocytes	6–25 ng/ml (bioassay) 150–600 ng/ml (bioassay)
Gamma globulin	Serum	0.5–1.6 g/dl
Globulins, total	Serum	2.3–3.5 g/dl
Glucose, fasting	Serum or plasma	70–110 mg/dl
Glucose tolerance		
Oral	Serum or plasma	Fasting: 70–110 mg/dl 30 min.: 30–60 mg/dl above fasting 60 min.: 20–50 mg/dl above fasting 120 min.: 5–15 mg/dl above fasting 180 min.: fasting level or below
Intravenous	Serum or plasma	Fasting: 70–110 mg/dl 5 min.: maximum of 250 mg/dl 60 min.: significant decrease 120 min.: below 120 mg/dl 180 min.: fasting level
Glucose-6-phosphate dehydrogenase (G6PD)	Erythrocytes	140–280 units/10^9 cells
Glutathione	Whole blood	24–37 mg/dl
Growth hormone	Serum	1–15 ng/ml
Guanase	Serum	<3 nmole/ml/min.
Hemoglobin	Serum or plasma Whole blood	0.5–5.0 mg/dl Women: 12.6–14.2 g/dl Men: 14.0–16.5 g/dl Pregnancy: >10.6 g/dl
α-Hydroxybutyric dehydrogenase	Serum	140–350 units/ml
Immunoglobulins	Serum, adults	
IgG		800–1,600 mg/dl, 80%
IgA		50–250 mg/dl, 15%
IgM		40–120 mg/dl, 0.5%
IgD		0.5–3.0 mg/dl, 0.2%
IgE		0.01–0.04 mg/100 dl, 0.0002%
Insulin	Plasma	11–240 μIU/ml (bioassay) 4–24 μunits/ml (radioimmunoassay)
Insulin tolerance	Serum	Fasting: glucose of 7–110 mg/dl 30 min.: fall to 50% of fasting level 90 min.: fasting level
Iron, total	Serum	60–200 μg/dl
Iron-binding capacity	Serum	250–450 μg/dl
Ketone bodies	Serum	Negative or 2–4 μg/dl
Lactic acid	Whole blood, venous Whole blood, arterial	5–20 mg/dl 3–7 mg/dl
Lactic dehydrogenase (LDH)	Serum	80–120 Wacker units 150–450 Wroblewski units 71–207 IU/L

(continued)

Appendix D. (continued)

Test	Material	Normal Value
Lactic dehydrogenase (heat stable)	Serum	30–60% of total LDH
Lactose tolerance	Serum	Serum glucose changes are similar to those seen in a glucose tolerance test
Lipase	Serum	0–1.5 Cherry-Crandall units/ml
Lipids, total	Serum	400–800 mg/dl
Cholesterol		120–260 mg/dl
Triglycerides		0–190 mg/dl
Phospholipids		150–380 mg/dl
Fatty acids, free		25 mg/dl
Neutral fat		0–200 mg/dl
Macroglobulins, total	Serum	70–430 mg/dl
Magnesium	Serum	1.5–2.5 mEq/L
Niacin	Whole blood	3.5–710 μg/ml
Nonprotein nitrogen (NPN)	Serum or plasma	20–35 mg/dl
	Whole blood	25–50 mg/dl
Osmolality	Serum	280–295 mOsm/kg
Oxygen		
Pressure (Pco_2)	Whole blood, arterial	95–100 mm Hg
Content	Whole blood, arterial	15–23 vol/dl
Saturation	Whole blood, arterial	96–100%
Pantothenic acid	Whole blood	20–80 pg/ml
pH	Whole blood, arterial	7.35–7.45
Phenylalanine	Serum	Adults: <3.0 mg/dl Newborns (term): 1.2–3.5 mg/dl
Phosphatase, acid, total	Serum	0–1.1 units/ml (Bodansky) 1–4 units/ml (King-Armstrong) 0.13–0.63 units/ml (Bessey-Lowry) 1.4–5.5 units/ml (Gutman-Gutman) 0–0.56 units/ml (Roy) 0–6.0 units/ml (Shinowara-Jones-Reinhart)
Phosphatase, alkaline, total	Serum	Adults: 1.5–4.5 units/dl (Bodansky) 4–13 units/dl (King-Armstrong) 0.8–2.3 units/ml (Bessey-Lowry) 15–35 units/ml (Shinowara-Jones-Reinhart) 30–85 IU Children: 5.0–14.0 units/dl (Bodansky) 3.4–9.0 units/ml (Bessey-Lowry) 15–30 units/dl (King-Armstrong)
Phospholipids	Serum	150–380 mg/dl
Phosphorus, inorganic	Serum	Adults: 1.8–2.6 mEq/L 3.0–4.5 mg/dl Children: 2.3–4.1 mEq/L 4.0–7.0 mg/dl
Potassium	Plasma	3.5–5.0 mEq/L
Proteins, total	Serum	6.0–8.0 g/dl
Albumin		3.5–5.5 g/dl
Globulin		2.3–3.5 g/dl

Test	Material	Normal Value
Riboflavin	Whole blood	100–500 pg/ml
Sodium	Plasma	135–148 mEq/L
Sulfates, inorganic	Serum	0.2–1.3 mEq/L 0.9–6.0 mg/dl
Thiamine	Whole blood	25–72 pg/ml
Transaminase		
Glutamic oxaloacetic	Serum (SGOT)	8–40 units/ml
Glutamic pyruvic	Serum (SGPT)	5–35 units/ml
Triglycerides	Serum	40–150 mg/dl
Urea clearance	Serum and urine	Maximum clearance: 60–99 ml/min. Standard clearance: 41–65 ml/min. or more than 75% of normal clearance
Urea nitrogen	Blood (BUN) Serum (SUN)	5–20 mg/dl 6–20 mg/dl
Uric acid	Serum	Men: 3.0–7.0 mg/dl Women: 2.0–6.0 mg/dl
Vitamin A	Serum	50–100 μg/dl
Vitamin B_6 (pyridoxine)	Plasma	30–80 ng/ml
Vitamin B_{12}	Serum	160–1,000 pg/ml
Vitamin C	Plasma	0.6–1.6 mg/dl
Vitamin E	Plasma	0.6 mg/dl
Zinc	Plasma	75–125 μg/dl

[a] The following works provide useful information on interpretation of tests: Bennington, J.L., Fouty, R.A., and Hougie, C., *Laboratory Diagnosis.* Toronto, Ont.: Macmillan, 1970; Byrne, C.J., Saxton, D.F., Pelikan, P.K., and Nugent, P.M., *Laboratory Tests. Implications for Nurses and Allied Health Professionals.* Menlo Park, Calif.: Addison-Wesley, 1981; Halsted, J.A., and Halsted, C.H., Eds., *The Laboratory in Clinical Medicine. Interpretation and Application,* 2nd ed. Philadelphia: W.B. Saunders, 1981; Ravel, R., *Clinical Laboratory Medicine,* 3rd ed. Chicago: Year Book Medical Publishers, 1978; Tilkian, S.M., and Conover, M.H., *Clinical Implications of Laboratory Tests.* St. Louis: C.V. Mosby, 1975; and Wallach, J., *Interpretation of Diagnostic Tests,* 2nd ed. Boston: Little, Brown, 1974.

Note: This list is not exhaustive but contains those values most likely to be useful to nutritionists. The values were compiled from a number of sources which did not always agree; therefore, values given are representative.

Appendix E. Normal Laboratory Values: Urine

Test	Type of Specimen	Normal Value
Acetoacetic acid	Random	Negative
Acetone	Random	Negative
Albumin	Random	Negative
Aldosterone	24 hr	2–26 μg/24 hr
Alpha-amino acid nitrogen	24 hr	100–290 mg/24 hr
Ammonia nitrogen	24 hr	500–1,200 mg/24 hr 20–70 mEq/24 hr
Amylase	24 hr	80–5,000 Somogyi units/24 hr
Ascorbic acid	Random 24 hr	1–7 mg/dl >50 mg/24 hr
Bence Jones protein	Random	Negative
Bilirubin	Random	Negative
Blood, occult	Random	Negative, 0.02 mg/dl
Chloride	24 hr	110–250 mEq/24 hr
Cortisol	24 hr	<150 μg/24 hr
Creatine	24 hr	Men: 0–40 mg/24 hr Women: 0–100 mg/24 hr Higher in children and during pregnancy
Creatinine	24 hr	Men: 20–26 mg/kg/24 hr 1.0–2.0 g/24 hr Women: 14–22 mg/kg/24 hr 0.8–1.8 g/24 hr
Cystine	24 hr	<100 mg/24 hr
Glucose	Random 24 hr	Negative 130 mg/24 hr
Hemoglobin	Random	Negative
Homogentisic acid	Random	Negative
Homovanillic acid (HVA)	24 hr	<15 mg/24 hr
5-Hydroxyindoleacetic acid (5-HIAA)	Random 24 hr	Negative <10 mg/24 hr
Ketone bodies	Random	Negative
Lactose	24 hr	12–40 mg/24 hr
Magnesium	24 hr	6.0–8.5 mEq/24 hr
Osmolality	Random	Men: 390–1,090 mOsm/L Women: 300–1,090 mOsm/L
Oxalic acid	24 hr	10–55 mg/24 hr
pH	Random	4.6–8.0
Phenolsulfonphthalein (PSP)	Urine, timed after 6 mg PSP IV 15 min. 30 min.	 28–50% dye excreted 16–24% dye excreted

Test	Type of Specimen	Normal Value
Phenolsulfonphthalein (PSP)	60 min. 120 min.	9–17% dye excreted 3–10% dye excreted
Phenylpyruvic acid	Random	Negative
Phosphorus	Random	0.9–1.3 g/24 hr 0.2–0.6 mEq/24 hr
Potassium	24 hr	25–100 mEq/24 hr
Reducing substances, total	24 hr	0.5–1.5 mg/24 hr
Sodium	24 hr	40–180 mEq/24 hr
Specific gravity	Random	1.016–1.022 (normal fluid intake) 1.001–1.040 (range)
Sugars (excluding glucose)	Random	Negative
Titratable acidity	24 hr	20–40 mEq/24 hr
Urea nitrogen	24 hr	6–17 g/24 hr
Uric acid	24 hr	250–750 mg/24 hr
Urobilinogen	2 hr 24 hr	0.3–1.0 Ehrlich units 0.05–2.5 mg/24 hr, or 0.5–4.0 Ehrlich units/24 hr
Vanillylmandelic acid (VMA)	24 hr	<8 mg/24 hr (adults)
Volume, total	24 hr	600–1,600 ml/24 hr
Zinc	24 hr	0.15–1.2 mg/24 hr

Note: This list is not exhaustive but contains those values most likely to be useful to nutritionists. The values were compiled from a number of sources which did not always agree; therefore, values given are representative. Further information on interpretation of tests is available (see footnote a, Appendix D).

Appendix F. Normal Laboratory Values: Hematology*

Test	Value
Red blood cell count	Men: 4.6–6.2 × $10^6/mm^3$ Women: 4.0–5.5 × $10^6/mm^3$ Pregnancy: >3.6 × $10^6/mm^3$
White blood cell count	4,500–11,000/ml
Differential white blood cell count	
Segmented neutrophils	54–75%, 3,000–7,500/ml
Bands	0–8%, 0–700/ml
Lymphocytes	25–40%, 1,500–4,500/ml
Monocytes	2–8%, 100–500/ml
Eosinophils	0.5–4%, 50–450/ml
Basophils	0–1%, 0–200/ml
Platelet count	150,000–400,000/ml
Hemoglobin	Men: 14.0–18.0 g/dl Women: 12.0–16.0 g/dl Pregnancy: >10.6 g/dl
Hematocrit (packed cell volume [PCV])	Men: 42–52% Women: 37–47% Pregnancy: >34%
Reticulocyte count	0.2–2.0%
Red blood cell indexes	
Mean corpuscular volume (MCV)	82–92 μ^3
Mean corpuscular hemoglobin (MCH)	27–35 pg
Mean corpuscular hemoglobin concentration (MCHC)	30–38%
Blood volume (7–8% of body weight in kilograms)	Men: 69 ml/kg Women: 65 ml/kg
Plasma volume	Men: 44 ml/kg Women: 40 ml/kg
Red blood cell volume	Men: 26 ml/kg Women: 21 ml/kg

* This list is not exhaustive but contains those values most likely to be useful to nutritionists. The values were compiled from a number of sources which did not always agree; therefore, values given are representative. Further information on interpretation of tests is available (see footnote a, Appendix D).

Appendix G. Normal Laboratory Values: Tests Used in Gastroenterology*

Test	*Value*
Hydrochloric acid output (mEq/hr)	
Men	Basal: 0 – 17 Histalog stimulation: 0 – 48
Women	Basal: 0 – 15 Histalog stimulation: 0 – 25
Gastric contents (fasting, 12-hr overnight specimen)	25 – 100 ml
Serum gastrin, normal	<200 pg/ml
Intestinal absorption	
Fecal fat	<6.0 g lipid per day
Fecal nitrogen	<2.0 g N/day
D-Xylose absorption, 25-g oral dose	>4.5 g/5-hr urine
Lactose tolerance, 100-g oral dose	>20 mg/dl rise in blood glucose
Schilling test	>7% radioactivity in 24-hr urine
Pancreatic function	
Serum amylase	50 – 200 Somogyi units/dl
Urinary amylase/24 hr	800 – 5,000 Somogyi units
Serum lipase	<1.5 Cherry-Crandall units/ml
Duodenal drainage (pancreatic secretion)	
Volume	>2 ml/kg/80 min.
Bicarbonate	> 90 mEq/L
Amylase	>6 units/kg/80 min.
Trypsin	160 – 600 μg/ml 20 min. after Lundh meal of corn oil and dextrose
Sweat chloride, normal	10 mEq/L

* This list is not exhaustive but contains those values most likely to be useful to nutritionists. The values were compiled from a number of sources which did not always agree; therefore, values given are representative. Further information on interpretation of tests is available (see footnote a, Appendix D).

Appendix H. Osmolality and Specific Gravity

Osmosis is the movement of fluid across a semipermeable membrane from an area of lower concentration of solutes to an area of higher concentration. Osmotic pressure is the difference in the concentration of the number of particles of solutes. It is expressed in terms of *osmols* or *milliosmols* (mOsm). One millimole (mmole) of a substance that does not dissociate in solution equals 1 mOsm. If a substance dissociates, it contains milliosmoles equivalent to the number of particles produced. Sodium chloride dissociates into sodium ion (Na^+) and chloride ion (Cl^-), so 1 mmole equals 2 mOsm. One millimole of sodium phosphate (Na_2HPO_4) dissociates into two Na ions and one HPO_4 ion, making 3 mOsm.

Osmolality is measured in milliosmoles of solute per *kilogram* of solvent, whereas *osmolarity* is defined as milliosmoles of solute per liter of solution (solute plus solvent). When the solvent is water, as it is in most biologic systems, osmolarity is approximately 80 percent of osmolality.

Normal osmolality of serum is 280 to 295 mOsm/kg. It is determined mainly by the concentrations of sodium, urea, and glucose. Amino acids, small peptides, and other electrolytes also have an osmotic effect, whereas starch, whole protein, and long-chain fat have a low osmolality. Serum osmolality can be estimated using the formula:

$$\text{mOsm/kg} = 2(\text{Na}^+ + \text{K}^+) + \frac{\text{Serum urea nitrogen}}{3} + \frac{\text{glucose}}{18}$$

where Na^+ and K^+ (potassium ion) are given in milliequivalents per liter; serum urea nitrogen and glucose are given in milligrams per deciliter.

Specific gravity sometimes is used to measure urine concentrations. Specific gravity differs from osmolality in that it depends on the size and weight of dissolved particles in addition to the number of particles. Distilled water has a specific gravity of 1 g/ml. Normal range for urine is 1.001 to 1.025.

Appendix I. Caffeine*

RELATED COMPOUNDS

Compound	*Formula*	*Source*
Caffeine	1,3,7 trimethylxanthine	Coffee, tea, cocoa beans, kola nuts
Theobromine	3,7 dimethylxanthine	Cocoa
Theophylline	1,3 dimethylxanthine	Tea

ABSORPTION, METABOLISM, AND EXCRETION OF CAFFEINE

Absorbed rapidly
Distributed throughout body water within 1 hr
Readily transferred across placenta
Metabolic half-life ≅ 3 hr
Excreted in urine as methylxanthine derivatives, small amount of unchanged caffeine in urine; some fecal excretion; primary excretion product is 1-methyl uric acid

PHYSIOLOGIC EFFECTS OF CAFFEINE

Cardiac muscle stimulant
Smooth muscle relaxant
Central nervous system stimulant
Diuretic
Stimulates gastric acid secretion
Increases plasma glucose and free fatty acid concentrations

WITHDRAWAL SYMPTOMS

Nausea
Vomiting
Irritability

TOXICITY

Can cause vomiting and convulsions
Acute human fatal dose ≅ 170 mg/kg body weight

PHARMACOLOGIC USES OF METHYLXANTHINES

Caffeine: Cerebral stimulant; respiratory stimulant (in premature infants); chronic use does not decrease effect; pharmacologic dose for adult ≅ 200 mg
Theobromine: Diuresis
Theophylline: Coronary dilation

* The material in this appendix has been compiled from the following sources: Graham, D.M., Caffeine—its identity, dietary sources, intake and biological effects. *Nutr. Rev.* 36:97, 1978; Coffee drinking and peptic ulcer disease. *Nutr. Rev.* 34:167, 1976; Stephenson, P., Physiologic and psychotropic effects on man. *J. Am. Diet. Assoc.* 7:240, 1977; Hospital Food Service, Clinical Dietetic Section, *Manual of Clinical Dietetics.* Los Angeles: University of California, 1977; Bunker, M.L., and McWilliams, M., Caffeine content of common beverages. *J. Am. Diet. Assoc.* 74:28, 1979; Nazy, M., Caffeine content of beverages and chocolate. *J.A.M.A.* 229:337, 1974; and American Dietetic Association, *Handbook of Clinical Dietetics.* New Haven, Conn.: Yale University Press, 1981.

METHYLXANTHINES IN FOOD AND DRINK

Food or Beverage	*Caffeine (mg/6-oz. cup)*	*Theophylline (mg/6-oz. cup)*	*Theobromine (mg/6-oz. cup)*
Roasted and ground coffee, brewed to varying strengths	60–150		
Instant coffee	60		
Nescafé	7		
Decaffeinated coffee	3		
Decaf	0.18		
Sanka	3.3		
Tea, brewed to varying strengths	18–107	2	1
Instant tea	55		2
Cocoa (mean, all types)	13		250
African			272
South American			232
Cola beverages			
Coca-Cola	64.7		
Diet Pepsi-Cola	36		
Diet-Rite Cola	31.7		
Dr. Pepper	60.9		
Diet Dr. Pepper	54.2		
Pepsi-Cola	43.1		
Royal Crown Cola	33.7		
Diet RC Cola	30.0		
Tab	49.4		
Mountain Dew	54.7		

DRUG SOURCES OF CAFFEINE

Drug	*Usual Purpose for Use*	*Caffeine Content (mg/tablet)*
Anacin	Headache relief	32
A.P.C.	Analgesic	32
Bromoquinine	Cold tablet	15
Cope	Headache relief	32
Darvon	Prescription drug	32
Dristan	Allergy relief	30
Excedrin	Headache relief	32
Fiorinal	Prescription drug	40
Migral	Prescription drug	50
No Doz	Keep awake	100–200
Sinarest	Allergy relief	31
Vivarin	Keep awake	100–200

Appendix J. Oral Supplementary Feedings

Appendix J. Oral Supplementary Feedings

Product	Composition (Source)			Caloric Density	Lactose	Residue	Notes
	Carbohydrate (g/100 kcal)	Protein (g/100 kcal)	Fat (g/100 kcal)				
Citrotein[a]	18.42 (Maltodextrins, sucrose, glucose)	6.05 (Egg albumin)	0.26 (Soy oil, monoglycerides, diglycerides)	0.66 kcal/ml	No	Low	Protein and vitamin supplement to clear liquid diet
Delmark Eggnog[b]	13 (Nonfat dry milk, maltodextrin, sugar)	5.25 (Nonfat dry milk, egg white, egg yolk solids)	3.0 (Cottonseed oil, soy oil, egg yolk)	1.16 kcal/ml	Yes		
Delmark Milkshake[b]	12.5 (Sugar, maltodextrins, ice cream mix)	3.8 (Egg, milk)	3.85 (Vegetable oil)	0.95 kcal/ml	Yes		
Dietene[a]	15.75 (Nonfat milk, sucrose)	8.75 (Nonfat milk)	0.2	0.8 kcal/ml	Yes		Add powder to milk
dp High p.e.r. Protein[c]	2.0	20.6	1.0	2.58 kcal/g			Protein supplement; low electrolyte
Gevral[d]	6.68 (Lactose, sucrose)	17.1 (Calcium caseinate)	0.57 (Milk fat)	0.653 kcal/ml	Yes	Low	Protein-calorie supplement; artificial flavors
Lolactene[a]	13 (Corn syrup solids, sucrose)	6.6 (Caseinate)	2.3 (Vegetable oil, monoglycerides, diglycerides)	0.8 kcal/ml	Low	None	
Lonalac[e]	30 (Lactose)	21 (Casein)	49 (Coconut oil)	0.67 kcal/ml	High	Low	Low sodium, high potassium

Note: The composition of these products is subject to change. Current product literature should be consulted before use. This table is not intended to be comprehensive.

[a] Doyle Pharmaceutical.
[b] Delmark.
[c] General Mills.
[d] Lederle Laboratories.
[e] Mead Johnson Nutritional.

Appendix K. Sources of Single Nutrients

Appendix K. Sources of Single Nutrients

Product (Form)	Composition (Source)			Caloric Density	Osmolality (mOsm/kg)	Lactose	Residue	Notes
	Carbohydrate (g/100 kcal)	Protein (g/100 kcal)	Fat (g/100 kcal)					
Protein sources								
Casec[a] (powder)	0	23.78 (Calcium caseinate)	0.54 (Butterfat	3.7kcal/g		No	Low	Add to liquid or food; provides no vitamins
Promix[b] (powder)	2.27	22.7 (Whey protein)	1.1	3.52 kcal/g		No		Add to liquid foods; provides no vitamins
Propac[c] (powder)	1.25	19.2 (Whey protein)	4.5	4.0 kcal/g		Yes		Add to liquid foods; provides no vitamins
Carbohydrate sources								
Cal-Power[d] (liquid)	27.2 (Deionized corn syrup)	0.06	0	1.8 kcal/ml		No		Low electrolyte; high osmolality; for oral or tube feedings
Controlyte[e] (powder)	14.3 (Cornstarch hydrolysate)	Trace	4.8 (Soy oil)	2.0 kcal/ml (or 5.0 kcal/g)	598	No	Low	For oral or tube feedings; calorie source; add to liquid or food; high osmolality; low protein; low electrolyte
Hy-Cal[f] (liquid)	24.41 (Liquid glucose)	0.01	0.01	2.5 kcal/ml	2,781	No	Low	Oral supplement; low electrolyte; high osmolality
Lytren[a] (powder)	25.3	0	0	0.333 kcal/g	290	No	Low	Electrolyte source; provides some kilocalories; useful in prevention of metabolic defects due to diarrhea
Moducal[a] (liquid or powder)	25 (Maltodextrins)	0	0	2.0 kcal/ml (liq.) 4.0 kcal/g (powd.)	725 (liq.)	No	Low	Calorie source

Pedialyte[g]	25	0	0	0.2 kcal/ml				Calorie and electrolyte source
Polycose[g] (liquid or powder)	25	0	0	2.0 kcal/ml 4.0 kcal/g	570	No	Low	Caloric supplement; low electrolyte
Sumacal[c] (powder)	25 (Maltodextrins)	0	0	4.0 kcal/g	680 (Cherry, lemon, lime)	No	Low	Caloric supplement; low electrolyte
Sumacal Plus[c] (powder)	3.2	0	0	2.5 kcal/g	890		Low	Caloric supplement; low electrolyte
Lipid sources								
Lipomul-Oral[h]	0.11	0.01	11.11 (Corn oil)	6.0 kcal/ml		No	Low	Oral supplement; low electrolyte
MCT Oil[a]	0	0	12.05 (Coconut oil fraction)	7.7 kcal/ml	Negligible	No		Oral supplement; 60% C8 and 24% C10 fatty acids; low electrolyte
Microlipid[c]	0	0	11.11 (Soy, corn, or safflower oil)	4.5 kcal/ml	80	No	Low	Oral supplement; low electrolyte

Note: The composition of these products changes frequently. Current product literature should be consulted before use. This table is not intended to be comprehensive.
[a] Mead Johnson Nutritional.
[b] Navaco Laboratories.
[c] Organon Pharmaceuticals.
[d] General Mills.
[e] Doyle Pharmaceutical.
[f] Beecham Laboratories.
[g] Ross Laboratories.
[h] The Upjohn Company.

Appendix L. Complete Liquid Formula Diets

Appendix L. Complete Liquid Formula Diets

Product	Composition (Source): Carbohydrate (% of kcal)	Composition (Source): Protein (% of kcal)	Composition (Source): Lipid (% of kcal)	Electrolytes (mEq/100 ml at usual dilution): Sodium	Electrolytes (mEq/100 ml at usual dilution): Potassium	Caloric Density (kcal/ml at usual dilution)	Osmolality (mOsm/kg); (Flavors)	Lactose (g/100 ml)	Residue	Notes
Hydrolyzed protein – based										
Criticare[a]	82.8 (Maltodextrin; modified cornstarch)	14.4 (30% Small peptides; 70% amino acids)	2.8 (Sunflower oil)	2.7	3.4	1.06	650	0	Low	For oral or tube feeding
Nutramigen[a]	52 (Sucrose; tapioca starch)	13 (Hydrolyzed casein)	35 (Corn oil)	1.38	1.76	0.68	479	0	Low	For oral or tube feeding; infant formula; galactose-free; useful in management of allergy, galactosemia; renal solute load 13 mOsm/dl
Pregestimil[a]	54 (Corn syrup solids; tapioca starch)	11 (Hydrolyzed casein; amino acids)	35 (Corn oil; MCT Oil)	1.38	1.9	0.65 (Infants) 1.5 (Adult formulation)	348	0	Low	For oral feeding; powder; infant feeding; renal solute load 13 mOsm/dl in formulas containing 20 kcal; useful in management of malabsorption disorders
Travasorb STD[b]	76 (Oligosaccharides)	12 (Hydrolyzed lactalbumin; L-methionine)	12 (MCT; sunflower oil)	4.0	2.99	0.45	450 (Unflavored) 500 (Orange) 600 (Beef broth)	0	Low	For oral or tube feeding
Travasorb HN[b]	70 (Oligosaccharides)	18 (Hydrolyzed lactalbumin; L-methionine)	12 (MCT; sunflower oil)	4.0	2.99	1.0	400	0	Low	For oral or tube feeding
Vipep[c]	68 (Corn syrup solids; sucrose; cornstarch; potassium gluconate; tapioca flour)	10 (20% Amino acids; 80% short-chain peptides)	22 (MCT Oil; corn oil)	3.26	2.18	1.0	520	0	Low	
Vital HN[d]	74 (Sucrose; hydrolyzed cornstarch)	16.7 (Partially hydrolyzed whey, meat, soy; amino acids)	9.3 (Safflower oil; MCT Oil)	1.7	3.0	1.0	450 (Various flavors)	0	Low	
Vivonex Standard[e]	90.2 (Glucose and oligosaccharides)	8.5 (Crystalline L-amino acids)	1.3 (Safflower oil)	2.0	3.0	1.0	550 (Unflavored) 678 (Beef broth) 610 (Orange, grape, strawberry) 580 (Tomato)	0	Low	For oral or tube feeding
Vivonex HN[e]	80.96 (Glucose and oligosaccharides)	18.26 (Crystalline L-amino acids)	0.78 (Safflower oil)	2.3	3.0	1.0	810 (Unflavored) 920 (Beef broth) 850 (Orange, grape, strawberry) 910 (Tomato)	0	Low	For oral or tube feeding
Isolates of intact protein: Non-milk-based										
Ensure[d]	54.5 (Corn syrup solids; sucrose)	14 (Sodium and calcium caseinate; soy isolate)	31.5 (Corn oil)	3.7	4.0	1.06	450 (Flavor packets available)	0	Low	For oral or tube feeding
Ensure Plus[d]	53.3 (Corn syrup solids; sucrose)	14.7 (Sodium and calcium caseinate; soy isolate)	32 (Corn oil)	5.0	6.0	1.5	600 (Flavor packets available)	0	Low	For oral feeding; for tube feeding with caution only
Isocal[a]	50 (Corn syrup [illegible]	12.5 (Sodium and [illegible]	37.5 (Soy oil; MCT)	2.2	3.2	1.04	300	0	Low	For tube feeding; renal solute load [illegible]

Isomil[d]	40 (Corn syrup; sucrose)	12 (Soy isolate; L-methionine)	48 (Coconut oil; soy oil)	1.3	1.8	0.67	250	0	Low	Infant formula
Magnacal[f]	50 (Maltodextrin; corn syrup; sucrose)	14 (Sodium and calcium caseinate; soy)	36 (Soy oil; monoglycerides; diglycerides)	4.3	3.2	2.0	520	0	Low	For tube feeding
Mull-soy[g]	32.7 (Sucrose)	17.8 (Soy flour)	49.5 (Soy oil)	1.3	1.8	0.74	252	0		For oral feeding; infant formula
Neo-Mull-soy[g]	40.1 (Sucrose)	11.4 (Soy isolate; L-methionine)	49.5 (Soy oil)			0.66	275	0		Infant formula
Nutri-1000 LF[c]	38 (Sucrose; corn syrup)	15 (Caseinate; soy isolate)	47 (Corn oil)	2.3	3.9	1.0	380 (Chocolate; vanilla)	0	Low	For tube feeding
Osmolite[d]	54.6 (Corn syrup solids; glucose polymers)	14.0 (Sodium and calcium caseinate; soy isolate)	31.4 (MCT Oil; corn oil; soy oil)	2.3	2.6	1.06	300	0	Low	For tube feeding
Portagen[a] (powder)	45 (Corn syrup solids; sucrose; lactose)	14 (Sodium caseinate)	41 (95% MCT Oil; 5% corn oil)	2.0	3.2	0.68 (Infants) 1.00 (Adult formulation)	158	<0.3/qt.	Low	For oral or tube feeding; useful in fat malabsorption; renal solute load 15 mOsm/dl
Precision High Nitrogen[h]	82.2 (Sucrose; maltodextrins)	16.7 (Egg albumin)	1.1 (Soy oil; MCT Oil; monoglycerides; diglycerides)	4.3	2.3	1.05	557 (Citrus)	0	Low	For oral or tube feeding
Precision Isotein HN[h]	52 (Maltodextrin; fructose)	23 (Lactalbumin; caseinate)	25 (Soy oil; MCT)	3.5	2.5	1.2	300	0	Low	For oral or tube feeding
Precision Isotonic[h]	60 (Sucrose; glucose oligosaccharides)	11.8 (Egg albumin)	28.2 (Soy oil; monoglycerides; diglycerides)	3.3	2.5	0.96	300 (Vanilla; orange)	0	Low	For oral or tube feeding
Precision LR[h]	89.2 (Sucrose; maltodextrins)	9.5 (Egg albumin)	1.3 (Soy oil)	3.0	2.2	1.11	500–545 (Cherry; lemon; lime; orange)	0	Low	For oral or tube feeding
Precision Moderate Nitrogen[h]	59.5 (Sucrose; maltodextrins)	12.9 (Egg albumin)	27.6 (Soy oil)	4.5	2.3	1.21	395 (Vanilla; citrus)	0	Low	For oral or tube feeding
ProSobee[a]	40 (Glucose polymers)	12 (Soy isolate; L-methionine)	48 (Soy oil; coconut oil)	1.3	2.1	0.68	200	0	Low	For oral feeding; ready to use or concentrated; infant formula; lactosefree; sucrosefree; useful in management of allergy, lactose or sucrose intolerance, galactosemia, gluten sensitivity; renal solute load 13 mOsm/dl
Renuf	50 (Corn syrup solids; sucrose; oat powder)	14 (Soy isolate; L-methionine)	36 (Soy oil)	2.2	3.2	1.0	345	0	Low	For oral or tube feeding
Travasorb[b]	54.5 (Sucrose; corn syrup solids)	14 (Caseinate; soy isolate)	31.5 (Corn oil; soy oil; monoglycerides; diglycerides)	3.22	3.24	1.06	450 (Vanilla; black walnut; eggnog)	0	Low	For oral or tube feeding
Travasorb MCT[b]	50 (Corn syrup solids)	20 (Lactalbumin; casein)	30 (80% MCT Oil; 20% sunflower oil)	1.52	4.45	1.0 or 2.0	250 or 475	0	Low	

(continued)

Appendix L (continued)

Product	Composition (Source): Carbohydrate (% of kcal)	Composition (Source): Protein (% of kcal)	Composition (Source): Lipid (% of kcal)	Electrolytes (mEq/100 ml at usual dilution): Sodium	Electrolytes (mEq/100 ml at usual dilution): Potassium	Caloric Density (kcal/ml at usual dilution)	Osmolality (mOsm/kg); (Flavors)	Lactose (g/100 ml)	Residue	Notes
Isolates of intact protein: Milk-based										
Carnation Instant Breakfast[i] (+8 oz. whole milk)	49.9 (Corn syrup solids; sucrose; lactose)	22.1 (Milk; nonfat dry milk; sodium caseinate; soy isolate)	28 (Milk fat)	4.2	7.2	1.22	560	9.51	Low	For oral feeding; powdered
Meritene Liquid[h]	46 (Lactose; corn syrup solids; sucrose)	24 (Milk; sodium caseinate)	30 (Vegetable oil; monoglycerides; diglycerides)	4.0	4.3	1.02	560 (Vanilla) 610 (Chocolate)	5.7	Low	For oral or tube feeding; also available as powder
Nutri-1000[c]	38 (Sucrose; lactose; corn syrup solids)	15 (Milk; caseinate; soy isolate)	47 (Corn oil)	2.3	3.9	1.06	500 (Chocolate; vanilla)	Milk-based	Low	
Nutri-1000 LF[c]	38 (Corn syrup solids; sucrose)	15 (Calcium and sodium caseinate; soy isolate)	47 (Corn oil; soy oil)	3.13	4.06	1.06		1	Low	
Sustacal Liquid[a]	55 (Sucrose; corn syrup solids)	24 (Skim milk; sodium and calcium caseinate; soy isolate)	21 (Soy oil)	4.0	5.3	1.0	625 (Vanilla) 697 (Chocolate)	0	Low	For oral feeding; for tube feeding with caution; renal solute load 364 mOsm/qt; also available as powder or pudding
Sustacal HC[a]	50 (Corn syrup solids; sucrose)	16 (Caseinates)	34 (Soy oil)	3.6	3.8	1.5	650 (Vanilla; eggnog)	0		For oral feeding
Blenderized diets										
Compleat-B[h]	48 (Maltodextrins; lactose; sucrose; vegetable and fruit purée; orange juice)	16 (Beef purée; milk)	36 (Corn oil; beef; milk)	5.2	3.4	1.07	390	2.4	Moderate	For tube feeding
Compleat Modified[h]	53 (Hydrolyzed cereal solids; fruit purées; vegetable purée)	16.0 (Beef; calcium caseinate)	31.0 (Corn oil)	2.9	3.6	1.07	300	0	Moderate	For tube feeding
Formula 2[c]	49 (Lactose; sucrose; vegetable; orange juice; farina)	15 (Nonfat dry milk; beef; egg yolks; casein)	36 (Beef; corn oil; egg yolk)	2.6	4.5	1.0	435–510	3.75	Moderate	For tube feeding; orange flavor
Vitaneed[f]	51 (Corn syrup solids; puréed vegetables and fruit; sucrose)	14 (Puréed beef; soy isolate)	35 (Puréed beef; soy oil)	2.3	3.2	1.02	435	0	Moderate	For oral or tube feeding
Special purpose formulas										
Amin-Aid[j]	74.8 (Maltodextrins; sucrose)	4.0 (Essential amino acids; histidine)	21.2 (Soy oil; monoglycerides; diglycerides)	<0.5	<0.2	1.95	850 (Orange; lemon-lime; berry; strawberry)	0	Low	Indicated for renal disease; also available as pudding; no added vitamins
Hepatic Aid[j]	69.8 (Maltodextrins; sucrose)	10.4 (High ratio of BCAA to AAA)	19.8 (Soy oil; monoglycerides;	<0.5	<0.2	1.65	900 (Chocolate; chocolate-mint;	0	Low	Indicated for hepatic disease; also available as pudding; no added

TraumaCal[a]	38 (Corn syrup)	22 (Calcium and sodium caseinate)	40 (Soy oil; MCT Oil)	5.2	3.6	1.5	500	0	Low	For oral or tube feeding. High in BCAA (1.25 g / 100 kcal).
Travasorb Hepatic[b]	77.4 (Glucose oligosaccharides; sucrose)	10.6 (Crystalline amino acids; 50% BCAA; low in AAA)	12.0 (MCT Oil; sunflower oil)			1.1	690 (Eggnog; custard; chocolate; apricot; strawberry	0	Low	For hepatic disease
Travasorb Renal[b]	81.1 (Glucose oligosaccharides; sucrose)	6.9 (Crystalline amino acids; EEA, histidine, arginine, and others)	12.0 (MCT Oil; sunflower oil)	0 (approx.)	0 (approx.)	1.35	590 (Apricot; strawberry)	0	No	For renal disease
MSUD Diet Powder[a]	54	8	38	1.15	1.79	0.68				Free of BCAA, for use in management of maple syrup urine disease
Product 3200 AB[a] (powder)	52	13 (Casein hydrolysate)	35	1.38	1.76	0.68				Low-phenylalanine, low-tyrosine food powder for management of tyrosinemia; contains 16 mg phenylalanine / 100 kcal and 9 mg tyrosine / 100 kcal; further details in Table 10-1
Product 3200 K[a] (powder)	39	12 (Soy protein isolate)	49	1.15	1.49	0.68				Infant formula for management of homocystinuria; contains 34 mg methionine / kcal; further details in Table 10-1
Product 80056[a] (powder)	59	0	41		1.02					A protein-free formula base providing carbohydrate and fat to which amino acids and sodium must be added; for management of rare amino acid metabolic disorders; further details in Table 10-1
Product 3232 A[a]	52 (Tapioca starch as stabilizer; add 59 g carbohydrate / qt)	13 (Casein hydrolysate)	35 (MCT Oil)	1.38	1.76	0.68				A protein hydrolysate formula base to be used in management of disaccharidase deficiency, impaired glucose transport, or impure fructose utilization; values given assume addition of 59 g carbohydrate / qt

Note: The composition of these products changes frequently. Current product literature should be consulted before use. This table is not intended to be comprehensive.

MCT = medium-chain triglycerides; BCAA = branched-chain amino acids; AAA = aromatic amino acids; EAA = essential amino acids.

[a] Mead Johnson Nutritional.

[b] Travenol Laboratories.

[c] Cutter Laboratories.

[d] Ross Laboratories.

[e] Norwich-Eaton Pharmaceuticals.

[f] Organon Pharmaceuticals.

[g] Syntex Laboratories.

[h] Doyle Pharmaceutical.

[i] Carnation.

[j] American McGaw.

Appendix M. Modified Diet Products

CEREAL PRODUCTS

Product	*Indications*
Aproten Macaroni Products (General Mills)	Low-protein or low-phenylalanine diet. Contains 0.14 g of protein and 4.00 mg of phenylalanine per 100 g of cooked weight
Aproten Rusks (General Mills)	Low protein or low-phenylalanine diet. Contains 0.1 g of protein per 10 g of Rusk
Wheat starch (Chicago Dietetic Supply)	Protein-restricted diet. Contains 0.5% protein
Cellu Dietetic Paygel P (General Mills)	
Low Pro Bread (General Mills Energ-G Foods)	Low-protein or low-phenylalanine diet
Baking Mix, Dietetic Paygel P (General Mills)	Low-protein, low-gluten, low-phenylalanine diet
Low Pro Cookies (Henkel Corp.)	Low-protein, low-phenylalanine, gluten-restricted diet. Contains 0.1 g of protein, 2 mg of phenylalanine, and 0.1 g of gluten
Prono (Henkel Corp.)	Low-protein, low-phenylalanine diet. Contains 0.02 g of protein, no phenylalanine (gelatin dessert)
Low-sodium breads and cereals (Chicago Dietetic Supply; Devonsheer Melba Corp.; New Vita Foods; Zinsmaster Baking Company; Van Brode Milling Co.; Venus Wafer Inc.)	Low-sodium diet

PROTEIN PRODUCTS

Product	*Indications*
Egg substitutes	Low-cholesterol diet
Egg Beaters (Standard Brands); Eggstra (Tillie Lewis Foods); Scramblers (Morningstar Farms); Second Nature (Avoset Food)	
Sausage and bacon substitutes	Low-cholesterol diet
Breakfast Strips and Grillers (Morningstar Farms)	
Low-sodium meats and fish—Cellu and Chicken-of-the-Sea (Chicago Dietetic Supply; Ralston Purina; Van Camp Seafood)	Low-sodium diet

FAT PRODUCTS

Product	*Indications*
Coffee Rich Non-Dairy Creamer (Rich Products Corp.)	Protein-restricted diet; is a concentrated source of energy
Poly Perx Cream substitute (Mitchell Foods, Inc.)	Low-cholesterol, high-polyunsaturated-fat diet

OTHER MODIFIED DIET PRODUCTS

Product	*Indications*
Low-sodium soups (Campbell Soup; Chicago Dietetic Supply; Clayco Foods)	Low-sodium diet
Low-sodium peanut butter (Organic Foods Corp.; Hollywood Health Foods; Derby Foods, Inc.; Chicago Dietetic Supply; Swift)	Low-sodium diet
Low-sodium canned vegetables (California Canners and Growers; Chicago Dietetic Supply; Libby, McNeill & Libby; S&W Fine Foods)	Low-sodium diet
Low-sodium milk (Canned Dairy Products Inc. [*LSM*]; Mead Johnson Nutritional [*Lonalac*])	Low-sodium diet
High-carbohydrate spreads and toppings	Calorie-restricted or carbohydrate-restricted diet
Fruit "spreads" (California Canners and Growers)	
Pancake and waffle topping (California Canners and Growers)	
Gelatin dessert (D-Zerta; unsweetened [General Foods])	Diabetic or calorie-restricted diet

Appendix N. Appropriate Serving Sizes of Usual Foods for Infants and Children

A. Dietary Evaluation Guidelines (0–12 months)

<table>
<tr><td>Age (months)</td><td>0</td><td>1</td><td>2</td><td>3</td><td>4</td><td>5</td><td>6</td><td>7</td><td>8</td><td>9</td><td>10</td><td>11</td><td>12</td></tr>
<tr><td>Average weight for NCHS 50th percentile
kg
1 lb</td><td>3.3
7.3</td><td>4.1
9.0</td><td>5.0
11.0</td><td>5.7
12.5</td><td>6.4
14.1</td><td>7.0
15.4</td><td>7.5
16.5</td><td>8.0
17.6</td><td>8.5
18.7</td><td>8.9
19.6</td><td>9.2
20.2</td><td>9.6
21.1</td><td>9.9
21.8</td></tr>
<tr><td>Calories per 24 hr</td><td colspan="7">Range: 95–145 kcal / kg; Average = 115 kcal / kg
43–66 kcal / lb; Average = 52 kcal / lb</td><td colspan="6">Range: 80–135 kcal / kg; Average = 105 kcal / kg
36–61 kcal / lb; Average = 48 kcal / lb</td></tr>
<tr><td>Fluid per 24 hr (ml)</td><td colspan="13">125–145 cc / kg body weight; 4.2–4.8 oz / kg / 24 hr; 2–2½ oz / lb / 24 hr</td></tr>
<tr><td>Number of milk feedings per 24 hr</td><td>8 or more</td><td>7–8</td><td>6–7</td><td colspan="3">4 or 5</td><td colspan="5">3 or 4</td><td colspan="2">3</td></tr>
<tr><td>Ounces formula per feeding</td><td>2½–4</td><td>3½–5</td><td>4–6</td><td>5–7</td><td>6–8</td><td colspan="2">7–8</td><td colspan="4">6–8</td><td colspan="2">7–6</td></tr>
<tr><td rowspan="5">Solids</td><td colspan="5" rowspan="5">No solid foods until:
a. 4–6 mos.
or
b. 6–7 kg</td><td colspan="8">Iron-fortified cereal (rice)
Teething biscuit
Iron-fortified mixed-grain cereals</td></tr>
<tr><td rowspan="3"></td><td colspan="4">Vegetables: carrots, squash, beans, peas</td><td colspan="3" rowspan="3"></td></tr>
<tr><td colspan="4">Fruits / juices: applesauce, pears, peaches, banana</td></tr>
<tr><td colspan="4">Strained meats, cheese, yogurt, cooked beans, egg yolk</td></tr>
<tr><td colspan="5">6–8 mos.: strained (puréed) foods
7–10 mos.: junior (chopped) foods
10–12 mos.: table foods</td><td colspan="3">Table foods (whole egg, orange juice, and whole milk at 12 mos.)</td></tr>
<tr><td>Age (months)</td><td>0</td><td>1</td><td>2</td><td>3</td><td>4</td><td>5</td><td>6</td><td>7</td><td>8</td><td>9</td><td>10</td><td>11</td><td>12</td></tr>
</table>

Note: By 12 months most infants consume two small jars of baby food or approximately 1 cup of solids per day.
Breast milk or infant formula is preferred during the first 12 months of life.
Whole milk (cow's) is recommended starting at approximately 1 year of age.

B. Dietary Evaluation Guidelines (1–12 years)

	Recommended Servings Per Day	Servings Eaten Per Day	Difference	Average Size of Servings				
				1 Year (100 kcal / kg / day)[a]	2–3 Years (90 kcal / kg / day)	4–5 Years (75 kcal / kg / day)	6–9 Years (60 kcal / kg / day)	10–12 Years (55 kcal / kg / day)
Milk and cheese	4			1 / 2 C	1 / 2–3 / 4 C	1 / 2–3 / 4 C	3 / 4–1 C	1 C
1 C milk =								
1.5 C cheese								
1.5 C ice cream								
1 C yogurt								
Meat group and meat	2–3							
Alternates								
Egg				1	1	1	1	1
Meat, poultry, fish				2 T	3 T	2–3 oz (4–6 T)	3–4 oz	4–5 oz
Peanut butter					1 T	2 T	2–3 T	3 T
Dried beans / peas				4 T	4 T	1 / 2 C	3 / 4 C	1 C
Fruits and vegetables	4 to include:							
Vitamin C (citrus, berries, tomatoes, etc.)	1			4 T (1 / 4 C)	8 T (1 / 2 C)	1 / 2 C	1 C	1 C
Vitamin A source (green or yellow fruits and vegetables)	1			2 T	3 T (2–3 times wk)	1 / 4 C	1 / 4 C	1 / 3 C
Others	2			2 T	3 T	1 / 2 C	1 / 2 C	1 / 2 C
Bread and cereals	4							
Bread				1 / 2 slice	1 slice	1-1 / 2 slices	1–2 slices	2 slices
Cold cereal				1 / 2 C	3 / 4 C	1 / 2 C	1 / 2 C	1-1 / 2 C
Cooked cereal / pasta				4 T	5 T (1 / 3 C)	1 / 2 C	1 / 2 C	3 / 4 C
Fats and carbohydrates								
Butter, margarine, mayonnaise or oil (100 kcal / T)	To meet caloric needs			1 T	1 T	1 T	2 T	2 T
Desserts / sweets (100 calories each):								
1 / 2 C pudding or ice cream								
2–3 cookies; 1 oz cake								
2 T sugar, honey or jam								

Adapted from Nelson, Waldo E., Vaughn, V. C., *Nelson Textbook of Pediatrics*, 11th ed. Philadelphia: W. B. Saunders, 1979, pp. 187, 189.

C = cup = 8 oz; T = tablespoon; 1 small jar baby food = 7 T.

[a] As a general rule of thumb, 1000 calories plus 100 calories for each year of life.

From San Diego Pediatric Nutrition Group; *Pediatric Nutrition Manual*. San Diego, Calif., 1981. Reprinted courtesy of Denise Ney, R.D. Not copyrighted.

Index